Anesthesia for Genetic, Metabolic, and Dysmorphic Syndromes of Childhood

Anesthesia for Genetic, Metabolic, and Dysmorphic Syndromes of Childhood

SECOND EDITION

Victor C. Baum, MD

Professor of Anesthesiology and Pediatrics
Executive Vice-Chair
Director, Cardiac Anesthesia
University of Virginia
Charlottesville, Virginia

Jennifer E. O'Flaherty, MD, MPH

Associate Professor of Anesthesiology and Pediatrics
Dartmouth-Hitchcock Medical Center
Lebanon, New Hampshire

Lippincott Williams & Wilkins
a Wolters Kluwer business
Philadelphia · Baltimore · New York · London
Buenos Aires · Hong Kong · Sydney · Tokyo

Acquisitions Editor: Brian Brown
Developmental Editor: Louise Bierig
Managing Editor: Nicole T. Dernoski
Project Manager: Nicole Walz
Senior Manufacturing Manager: Ben Rivera
Marketing Manager: Angela Panetta
Design Coordinator: Stephen Druding
Cover Designer: Stephen Druding
Production Services: Laserwords Private Limited, Chennai, India
Printer: Edwards Brothers

Library of Congress Cataloging-in-Publication Data

Baum, Victor C.
   Anesthesia for genetic, metabolic, and dysmorphic syndromes of childhood / Victor C. Baum, Jennifer E. O'Flaherty.—2nd ed.
      p. ; cm.
   Includes bibliographical references.
   ISBN-13: 978-0-7817-7938-8
   ISBN-10: 0-7817-7938-3
   1. Pediatric anesthesia. 2. Genetic disorders in children. 3. Metabolic disorders in children. I. O'Flaherty, Jennifer E. II. Title.
   [DNLM: 1. Anesthesia. 2. Abnormalities. 3. Child. 4. Genetic Diseases, Inborn. 5. Infant. 6. Metabolic Diseases. WO 440 B347a 2007]
   RD139.B38 2007
   617.9'6083—dc22

                                                                 2006020572

To the bookends of my life: my children Emily and Sophie,
and my parents Milton and Selma.
Sorry, there just wasn't room in the first edition.

V.C.B.

To my family: Beth, Katie, Liam, and Molly.
To my grandmother and my mother, who published first.

J.E.O.

Contents

Preface

Because both of us are anesthesiologists who are also pediatricians and who have practiced in a variety of general hospital settings, it has been a common experience for both of us to be stopped by a somewhat harried-appearing nonpediatrician colleague with the lament "I'm scheduled to anesthetize a patient with X syndrome. Quick, what do I need to know about X syndrome?" Such encounters formed the genesis of this book. Originally, the book was to be one of anesthesia and eponymous diseases. However, it quickly became apparent that many syndromes are not eponyms, and so the book grew into the current format. Although this book was written primarily for anesthesiologists who do not practice in large pediatric centers, we hope that it will also be of use to our colleagues who do have this luxury. Certainly, any clinician who graduated from medical school more than a few years ago will be amazed, as were we, at the large number of syndromes that we had thought of as "dysmorphic" but are now clearly "genetic" with the responsible genes and, often, gene products already identified. This trend has if anything accelerated in the years after the first edition. We hope that even colleagues who have an extensive knowledge of these syndromes will enjoy some of the miscellanea we have found and enjoyed collecting.

This book's approach is to assume the typical anesthesia scenario, namely a patient who arrives already carrying a diagnosis, rather than a patient with a constellation of signs and symptoms in search of a unifying diagnosis. Because of this, we have not used excessive space addressing the exact incidences of various findings. We subscribe to the school that says that if a finding is present in your patient, the incidence is 100%. We have elected to include all findings of the syndrome, even if uncommon, although we have tried to indicate when such findings are uncommon or rare, typically by the use of "may have" or the more grammatically correct "can have." Because of the small number of patients with certain uncommon syndromes, it can be hard to separate findings due to the syndrome and findings that were merely coincidental.

We appreciate the request of some readers of the first edition that we include either an index or an appendix of physical findings and which syndromes would include each finding, as an aid in diagnosis. However, anesthesiologists are rarely called upon to make a genetic diagnosis. Such a table would be frightfully complicated, would be ungainly, and would be in the end unhelpful. Craniosynostosis, for example, has been described as a component of more than 100 distinct syndromes.

Osler wrote, "The greater the ignorance, the greater the dogma." We might add as a corollary, "Once the pathologic anatomy and physiology are understood, an appropriate anesthetic plan naturally follows." This text is not meant to be a textbook of pediatric anesthesia. This book assumes that the anesthesiologist or anesthetist is competent, and when presented with the facts will arrive at an appropriate anesthetic plan. Because of this, specific anesthetic management is not discussed at length, and we have tried to be as nonjudgmental as possible in terms of clinical management, offering only suggestions not to be construed as standard of care. As an example, when presented with the clinical scenario of a potentially difficult airway, we do not provide a detailed description of the management of the patient with a difficult airway. We do, however, report techniques successfully used in the management of the difficult airway for a specific syndrome if they have appeared in the literature.

We have included only syndromes that are present during childhood. However, these children grow up and require surgery or anesthesia as adults. They may be cared for by anesthesiologists not accustomed to these disorders. For this reason we have chosen to title this book. . . *of childhood,* rather than. . . *in children.* Whenever possible, we have included relevant discussions of these syndromes in adults.

We have been admittedly arbitrary in several aspects of the book. We could not possibly make the text inclusive. The last edition of the inclusive McKusick's *Mendelian Inheritance in Man* was more than 2,600 pages of very small print. Scriver et al.'s *The Metabolic & Molecular Bases of Inherited Disease* is currently more than 6,300 pages in four volumes. If we could not find a syndrome discussed in a general pediatric text or in the anesthesia literature, generally we did not include it. When syndromes are known by a variety of names, we sometimes arbitrarily chose which would be listed as the primary name and which would be listed as the synonym(s). We chose as the primary identifier the name that we thought would be most widely known to anesthesiologists. We have also limited our search of the anesthesia literature to 1975 and later, and have generally limited it to the English language. We chose to include all anesthesia references, because we felt that different anesthesia departments might have different journals available to them. However, we have not included a small number of relatively recent brief communications, such as letters, which did not contribute significant new information. We did not include a small number of selected references from the 1970s and early 1980s which were limited in scope, or which utilized now obsolete techniques or drugs, particularly for syndromes with numerous recent references. Readers should be aware that many reports in the anesthesia literature are based on only a single case, and so must be interpreted judiciously. In cases where there were few or no relevant references in the anesthesia literature, we concentrated on providing general clinical review papers. This was sometimes difficult to do, particularly for some of the older, well-described syndromes, where references in the past 20 years were predominantly or exclusively at the biochemical or genetic level.

We have included syndromes for which there are no specific anesthetic implications or considerations. This information is important for the clinician to know.

For those interested in more information on the various syndromes, there are many available sources. We highly recommend McKusick's *Mendelian Inheritance in Man*, available online at http://www.ncbi.nlm.nih.gov/omim/. We also recommend *Recognizable Patterns of Human Malformation* [Jones, KL: *Smith's Recognizable Patterns of Human Malformation*. Philadelphia: Elsevier Saunders, 2006 (6th edition)]. Finally, we recommend *The Metabolic & Molecular Bases of Inherited Disease* [Scriver RC et al., eds.: *The Metabolic Basis of Inherited Disease*. New York: McGraw-Hill 2001 (8th edition)]. These texts cover the history, morphology, physiology, biochemistry, and genetics of these syndromes in exquisite detail.

We would like to thank the following physicians for supplying expertise on specific syndromes: Phil Morgan (Case Western Reserve University), Joseph Wagstaff (Carolinas Medical Center), Joe Kitterman (UCSF), Craig Langman (Feinberg School of Medicine, Northwestern University) and our colleagues Gary Kupfer, Kimberly Dunsmore, Peter Waldron, and Frank Saulsbury at the University of Virginia. We also particularly thank those parents from around the world who graciously offered to let us use photographs of their children and who shared their stories with us.

Finally, we enjoyed hearing from readers after publication of the first book. We were delighted that the book seemed to fulfill the purpose for which it was designed. Let us know how we did this time.

Victor C. Baum, MD
Jennifer E. O'Flaherty, MD, MPH

Introduction: How to Use This Book

This book is intended to be used like an encyclopedia, and for this reason there is no index. We use a uniform format to present information on all of the various syndromes. A complete list of subheadings follows. If there is no relevant information for one or more of the subheadings for a given syndrome, the heading is excluded. The only exception is the subheading **"Anesthetic Considerations,"** which is included even when there are no apparent anesthetic implications. This information is important for the clinician to know. "MIM #" refers to the listing number(s) of the syndrome in McKusick's *Mendelian Inheritance in Man* (see Preface). We have tried to list all possible findings associated with a particular syndrome. This might include findings noted in a small number of patients, which might not be a consequence of the syndrome, but which have been reported. In addition, not all patients with a specific syndrome are expected to have all, or even most, of the possible findings. We list these as things to be aware of and to look for, not necessarily things that will be found. When preceded by "occasional," "can have," or a similar notation, the implication is that this is a particularly uncommon finding. The references are a bibliography and may or may not be directly referred to in the text. Sources in the bibliography are listed in reverse chronologic order.

Name
Synonym(s)
MIM #
HEENT/Airway
Chest
Cardiovascular
Neuromuscular
Orthopedic
GI/GU
Other
Miscellaneous
Anesthetic Considerations
Bibliography

Glossary

Aclasis: Pathologic tissue originates from, and is continuous with, normal tissue, providing continuity of structure.

Acro-:   Refers to distal or extreme.

Acrocephaly: Pointed cranium, secondary to coronal and lambdoidal synostosis.

Acrodysostosis: Congenital malformation of the distal bones of the extremities.

Acromelic: Pertaining to the distal segment of long bones.

Adactyly: A developmental anomaly characterized by absence of the fingers or the toes.

Allele: One of two or more alternative forms of a gene which occupy corresponding loci on homologous chromosomes. More than two alternative forms of a gene are known as multiple alleles.

Ankylosis: Stiffening or fixation of a joint, due to injury, disease, or surgical intervention.

Anosmia: The inability to smell.

Apoptosis: Programmed cell death.

Arhinencephaly: Absence of the rhinencephalon (primarily involves olfactory nerves, bulbs, and tracts).

Arthrogryposis: A fixed flexion or contracture deformity of a joint. May be congenital.

Bathrocephaly: "Step" cranium, secondary to excessive bone formation at the lambdoid suture. There is a deep groove at the lambdoid suture between the occipital and parietal bones.

Blepharophimosis: Inability to open the eyelids to their full extent secondary to lateral displacement of the inner canthi.

Brachycephaly: Broad cranium, secondary to coronal synostosis which prevents anteroposterior skull growth.

Brachydactyly: A developmental anomaly characterized by short fingers and toes.

Camptodactyly: Permanent flexion deformity of one or both interphalangeal joints of a finger.

Camptomelic: Pertaining to the permanent bending or bowing of one or more limbs.

Cleido-:   Refers to the clavicle (from the Greek, for hook).

Clinodactyly: A developmental anomaly characterized by permanent lateral or medial deflection of a finger.

Coxa plana: Osteochondrosis of the capital femoral epiphysis (head of the femur).

Coxa valga: A hip deformity due to abnormal angulation of the femoral head such that the thigh is kept abducted (from the Latin for bowlegged). The angle between the femoral neck and the shaft is more obtuse than normal. The opposite of coxa vara.

Coxa vara: A hip deformity due to abnormal angulation of the femoral head such that the thigh is kept in a state of adduction (from the Latin for crooked), and the leg appears shortened. The angle between the femoral neck and the shaft is more acute than normal. The opposite of coxa valga.

Craniosynostosis: Premature closure of one or more cranial sutures.

Crus: A general term used to refer to anything resembling a leg. For example, the depression of the external ear, paralleling the posterior border, between the helix and the antihelix.

Cryptophthalmos: A developmental anomaly characterized by skin which is continuous over the eyeballs, without any evidence of eyelid formation.

Cryptorchidism: A developmental defect characterized by full or partial failure of the normal descent of a testis from its fetal position in the abdomen to its postnatal position in the scrotum.

Cubitus valgus: Lateral deviation of the extended forearm at the elbow.

Cubitus varus: Medial deviation of the extended forearm at the elbow.

Cutis marmorata: A transitory mottling of the skin, which is sometimes associated with exposure of the skin to cold.

Cyclopia: Merging of both orbits into a single orbit containing one eye.

Diaphysis: The shaft of a long bone.

Dolichocephaly: Long, narrow cranium, secondary to sagittal synostosis, which prevents lateral skull growth.

Dwarf: An abnormally small person. Dwarfism can be proportionate or disproportionate.

Dysostosis: A defect in the ossification of (fetal) cartilage leading to malformation of individual bones.

Ectopia cordis: Congenital displacement of the heart outside of the thoracic cavity.

Ectrodactyly: ("Lobster claw" deformity) A congenital deformity in which the hand, and less frequently the foot, is split down the middle and thus resembles a lobster claw.

Epiphysis: The part of a long bone derived from an ossification center, located at the end of a long bone and usually wider than the shaft (the diaphysis). It is originally separated from the shaft of the bone by cartilage.

Equinovarus: See talipes equinovarus.

Exostosis: A benign bony tumor or growth arising from the surface of a bone, characteristically capped by cartilage.

Genu valgum: "Knock-knees." A knee deformity in which there is abduction of the lower leg in relation to the thigh.

Genu varum: "Bowlegs." A knee deformity in which there is adduction of the lower leg in relation to the thigh.

Gibbus: A general term meaning hump. Often used to refer to a deformity of the spine.

Glossoptosis: Downward displacement or retraction of the tongue.

Heterochromia: A different color in two similar structures. Typically used to describe the situation of one brown eye and one blue eye.

Hydromelia: An increase in fluid in a dilated central canal of the spinal cord.

Hyperkeratosis: Hypertrophy of the stratum corneum layer of skin.

Hyperostosis: Hypertrophy of bone.

Hypertelorism: Abnormally increased distance between two paired organs or parts. Used almost exclusively to describe ocular hypertelorism, where the eyes are abnormally far apart.

Hypertrichosis: Excessive growth of hair, typically in places which normally have minimal or no hair.

Hypotelorism: Abnormally decreased distance between two paired organs or parts. Used almost exclusively to describe ocular hypotelorism, where the eyes are abnormally close together.

Keratoconus: A noninflammatory, abnormal protrusion of the cornea.

Keratosis pilaris: Development of keratotic plugs in hair follicles causing discrete follicular papules, usually occurring on the arms and thighs.

Lissencephaly: Smooth brain with lack of normal sulci and gyri.

Livedo reticularis: A diffuse flat purple to red vascular discoloration of the skin. It is lacy, in the form of a reticulum ("net-like").

Macrocephaly: Abnormally large head.

Megalencephaly: Abnormally large brain. This is in contradistinction to hydrocephalus in which the intracranial volume is enlarged, but due to excessive cerebrospinal fluid rather than overgrowth of neural tissue.

Mesomelic: Pertaining to the middle segment of long bones.

Metaphysis: The part of the shaft of a long bone (the diaphysis) where it joins the epiphysis.

Metatarsus varus: Inward deviation of the sole of the foot, such that the individual must walk on the outer border of the foot.

Microcephaly: Abnormally small head, usually associated with mental retardation.

Micrognathia: Abnormally small mandible.

Micromelia: A developmental anomaly characterized by abnormally short limbs.

Mosaicism: A situation in which two or more cell lines are derived from a single zygote, but are genotypically distinct.

Oligodactyly: A developmental anomaly characterized by the presence of fewer than five digits on an extremity.

Opisthotonos: A form of spasm in which the body arches backward.

Osteochondrodysplasia: Abnormal development of bone or cartilage.

Osteochondrosis: Degeneration of the ossification centers in children, followed by regeneration or recalcification.

p: Symbol for the short arm of a chromosome.

Pachygyria: Abnormal brain development resulting in thickened convolutions (gyri) and fewer sulci.

Periostosis: Abnormal deposition of periosteal bone.

Pes cavus: Exaggeration of the height of the longitudinal arch of the foot.

Pes planus: "Flatfoot." Flattening of the longitudinal arch of the foot.

Phocomelia: A developmental anomaly characterized by proximal segment shortening of the long bones, such that the hands and feet are attached close to the trunk. A classic example is the "thalidomide baby."

Pinguecula: A yellowish fibrous thickening of the cornea, usually located on the medial side. Occurs often in the elderly.

Plagiocephaly: Slanted cranium, secondary to unilateral coronal synostosis.

Platyspondyly: Flattened vertebral bodies.

Poikiloderma: An atrophic skin condition in which there are also pigmentary changes, giving the skin a mottled appearance.

Polydactyly: A developmental anomaly characterized by extra digits (fingers or toes). Polydactyly may be preaxial or postaxial (see below).

Porencephaly: The presence of one or more cavities (cysts) in the brain which may or may not communicate with the subarachnoid space.

Postaxial: Posterior to the axis of the body or a limb—specifically the medial (ulnar) side of the upper extremities and the lateral (fibular) side of the lower extremities.

Preaxial: Anterior to the axis of the body or a limb—specifically the lateral (radial) side of the upper extremities and the medial (tibial) side of the lower extremities.

Prognathia: Large and/or protruding mandible.

Pseudoarthrosis: A "false joint" as a result of a pathologic fracture in a long bone such that there is movement at a point along the diaphysis of the long bone.

Pseudocamptodactyly: A flexion deformity of the fingers that occurs only with wrist extension. A result of short flexor muscles and tendons rather than a fixed flexion deformity.

Pseudohermaphrodite: An individual whose gonads are definitively male or female, but whose external genitalia are ambiguous, indeterminate, or inconsistent. Female pseudohermaphrodites have ovaries and male pseudohermaphrodites have testes.

Pterygium: An abnormal skin web.

q: Symbol for the long arm of a chromosome.

Rachitic: Bony changes similar to those seen with rickets.

Retrognathia: Abnormally positioned mandible, such that the mandible is behind the frontal plane of the forehead.

Rhizomelic: Pertaining to the hip or shoulder joints (from the Greek, referring to the root of a limb).

Scaphocephaly: "Boat-shaped" cranium, secondary to sagittal synostosis which prevents lateral skull growth.

Schizencephaly: Abnormal clefts in the brain.

Spondylo-:   Refers to the vertebrae or spinal column.

Symphalangism: Congenital end-to-end fusion of contiguous phalanges of a digit.

Syndactyly: Webbing together of adjacent fingers or toes.

Synophrys: Eyebrows that overgrow and fuse in the midline.

Synostosis: The osseous union of bones that are normally distinct.

Talipes equinovarus: One of the most common of the clubfoot deformities. There is a combination of an equinus deformity (plantar extension) and a varus deformity (inversion of the foot).

Telecanthus: Abnormally increased distance between the medial canthi of the eyelids.

Torticollis: "Wry-neck." Cervical muscle contracture leading to twisting of the neck so that the head is pulled to one side with the chin pointing to the opposite side.

Trident hand: A congenital deformity in which the hand is three-pronged.

Trigonocephaly: Triangular cranium, secondary to metopic synostosis.

Turricephaly: Tower shaped cranium, secondary to coronal and lambdoidal synostosis.

Syndromes Starting with Numerals

2-Methylacetoacetyl-CoA Thiolase Deficiency

See Beta-ketothiolase deficiency

3β-Hydroxysteroid Dehydrogenase Deficiency

Included in Congenital adrenal hyperplasia

3-Hydroxy-3-Methylglutaryl-CoA Lyase Deficiency

See Hydroxymethylglutaric aciduria

3-Oxothiolase Deficiency

See Beta-ketothiolase deficiency

4-Hydroxyphenylpyruvic Acid Dioxygenase (Oxidase) Deficiency

See Tyrosinemia III

4p- Syndrome

SYNONYM: Wolf-Hirschhorn syndrome

MIM #: 194190

This syndrome is due to a deletion of the short arm of chromosome 4. It is marked by a variety of midline fusion defects, and about one-third die by 2 years of age. Deletions are of variable sizes. Deletions tend to be paternally derived while translocations tend to be maternally derived.

HEENT/AIRWAY: Microcephaly, prominent glabella (area of the forehead just above the nose—"Greek helmet facies"), midline scalp defects. Hypertelorism, epicanthal folds, strabismus, iris coloboma, high arched eyebrows. Simple, low-set ears with preauricular pits or tags. Short upper lip and philtrum, downturned fish-like mouth, fused teeth, delayed tooth eruption and shedding of deciduous teeth, bilateral cleft lip and cleft palate. Micrognathia. Webbed neck.

CHEST: Patients often have recurrent aspiration secondary to severe neurologic disability. Recurrent respiratory tract infections. May have diaphragmatic hernia, pulmonary isomerism (symmetric right and left lung).

CARDIOVASCULAR: Atrial and ventricular septal defects.

NEUROMUSCULAR: Severe mental and motor retardation. Hypotonia, seizures. Seizures often severe in infancy, and decrease in frequency after 5 years of age. May have absent septum pellucidum, interventricular cysts, agenesis of the corpus callosum.

ORTHOPEDIC: Scoliosis. Simian crease, hyperconvex nails, polydactyly. Absent pubic rami, congenital hip dislocation,

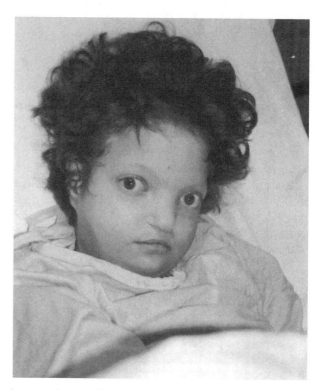

4p- syndrome. This 10-year-old girl with 4p- syndrome has characteristic facies. She has profound psychomotor retardation. She does not walk or talk.

1

metatarsus adductus, clubfoot deformity. Fused or bifid vertebrae. Short stature.

GI/GU: Malrotation of the gut. Hypospadias, cryptorchidism, absent uterus. Renal hypoplasia.

OTHER: Intrauterine growth retardation. Precocious puberty. May have variable deficiency of one of several immunoglobulins.

ANESTHETIC CONSIDERATIONS
Micrognathia may make direct laryngoscopy and tracheal intubation difficult. Stable fixation of an orotracheal tube may be problematic (5). A single case of malignant hyperthermia in a young child with Wolf-Hirschhorn syndrome has been reported (4), but there is no other evidence that malignant hyperthermia is associated with this syndrome. Chronic use of anticonvulsant medications may affect the metabolism of some anesthetic drugs. Children with congenital heart disease require perioperative antibiotic prophylaxis as clinically indicated.

Bibliography:
1. Iacobucci T, Nani L, Picoco F, et al. Anesthesia for a child with Wolf-Hirshhorn [sic] syndrome [Letter]. *Paediatr Anaesth* 2004;14:969.
2. Battaglia A, Carey JC, Wright TJ. Wolf-Hirschhorn (4p-) syndrome. *Adv Pediatr* 2001;48:75–113.
3. Marcelis C, Schrander-Stumpel C, Engelen J, et al. Wolf-Hirschhorn (4p-) syndrome in adults. *Genet Couns* 2001;12:35–48.
4. Ginsburg R, Purcell-Jones G. Malignant hyperthermia in the Wolf-Hirschhorn syndrome. *Anaesthesia* 1988;43:386–388.
5. Jobes DR, Nicolson SC. An alternative method to secure an endotracheal tube in infants with midline facial defects. *Anesthesiology* 1986;64:643–644.

5α-Reductase Deficiency

SYNONYM: Pseudovaginal perineoscrotal hypospadias; Steroid 5α-reductase 2 deficiency

MIM #: 264600

This male-limited autosomal recessive disease is another cause of male pseudohermaphroditism. The defect results in defective conversion of testosterone to dihydrotestosterone. Thus, levels of testosterone are normal. At least 45 distinct mutations have been described. Masculinization at puberty is due to retained activity of the 5α-reductase 1 gene.

GI/GU: Ambiguous genitalia. Small phallus, a bifid scrotum, and perineal hypospadias. Histologically normal testes, epididymides, and vasa deferentia. Underdeveloped seminal vesicles that lead into a vagina, which usually ends blindly. Absent or rudimentary prostate. Can have a urogenital sinus. Sperm production is minimal or absent, and fertility usually requires *in vitro* intervention.

OTHER: With puberty, there is masculinization with deepening voice, phallic enlargement, and a scanty beard.

Affected 46, XY males raised as females often revert to male gender identity at the time of expected puberty.

MISCELLANEOUS: Inhibition of 5α-reductase has been suggested for the prevention of male pattern baldness, and for the treatment of resistant acne, benign prostatic hypertrophy and idiopathic hirsutism. *Middlesex*, by Jeffrey Eugenides, the winner of the 2003 Pulitzer prize for fiction, is told from the perspective of the protagonist, who had 5α-reductase deficiency. In a New Guinea population the disorder is common enough that affected individuals are recognized early and assigned to a third sex. However, they face the same problems when forced to adjust to adult gender roles.

ANESTHETIC CONSIDERATIONS
A certain degree of sensitivity is required when speaking with patients, or families of patients, with intersex disorders.

FIGURE: See **Appendix A**

Bibliography:
1. Sultan C, Lumbroso S, Paris F, et al. Disorders of androgen action. *Sem Rep Med* 2002;20:217–228.
2. Hochberg Z, Chayen R, Reiss N, et al. Clinical, biochemical, and genetic findings in a large pedigree of male and female patients with 5-alpha-reductase 2 deficiency. *J Clin Endocrinol Metab* 1996;81:2821–2827.
3. Wilson JD, Griffin JE, Russel DW. Steroid 5 alpha-reductase 2 deficiency. *Endocr Rev* 1993;14:577–593.
4. Tenover JS. Prostates, pates, and pimples: the potential medicinal uses of steroid 5 alpha reductase inhibitors. *Endocrinol Metab Clin North Am* 1991;20:893–909.

5p- Syndrome

See Cri du chat syndrome

5,10-Methylene Tetrahydrofolate Reductase Deficiency

MIM #: 236250

This autosomal recessive disorder is due to a defect in 5,10-methylene tetrahydrofolate reductase (MTHFR), a cytoplasmic enzyme that is involved in the metabolism of the sulfur-containing amino acids. Specifically, it catalyzes the conversion of 5,10-methylene tetrahydrofolate to 5-methyl tetrahydrofolate. The methyl group is donated to homocysteine (catalyzed by methionine synthase) to form methionine. The clinical severity mirrors the degree of enzyme activity deficiency, and the age of onset varies from infancy to adulthood. Two-thirds of patients are female. The disease can have findings similar to homocystinuria. The disease is generally very difficult to treat. Certain specific mutations can be a risk factor for spina bifida and anencephaly. The C667T single nucleotide polymorphism (SNP) (the thermolabile variant) is relatively common and associated with a hypercoagulable state. Most patients are heterozygous for several substitutions in the gene (compound heterozygotes).

HEENT/AIRWAY: Microcephaly.

CARDIOVASCULAR: High levels of homocysteine have been implicated as a cardiovascular risk factor. MTHFR deficiency may be implicated in the development of coronary artery disease. The C667T SNP, which is relatively common in the population, has been shown to be associated with increased risk of asymptomatic carotid artery disease in postmenopausal women.

NEUROMUSCULAR: Mild developmental delay and mental retardation. Hallucinations, delusions, catatonia. Waddling gait, seizures. Proximal muscle weakness. The neuropathologic findings include dilated ventricles, microgyria, demyelination, macrophage infiltration, and gliosis. Arterial and venous cerebrovascular thrombosis can be fatal. Risk of spina bifida and anencephaly. There is variability in the age of onset of symptoms and the severity of symptoms.

OTHER: Vascular thrombosis and vascular changes similar to those of homocystinuria (see later). The prothrombotic state can result in both arterial and venous thromboses. Patients have elevated homocysteine levels and homocystinuria, although to a far lesser degree than in the disease homocystinuria. A megaloblastic anemia only rarely develops in these patients. This defect may predispose to preeclampsia.

MISCELLANEOUS: The increased risk of spina bifida and anencephaly with certain mutations may account, at least in part, for the effect of maternal dietary folate supplementation in decreasing the risk of these defects in fetuses of normal women. Because arsenic is detoxified by demethylation, the decreased availability of methyl donors in this disease has been suggested to increase the neurotoxicity of arsenic.

ANESTHETIC CONSIDERATIONS

5,10-methylene tetrahydrofolate reductase immediately precedes methionine synthetase in the pathway involved with methionine synthesis. Given the inhibitory effect of nitrous oxide on the latter enzyme (via irreversible oxidation of the cobalt atom of vitamin B_{12}), nitrous oxide is contraindicated in these patients, and neurologic deterioration with death has been reported after anesthesia with nitrous oxide (1).

Bibliography:
1. Selzer RR, Rosenblatt DS, Laxova R, et al. Adverse effect of nitrous oxide in a child with 5,10-methylenetetrahydrofolate reductase deficiency. *N Engl J Med* 2003;349:49–50.
2. Grandone E, Margaglione M, Colaizzo D, et al. Factor V Leiden, C>T MTHFR polymorphism and genetic susceptibility to preeclampsia. *Thromb Haemost* 1997;77:1052–1054.
3. Beckman DR, Hoganson G, Berlow S, et al. Pathologic findings in 5,10-methylene tetrahydrofolate reductase deficiency. *Birth Defects Orig Artic Ser* 1987;23:47–64.

9p- Syndrome

MIM #: 158170

This syndrome is due to a deletion of the short arm of chromosome 9. The clinical picture is variable, but craniosynostosis, a long philtrum, hernias, and digital abnormalities are always present.

HEENT/AIRWAY: Craniosynostosis (particularly of metopic suture), flat occiput. Trigonocephaly. Upward-slanting palpebral fissures, epicanthal folds, prominent eyes due to hypoplastic supraorbital ridges, highly arched eyebrows. Poorly formed, posteriorly rotated ears with adherent earlobes. Midface hypoplasia with short nose, flat nasal bridge, and anteverted nostrils. Choanal atresia. Long philtrum, small mouth, cleft palate, high-arched palate. Micrognathia. Short, broad neck with low posterior hairline.

CHEST: Diaphragmatic hernia.

CARDIOVASCULAR: Congenital cardiac defects, most frequently ventricular septal defect, patent ductus arteriosus, or pulmonic stenosis.

NEUROMUSCULAR: Moderate to severe mental retardation, but often with good social adaptation, and psychological similarities to those of Williams syndrome (see later) have been noted. Poor memory, visual-motor skills, and visual-spatial skills.

ORTHOPEDIC: Normal growth, scoliosis. Long middle phalanges, short distal phalanges, simian crease, postaxial polydactyly. Foot positioning defects. Long fingers and toes.

GI/GU: Diastasis recti, inguinal and umbilical hernias. Micropenis, cryptorchidism, hypoplastic labia majora. Hydronephrosis.

OTHER: Nonketotic hyperglycinemia (see later) has been observed in a patient with 9p- syndrome, suggesting at least one of the genes for that syndrome resides on the short arm of chromosome 9.

MISCELLANEOUS: Acute leukemia has been associated with partial deletion of the short arm of chromosome 9, and the affected gene is usually maternally derived. 9p deletion has also been implicated with other cancers.

ANESTHETIC CONSIDERATIONS

Although not reported, the small mouth and micrognathia may make direct laryngoscopy and tracheal intubation difficult. Choanal atresia precludes placement of a nasal airway, nasal intubation, or placement of a nasogastric tube. Consider preoperative evaluation of renal function in patients with a history of renal abnormalities which predispose to renal insufficiency. Patients with congenital heart disease require perioperative antibiotic prophylaxis as indicated.

Bibliography:
1. Huret JL, Leonard C, Forestier B, et al. Eleven new cases of del(9p) and features from 80 cases. *J Med Genet* 1988;25:741–749.

10 qter Deletion Syndrome

MIM #: None

This syndrome involves a deletion of the terminal portion of the long arm of chromosome 10. Most patients have been female.

HEENT/AIRWAY: Microcephaly. Upward-slanting palpebral fissures, hypertelorism. Broad, beak-like nose. Micrognathia. Short neck.

CARDIOVASCULAR: Congenital cardiac defects of a wide variety of types.

NEUROMUSCULAR: Variable mental retardation.

ORTHOPEDIC: Growth retardation.

GI/GU: Can have bladder obstruction and urethral reflux, and secondary urinary tract infections.

ANESTHETIC CONSIDERATIONS
Micrognathia and short neck may make laryngoscopy and tracheal intubation difficult. Patients with congenital heart disease require perioperative antibiotic prophylaxis as clinically indicated.

Bibliography:
1. Costakos DT, Love LA, Josephson K, et al. Pathological case of the month. Chromosome 10 qter deletion syndrome. *Arch Pediatr Adolesc Med* 1998;152:507–508.
2. Davis ST, Ducey JP, Fincher CW, et al. The anesthetic management of a patient with chromosome 10qter deletion syndrome. *J Clin Anesth* 1994;6:512–514.

11β-Hydroxylase Deficiency

Included in Congenital adrenal hyperplasia

11β-Hydroxysteroid Dehydrogenase Deficiency

SYNONYM: 11β-ketoreductase deficiency; Apparent mineralocorticoid excess

MIM #: 218030

This autosomal recessive defect in 11β-hydroxysteroid dehydrogenase results in low renin hypertension and hypokalemia. This enzyme has two functional isoforms, one of which catalyzes the conversion of cortisol to cortisone (dehydrogenase activity) and the conversion of cortisone to cortisol (oxoreductase activity). The other isoform catalyzes just the conversion of cortisol to cortisone. In this disease, there is decreased conversion of cortisol to cortisone. Other features of the defect suggest a primary mineralocorticoid excess, which cannot be documented, and the defect is also known as the syndrome of apparent mineralocorticoid excess (AME) because of a defect in the first isoform type. Apparently the defect prevents cortisol from acting as a ligand for the mineralocorticoid receptor.

HEENT/AIRWAY: Hypertensive retinopathy.

CARDIOVASCULAR: Low renin hypertension. Left ventricular hypertrophy from systemic hypertension.

OTHER: Hypokalemia. Low aldosterone levels.

MISCELLANEOUS: Inhibition of this enzyme may be the mechanism of licorice-induced hypertension (very uncommon in the United States, where almost all domestic licorice is artificially flavored) (2). Similar inhibition can be caused by compounds in grapefruit juice. Activity of this enzyme may be related to the development of the metabolic syndrome, obesity, and type 2 diabetes.

ANESTHETIC CONSIDERATIONS
Patients may have significant hypertension with end-organ involvement. Blood pressure must be controlled before elective surgery. Serum potassium level should be determined preoperatively. Steroid replacement therapy should be continued perioperatively.

FIGURE: See **Appendix A**

Bibliography:
1. Stewart PM, Corrie JET, Shackleton CHL, et al. The syndrome of apparent mineralocorticoid excess: a defect in the cortisol-cortisone shuttle. *J Clin Invest* 1988;82:340–349.
2. Stewart PM, Wallace AM, Valentino R, et al. Mineralocorticoid activity of licorice: 11-beta-hydroxysteroid dehydrogenase comes of age. *Lancet* 1987;2:821–824.

11β-Ketoreductase Deficiency

See 11β-hydroxysteroid dehydrogenase deficiency

11q- Syndrome

SYNONYM: Jacobsen syndrome

MIM #: 147791

This syndrome is due to deletion of the terminal band of the long arm of chromosome 11. This fragment of the

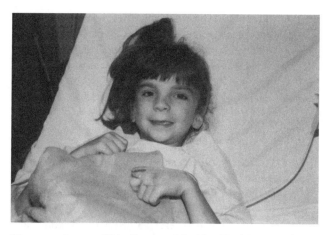

11q- syndrome. This 8-year-old girl with 11q- syndrome has thrombocytopenia as well as a chronic low white blood cell count. She has dysmorphic facies, mild mental retardation and congenital heart disease (parachute mitral valve and bicuspid aortic valve). She also has decreased pain sensation.

chromosome is known to contain a fragile site. Seventy-five percent of affected children are girls. The syndrome is characterized by trigonocephaly, carp-shaped mouth, and mental retardation.

HEENT/AIRWAY: Trigonocephaly (see C syndrome for illustration). Microcephaly, less commonly macrocephaly. Epicanthal folds, telecanthus, hypertelorism, ptosis, strabismus, coloboma of iris or retina, retinal dysplasia. Low-set or malformed ears. Flat nasal bridge, short nose with upturned tip. Carp-shaped mouth. Micrognathia. Short neck.

CHEST: Frequent respiratory infections. Pectus excavatum. Missing ribs.

CARDIOVASCULAR: A variety of congenital cardiac defects.

NEUROMUSCULAR: Moderate to severe mental retardation. Hypotonia in infancy, hypertonicity when older.

ORTHOPEDIC: Growth retardation. Joint contractures. Fifth finger clinodactyly, brachydactyly. Hammer toe. Bilateral camptodactyly. Short fingers.

GI/GU: Pyloric stenosis, inguinal hernia. Annular pancreas. Hypospadias, cryptorchidism, hypoplasia of labia and clitoris, vesicoanal fistula.

OTHER: Intrauterine growth retardation, failure to thrive. Isoimmune thrombocytopenia is common.

ANESTHETIC CONSIDERATIONS
Tracheal intubation may be difficult due to the short neck and micrognathia. Contractures may make optimal positioning difficult. Baseline platelet count should be obtained. Bleeding from thrombocytopenia is a very real concern. In addition to platelet transfusion, DDAVP has been suggested for minor surgery. Patients with structural cardiac defects need perioperative antibiotic prophylaxis as indicated.

Bibliography:
1. Easley RB, Sanders D, McElrath-Schwartz J, et al. Anesthetic implications of Jacobsen syndrome. *Paediatr Anaesth* 2006;16:66–71.
2. Grossfeld PD, Mattina T, Lai Z, et al. The 11q terminal deletion disorder: a prospective study of 110 cases. *Am J Med Genet A* 2004;129:51–61.

13q- Syndrome

MIM #: None

The phenotype and natural history of this syndrome is variable, based on the specific chromosomal section deleted. It can be associated with the development of retinoblastoma.

HEENT/AIRWAY: Microcephaly. May have trigonocephaly or facial asymmetry. Hypertelorism, ptosis, epicanthal folds, microphthalmia. May have colobomas. Retinoblastomas, often bilateral. May have dysplastic retina or optic nerve. Prominent, low placed ears. Prominent nasal bridge. Prominent maxilla. Micrognathia. May have narrow palate. Short webbed neck.

CARDIOVASCULAR: Cardiac defects.

NEUROMUSCULAR: Mental retardation. May have holoprosencephalic type of brain defects.

ORTHOPEDIC: Growth deficiency, often of prenatal onset. Small or absent thumbs, clinodactyly of fifth finger, fused fourth and fifth metacarpals. Talipes equinovarus, short hallux. Focal lumbar agenesis.

GI/GU: May have imperforate anus or Hirshsprung disease. Hypospadias, cryptorchidism. May have bifid scrotum or renal anomalies.

ANESTHETIC CONSIDERATIONS
Tracheal intubation may be difficult due to prominent maxilla, micrognathia and short neck. May come to the operating room for Hirshsprung disease or the development of retinoblastoma requiring enucleation. In two case reports, tracheal intubation was not difficult.

Bibliography:
1. Mayhew JF, Fernandez M, Wheaton M. Anesthesia in a child with deletion 13q syndrome [Letter]. *Paediatr Anaesth* 2005;15:350.
2. Inada T, Matsumoto H, Shingu K. Anaesthesia in a child with deletion 13q syndrome [Letter]. *Paediatr Anaesth* 1998;8:441.

17α-Hydroxylase Deficiency

Included in Congenital adrenal hyperplasia

17β-Hydroxysteroid Dehydrogenase Deficiency

See 17-ketosteroid reductase deficiency

17-Ketosteroid Reductase Deficiency

SYNONYM: 17β-hydroxysteroid dehydrogenase deficiency; Pseudohermaphroditism, male

MIM #: 264300

This autosomal recessive disorder, due to inadequate function of the gene for 17-ketosteroid reductase, results in male pseudohermaphroditism. This enzyme is required for the final step in androgen production. These children are XY males, with testes, but have female external genitalia. There is virilization with normal male secondary sex characteristics at puberty. Of interest, this enzyme is nonfunctional until puberty, when there is a progressive increase in activity, with increase in testosterone to almost normal levels. Children are usually raised as girls, and removal of the testes can prevent the pubertal masculinization. In genetic females, this defect can result in polycystic ovaries and hirsutism. The findings in this disorder are very similar to those of 5α-reductase deficiency.

GI/GU: Male pseudohermaphroditism—there are female-appearing external genitalia at birth, though the genitalia may be somewhat ambiguous. Inguinal testes, with normal virilization at puberty.

OTHER: Gynecomastia, infertility, hypothyroidism.

ANESTHETIC CONSIDERATIONS
Patients may be hypothyroid. Otherwise, there are no metabolic consequences of particular importance to anesthesia. However, a particular degree of sensitivity is needed when speaking to girls and boys with gender ambiguity.

FIGURE: See Appendix A

Bibliography:
1. Castro-Magana M, Anguo M, Uy J. Male hypogonadism with gynecomastia caused by late-onset deficiency of testicular 17-ketosteroid reductase. N Engl J Med 1993;328:1297–1301.
2. Pang S, Softness B, Sweeney WJ, et al. Hirsutism, polycystic ovarian disease, and ovarian 17-ketoreductase deficiency. N Engl J Med 1987;316:1295–1301.

17,20-Desmolase (Lyase) Deficiency

SYNONYM: Desmolase deficiency

MIM #: 309150

This X-linked (probably recessive) disorder is due to absence of the enzyme 17,20-desmolase, which is involved in steroid biosynthesis. Because this enzyme is not involved in the pathway for hydrocortisone, the adrenogenital syndrome does not occur. This enzyme, as well as other enzymes of steroidogenesis, is a cytochrome P450 oxidase, and is also known as P450c17. Absence of the desmolase activity results in deficient gonadal sex hormone production. Genetic boys have female external genitalia (male pseudohermaphroditism), and girls are phenotypically normal but fail to undergo adrenarche and puberty.

Although deficient 17,20-desmolase and 17α-hydroxylase activities can occur separately and were thought to represent two distinct enzymes, they are currently known to reside in a single protein. The gene for this protein has been localized to chromosome 10, and at least 16 distinct mutations have been described.

GI/GU: Ambiguous genitalia in boys and pubertal developmental failure in girls. Adrenal hyperplasia.

ANESTHETIC CONSIDERATIONS
There are no metabolic consequences of particular importance to anesthesia. However, a particular degree of sensitivity is needed when speaking to girls and boys with gender ambiguity.

FIGURE: See Appendix A

Bibliography:
1. Zachmann M. Prismatic cases: 17,20-desmolase (17,20-lyase) deficiency. J Clin Endocrinol Metab 1996;81:457–459.
2. Zachmann M, Vollmin JA, Hamilton W, et al. Steroid 17,20-desmolase deficiency: a new cause of male pseudohermaphroditism. Clin Endocrinol 1972;1:369–385.

18-Hydroxylase Deficiency

SYNONYM: Corticosterone methyl oxidase I deficiency

MIM #: 203400

This autosomal recessive disorder in steroid biosynthesis results in aldosterone deficiency. This enzyme (possibly part of a multifunctional enzyme P450C11) is responsible for the conversion of corticosterone to aldosterone.

GI/GU: Poor feeding with occasional vomiting.

OTHER: Failure to thrive, dehydration, and intermittent fever. Hypernatremia. Hypokalemia.

ANESTHETIC CONSIDERATIONS
Patients should have baseline electrolyte and hydration status evaluated. Patients with a history of poor feeding and vomiting are at increased risk for perioperative aspiration. Patients should receive stress dose steroids perioperatively, and then continue on steroid replacement therapy.

FIGURE: See Appendix A

Bibliography:
1. White PC, New MI, Dupont B. Congenital adrenal hyperplasia. *N Engl J Med* 1987;316:1580–1586.
2. Yanagibashi K, Haniu M, Shively JE, et al. The synthesis of aldosterone by the adrenal cortex: two zones (fasciculata and glomerulosa) possess one enzyme for 11 beta-18-hydroxylation, and aldehyde synthesis. *J Biol Chem* 1986;261:3556–3562.

18p- Syndrome

MIM #: None

This syndrome is due to deletion of the short arm of chromosome 18. The hallmark findings are mental retardation, growth deficiency, and prominent ears. However, there may be significant variability in expression.

HEENT/AIRWAY: Microcephaly, rounded face. Ptosis, epicanthal folds, loss of hair of outer eyebrows, hypertelorism, cataracts, strabismus. Large, protruding ears. Low nasal bridge. Wide mouth with downturned corners, dental caries, cleft palate. Micrognathia. Webbed neck.

CHEST: Pectus excavatum, broad chest.

CARDIOVASCULAR: Congenital heart disease.

NEUROMUSCULAR: Mild to severe mental retardation, particularly poor language skills. Restlessness, emotional lability, fear of strangers. May be hypotonic. May have holoprosencephaly.

ORTHOPEDIC: Mild to moderate growth deficiency. Kyphoscoliosis. Small hands and feet, clinodactyly of fifth finger, simian crease. Cubitus valgus, dislocated hip, clubfoot deformity. Rheumatoid arthritis-like picture, polymyositis.

GI/GU: Inguinal hernia. Genital anomalies.

OTHER: Immunoglobulin A (IgA) deficiency. Alopecia, hypopigmentation.

ANESTHETIC CONSIDERATIONS
Although not reported, micrognathia might make direct laryngoscopy and tracheal intubation difficult. Behavioral problems may complicate preoperative management. Patients with IgA deficiency may have allergic reactions to the IgA found in transfused blood. Patients with congenital heart disease may require perioperative antibiotic prophylaxis as clinically indicated.

Bibliography:
1. Movahhedian HR, Kane HA, Borgaonkar D, et al. Heart disease associated with deletion of the short arm of chromosome 18. *Del Med J* 1991;63:285–289.
2. Kane HA, Borgaonkar D, McDermott M, et al. 18p monosomy syndrome [Letter]. *Pediatr Cardiol* 1991;12:133.

18q- Syndrome

MIM #: 601808

This syndrome is due to a deletion of the long arm of chromosome 18. There is significant clinical variability. In general, the size of the deletion correlates with the severity of the disease. The primary finding is midface hypoplasia.

HEENT/AIRWAY: Microcephaly, midface hypoplasia. Deep-set eyes, epicanthal folds, slanted palpebral fissures, hypertelorism, microphthalmia, hypoplasia of iris, cataracts, retinal defect, myopia, nystagmus. Prominent antihelix or antitragus, narrow or atretic external auditory canal with conductive deafness. Can have sensorineural hearing loss. Carp-shaped mouth. Narrow palate, cleft lip or palate.

CHEST: Extra rib. Widely spaced nipples.

CARDIOVASCULAR: Cardiac defects.

NEUROMUSCULAR: Moderate to severe mental retardation. Hypotonia, poor coordination. May have seizures, choreoathetosis, atrophy of olfactory and optic tracts, poorly myelinated central white matter tracts, hydrocephalus, porencephalic cysts, cerebellar hypoplasia. Behavioral problems described as "obnoxious or autistic."

ORTHOPEDIC: Small stature. Long hands, tapered fingers, short first metacarpals, simian crease. Hypoplastic tapering of distal legs, abnormal placement of toes, clubfoot deformity. Dimpled skin over acromion and knuckles.

GI/GU: Horseshoe kidney. Hypoplastic labia majora. Cryptorchidism, micropenis.

OTHER: Eczema. Hypothyroidism.

ANESTHETIC CONSIDERATIONS
Behavioral problems may complicate preoperative care. The anesthesiologist should be sensitive to possible hearing or visual deficits. Patients with congenital heart disease require perioperative antibiotic prophylaxis as indicated.

Bibliography:
1. Chudley AE, Kovnats S, Ray M. Recognizable behavioral and somatic phenotype in patients with proximal interstitial 18q deletion: report on a new affected child and follow-up on the original reported familial cases. *Am J Med Genet* 1992;43:535–538.

21-Hydroxylase Deficiency

Included in Congenital adrenal hyperplasia

22q11.2 Deletion Syndrome

See DiGeorge syndrome

Syndromes Listed Alphabetically

A

AADC Deficiency

See Aromatic L-amino acid decarboxylase deficiency

Aarskog Syndrome

SYNONYM: Aarskog-Scott syndrome; Faciodigitogenital syndrome

MIM #: 305400

This syndrome is characterized by short stature, hypertelorism, and shawl scrotum. It appears to be inherited in an X-linked recessive pattern, with female carriers expressing mild features of the syndrome in their face and hands. However, there is some evidence of autosomal dominant inheritance, with a strong sex influence accounting for the preponderance of affected boys. This syndrome is caused by a mutation in the *FDG1* (faciodigitogenital) gene, which encodes the FDGY protein. This protein is a guanine nucleotide exchange factor. By activating a GTPase it stimulates fibroblasts to form filopodia, the cellular elements involved in signaling, adhesion, and migration. It also activates a kinase pathway that regulates cell growth, apoptosis, and cellular differentiation.

HEENT/AIRWAY: Normocephalic. Rounded facies. Hypertelorism with possible ptosis of eyelids and downward slant of palpebral fissures. Widow's peak. Upper helices of ears overfolded. Small nose, anteverted nares. Long philtrum. Maxillary hypoplasia. Slight crease below the lower lip. Retarded dental eruption. Permanent teeth characterized by broad central incisors. Short neck, occasionally with webbing. May have cleft lip and cleft palate.

CHEST: Pectus excavatum.

CARDIOVASCULAR: Congenital heart disease (small ventricular septal defect) has been reported but is uncommon.

NEUROMUSCULAR: Occasional mild to moderate mental retardation. Attention deficit and hyperactivity disorder (ADHD) common. Hypermobility of the cervical spine in association with ligamentous laxity or odontoid hypoplasia can result in neurologic deficit.

ORTHOPEDIC: Ligamentous laxity. Short stature with distally shortened limbs. Possible hypoplasia or synostosis of one or more cervical vertebrae. Brachydactyly with clinodactyly of the fifth finger, simian crease, interdigital webbing, and hyperextensible fingers. Broad thumbs and great toes, flat feet. Possible spina bifida occulta. Calcified intervertebral disks. Retarded bone age.

GI/GU: "Shawl" scrotum. Cryptorchidism. Umbilical and inguinal hernias common.

OTHER: Isolated growth hormone deficiency. Delayed puberty.

MISCELLANEOUS: Dagfinn Aarskog is a Norwegian pediatric endocrinologist.

ANESTHETIC CONSIDERATIONS
Although perioperative complications have not been described, the presence of vertebral laxity and/or odontoid abnormalities suggests that care should be taken to prevent excessive neck manipulation during positioning and laryngoscopy. Children with congenital heart disease will require appropriate antibiotic prophylaxis. The presence of ADHD requires additional attention in the preinduction period.

Bibliography:
1. Teebi AS, Rucquoi JK, Meyn MS. Aarskog syndrome: report of a family with review and discussion of nosology. *Am J Med Genet* 1993;46: 501–509.
2. Berry C, Cree J, Mann T. Aarskog's syndrome. *Arch Dis Child* 1980;55: 706–710.

Aarskog-Scott Syndrome

See Aarskog syndrome

Aase Syndrome

MIM #: 105650

This likely autosomal recessive, but possibly autosomal dominant, disease involves congenital anemia and radial/thumb anomalies. This is probably a variant of Blackfan-Diamond syndrome (see later) rather than a distinct syndrome and is now categorized as such.

HEENT/AIRWAY: Late closure of fontanelles.

CARDIOVASCULAR: Possible ventricular septal defect.

ORTHOPEDIC: Triphalangeal thumb. Mild radial hypoplasia. Narrow, sloping shoulders. There is mild growth deficiency.

OTHER: Congenital hypoplastic anemia that tends to improve with age. Anemia is responsive to prednisone therapy.

ANESTHETIC CONSIDERATIONS
The patient's hematocrit should be evaluated preoperatively. Radial anomalies may limit peripheral vascular access and make placement of a radial arterial catheter more difficult.

Bibliography:
1. Hurst JA, Baraitser M, Wonke B. Autosomal dominant transmission of congenital erythroid hypoplastic anemia with radial abnormalities. *Am J Med Genet* 1991;40:482–484.
2. Muis N, Beemer FA, van Dijken P, et al. The Aase syndrome: case report and review of the literature. *Eur J Pediatr* 1986;145:153–157.

Aase-Smith Syndrome

MIM #: 147800
This autosomal dominant syndrome is characterized by severe joint contractures and other joint abnormalities, including limited ability to open the mouth. The infants can be stillborn or die in infancy. There is also an Aase-Smith syndrome II, which is the same as Blackfan-Diamond syndrome (see later).

HEENT/AIRWAY: May have ptosis. External ear abnormalities. Cleft palate. Limited ability to open the mouth.

CARDIOVASCULAR: May have ventricular septal defect or multiple ventricular septal defects.

NEUROMUSCULAR: Dandy-Walker malformation with associated hydrocephalus.

ORTHOPEDIC: Severe joint contractures. Thin fingers. Absent knuckles with reduced interphalangeal creases. Inability to make a complete fist. Hypoplastic dermal ridges. Limited extension of the elbows and knees. Clubfoot deformity.

OTHER: Congenital neuroblastoma has been reported.

ANESTHETIC CONSIDERATIONS
Limitations in opening the mouth persist after the induction of anesthesia (1) and may make direct laryngoscopy and tracheal intubation difficult. Patients must be carefully positioned and padded intraoperatively secondary to joint contractures and other joint abnormalities. Patients with congenital cardiac defects will require appropriate antibiotic prophylaxis.

Bibliography:
1. Patton MA, Sharma A, Winter RM. The Aase-Smith syndrome. *Clin Genet* 1985;28:521–525.

Abetalipoproteinemia

SYNONYM: Acanthocytosis

MIM #: 200100
This autosomal recessive disease is due to the absence of apolipoprotein B, secondary to a deficiency in the microsomal triglyceride transfer protein. This is the sole apoprotein of low-density lipoproteins and one of the components of very low density lipoproteins. The classic finding is the presence of acanthocytes on a blood smear (from the Greek word *acanthi*, for thorn).

HEENT/AIRWAY: Pigmentary degeneration of the retina. Ophthalmoplegia, ptosis, and anisocoria, presumably secondary to neuropathy, have been described.

CARDIOVASCULAR: Fatal cardiomyopathy has been described in a patient.

NEUROMUSCULAR: Ataxia, demyelination, and decreased deep tendon reflexes in adolescents and adults. Neurologic findings may be severe in untreated patients, with eventual inability to stand unaided. Peripheral sensory neuropathy. In general, the cranial nerves are spared, but involvement of oculomotor nerves and degeneration of the tongue have been reported. There may be muscle weakness, which can be difficult to appreciate in the presence of denervation.

ORTHOPEDIC: Untreated patients can have muscle contractures, pes cavus, clubfoot deformity, and kyphoscoliosis.

GI/GU: Vomiting and the celiac syndrome with defective absorption of lipids. The intestinal villi are normal. Malabsorption symptoms tend to diminish with age, probably reflecting, at least in great part, the aversion of these patients to dietary fat.

OTHER: Poor weight gain. Examination of a blood smear shows acanthocytes, a particular type of burr cell with protuberances. These cells do not easily form rouleaux, and the sedimentation rate is very low. Red blood cell survival is shortened, and there may be hyperbilirubinemia. Anemia, which has been described, is probably secondary to fat malabsorption. Fat-soluble vitamin malabsorption (vitamins A, D, E, and K). Many of the findings of the disease are due to secondary vitamin E deficiency. Vitamin K malabsorption can result in prothrombin deficiency. Serum cholesterol is very low and serum beta lipoprotein is absent.

MISCELLANEOUS: Acanthocytes, although constituting 50% to 100% of peripheral red blood cells, are absent in the marrow, suggesting that their formation requires exposure to plasma. The defect in the red blood cell membrane morphology can be reversed by chlorpromazine.

ANESTHETIC CONSIDERATIONS
Fat-soluble vitamins may be deficient secondary to malabsorption. The prothrombin time may be abnormal secondary to vitamin K deficiency. Patients reportedly show diminished response to local anesthetics. There are no reports of the efficacy of neuraxial blockade. The presence of denervation is a likely contraindication for succinylcholine, secondary to the risk of exaggerated hyperkalemia.

Bibliography:
1. Rampoldi L, Danek A, Monaco AP. Clinical features and molecular bases of neuroacanthocytosis. *J Mol Med* 2002;80:475–491.
2. Rader DJ, Brewer HB. Abetalipoproteinemia: new insights into lipoprotein assemble and vitamin E metabolism from a rare genetic disease. *JAMA* 1993;270:865–869.
3. Azizi E, Zaidman JL, Eschar J, et al. Abetalipoproteinaemia treated with parenteral and oral vitamins A and E, and with medium chain triglycerides. *Acta Paediatr Scand* 1978;67:797–801.

Absent Pulmonary Valve Syndrome

MIM #: None

This syndrome has findings that are limited to the heart and chest. The pulmonary valve leaflets are absent, and there is almost always an associated ventricular septal defect.

CHEST: There can be compression of the trachea and bronchi by the massively dilated main pulmonary arteries and their branches. In some patients, the smaller intrapulmonary bronchi are obstructed by abnormally branching segmental pulmonary arteries, which is not relieved by surgical correction of the proximal pulmonary arterial dilatation. There can be unilateral obstructive emphysema and segmental atelectasis visible on chest radiographs. Airway obstruction tends to improve over the first year because of factors including maturation and stiffening of the airways, smaller pulmonary arteries with the postnatal fall in pulmonary vascular resistance, and possibly, the development of obstruction to outflow at the level of the pulmonary valve annulus. Bronchial obstruction has been treated by endobronchial stents. Patients with an intact ventricular septum often have less severe respiratory involvement that presents later in life than those with a ventricular septal defect.

CARDIOVASCULAR: Absent pulmonary valve leaflets. There is almost always an associated ventricular septal defect, but a variety of other cardiac lesions have also been described. The pulmonary valve annulus can be obstructive, and there is massive dilatation of the pulmonary arteries. These findings are often known as "tetralogy of Fallot with absent pulmonary valve." An obligate consequence of the absence of pulmonary valve tissue is massive pulmonary insufficiency. The right ventricle is dilated. There can be transient cyanosis in the neonate, which usually resolves as pulmonary vascular resistance falls over the first weeks of life. Surgical repair is by insertion of a prosthetic pulmonary valve, with closure of the ventricular septal defect.

GI/GU: Hepatomegaly may be present in infants with profound heart failure.

ANESTHETIC CONSIDERATIONS
Respiratory obstruction in the spontaneously breathing infant may be overcome by placing the infant prone. The addition of continuous positive airway pressure may help keep the major airways patent. Care should be taken to avoid stacking of breaths and overdistention in children with obstructive disease. Patients should receive perioperative antibiotic prophylaxis as indicated.

Bibliography:
1. Zucker N, Rozin I, Levitas A, et al. Clinical presentation, natural history, and outcome of patients with the absent pulmonary valve syndrome. *Cardiol Young* 2004;14:402–408.
2. Kirshbom PM, Kogon BE. Tetralogy of Fallot with absent pulmonary valve syndrome. Sem Thorac Cardiovasc surg. *Pediatr Card Surg Ann* 2004;7:65–71.
3. Stayer SA, Shetty S, Andropoulos DB. Perioperative management of tetralogy of Fallot with absent pulmonary valve. *Paediatr Anaesth* 2002;12:705–711.
4. Horigome H, Sakakibara Y, Atsumi N, et al. Absent pulmonary valve with intact ventricular septum presenting as cardiorespiratory failure at birth. *Pediatr Cardiol* 1997;18:136–138.
5. Godart F, Houyel L, Lacour-Gayet F, et al. Absent pulmonary valve syndrome: surgical treatment and considerations. *Ann Thorac Surg* 1996;62:136–142.

Acanthocytosis

See Abetalipoproteinemia

Acetylaspartic Aciduria

See Canavan disease

Acetyl-CoA Acetyltransferase-1 Deficiency

See Beta-ketothiolase deficiency

Achondrogenesis

Includes Parenti-Fraccaro achondrogenesis and Langer-Saldino achondrogenesis

MIM #: 200600, 200610, 200710, 200720, 600972

This early lethal chondrodystrophy has been described in two forms (type I and type II). Type I achondrogenesis is also known as **Parenti-Fraccaro achondrogenesis** and has two distinct subtypes, type IA and type IB. Type II achondrogenesis is also known as **Langer-Saldino achondrogenesis**. A nonlethal form of chondrodystrophy that was called **achondrogenesis** by Grebe is now referred to as Grebe syndrome (see later).

All patients with achondrogenesis die *in utero* or shortly after birth. Types IA, IB, and II can be distinguished on the grounds of clinical, radiologic, and histopathologic examination, but all involve severe defects in the development of cartilage and bone.

Types IA and IB achondrogenesis are inherited in an autosomal recessive manner. A mutation in the diastrophic dysplasia sulfate transporter gene (*DTDST*) has been shown to be the cause of type IB achondrogenesis. Therefore, type IB achondrogenesis and diastrophic dysplasia (see later) are allelic disorders. Type II achondrogenesis is likely inherited in an autosomal dominant manner, although most of the reported cases have occurred in otherwise normal families, presumably reflecting fresh mutations. A mutation in the *COL2A1* gene, leading to abnormal type II collagen, causes type II achondrogenesis. Mutations in the *COL2A1* gene are also responsible for Kniest syndrome, spondyloepiphyseal dysplasia congenita, and Stickler syndrome (see later).

HEENT/AIRWAY

Types IA/IB: Large poorly ossified cranium, maxillary hypoplasia or high palate, low nasal bridge, micrognathia.

Type II: Large cranium with particularly large anterior and posterior fontanelles, prominent forehead, maxillary hypoplasia or high palate, flat nasal bridge, small anteverted nares, and micrognathia.

CHEST

Type IA: Barrel chest. Multiple broken ribs. Hypoplastic scapulae.

Type II: Pulmonary hypoplasia.

ORTHOPEDIC

Types IA/IB: Extreme short stature. Micromelia. Short ribs. Bony ossification clearly abnormal, especially in the hands, feet, lower spine, and pelvic bones. Types IA and IB can be distinguished by radiographic features. For example, type IA involves multiple rib fractures, whereas type IB does not.

Type II: Extreme short stature. Micromelia. Short ribs, without fractures. Short, broad long bones. Bony ossification varies from normal to virtually absent in the lower spine and pelvis.

MISCELLANEOUS: A form of type I achondrogenesis was described in 1986 and is referred to as "schneckenbecken dysplasia" (German for "snail's pelvis"; *MIM* # 269250). It is unclear whether the screenwriter of the film *The Birdcage*, who penned the line "When the schnecken beckons," was aware of this entity (*schnecken* is a type of sweet roll).

ANESTHETIC CONSIDERATIONS
Patients are unlikely to benefit from surgery/anesthesia because of the early lethality of this disorder. Direct laryngoscopy and tracheal intubation may be difficult because of

micrognathia. Care must be taken in positioning because of the severe chondrodysplasia and possibility of fractures.

Bibliography:
1. Superti-Furga A, Hastbacka J, Wilcox WR, et al. Achondrogenesis type IB is caused by mutations in the diastrophic dysplasia sulfate transporter gene. *Nat Genet* 1996;2:100–102.
2. Borochowitz Z, Lachman R, Adomian GE, et al. Achondrogenesis type I: delineation of further heterogeneity and identification of two distinct subgroups. *J Pediatr* 1988;112:23–31.
3. Borochowitz Z, Jones KL, Silbey R, et al. A distinct lethal neonatal chondrodysplasia with snail-like pelvis: schneckenbecken dysplasia. *Am J Med Genet* 1986;25:47–59.
4. Borochowitz Z, Ornoy A, Lachman R, et al. Achondrogenesis II-hypochondrogenesis: variability versus heterogeneity. *Am J Med Genet* 1986;24:273–288.
5. Chen H, Lin CT, Yang SS. Achondrogenesis: a review with special consideration of achondrogenesis type II (Langer-Saldino). *Am J Med Genet* 1981;10:379–394.

Achondroplasia

MIM #: 100800

The most common type of short-limbed dwarfism (1 in 15,000 births), this autosomal dominant disease results from the failure in development of endochondral bone, primarily at the epiphyseal growth plates and the base of the skull. There is premature fusion of bones. The underlying defect is a mutation in the gene encoding fibroblast growth factor receptor-3 (*FGFR3*). Histologic evaluation at the epiphyseal line shows short cartilaginous columns that lack the usual linear arrangement, and some cartilage cells that appear to be undergoing a mucinoid degeneration. Close to 90% of cases represent spontaneous gene mutations (affected children are born to parents without achondroplasia), with advanced paternal age an increased risk for gene mutation. The homozygous form is usually fatal within the first few weeks of life secondary to respiratory insufficiency or severe neurologic impairment from hydrocephalus. People with the heterozygous form have normal intelligence and life expectancy. Surgical decompression of the cervicomedullary junction may be performed during the first few years of life, although the timing and necessity of such intervention is still debated.

HEENT/AIRWAY: Macrocephaly, short cranial base with small foramen magnum, prominent forehead, and flattened midface. Short eustachian tubes can lead to conductive hearing loss secondary to chronic recurrent otitis media. Saddle nose, narrow nasal passages, choanal stenosis. Long, narrow mouth with high-arched palate, macroglossia, prominent mandible. Tonsillectomy and adenoidectomy can improve symptoms of sleep apnea.

CHEST: Chest wall deformities in children include abnormal spinal curvature and a small rib cage that can lead to impaired respiratory function secondary to a constrictive thoracic cage. Restrictive lung disease can be severe enough to cause

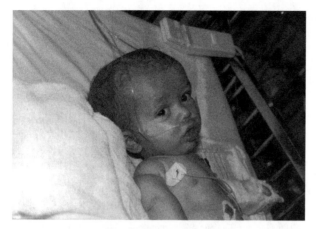

Achondroplasia. FIG. 1. A young infant with achondroplasia. His head and ventricles are large, although his head circumference is within normal limits for a child with achondroplasia. He had a history of apneic spells and had "trimming" of his epiglottis. During a later tonsillectomy he presumably had a vagally-mediated asystolic arrest.

hypoxemia or hypercapnia and can be present in childhood. Thoracic cage constriction improves over time, and adults have an almost normal chest wall configuration. Obstructive sleep apnea can occur. There can also be a component of central respiratory dysfunction (see *Neuromuscular*).

CARDIOVASCULAR: Patients can develop pulmonary artery hypertension and right ventricular hypertrophy with strain.

NEUROMUSCULAR: Foramen magnum is small and funnel shaped. Brainstem compression at the level of the foramen magnum can cause central apnea. Multiple cervical spine abnormalities, including instability, stenosis, and fusion. Persistent thoracolumbar kyphosis can compress the spinal cord. Small intervertebral foramina can cause compression of individual nerve roots. There is progressive narrowing of the spinal canal caudally. Possible cauda equina syndrome. Spinal cord or root compression can occur at any level and can result in hyperreflexia, sustained clonus, hypertonia, paresis, or asymmetry of movement or strength. Narrowed foramen magnum can result in hydrocephalus. Motor development is often delayed.

ORTHOPEDIC: Short stature, secondary to rhizomelic shortening of arms and legs. Trunk length is normal. Long bones are shortened. Incomplete extension at the elbow. Hyperextensibility of other joints, especially the knees. Trident hands. Thoracolumbar kyphosis and severe lumbar lordosis. Small pelvis. Bowing of the lower extremities. Occipitalization of C1. Patients can have a variety of spine abnormalities (see *Neuromuscular*).

OTHER: Obesity is often present in both sexes. Glucose intolerance is common. The small maternal pelvis, exaggerated lumbar lordosis, and near-normal fetal size make delivery in

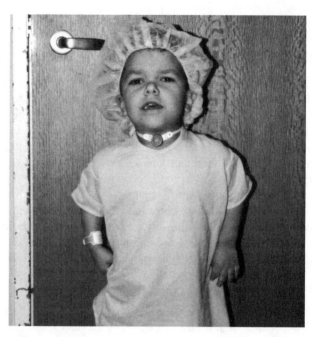

Achondroplasia. FIG. 2. The same patient at 7 years of age. He has had a tracheostomy in the interval, as well as surgical straightening of his tibias and fibulae.

women with achondroplasia by cesarean section preferable. The relatively large fetus causes more than usual impingement of the uterus on the diaphragm during pregnancy, with reduction in functional residual capacity.

ANESTHETIC CONSIDERATIONS
Recall that despite the child-sized stature, patients have intelligence and social skills normal for their chronologic age.

Instability of the cervical spine is rare, but possible. Compression at the cervicomedullary junction can occur in the supine position when the large occiput displaces the head sufficiently forward so that the prominent posterior margin of the foramen magnum impinges on the upper spinal cord or medulla. This can be prevented by placing a bolster under the shoulders. Forty-six percent of patients have spinal involvement, so perioperative neurologic and orthopedic examinations are critical. Monitoring somatosensory evoked potentials may help identify early cord compression in surgery requiring abnormal positioning (4), but false-negative results with a brainstem infarction and a C1 sensory level have been reported (12), although the data in this case may have been corrupted by the use of excessive isoflurane.

Visualization of the larynx is usually uncomplicated but may be difficult if there is limited cervical extension. Patients can usually be ventilated by a mask, but a good mask fit may be difficult to obtain. The narrow nasopharynx or choanal stenosis can preclude placement of a nasal airway, nasal intubation, or placement of a nasogastric tube. Macroglossia can obstruct the airway, and obstruction can resolve with an oropharyngeal airway. Endotracheal tubes smaller than those estimated on the basis of age are often needed, and an approximation based on weight may be more appropriate (12).

Low functional residual capacity can lead to rapid desaturation with the induction of anesthesia. Respiratory status could require an arterial catheter. Patients can require postoperative ventilation, and pain control is critical to postoperative respiratory status.

Obesity can predispose to gastroesophageal reflux. Excess skin and subcutaneous tissue may make placement of venous catheters more difficult. Careful positioning is required because of the hyperextensibility of most joints, especially the knee. Short, thick upper arms can make fixation of an appropriate-sized blood pressure cuff difficult, and falsely high pressures can be displayed by noninvasive monitors. An appropriate blood pressure cuff should cover two thirds of the upper arm length.

A retrospective study reported very few problems in the management of general anesthesia for patients with achondroplasia (3). Despite spinal abnormalities and possible technical difficulties, regional anesthesia for cesarean section has been reported, although lower-than-normal volumes of anesthetic are required because of the short stature of these patients (approximately 5 to 12 mL) (2,6,7,9,10,15). Given this range, incremental dosing is important.

Bibliography:
1. Krishnan BS, Eipe N, Korula G. Anaesthetic management of a patient with achondroplasia. *Paediatr Anaesth* 2003;13:547–549.
2. Morrow MJ, Black IH. Epidural anaesthesia for Caesarean section in an achondroplastic dwarf. *Br J Anaesth* 1998;81:619–621.
3. Monedero P, Garcia-Pedrajas F, Coca I, et al. Is management of anesthesia in achondroplastic dwarfs really a challenge? *J Clin Anesth* 1997;9:208–212.
4. Cunningham MJ, Ferrari L, Kearse LA Jr, et al. Intraoperative somatosensory evoked potential monitoring in achondroplasia. *Paediatr Anaesth* 1994;4:129–132.
5. Shiang R, Thompson LM, Zhu YZ, et al. Mutations in the transmembrane domain of FGFR3 causes the most common genetic form of dwarfism, achondroplasia. *Cell* 1994;78:335–342.
6. Carstoniu J, Yee I, Halpern S. Epidural anaesthesia for Caesarean section in an achondroplastic dwarf. *Can J Anaesth* 1992;39: 708–711.
7. McArthur RDA. Obstetric anaesthesia in an achondroplastic dwarf at a regional hospital. *Anaesth Intensive Care* 1992;20:376–378.
8. Berkowitz I, Raja S, Bender K, et al. Dwarfs: pathophysiology and anesthetic implications. *Anesthesiology* 1990;73:39–59.
9. Wardall GJ, Frame WT. Extradural anaesthesia for cesarean section in achondroplasia. *Br J Anaesth* 1990;64:367–370.
10. Brimacombe JR, Caunt JA. Anaesthesia in a gravid achondroplastic dwarf. *Anaesthesia* 1990;45:132–134.
11. Hall JG. The natural history of achondroplasia. In: Nicoletti B, Kopits SE, Ascani E, et al., eds. *Human achondroplasia: a multidisciplinary approach*, New York: Plenum Press, 1988:3–10.
12. Mayhew JF, Katz J, Miner M, et al. Anaesthesia for the achondroplastic dwarf. *Can Anaesth Soc J* 1986;33:216–221.
13. Kalla GN, Fening E, Obiaya MO. Anaesthetic management of achondroplasia. *Br J Anaesth* 1986;58:117–119.
14. Stokes DC, Phillips JA, Leonard CO, et al. Respiratory complications of achondroplasia. *J Pediatr* 1983;102:534–541.
15. Cohen SE. Anesthesia for cesarean section in achondroplastic dwarfs. *Anesthesiology* 1980;52:264–266.

Acid Maltase Deficiency

See Pompe disease

Acroosteolysis Syndrome

See Hajdu-Cheney syndrome

Acrocallosal Syndrome

MIM #: 200990

This autosomal recessive disorder is marked by polydactyly, mental retardation, and agenesis of the corpus callosum. The syndrome is caused by mutations in the gene *GLI3*.

HEENT/AIRWAY: Macrocephaly, protruding occiput and forehead, large anterior fontanelle, defect in the calvarium. Hypoplastic midface. Strabismus, hypertelorism, downslanting palpebral fissures, nystagmus, decreased retinal pigmentation. Small nose. Malformed ears. Cleft lip, cleft palate, high-arched palate.

CARDIOVASCULAR: Congenital heart defects.

NEUROMUSCULAR: Severe mental retardation, agenesis of the corpus callosum, hypotonia, arachnoid cysts, seizures.

ORTHOPEDIC: Postaxial polydactyly, duplication of hallux. Tapered fingers. Toe syndactyly. Bipartite clavicle.

GI/GU: Umbilical and inguinal hernias. Hypospadias, cryptorchidism, micropenis. Rectovaginal fistula.

OTHER: Postnatal growth retardation.

MISCELLANEOUS: The gene *GLI3* is analogous to a gene in *Drosophila* that regulates, among other genes, the gooseberry gene.

ANESTHETIC CONSIDERATIONS

Clavicular anomalies may make placement of a subclavian venous catheter more difficult. Patients with congenital heart disease require perioperative antibiotics as indicated. Anticonvulsant medications should be continued through the perioperative period. Long-term use of anticonvulsant medications, as well as abnormal liver function, may affect the metabolism of some anesthetic medications and other drugs.

Bibliography:
1. Koenig R, Bach A, Woelki U, et al. Spectrum of the acrocallosal syndrome. *Am J Med Genet* 2002;108:7–11.
2. Gelman-Kohan Z, Antonelli J, Ankori-Cohen H, et al. Further delineation of the acrocallosal syndrome. *Eur J Pediatr* 1991;150:797–799.
3. Casamassima AC, Beneck D, Gewitz MH, et al. Acrocallosal syndrome: additional manifestations. *Am J Med Genet* 1989;32:311–317.

Acrocephalosyndactyly Type I

See Apert syndrome

Acrocephalosyndactyly Type II

See Carpenter syndrome

Acrocephalosyndactyly Type III

See Saethre-Chotzen syndrome

Acrocephalosyndactyly Type IV

See Goodman syndrome

Acrocephalosyndactyly Type V

See Pfeiffer syndrome

Acrodysostosis

MIM #: 101800

This autosomal dominant disorder is characterized by mental retardation, short hands and feet with acrodysostosis (progressive defects in ossification distally) and distinctive facies, including a small nose and prominent mandible. The gene defect responsible for this disorder is not known. Although it had been suggested that this disorder is a variant of pseudohypoparathyroidism (see later), recent genetic studies have shown that the two disorders are distinct (1).

HEENT/AIRWAY: Brachycephaly. Hypertelorism, optic atrophy, strabismus. Blue eyes have been described in Japanese patients. Small, broad, upturned nose with a low nasal bridge. Hearing deficit common. Flat midface and prominent mandible.

NEUROMUSCULAR: Mental retardation common. Occasional hydrocephalus.

ORTHOPEDIC: Mild to moderate short stature is common. Advanced bone age. Upper limbs relatively shorter than lower limbs. Abnormally small vertebrae are susceptible to compression. Scoliosis. Spinal canal stenosis. Short limbs with acrodysostosis. Epiphyses are cone shaped. Short and broad hands, feet, fingers, and toes. Short metatarsals.

GI/GU: Rare renal anomalies. Cryptorchidism. Hypogonadism.

OTHER: Wrinkling of the dorsum of the hands. Pigmented nevi.

ANESTHETIC CONSIDERATIONS

Restriction of movement in the hands and spine may present problems in positioning the patient, and wrinkling of the skin of the hands could make intravenous catheter placement more difficult.

Bibliography:

1. Wilson LC, Oude Luttikhuis ME, Baraitser M, et al. Normal erythrocyte membrane Gs-alpha bioactivity in two unrelated patients with acrodysostosis. *J Med Genet* 1997;34:133–136.
2. Steiner RD, Pagon RA. Autosomal dominant transmission of acrodysostosis. *Clin Dysmorphol* 1992;1:201–206.
3. Butler MG, Rames LJ, Wadlington WB. Acrodysostosis: report of a 13 year old boy with a review of the literature and metacarpophalangeal pattern profile analysis. *Am J Med Genet* 1988;30:971–980.

Acromesomelic Dwarfism

See Acromesomelic dysplasia

Acromesomelic Dysplasia

SYNONYM: Acromesomelic dwarfism. (Includes Hunter-Thompson and Maroteaux types)

MIM #: 201250, 602875

These autosomal recessive disorders are characterized by short-limbed dwarfism, a prominent forehead, and lower thoracic kyphosis. The **Hunter-Thompson type** is caused by a defect in the gene that encodes cartilage-derived morphogenetic protein 1 (*CDMP1*), a member of the transforming growth factor—beta superfamily. The **Maroteaux type** is caused by a defect in the natriuretic peptide receptor B gene. Acromesomelic disorders have disproportionate shortening of the middle (forearms and lower legs) and distal (hands and feet) skeleton. In the Hunter-Thompson form skeletal elements of the hands or feet are fused, while in the Maroteaux type all elements are present but have abnormal growth. A third acromesomelic dysplasia is Grebe syndrome (see later).

HEENT/AIRWAY: Macrocephaly, prominent forehead. May have corneal opacities. May have a short nose.

CHEST: Lower thoracic kyphosis. Clavicles are curved superiorly and thus appear high.

NEUROMUSCULAR: Intelligence is normal. Motor development is often delayed.

ORTHOPEDIC: Extreme short stature. Short limbs, which are more pronounced distally—forearms and hands are relatively shorter than upper arms, and lower legs are shorter than upper legs. Short and broad metacarpals, metatarsals, and phalanges. Bowed radius, dislocation of the radial head, limited elbow extension. Joint laxity. Epiphyses are cone shaped. Metaphyses of long bones are flared. Hypoplasia of the ilia and acetabular region in childhood may lead to early osteoarthritis of the hip. Lumbar lordosis. Gibbus deformity.

MISCELLANEOUS: This Hunter and Thompson do not presumably refer to Hunter Thompson, the recently deceased "gonzo" journalist.

ANESTHETIC CONSIDERATIONS

Recall that despite the child-sized stature, patients have intelligence that is normal for their chronologic age. Might require a smaller-than-expected endotracheal tube if sized according to age. Clavicular anomalies may make placement of a subclavian venous catheter more difficult. Radial anomalies may make placement of a radial arterial catheter more difficult. Careful positioning is required secondary to limited elbow extension and hyperextensibility of most other joints. Spine deformities might make neuraxial techniques more difficult.

Bibliography:

1. Thomas IT, Lin K, Nandekar M, et al. A human chondrodysplasia due to a mutation in a TGF-beta superfamily member. *Nat Genet* 1996; 12:315–317.
2. Fernandez del Moral R, Sontolaya Jimenez JM, Rodriguez Gonzalez JI, et al. Report of a case: acromesomelic dysplasia: radiologic, clinical and pathological study. *Am J Med Genet* 1989;33:415–419.
3. Langer LO, Beals RK, Solomon IL, et al. Acromesomelic dwarfism: manifestations in childhood. *Am J Med Genet* 1977;1:87–100.

Acyl-CoA Dehydrogenase Deficiency

See Glutaric aciduria type II

ADA Deficiency

See Adenosine deaminase deficiency

Adams-Oliver Syndrome

SYNONYM: Aplasia cutis congenita

MIM #: 100300

This autosomal dominant disorder involves failure of skin development over an area of the scalp (aplasia cutis congenita) and various limb reduction defects. There is wide variability in expression, with some affected people showing only subclinical (i.e. radiographic) evidence of the disease. The gene defect responsible for this disorder is not known.

HEENT/AIRWAY: Failure of development of the skin overlying an area of the scalp (aplasia cutis congenita), usually in the parietal region. There may be single or multiple defects. Defects are usually covered by a thin membrane or scar tissue, or may be ulcerated. Skin grafting may be needed. Skull defects can underlie the scalp defect. Occasional microphthalmia. Occasional cleft lip or palate.

CARDIOVASCULAR: Occasional cardiac defects.

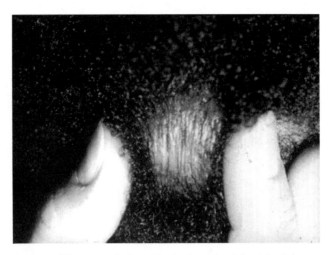

Adams-Oliver syndrome. Typical scalp defect in Adams-Oliver syndrome. (Courtesy of Dr. Neil Prose, Department of Dermatology, Duke University.)

NEUROMUSCULAR: There is a risk of hemorrhage or meningitis when the superior sagittal sinus or the dura is exposed by an overlying bony defect. Despite the sometimes large defects in the skull, underlying central nervous system abnormalities have only on occasion been associated with this syndrome. Intelligence is normal.

ORTHOPEDIC: Mild growth deficiency. Various limb reduction defects including absence of the lower extremity below midcalf. Absence or hypoplasia of the metacarpals, metatarsals, and phalanges. Short terminal phalanges, hypoplastic nails.

GI/GU: Occasional duplicated renal collecting system.

OTHER: Cutis marmorata. Dilated scalp veins.

MISCELLANEOUS: Cutis marmorata and dilated scalp veins suggest that vascular disruption may play a role in the pathogenesis of the Adams-Oliver syndrome. Aplasia cutis congenita and limb reduction defects are consistent with this hypothesis.

ANESTHETIC CONSIDERATIONS

Care should be taken to avoid hemorrhage or infection when the superior sagittal sinus or the dura is exposed by an overlying bony defect. Because of the abnormal local vascularity, skin grafts rather than flaps will be required to close scalp defects. Both scalp and limb reduction defects may make intravenous access more difficult. Patients with congenital cardiac defects will require appropriate antibiotic prophylaxis.

Bibliography:

1. Zapata HH, Sletten LJ, Pierpont ME. Congenital cardiac malformations in Adams-Oliver syndrome. *Clin Genet* 1995;47:80–84.

2. Bamforth JS, Kaurah P, Byrne J, et al. Adams-Oliver syndrome: a family with extreme variability in clinical expression. *Am J Med Genet* 1994;49:393–396.
3. Whitely CB, Gorlin RJ. Adams-Oliver syndrome revisited. *Am J Med Genet* 1991;40:319–326.

Addison-Schilder Disease

See Adrenoleukodystrophy

Adenosine Deaminase Deficiency

SYNONYM: ADA deficiency

MIM #: 102700

This autosomal recessive enzyme deficiency causes one type of severe combined immunodeficiency syndrome (SCIDS, see later) with combined B- and T-cell defects, and accounts for approximately one half of the autosomal recessive cases of SCIDS. Some mutations allow partial enzyme activity with later onset and survival into adulthood, although with an increased incidence of severe infections. Adenosine deaminase catalyzes the conversion of adenosine to inosine, and deoxyadenosine to deoxyinosine. In the absence of adenosine deaminase, the cell converts deoxyadenosine to deoxy-ATP, which is toxic to cells by activating enzymes that deplete ATP and other adenosine nucleotides from the cells. Lymphocytes are particularly efficient at this, and in essence, poison themselves.

HEENT/AIRWAY: Chronic or recurrent sinus infections.

CHEST: Chronic or recurrent pulmonary infections, asthma.

ORTHOPEDIC: Skeletal dysplasia.

GI/GU: Can have hepatic dysfunction—hepatitis with hyperbilirubinemia that resolves with enzyme treatment.

OTHER: Decreased B-, T-, and CD4 lymphocytes; recurrent candidiasis; warts; and herpes zoster. Severe susceptibility to disease from live virus immunizations (polio, measles) and bacille Calmette-Guérin (BCG) vaccine. Variable humeral immunity (normal, hyperactive, or reduced). Can have autoimmune hemolytic anemia. Can develop B-cell lymphoma.

MISCELLANEOUS: Adenosine deaminase has also been found to be lacking in patients with cartilage-hair hypoplasia syndrome (see later). Patients have been treated successfully with bone marrow transplantation, polyethylene glycol—modified adenosine deaminase (very expensive), and gene therapy with viral vectors. Adenosine deaminase is found in all mammals with the exception of the horse.

ANESTHETIC CONSIDERATIONS
Careful aseptic technique is particularly important. Transfusion of nonirradiated blood can cause graft versus host disease.

Bibliography:
1. Parkman R, Weinberg K, Crooks G, et al. Gene therapy for adenosine deaminase deficiency. *Annu Rev Med* 2000;51:33–47.
2. Rosen FS, Bhan AK. A 54-day old premature girl with respiratory distress and persistent pulmonary infiltrates. *N Engl J Med* 1998;338:1752–1758.
3. Ozsahin H, Arredondo-Vega FX, Santisteban I, et al. Adenosine deaminase deficiency in adults. *Blood* 1997;89:2849–2855.
4. Bollinger ME, Arredondo-Vega FX, Santisteban I, et al. Hepatic dysfunction as a complication of adenosine deaminase deficiency. *N Engl J Med* 1996;334:1367–1371.

Adrenogenital Syndrome

See Congenital adrenal hyperplasia

Adrenoleukodystrophy

SYNONYM: Addison-Schilder disease; Siemerling-Creutzfeldt disease. (Includes adrenomyeloneuropathy)

MIM #: 300100, 202370

There are two types of this disease: an X-linked recessive type and an autosomal recessive neonatal type. The X-linked recessive disorder is characterized by adrenal cortical insufficiency and central nervous system demyelination due to the accumulation of very long chain fatty acids. Presumably, accumulation of 24- to 30-carbon very long chain fatty acids interferes with both myelin formation and adrenal steroid synthesis. Significant phenotypic variation has been described in identical twins with adrenoleukodystrophy, suggesting that nongenetic factors are important in the phenotypic expression. At least seven phenotypic types have been described in males and five in female carriers. The responsible gene is *ABCD1*, which is a member of the ATP-binding cassette superfamily. These produce a variety of proteins that translocate a variety of proteins across intra- and extracellular membranes. The gene responsible for cystic fibrosis is another member of this family. The syndrome of **adrenomyeloneuropathy** occurs in some families with adrenoleukodystrophy and is presumably a phenotypic variant of the same mutation. These patients present with neurologic findings in adulthood, and with evidence of long-standing hypersecretion of adrenocorticotropic hormone (ACTH). The X-linked recessive type of adrenoleukodystrophy is one of the leukodystrophies, the others of which are metachromatic leukodystrophy, Krabbe disease, Canavan disease, Pelizaeus-Merzbacher disease, and Alexander disease.

The autosomal recessive neonatal type is a peroxisomal disorder, related to Zellweger syndrome and Refsum disease (see later). It has been suggested that the same gene [peroxin-1 (*PEX-1*), the functioning of which is required for transportation of proteins into peroxisomes] is involved in infantile Refsum disease, neonatal adrenoleukodystrophy, and Zellweger syndrome and that they represent a continuum, with Zellweger syndrome being the most severe, neonatal adrenoleukodystrophy having intermediate severity, and infantile Refsum disease being the least severe. The abnormality involves absent or almost absent peroxisomes, with a deficiency of all the peroxisomal β-oxidation enzymes. Mutations in several other peroxin genes have also been reported to result in this syndrome.

HEENT/AIRWAY

X-linked: Visual disturbances, including decreased acuity with or without visual field defects, optic atrophy. May have Balint syndrome (a psychic paralysis of visual fixation, optic ataxia, and relatively intact vision). There is an increased incidence of color blindness, presumably because of a close linkage with the color blindness gene(s). Cognitive hearing loss.

Neonatal: Retinopathy, impaired hearing. Neonatal cataracts. Esotropia. Broad nasal bridge. Low-set ears. High-arched palate.

NEUROMUSCULAR

X-linked: Severe mental and motor retardation, and patients may lose milestones between 3 and 5 years of age. Severe hypotonia. Enlarged ventricles, atrophy of the pons and cerebellum. May have seizures. May have behavioral disturbances, difficulty understanding speech in a noisy environment (impaired auditory discrimination), parietal disturbances (including dressing apraxia), poor body orientation in space, diminished graphesthesia. May have spastic paraplegia, peripheral neuropathy, and limb and truncal ataxia. Nerve conduction studies may be abnormal. Treatment of adrenal insufficiency with steroids does not affect the severity or progression of the neurologic disease.

Neonatal: Mental retardation, motor delay, seizures. Extent of neurologic involvement is variable, ranging from a stable handicap with some mental retardation to severe mental retardation, psychomotor delay, and seizures.

GI/GU: Liver function is typically abnormal (but not as abnormal as in the related Zellweger disease). Patients may have gastroesophageal reflux. Hypogonadism with impotence.

OTHER: The adrenal response to an ACTH challenge may be abnormal, but adrenal insufficiency is less common. Hyperpigmentation of the skin from oversecretion of ACTH.

MISCELLANEOUS: Disorders of peroxisomal function include autosomal recessive neonatal adrenoleukodystrophy,

Zellweger syndrome, and Refsum disease (see later). Functions of peroxisomes include synthesis of cell membrane components (particularly constituents of myelin), bile acid synthesis, and fatty acid metabolism. Purported success in treating this disease with a dietary supplement ("Lorenzo's oil") was the basis for a popular film (of the same name) several years ago. Although this therapy can normalize very long chain fatty acids in blood, it does not affect disease progression. It may, however, reduce the risk of developing brain abnormalities on magnetic resonance imaging in asymptomatic boys. Bone marrow transplantation has been suggested as therapy.

Thomas Addison (the same Addison of Addison's disease) committed suicide in 1860 at the age of 65 by jumping out of a window of his villa.

ANESTHETIC CONSIDERATIONS

Sedative premedication increases the risk of airway obstruction in patients with significant hypotonia. Patients are at risk for perioperative aspiration because of airway hypotonia and gastroesophageal reflux. The risk of excessive potassium release with succinylcholine is unknown but is theoretically possible in bedridden patients with atrophic muscles. Patients require careful perioperative positioning secondary to demineralization of bones and ligamentous laxity due to the hypotonia. Patients should be observed closely in the postanesthesia care unit for evidence of airway obstruction from residual anesthetic.

Phenothiazines, butyrophenones, metoclopramide, and other dopaminergic blockers may exacerbate movement disorders. Ondansetron is safe as an antiemetic because it does not have antidopaminergic effects. Anticonvulsant medications should be continued throughout the perioperative period. Long-term use of anticonvulsant medications and abnormal liver function may affect the metabolism of some anesthetics and other drugs. Perioperative stress-dose steroid treatment is probably reasonable if the patient's adrenal status is not known.

Because insults or injuries to the brain may accelerate demyelination and exacerbate neurologic symptoms, the risk of neurologic surgery is unknown. A teenage patient with only minimal symptoms experienced significant worsening of his disease after cardiopulmonary bypass to correct a ventricular septal defect (3). On the other hand, hemodynamic and hormonal responses to anesthesia and minor surgery were normal in an otherwise asymptomatic child (5).

Bibliography:
1. Moser H, Dubey P, Fatemi A. Progress in X-linked adrenoleukodystrophy. *Curr Opin Neurol* 2004;17:263–269.
2. Kindopp AS, Ashbury T. Anaesthetic management of an adult patient with X-linked adrenoleukodystrophy. *Can J Anaesth* 1998;45:990–992.
3. Luciani GB, Pessotto R, Mazzucco A. Adrenoleukodystrophy presenting as postperfusion syndrome [Letter]. *N Engl J Med* 1997;336:731–732.
4. Schwartz RE, Stayer SA, Pasquariello CA, et al. Anaesthesia for the patient with neonatal adrenoleukodystrophy. *Can J Anaesth* 1994;41:56–58.

5. Nishina K, Mikawa K, Maekawa N, et al. Anaesthetic considerations in a child with leukodystrophy. *Paediatr Anaesth* 1993;3:313–316.
6. Tobias JD. Anaesthetic considerations for the child with leukodystrophy. *Can J Anaesth* 1992;39:394–397.
7. Moser HW, Moser AE, Singh I, et al. Adrenoleukodystrophy: survey of 303 cases: biochemistry, diagnosis, and therapy. *Ann Neurol* 1984; 16:628–641.

Adrenomyeloneuropathy

Included in Adrenoleukodystrophy syndrome

AEC Syndrome

SYNONYM: Hay-Wells ectodermal dysplasia

MIM #: 106260

This autosomal dominant ectodermal dysplasia is associated with cleft lip and palate and congenital filiform fusion of the eyelids. AEC stands for **A**nkyloblepharon, **E**ctodermal defects, and **C**left lip and palate. The syndrome is due to defects in the gene *TP73L* (p63). This is an isoform of the p53 gene. Some patients with **E**ctrodactyly, **E**ctodermal dysplasia, and **C**lefting (EEC) syndrome (see later) have defects in the same gene. In AEC syndrome the mutation affects regions involved in protein–protein interaction, while the EEC mutations affect the DNA-binding domain. It has also been suggested that there is overlap with Rapp-Hodgkin ectodermal dysplasia (see later). There is marked variability of clinical expression.

HEENT/AIRWAY: Oval facies with flattened midface and broad nasal bridge. Scalp erosions. Congenital adhesions between the eyelids with filamentous bands (ankyloblepharon filiforme adnatum). Anomalies of the eye not associated with the tissue bands. Thin eyelashes. Photophobia common. Atretic lacrimal ducts. Otitis media is common. Conductive hearing loss, atretic external auditory canals. Cup-shaped ears. Abnormal dentition, including conical and widely spaced teeth, hypodontia, and anodontia. Cleft lip or palate.

CARDIOVASCULAR: Rare patent ductus arteriosus or ventricular septal defect.

GI/GU: Hypospadias, micropenis, vaginal dryness.

OTHER: Ectodermal defects including hyperkeratosis and palmar and plantar keratoderma. Red, cracking skin at birth. Hyperpigmentation; coarse, wiry, and sparse hair; dystrophic, hypoplastic, or absent nails; and sweat gland deficiency or dysfunction. Sparse body hair. Scalp infections are common. Supernumerary nipples.

ANESTHETIC CONSIDERATIONS
Heat intolerance is common because of poorly functioning sweat glands. There is some capacity to produce sweat, so hyperthermia is not usually a problem.

Bibliography:
1. Propst EJ, Campisi P, Papsin BC. Head and neck manifestations of Hay-Wells syndrome. *Otolaryngol Head Neck Surg* 2005;132:165–166.
2. Weiss AH, Riscile G, Kousseff BG. Ankyloblepharon filiforme adnatum. *Am J Med Genet* 1992;42:369–373.
3. Greene SL, Michels VV, Doyle JA. Variable expression in ankyloblepharon-ectodermal defects-cleft lip and palate syndrome. *Am J Med Genet* 1987;27:207–212.
4. Spiegel J, Colton A. AEC syndrome: ankyloblepharon, ectodermal defects, and cleft lip and palate. *J Am Acad Dermatol* 1985;12:810–815.

Aglossia-Adactyly Syndrome

See Oromandibular-limb hypogenesis

Aicardi Syndrome

MIM #: 304050

This syndrome is seen only in girls (with the exception of one boy with an XXY karyotype), suggesting an X-linked dominant mode of inheritance that is lethal in the hemizygous boy. The main features are infantile spasms, agenesis of the corpus callosum, and chorioretinopathy. The gene responsible for this disorder appears to be located on the short arm of the X chromosome. The gene product is unknown. Most patients die in adolescence or early adulthood. The Aicardi and Goltz syndromes (see later) may be contiguous gene syndromes on the short arm of the X chromosome.

HEENT/AIRWAY: Microcephaly. Facial asymmetry. Chorioretinopathy marked by chorioretinal holes. Microphthalmia, small optic nerves and chiasm. Retinal detachment. Cataracts. Coloboma. Nystagmus. Occasional cleft lip or palate.

CHEST: Kyphoscoliosis may adversely affect pulmonary status. Rib abnormalities include absent, extra, fused, or bifid ribs.

NEUROMUSCULAR: Microcephaly, severe mental retardation. Partial or total agenesis of the corpus callosum. Electroencephalographic evidence of independent activity of right and left hemispheres. Abnormalities of the cerebrum, cerebellum, and ventricles. Infantile spasms progressing to other seizure types by 2 years of age. Hypotonia. May be associated with the development of central nervous system tumors. Dandy-Walker or Arnold-Chiari malformations.

ORTHOPEDIC: Kyphoscoliosis. Vertebral anomalies include spina bifida, hemivertebrae, and abnormally shaped vertebrae. Scoliosis. Proximally placed thumbs.

GI/GU: Hiatal hernia.

OTHER: Scalp lipomas. Cavernous hemangiomas. Precocious puberty. A variety of tumors including hepatoblastoma, teratoma, embryonal carcinoma, and angiosarcoma.

ANESTHETIC CONSIDERATIONS

Because of their neurologic status, patients are at risk for aspiration. Recurrent pneumonia is common, and pulmonary status can be further compromised by kyphoscoliosis. Patients usually have significant visual impairment. In one reported case in the anesthesia literature, caudal block was impossible because of abnormal vertebral anatomy, and intravenous cannulation was not possible because of "generalized hypotropia" of subcutaneous tissues (4). Long-term use of anticonvulsant medications may affect the metabolism of some anesthetic drugs.

Bibliography:

1. Aicardi J. Aicardi syndrome. *Brain Dev* 2005;27:164–171.
2. Gooden CK, Pate VA, Kavee R. Anesthetic management of a child with Aicardi syndrome [Letter]. *Paediatr Anaesth* 2005;15:172–173.
3. Sutton VR, Hopkin BJ, Eble TN, et al. Facial and physical features of Aicardi syndrome: infants to teenagers. *Am J Med Genet A* 2005;138:254–258.
4. Iacobucci T, Galeone M, de Francisi G. Anaesthesia management in a patient with Aicardi's syndrome [Letter]. *Anaesthesia* 2003;58:95.
5. Trifiletti RR, Incorpora G, Polizzi A, et al. Aicardi syndrome with multiple tumors: a case report with literature review. *Brain Dev* 1995;17:283–285.
6. Menezes AV, MacGregor DL, Buncic JR. Aicardi syndrome: natural history and possible predictors of severity. *Pediatr Neurol* 1994;11:313–318.

Alagille Syndrome

SYNONYM: Arteriohepatic dysplasia

MIM #: 118450

This disease primarily involves the heart, pulmonary arteries, and liver. It is due to a defect in the human homolog of the rat gene jagged 1 (*JAG1*), which produces a ligand for the protein "Notch 1," a transmembrane receptor involved in cell fate decisions. *JAG1* is highly expressed in the developing heart and vascular structures, corresponding to the areas of observed clinical defects. The disease is presumably autosomal dominant, with marked variability in expression, and many cases are sporadic. A small number of patients will have the syndrome as the result of a microdeletion of chromosome 20 rather than a simple single gene defect. Liver transplantation has been used successfully.

HEENT/AIRWAY: Broad forehead. Long, thin face. Eccentric pupils, deep-set eyes, chorioretinal atrophy, and pigment clumping. Posterior embryotoxon of the eye. Bulbous tip of the nose. Pointed mandible.

CARDIOVASCULAR: Pulmonary valvar and peripheral pulmonary artery stenosis. Occasional tetralogy of Fallot, atrial septal defect, or ventricular septal defect. Abdominal coarctation has been reported.

NEUROMUSCULAR: Poor school performance. Absent deep tendon reflexes. Intracranial hemorrhage has been reported spontaneously or after minor trauma. Hepatic encephalopathy with severe hepatic disease. Can have carotid and intracranial artery aneurysms.

ORTHOPEDIC: Growth retardation. Butterfly vertebrae, decrease in the interpedicular distances of the lumbar spine. Foreshortening of the fingers. Recurrent and/or poorly healing long bone fractures.

GI/GU: Intrahepatic biliary hypoplasia or atresia with cholestasis. The absence of intrahepatic biliary ducts is not congenital. There appears to be early cholestasis, portal inflammation, and inflammation of intralobular bile ducts, followed by loss of biliary ducts. Patients can have cirrhosis with portal hypertension and hypersplenism. Hepatocellular carcinoma can develop. There can be renal dysplasia, or renal artery stenosis with systemic hypertension.

OTHER: Hypercholesterolemia and hyperlipidemia with xanthomas of the skin. Essential fatty acid deficiency and vitamin K deficiency from inadequate absorption. Pruritus from cholestasis. A bleeding dyscrasia is not limited solely to intracranial bleeding. Abnormal and excessive bleeding can occur spontaneously or can be intraoperative. Bleeding postoperatively, even after a minor procedure, is fatal. The etiology is unclear, and hemostatic test results are normal. The dyscrasia could be related to the defect in *JAG1*, which is widely expressed in endothelium and megakaryocytes.

ANESTHETIC CONSIDERATIONS

Baseline cardiac status should be evaluated preoperatively. Patients require perioperative antibiotic prophylaxis as indicated. Renal and hepatic function can be abnormal. Renal insufficiency has implications for perioperative fluid management and the choice of anesthetic drugs. Hepatic dysfunction can lead to abnormalities in the protein binding of some anesthetic drugs. Vitamin K deficiency (from malabsorption) can lead to clotting abnormalities. Esophageal varices can develop in patients with cirrhosis, so nasogastric tubes and transesophageal echocardiography probes should be passed with caution. Excessive perioperative bleeding is possible.

Bibliography:

1. Subramaniam K, Myers LB. Combined general and epidural anesthesia for a child with Alagille syndrome: a case report. *Paediatr Anaesth* 2004;14:787–791.
2. Lykavieris P, Crosnier C, Trichet C, et al. Bleeding tendency in children with Alagille syndrome. *Pediatrics* 2003;111:167–170.
3. Choudhry DK, Rehman MA, Schwartz RE, et al. The Alagille's syndrome and its anaesthetic considerations. *Paediatr Anaesth* 1998;8:79–82.
4. Hoffenberg EJ, Narkewicz MR, Sondheimer JM, et al. Outcome of syndromic paucity of intrahepatic bile ducts (Alagille syndrome) with onset of cholestasis in infancy. *J Pediatr* 1995;127:220–224.

Albers-Schönberg Disease

See Osteopetrosis

Albinism

MIM #: 203100, 203200

There are a variety of types of albinism because a variety of genes are involved in the full melanin biochemical and metabolic pathway. The most common forms are the types of oculocutaneous albinism, which are autosomal recessive. Type I oculocutaneous albinism is due to an abnormality in the gene encoding tyrosinase. Tyrosinase catalyzes the conversion of tyrosine into dopa (3,4-dihydroxyphenylalanine), which is a precursor of melanin. Patients with type IA disease never synthesize melanin in any tissue. Patients with type IB disease have a mutation that allows some residual synthetic activity. This form has more phenotypic variability, and in some people pigmentation can approach normal. One variant of type IB is temperature sensitive, with pigmented arm and leg hair, but white scalp and axillary hair. Type II disease is particularly common in equatorial Africa. It has been suggested that the gene responsible for type II disease is a human analog of the pink-eyed dilution gene of the mouse. There is phenotypic variation with type II disease, and the phenotype can also be affected by the underlying constitutional pigment background. Albinism occurs in all racial groups.

HEENT/AIRWAY: Absence of retinal pigment (producing a pronounced red reflex). The iris is blue, thin, without a cartwheel effect, and the lens can be seen through it. Some iris pigment can develop in type IB and in type II. Photophobia, nystagmus, strabismus, hypoplasia of the fovea, visual loss.

OTHER: The skin and hair lack pigmentation in type IA. In type IB there can be some pigment developing with time. The hair is white or, after prolonged exposure to sunlight, extremely light blond in type IA, and can become blond or brown in type IB. Hair can on occasion be reddish in type II and can also darken with age. Melanocytes are present but do not contain pigment. There is increased susceptibility to skin neoplasia, but less so in subtypes in which lentigines, or pigmented freckles, can develop.

MISCELLANEOUS: Well-known albinos include (purportedly) Noah, of flood fame (3), and the Reverend Dr. Spooner, who gave his name to the term "spoonerism." It is suggested that his speech aberration was related to his nystagmus, which caused a jumbling of information on the printed page. Albinism was one of the four inborn errors of metabolism (the others being cystinuria, alcaptonuria, and pentosuria) discussed by Garrod in his famous series of lectures in 1902 (4).

It is thought that the temperature-sensitive type IB disease is analogous to that in Siamese cats and the Himalayan mouse, which have tyrosinase mutations that make the enzyme sensitive to higher temperatures, such that melanin synthesis takes place in the cooler areas of the body.

ANESTHETIC CONSIDERATIONS
Consideration should be given to patients with photophobia in brightly lit operating rooms.

Bibliography:
1. Biswas S, Lloyd IC. Oculocutaneous albinism. *Arch Dis Child* 1999;80:565–569.
2. Sethi R, Schwartz RA, Janninger CK. Oculocutaneous albinism. *Cutis* 1996;57:397–401.
3. Sorsby A. Noah: an albino. *BMJ* 1958;2:1587–1589.
4. Garrod AE. The incidence of alkaptonuria: a study in individuality. *Lancet* 1902;2:1616–1620.

Albright Hereditary Osteodystrophy

See Pseudohypoparathyroidism
Note: This is a distinct entity from McCune-Albright syndrome.

Albright Syndrome

See McCune-Albright syndrome

Alcaptonuria

SYNONYM: Alkaptonuria; Ochronosis

MIM #: 203500

This autosomal recessive disease is due to an abnormality in the gene encoding homogentisic acid oxidase (homogentisate 1,2-dioxygenase). This enzyme is part of the tyrosine and phenylalanine degradation pathways and catalyzes the conversion of homogentisic acid to maleylacetoacetic acid. Deficiency of this enzyme causes accumulation of homogentisic acid ("alkapton"). There is abnormal pigmentation (ochronosis) of a variety of tissues. Pigmentary changes are probably due to a polymer derived from homogentisic acid, although its exact structure is not known.

HEENT/AIRWAY: Corneal pigmentation in older adults. One of the hallmarks of the early descriptions was dark (ochronotic) staining of the ear cartilage, also seen primarily in adults. Ear cartilage can calcify.

CARDIOVASCULAR: Ochronosis of the aortic valve has been described, and mitral involvement has also been described. Aortic staining. There is increased generalized atherosclerosis and coronary artery calcification, and aortic and mitral annular calcification.

ORTHOPEDIC: Osteoarthritis, including hips, knees, and spine, beyond the second or third decade. Arthritis is more severe, and appears at a younger age, in male patients. The radiographic changes in the spine are said to be almost

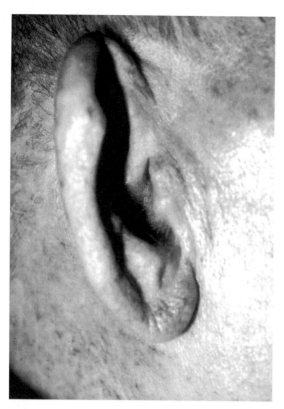

Alcaptonuria. FIG. 1. Ochronotic staining of the external ear in an adult with alcaptonuria. (Courtesy of Dr. Kenneth E. Greer, Department of Dermatology, University of Virginia Health System.)

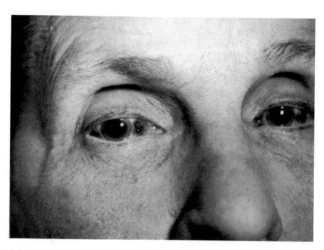

Alcaptonuria. FIG. 2. Ochronotic staining of the conjunctivae in an adult with alcaptonuria. (Courtesy of Dr. Kenneth E. Greer, Department of Dermatology, University of Virginia Health System.)

pathognomonic. There is an increased incidence of ruptured intervertebral discs. Patients requiring joint replacement do so at a mean age of 55 years. There is dark (ochronotic) pigmentation of cartilage.

GI/GU: Urine darkens with standing or at high pH, although some patients may not have this manifestation. Rarely, renal failure in adults. There is an increased incidence of prostatitis.

OTHER: The pigment also appears in sweat and can stain clothes.

MISCELLANEOUS: This disorder is of significant historical interest because it was one of the first four human disorders suggested by Garrod to be a recessive inborn error of metabolism (4). Alcaptonuria (with homogentisic acid pigmentation) has been described in an Egyptian mummy and has been diagnosed during coronary bypass surgery due to the observation of a black aorta. More patients with this disorder have been reported from Slovakia than anywhere else. Ochronosis is from the Greek word *ochros* ("sallow") and *nosos* ("disease"). It was so named by Virchow because, microscopically, the grossly bluish black pigmentation is ochre colored. **Alcaptonuria** is a term

derived from the alkaline urine's avid uptake of oxygen. A phenotypically similar disorder appears after prolonged application of carbolic acid surgical dressings. Urine turns darker with alkalinization—if soap is used to wash diapers of these infants, the discoloration worsens, rather than being removed. In older tests for urinary glucose (or, more correctly, reducing sugars) using Benedict reagent, this urine showed falsely elevated sugar levels.

ANESTHETIC CONSIDERATIONS

There are few specific anesthetic concerns. Laryngeal and tracheal cartilages can be heavily pigmented. One should not be alarmed when the urine in the Foley catheter collection bag turns dark. Lumbosacral arthritis and ankylosis may be a relative contraindication to regional anesthesia.

FIGURE: See **Appendix B**

Bibliography:

1. Phornphutkul C, Introne WJ, Perry MB, et al. Natural history of alkaptonuria. *N Engl J Med* 2002;347:2111–2121.
2. Scriver CR. Alkaptonuria: such a long journey. *Nat Genet* 1996;14:5–6.
3. Kenny D, Ptacin MJ, Bamrah VS. Cardiovascular ochronosis: a case report and review of the medical literature. *Cardiology* 1990;77:477–483.
4. Garrod AE. The incidence of alkaptonuria: a study in individuality. *Lancet* 1902;2:1616–1620.

Alcohol

See Fetal alcohol syndrome

Aldehyde Oxidase Deficiency

Included in Molybdenum cofactor deficiency

Alexander Disease

MIM #: 203450

This autosomal recessive leukodystrophy is characterized by megalencephaly (a large head) in infancy and progressive spasticity and dementia. Its features are similar to those of Canavan disease (see later). The responsible gene encodes glial fibrillary acidic protein. There are infantile, juvenile, and adult forms, all having defects in this gene. The infantile form is most common. Most patients die within 10 years of diagnosis. The juvenile form is more slowly progressive, and the adult form is more heterogeneous.

HEENT/AIRWAY: Megalencephaly in infancy. Copious oral secretions.

NEUROMUSCULAR: Seizures, choreoathetosis, progressive spasticity and dementia, demyelination. Can have hydrocephalus.

GI/GU: Increased incidence of gastroesophageal reflux.

MISCELLANEOUS: This disease is one of the leukodystrophies; the others are adrenoleukodystrophy, metachromatic leukodystrophy, Krabbe disease, Canavan disease, and Pelizaeus-Merzbacher disease. Leukodystrophies involve defective formation of myelin. Histologically, Alexander disease is characterized by the presence of Rosenthal fibers (tapered eosinophilic rods) in cortical white matter astrocytes.

ANESTHETIC CONSIDERATIONS

Gastroesophageal reflux, copious oral secretions, and poor airway tone increase the risk of perioperative aspiration. Consideration should be given to anticholinergic premedication to dry oral secretions. Careful intraoperative positioning and padding is important in these patients with poor nutrition. The risk of excessive potassium release with succinylcholine is unknown but is theoretically possible in bedridden patients with atrophic muscles. Anticonvulsant medications need to be continued (or a parenteral form substituted) in the perioperative period and may alter the metabolism of some anesthetic drugs. Copious secretions and airway hypotonia make close postoperative observation of airway adequacy particularly important.

Phenothiazines, butyrophenones, metoclopramide, and other dopaminergic blockers should be avoided because they may exacerbate movement disorders. Ondansetron ought to be safe as an antiemetic because it does not have antidopaminergic effects.

Bibliography:
1. Hanefeld FA. Alexander disease: past and present. *Cell Mol Life Sci* 2004;61:2750–2752.
2. Johnson AB, Brenner M. Alexander's disease: clinical, pathologic, and genetic features. *J Child Neurol* 2003;18:625–632.
3. Aicardi J. The inherited leukodystrophies: a clinical overview. *J Inherit Metab Dis* 1993;16:733–743.
4. Tobias JD. Anaesthetic considerations for the child with leukodystrophy. *Can J Anaesth* 1992;39:394–397.

Alkaptonuria

See Alcaptonuria

Alpers Disease

MIM #: 203700

Alpers disease is a progressive autosomal recessive neurologic disorder beginning with seizures and progressing to spasticity, myoclonus, and dementia. Clinical manifestations can be induced or exacerbated by concurrent infection or other stress. Death is usually by 3 years of age. The responsible gene is the nuclear gene encoding mitochondrial DNA polymerase gamma (*POLG*).

HEENT/AIRWAY: Progressive microcephaly. Cortical blindness. Micrognathia has been reported.

CHEST: Recurrent aspiration pneumonia.

CARDIOVASCULAR: Cardiorespiratory arrest may be a final outcome.

NEUROMUSCULAR: Intractable seizures, including epilepsia partialis continua. Status epilepticus is often the terminal event. Progressive spasticity, ataxia, hypotonia, myoclonus, and dementia.

ORTHOPEDIC: Prenatal onset of decreased mobility can result in postnatal joint limitation.

GI/GU: Swallowing difficulties. Hepatic cirrhosis with jaundice. Liver failure can be rapidly progressive and fatal in early childhood. Treatment of seizures with valproate can accelerate fulminant hepatic failure.

ANESTHETIC CONSIDERATIONS

Because of swallowing difficulties, patients are at increased risk for aspiration. Anticonvulsant medications should be continued perioperatively and may affect the metabolism of some anesthetic drugs. Hepatic dysfunction can lead to clotting abnormalities or abnormalities in the protein binding of anesthetic drugs. Stress (and presumably surgery) can exacerbate symptoms. Patients must be carefully positioned perioperatively secondary to hypotonia and, possibly, limited joint mobility.

Bibliography:
1. Harding BN, Alsanjari N, Smith SJ, et al. Progressive neuronal degeneration of childhood with liver disease (Alpers disease) presenting in young adults. *J Neurol Neurosurg Psychiatry* 1995;58:320–325.

2. Frydman M, Jager-Roman E, deVries L, et al. Alpers progressive infantile neuronal poliodystrophy: an acute neonatal form with findings of the fetal akinesia syndrome. *Am J Med Genet* 1993;47:31–36.
3. Narkewicz MR, Sokol RJ, Beckwith B, et al. Liver involvement in Alpers disease. *J Pediatr* 1991;119:260–267.

Alpha₁-Antitrypsin Deficiency

SYNONYM: Alpha₁-protease inhibitor deficiency

MIM #: 107400

This autosomal recessive (or autosomal codominant) disease is due to an abnormality in the gene for alpha₁-antitrypsin. This protein inhibits pancreatic trypsin, but it is far more effective in inhibiting other serine proteases. Its primary role is lung protection by inhibition of neutrophil elastase. Deficiency of alpha₁-antitrypsin leads primarily to pulmonary and hepatic abnormalities. A variety of different mutations (at least 60) have been described, with the subtypes exhibiting a spectrum of clinical manifestations. Specific treatment, in addition to transplantation, has been by parenteral alpha₁-antitrypsin prepared from pooled human plasma. It is extremely expensive. The inhalation of alpha₁-antitrypsin has been suggested.

CHEST: Emphysema, primarily of the lung bases. Homozygotes develop severe degenerative lung disease, primarily emphysema, but also chronic bronchitis and recurrent pneumonia. Heterozygotes with certain subtypes are predisposed to chronic obstructive lung disease. There is also an increased incidence of sclerosing alveolitis. Pulmonary degeneration is significantly exacerbated by smoking. Onset of dyspnea is at 45 to 55 years in nonsmokers and 35 years in smokers. Emphysema in childhood is extremely rare.

CARDIOVASCULAR: Cor pulmonale can develop secondary to pulmonary disease.

GI/GU: Hepatic involvement occurs with certain subtypes. There may be neonatal cholestasis, sometimes leading to infantile cirrhosis with eventual portal fibrosis and esophageal varices. Hepatic intracellular inclusions. There is an increased incidence of hepatocellular carcinoma. With some subtypes, heterozygotes can also have liver disease. Liver disease can be subclinical and can present in adults with no history of neonatal disease. A patient who also had pancreatic fibrosis (but without pancreatic exocrine dysfunction) has been reported and it has been suggested that one phenotype may make the pancreas more susceptible to chronic pancreatitis. Contrary to the earliest reports that suggested a poor outcome for children with liver disease, it appears that approximately two of three children will show some recovery. Panniculitis.

MISCELLANEOUS: One in ten people of European descent is a carrier of one of the two mutations that result in partial deficiency of this protein. Liver transplantation has been successful in patients, even children, who have terminal or preterminal hepatic disease without pulmonary emphysema. Similarly, single lung transplantation has been used successfully.

ANESTHETIC CONSIDERATIONS

Hemodynamically significant air trapping can occur in patients with severe emphysema. Hepatic dysfunction may lead to clotting abnormalities or abnormalities in the protein binding of anesthetic drugs. Patients with cirrhosis can develop esophageal varices, and nasogastric tubes or transesophageal echocardiography probes should be passed with caution. Levels of alpha₁-antitrypsin are normally increased during episodes of fever or inflammation because alpha₁-antitrypsin is an acute-phase reactant. Therefore, perioperative control of the patient's temperature and perioperative management of inflammation would seem to be reasonable goals.

Bibliography:
1. Stoller JK, Aboussouan LS. Alpha₁-antitrypsin deficiency. *Lancet* 2005; 365:2225–2236.
2. Carrell RW, Lomas DA. Alpha₁-antitrypsin deficiency—a model for conformational diseases. *N Engl J Med* 2002;346:45–53.
3. Stoller J. Clinical features and natural history of severe alpha₁-antitrypsin deficiency: Roger S. Mitchell lecture. *Chest* 1997;111:S123–S128.
4. Eriksson S. A 30-year perspective on alpha₁-antitrypsin deficiency. *Chest* 1996;110:237S–242S.
5. Perlmutter DH. Clinical manifestations of alpha₁-antitrypsin deficiency. *Gastroenterol Clin North Am* 1995;24:27–43.

Alpha-Galactosidase A Deficiency

See Fabry disease

Alpha-Galactosidase B Deficiency

See Schindler disease

Alpha-1,4-Glucan:alpha-1,4-Glucan-6-alpha-Glucosyltransferase Deficiency

See Brancher deficiency

Alpha-1,4-Glucosidase Deficiency

See Pompe disease

Alpha-N-Acetylgalactosaminidase Deficiency

See Schindler disease

α-Mannosidosis

See Mannosidosis

α₁-Protease Inhibitor Deficiency

See Alpha₁-antitrypsin deficiency

Alport Syndrome

SYNONYM: Progressive hereditary nephritis

MIM #: 301050, 104200, 203780

This syndrome involves progressive renal disease and hearing loss. X-linked dominant, autosomal dominant, and autosomal recessive forms have been described. There is significant variability in the age of onset and the severity of symptoms. Also, the extent of renal impairment does not correlate with the extent of auditory impairment. Up to 3% of children with chronic renal failure have Alport syndrome. This syndrome is caused by a defect in the glomerular basement membrane, which appears irregularly thickened on microscopy. Mutations in a variety of genes encoding type IV basement membrane specific collagen chains appear to be responsible for this syndrome.

HEENT/AIRWAY: Asymmetric progressive sensorineural hearing loss—usually not detected until midchildhood. May have cataracts, keratoconus, myopia, retinal detachment, and nystagmus.

CARDIOVASCULAR: Hypertension may occur in patients with renal failure.

NEUROMUSCULAR: Rarely, myopathy or polyneuropathy has been reported in association with Alport syndrome.

GI/GU: Progressive nephritis and eventual renal failure. Hematuria—either microscopic or gross. May have proteinuria, hypophosphatemia, or nephrocalcinosis. Nephrotic syndrome is rare. Alport syndrome lacks the glomerular basement membrane protein, which is the purported antigen for the autoimmune Goodpasture syndrome. A small number of patients will develop anti–basement membrane nephritis after renal transplantation and will reject the kidney.

OTHER: Rarely, thrombocytopenia has been reported in association with Alport syndrome, although this could represent Fechtner syndrome (see later). Diffuse leiomyomatosis has been reported.

MISCELLANEOUS: Arthur Cecil Alport owned a small gold mine near Johannesburg. Unlike the other Cecil (Rhodes), Alport's gold mine proved to be nonlucrative, so he had to persist with medicine. Later in his career, Alport resigned from the Royal College of Physicians because he felt that they were not supporting him in his efforts to reform rampant corruption in Cairo, where he had been chair of medicine in the mid-1940s.

ANESTHETIC CONSIDERATIONS
Renal disease affects intraoperative fluid management. Renally excreted drugs may be contraindicated. Patients with advanced renal disease may be hypertensive. Consider having an interpreter present perioperatively for patients who are deaf. Rarely have myopathy, polyneuropathy, or thrombocytopenia been reported in association with Alport syndrome. Myopathy would be a contraindication to the use of succinylcholine.

Bibliography:
1. Flinter F. Alport's syndrome. *J Med Genet* 1997;34:326–330.
2. Gubler MC, Knebelmann B, Beziau A, et al. Autosomal recessive Alport syndrome: immunohistochemical study of type IV collagen chain distribution. *Kidney Int* 1995;47:1142–1147.
3. M'Rad R, Sanak M, Deschenes G, et al. Alport syndrome: a genetic study of 31 families. *Hum Genet* 1992;90:420–426.

Alström Syndrome

MIM #: 203800

A distinct but clinically similar syndrome to Bardet-Biedl syndrome; the hallmarks of this autosomal recessive disorder are retinitis pigmentosa, hearing loss, obesity, diabetes, and renal insufficiency. Unlike the Bardet-Biedl syndrome, there is no mental retardation, polydactyly, or hypogenitalism. The defect is due to mutations in the gene *ALMS1*. The gene product and physiologic role of this gene are not yet known.

HEENT/AIRWAY: Retinitis pigmentosa, central vision loss, nystagmus, severe vision loss in the first decade with eventual blindness. Photophobia. Sensorineural hearing loss. Subcapsular cataracts.

CHEST: Chronic obstructive pulmonary disease. Recurrent pneumonia. Pulmonary fibrosis.

CARDIOVASCULAR: Dilated cardiomyopathy. Atherosclerosis. Hypertension.

NEUROMUSCULAR: Can have normal intelligence, but can have motor or language delay. Tics and absence seizures.

ORTHOPEDIC: Advanced bone age. Short adult height with pubertal onset of short stature. Kyphosis. Scoliosis.

GI/GU: Can have hepatic dysfunction. Chronic active hepatitis. Pancreatitis. Progressive nephropathy with nephritis and renal failure. Recurrent urinary tract infections and abnormal voiding patterns.

OTHER: Truncal obesity with childhood onset. Hyperinsulinism followed by insulin-resistant diabetes mellitus. There can be end-organ unresponsiveness to other polypeptide hormones, including hypergonadotropic hypogonadism in boys, menstrual irregularities in women, hypothyroidism, diabetes insipidus, and growth hormone deficiency. Gynecomastia. Hypertriglyceridemia. Acanthosis nigricans of skin. Alopecia.

MISCELLANEOUS: Carl Alström was a Swedish psychiatrist.

ANESTHETIC CONSIDERATIONS

Keep in mind that patients can have significant visual or hearing impairment. Patients with photophobia will be uncomfortable in a brightly lit operating room. Baseline cardiac status should be evaluated, as symptomatic cardiomyopathy can be of early or delayed onset. Baseline pulmonary and renal status should be evaluated. Renal disease can affect intraoperative fluid management and the use of renally excreted drugs. The presence of diabetes mellitus requires attention to glucose status. Venous access and identification of landmarks for regional anesthesia can be difficult secondary to obesity. Obesity can result in desaturation with the induction of anesthesia due to increased airway closure and decreased functional residual capacity. Obesity is also a risk factor for perioperative aspiration. Obese patients require lower than expected drug doses on a per kilogram basis. History should be reviewed for associated endocrinopathies, as delineated in the preceding text.

Bibliography:
1. Marshall JD, Bronson RT, Collin GB, et al. New Alström syndrome phenotypes based on the evaluation of 182 cases. *Arch Intern Med* 2005;165:675–683.
2. Awazu M, Tanaka T, Sato S, et al. Hepatic dysfunction in two sibs with Alström syndrome: case report and review of the literature. *Am J Med Genet* 1997;69:13–16.
3. Millay RH, Weleber RG, Heckenlively JR. Ophthalmologic and systemic manifestations of Alström's disease. *Am J Ophthalmol* 1986;102:482–490.

Amniotic Band Sequence

MIM #: 217100

This sequence occurs sporadically, with no discernible inheritance pattern. It is a consequence of amniotic membrane rupture after which loose bands of amnion wrap around parts of the developing fetus. Amniotic membrane rupture and subsequent amniotic band formation may occur at any time during gestation, but is most likely in the first trimester when the amniotic membrane is most fragile. Because amniotic bands occur as a random event, there is no pattern to the resulting deformations. Most commonly the fetal limbs are involved, but occasionally, bands of amnion encircle the umbilical cord and lead to constriction of umbilical blood flow. When bands of amnion encircle the fetal limbs, various limb

reduction defects can occur. Occasionally, amniotic bands lead to angulation deformities and other limb deformities by restricting normal fetal movement when a limb becomes tethered, although it is not actually constricted.

In addition to band formation, leakage of amniotic fluid after amniotic membrane rupture can lead to limb and even vertebral abnormalities secondary to limitation of the normal movements in the fetus. In addition, significant loss of amniotic fluid can lead to lung hypoplasia secondary to lack of fluid movement with fetal "respirations." However, most patients are normal except those with the typical band-related deformities.

HEENT/AIRWAY: Several cases involving cleft lip or palate have been reported.

ORTHOPEDIC: Evidence of amniotic bands constricting one or more limbs, with amputation of all or part of a limb, amputation of one or more digits, ring-like constriction defects without amputation, distal limb hypoplasia, distal limb edema or pseudosyndactyly (secondary to compression, which prevents separation of the digits), and angulation deformities.

ANESTHETIC CONSIDERATIONS

Limb reduction defects may make vascular access difficult.

Bibliography:
1. Muraskas JK, McDonnell JF, Chudik RJ, et al. Amniotic band syndrome with significant orofacial clefts and disruptions and distortions of craniofacial structures. *J Pediatr Surg* 2003;38:635–638.
2. Bamforth JS. Amniotic band sequence: Streeter's hypothesis reexamined. *Am J Med Genet* 1992;44:280–287.

Amylo-1,6-Glucosidase Deficiency

See Debrancher deficiency

Amyoplasia Congenita Disruptive Syndrome

MIM #: None

This sporadic disorder may be the result of an intrauterine vascular accident that affects the developing anterior horn cells of the fetal spinal cord. This results in a wide variety of joint flexure and contracture deformities (arthrogryposis) involving essentially all joints. Typically, patients exhibit fixed extension at the elbow, flexion of the hands and wrists, internal rotation of the shoulders, flexion or dislocation of the hips, and clubfeet. Fractures can occur during birth secondary to the unforgiving joints.

HEENT/AIRWAY: Round facies with capillary hemangioma on the forehead. In some patients, extraocular movements are limited or the electroretinogram is abnormal. Small, upturned nose. Micrognathia.

NEUROMUSCULAR: Intelligence is normal.

ORTHOPEDIC: Fixed extension at the elbow, flexion of the hands and wrists, internal rotation of the shoulders, flexion or dislocation of the hips, and clubfeet. Variable contractures of other major joints. Contractures are usually symmetric and involve all four extremities. Decreased muscle mass, which is replaced by fibrous bands and fatty tissue. Pterygia may develop at affected joints. Occasional scoliosis, but usually a very straight, immobile spine.

GI/GU: May have gastroschisis, bowel atresia, or hypertrophic pyloric stenosis.

ANESTHETIC CONSIDERATIONS
Care must be taken with positioning because these patients have fixed flexure and contracture deformities at most joints. Fractures secondary to the unforgiving joints occur during birth and could also occur during surgery unless the patient is properly positioned and padded.

Bibliography:
1. Schrander-Stumpel CT, Howeler CJ, Reekers AB, et al. Arthrogryposis, ophthalmoplegia, and retinopathy: confirmation of a new type of arthrogryposis. *J Med Genet* 1993;30:78–80.
2. Robertson WL, Glinski LP, Kirkpatrick SJ, et al. Further evidence that arthrogryposis multiplex congenita in the human sometimes is caused by an intrauterine vascular accident. *Teratology* 1992;45:345–351.
3. Hall JG, Reed DS, Driscoll EP. Part I: amyoplasia: a common sporadic condition with congenital contractures. *Am J Med Genet* 1983;15:571–590.

Andersen Disease

See Brancher deficiency
Note: There is also an Andersen syndrome and Anderson disease (see next entries).

Andersen Syndrome

Included in Long QT syndrome
Note: There is also an Andersen disease and an Anderson disease (see separate entries).

Anderson Disease

MIM #: 246700
Note: There is also an Andersen disease (see prior entry).
This autosomal recessive disease results in a defect of intestinal lipid transport with subsequent fat malabsorption. The gene and gene product responsible for the disorder are not known.

HEENT/AIRWAY: Mild color vision defect.

NEUROMUSCULAR: Mental retardation, decreased deep tendon reflexes, diminished vibratory sense.

GI/GU: Severe childhood diarrhea and steatorrhea. Steatorrhea can be treated by substituting medium-chain for long-chain triglycerides in the diet.

OTHER: Growth retardation and malnutrition. Hypoalbuminemia. Absent chylomicron formation. Vitamin A and E deficiencies have been documented. Recurrent infections.

ANESTHETIC CONSIDERATIONS
Hypoalbuminemia can affect the binding of some anesthetic drugs. Vitamin A and E deficiencies have been documented. One can only speculate about other fat-soluble vitamin deficiencies—in particular, vitamin K deficiency with an attendant risk of bleeding.

Bibliography:
1. Roy CC, Levy E, Green PHR, et al. Malabsorption, hypocholesterolemia, and fat-filled enterocytes with increased intestinal apoprotein B: chylomicron retention disease. *Gastroenterology* 1987;92:390–399.

Anderson-Fabry Disease

See Fabry disease

Angelman Syndrome

SYNONYM: Happy puppet syndrome

MIM #: 105830
This syndrome, which usually occurs sporadically, is distinguished by characteristic facies, fits of laughter, and a puppet-like gait, hence the designation "happy puppet." Laughter is generally in response to an appropriate stimulus, but the response is disproportionate. Most patients with the syndrome have a chromosomal deletion between 15q11 and 15q13. Similar deletions are present in the Prader-Willi syndrome (see later); however, the origin of the chromosomal deletion is maternal in Angelman syndrome and paternal in Prader-Willi syndrome. The specific gene responsible for Angelman syndrome is the gene encoding ubiquitin-protein ligase (*UBE3A*). *UBE3A* has biparental expression in most tissues, but maternal expression in the brain. Approximately 70% of patients will have several gamma-aminobutyric acid (GABA) receptor subunits included in the deletion. Loss of these receptor subunits increases the severity of seizures and other neurologic deficits.

HEENT/AIRWAY: Brachycephaly. Occipital depression or groove. Flat midface with deep-set eyes. Decreased pigmentation of the iris that gives rise to blue eyes in most patients.

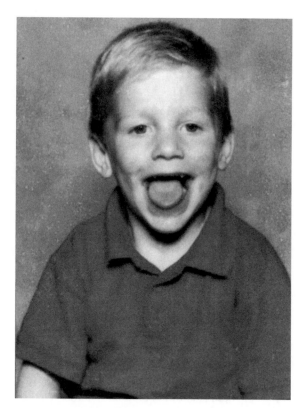

Angelman syndrome. A happy young boy with Angelman syndrome.

Occasional strabismus. Wide mouth (macrostomia), characteristically open with a protruding tongue. Widely spaced teeth. Prognathia.

NEUROMUSCULAR: Mental retardation. Marked motor and speech delay. Recurrent fits of laughter, which are not necessarily a reflection of the patient's mood, but are more likely due to a defect at the level of the brainstem. Dominant vagal tone. Wide-based gait with ataxic arm and leg movements resulting in a puppet-like gait. Abnormal electroencephalogram. Seizures in the vast majority. Hypotonia. Occasional hyperreflexia. Cerebral or cerebellar atrophy on computed tomography scan.

ORTHOPEDIC: Occasional scoliosis.

OTHER: Often have blond hair and hypopigmentation.

MISCELLANEOUS: Pronounced "Angel man." The French refer to this syndrome as *marionette joyeuse*. Because Angelman was unable to establish scientific proof that all the three children he had seen had the same condition, he was reluctant to publish an article about them. However, when on holiday in Italy, Angelman saw an oil painting in the Castelvecchio museum in Verona called "Boy with a Puppet." The boy's laughing face and the fact that Angelman's patients exhibited jerky movements gave him the idea of writing an article about the three children with a title of "*Puppet Children.*"

ANESTHETIC CONSIDERATIONS
Severe intellectual impairment and speech delay present a challenge perioperatively, particularly at the time of induction. Induction through an intramuscular injection of ketamine may be the best option in many cases. Long-term use of anticonvulsant medications can affect the metabolism of some anesthetic drugs. Intraoperative bradycardia for no apparent reason has been reported. This might be due to the increased vagal tone. Although theoretically the use of benzodiazepines could be problematic with GABA dysregulation, these patients generally respond well to these drugs.

Bibliography:
1. Bujok G, Knapik P. Angelman syndrome as a rare anaesthetic problem [Letter]. *Paediatr Anaesth* 2004;14:281–283.
2. Cassidy SB, Schwartz S. Prader-Willi and Angelman syndromes. Disorders of genomic imprinting. *Medicine (Baltimore)* 1998;77:140–151.
3. Kishino T, Lalande M, Wagstaff J. UBE3A/E6-AP mutations cause Angelman syndrome. *Nat Genet* 1997;15:70–73.
4. Buntinx IM, Hennekam RCM, Brouwer OF, et al. Clinical profile of Angelman syndrome at different ages. *Am J Med Genet* 1995;56:176–183.
5. Saitoh S, Harada N, Jinno Y, et al. Molecular and clinical study of 61 Angelman syndrome patients. *Am J Med Genet* 1994;52:158–163.
6. Clayton-Smith J. Clinical research on Angelman syndrome in the United Kingdom: observations on 82 affected individuals. *Am J Med Genet* 1993;46:12–15.
7. Robb SA, Pohl KRE, Baraitser M, et al. The "happy puppet" syndrome of Angelman: review of the clinical features. *Arch Dis Child* 1989;64:83–86.

Aniridia-Wilms Tumor Association

SYNONYM: WAGR syndrome

MIM #: 194072

The association between aniridia and Wilms tumor has been recognized for many years. It is currently estimated that 1% to 2% of patients with aniridia also have Wilms tumor. Aniridia and Wilms tumor have also been associated with genitourinary anomalies and mental retardation, which has been termed WAGR syndrome, which is autosomal dominant: **W**ilms tumor, **A**niridia, **G**enitourinary anomalies or gonadoblastoma, and **R**etardation. Hemihypertrophy has also been described in some of these patients. The WAGR syndrome is a classic example of a contiguous gene syndrome. Aniridia, Wilms tumor/other genitourinary abnormalities, and mental retardation are all due to mutations in separate, but contiguous, genes in the region of 11p13. For example, Wilms tumor and other genitourinary abnormalities are probably due to a mutation in the Wilms tumor suppressor gene (*WT1*).

HEENT/AIRWAY: May have microcephaly. Aniridia, cataracts, nystagmus, ptosis, blindness. Hypoplastic ears. Protuberant lips. Micrognathia.

CARDIOVASCULAR: Occasional ventricular septal defect.

NEUROMUSCULAR: Moderate to severe mental retardation.

ORTHOPEDIC: May have hemihypertrophy. May have short stature.

GI/GU: Wilms tumor. Renal failure. Genitourinary anomalies including ambiguous genitalia, cryptorchidism, and hypospadias. Gonadoblastoma also reported. Uterine malformations. Streak ovaries.

OTHER: Obesity

MISCELLANEOUS: Max Wilms was an early 20th century German surgeon. He died of diphtheria at the age of 51.

ANESTHETIC CONSIDERATIONS
When meeting the patient before surgery, recall that he or she may have significant visual impairment. Micrognathia is usually mild but can make tracheal intubation more difficult. Patients may be receiving chemotherapeutic agents for either Wilms tumor or gonadoblastoma. Patients with cardiac defects need appropriate perioperative antibiotic prophylaxis as indicated.

Bibliography:
1. Fischbach BV, Trout KL, Lewis J, et al. WAGR syndrome: a clinical review of 54 cases. *Pediatrics* 2005;116:984–988.
2. Pavilack MA, Walton DS. Genetics of aniridia: the aniridia-Wilms tumor association. *Int Ophthalmol Clin* 1993;33:77–85.

Anomalous Origin, Left Coronary Artery

SYNONYM: Bland-White-Garland syndrome

MIM #: None

In this disorder, the left main coronary artery has its origin from the pulmonary artery rather than the aorta. Blood in the left main coronary artery is therefore desaturated. The pathogenesis of this anomaly is unknown.

CARDIOVASCULAR: Impressively, the left ventricular function is adequate during the first weeks of life when pulmonary vascular resistance is normally elevated, despite the fact that the left main coronary artery is delivering desaturated blood. It is only when pulmonary vascular resistance (and, therefore, the left main coronary artery perfusion pressure) falls that left ventricular ischemia develops. Very rarely can patients sustain a precarious balance in which ischemia increases left ventricular end-diastolic pressure, which in turn increases pulmonary arterial pressure and coronary perfusion pressure, maintaining coronary flow.

There can be mitral insufficiency secondary to ischemia and ventricular dilatation. The cardiac silhouette is markedly

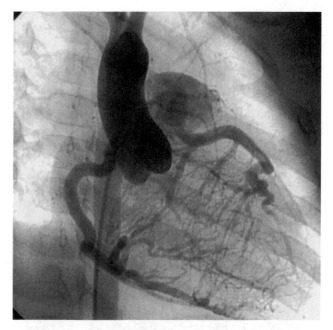

Anomalous origin, left coronary artery. FIG. 1. This aortogram in a 3-year-old with anomalous origin of the left coronary artery shows only a single, large right coronary artery originating from the aortic root. The left coronary artery (to the right side of the photo) fills through the collaterals and contrast can be seen filling the pulmonary artery through retrograde flow from the left coronary artery.

enlarged on chest radiographs, and the electrocardiogram shows anterolateral ischemia. Patients can present with congestive failure or signs of ischemia and angina. Ischemia in infants is often marked by crying, pallor, and diaphoresis during periods of increased activity such as eating. At first such ischemia is transient, but will worsen over time, eventually resulting in an anterolateral infarction. Unrepaired, there is a 90% mortality rate by 1 year. Surgical repair is undertaken when the diagnosis is made and is currently most often accomplished by reimplanting the anomalous coronary artery in the aorta.

MISCELLANEOUS: This defect was actually first described pathologically by Brooks. Bland, White, and Garland described the clinical features and correctly ascribed the findings to angina. The "White" in this syndrome is Dr. Paul Dudley White (of Wolff-Parkinson-White syndrome, and the Lee-White clotting time).

ANESTHETIC CONSIDERATIONS
Anesthetic management is not that dissimilar from the management of adults with coronary ischemia, with or without cardiomyopathy. However, because there is a coronary steal through coronary collaterals into the left main coronary artery and pulmonary artery, maneuvers to transiently increase pulmonary vascular resistance will both increase coronary perfusion pressure in the left coronary artery and also decrease the degree of coronary steal.

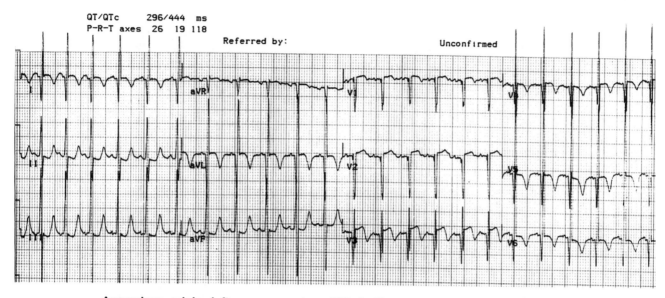

QT/QTc 296/444 ms
P-R-T axes 26 19 118
Referred by: Unconfirmed

Anomalous origin, left coronary artery. FIG. 2. Electrocardiogram of a 3-month-old infant with anomalous origin of the left coronary artery. Note Q waves in leads I, aVL and the left precordial leads.

Bibliography:
1. Kleinschmidt S, Grueness V, Molter G. The Bland-White-Garland syndrome: clinical picture and anaesthesiological management. *Paediatr Anaesth* 1996;6:65–68.
2. Sheinbaum RJ. Cardiac arrest and resuscitation in a child with undetected anomalous left coronary artery. *Anesthesiology* 1990;72:1091–1093.

Antithrombin III Deficiency

MIM #: 107300

Antithrombin III deficiency is one of the causes of hereditary thrombophilia, a familial propensity to develop venous thromboembolism. Antithrombin III deficiency is inherited in an autosomal dominant manner. Antithrombin III inactivates thrombin and factor Xa by binding to them and forming thrombin–antithrombin III and factor Xa—antithrombin III complexes, thereby permitting fibrinolysis. Two major subtypes of antithrombin III deficiency have been described. Type I deficiency is characterized by diminished synthesis of normal antithrombin III. Type II deficiency is characterized by near-normal levels of dysfunctional antithrombin III. Type II deficiency is associated with a lower risk of thrombosis. Thrombotic events are rare in affected children, which may be due in part to a protective effect of elevated levels of alpha-2-macroglobulin during childhood. Acquired deficiencies of antithrombin III are very common; therefore, the definitive diagnosis of a hereditary deficiency of antithrombin III is often difficult to make. Often the diagnosis is dependent on finding the disorder in multiple family members.

CARDIOVASCULAR: Recurrent thrombosis of the deep veins of the legs and the mesenteric veins. Approximately 40%

will develop pulmonary emboli. Infants can rarely develop cerebral venous thrombosis. The onset of thrombotic events is usually after puberty.

MISCELLANEOUS: First described in 1965 by Egeberg, who presented a Norwegian family in which members of three consecutive generations exhibited recurrent thromboembolic events and had plasma concentrations of antithrombin III that were approximately 50% of normal.

ANESTHETIC CONSIDERATIONS
Routine preoperative screening for hypercoagulable states such as antithrombin III deficiency is not necessary. Prophylactic perioperative anticoagulation is recommended for all patients where warranted, and identification of a hypercoagulable state would not alter this recommendation. Neuraxial anesthesia should be avoided in patients who are anticoagulated. Hypovolemia, hypotension, and hypothermia should be avoided because they may increase the risk of thrombosis. Antithrombin III concentrates or recombinant human antithrombin III can be used during periods of acute thromboembolism. Patients who are deficient in antithrombin III will have incomplete anticoagulation from heparin before cardiopulmonary bypass. This is resolved with exogenous antithrombin III, through an infusion of either fresh frozen plasma or recombinant antithrombin III.

Bibliography:
1. Johnson CM, Mureebe L, Silver D. Hypercoagulable states: a review. *Vasc Endovascular Surg* 2005;39:123–133.
2. Baglin T, Luddington R, Brown K, et al. Incidence of recurrent venous thromboembolism in relation to clinical and thrombophilic risk factors: prospective cohort study. *Lancet* 2003;362:523–526.
3. Takahashi J, Ito M, Okude J, et al. Pulmonary thromboembolectomy in congenital antithrombin III deficiency associated with acute

pulmonary embolism- report of a case. *Ann Thorac Cardiovasc Surg* 2003;9:192–196.

4. Okamoto T, Minami K. Anesthesia for a child with a congenital antithrombin deficiency [Letter]. *Can J Anaesth* 2003;50:311.

5. Crowther MA, Kelton JG. Congenital thrombophilic states associated with venous thrombosis: a qualitative overview and proposed classification system. *Ann Intern Med* 2003;138:128–134.

6. Levy JH, Despotis GJ, Szlam F, et al. Recombinant human transgenic antithrombin in cardiac surgery: a dose-finding study. *Anesthesiology* 2002;96:1095–1102.

7. Baud O, Picard V, Durand P, et al. Intracerebral hemorrhage associated with a novel antithrombin gene mutation in a neonate. *J Pediatr* 2001;139:741–743.

8. Shinozaki M, Yamaguchi S, Mishio M, et al. Anesthetic management of a patient with congenital antithrombin III Deficiency using temporal inferior vena cava filter [Japanese]. *Masui* 2001;50:648–650.

9. Brinks HJ, Weerwind PW, Verkroost MW, et al. Familial antithrombin III deficiency during cardiopulmonary bypass: a case report. *Perfusion* 2000;15:553–556.

10. Lane DA, Kunz G, Olds RJ, et al. Molecular genetics of antithrombin deficiency. *Blood Rev* 1996;10:59–74.

11. Rowbottom SJ. Epidural caesarean section in a patient with congenital antithrombin III deficiency. *Anaesth Intensive Care* 1995;23:493–495.

12. Levy JH. Antithrombin deficiency in special clinical syndromes—Part II: cardiovascular surgery. *Semin Hematol* 1995;32:49–55.

13. Jackson MR, Olsen SB, Gomez ER, et al. Use of antithrombin III concentrates to correct antithrombin III deficiency during vascular surgery. *J Vasc Surg* 1995;22:804–807.

14. Kelly MD, Rosenfeld D, Leslie GJ. Venous surgery in patients with congenital antithrombin III deficiency. *ANZ J Surg* 1994;64:865–868.

15. De Stefano V, Leone G, Mastrangelo S, et al. Thrombosis during pregnancy and surgery in patients with congenital deficiency of antithrombin III, protein C, protein S [Letter]. *Thromb Haemost* 1994;71:799–800.

16. Shichino T, Omatsu Y. Perioperative management of congenital antithrombin III deficiency [Japanese]. *Masui* 1989;38:1638–1640.

Antley-Bixler Syndrome

SYNONYM: Multisynostotic osteodysgenesis; Trapezoidocephaly-synostosis syndrome

MIM #: 207410

This autosomal recessive disorder is characterized by trapezoidocephaly, choanal atresia, and radiohumeral synostosis. The defect is due to mutations in a fibroblast growth factor receptor gene (*FGFR2*). Mutations in this gene are also responsible for Apert syndrome, Crouzon syndrome, Beare-Stevenson syndrome, and some cases of Pfeiffer syndrome, which have many phenotypic similarities.

A phenotypically similar syndrome with ambiguous genitalia and abnormal steroidogenesis is due to abnormalities in the gene encoding cytochrome P-450 oxidoreductase (*MIM # 201750*).

HEENT/AIRWAY: Trapezoidocephaly with severe frontal bossing. Coronal and lambdoidal craniosynostosis. Large anterior fontanelle. Brachycephaly. Proptosis. Depressed nasal bridge and maxillary hypoplasia. Long philtrum. Dysplastic ears with stenotic external auditory canals. Choanal stenosis or atresia.

Many patients exhibit severe upper airway obstruction secondary to choanal stenosis or atresia immediately after birth. Without a tracheostomy, more than half the patients

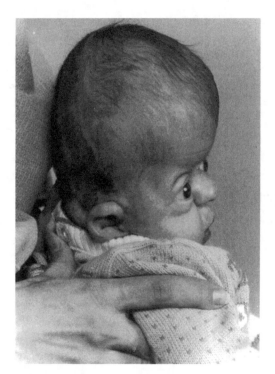

Antley-Bixler syndrome. A 6-week-old boy with Antley-Bixler syndrome. Craniosynostosis and midface hypoplasia are evident. (From LeBard SE, Thiemann LJ. Antley-Bixler syndrome: a case report and discussion. *Paediatr Anaesth* 1998;8:89–91, with permission.)

die before 3 months of age secondary to airway obstruction and associated apnea.

CHEST: May have a narrow chest.

CARDIOVASCULAR: Occasional atrial septal defect.

NEUROMUSCULAR: Occasional hydrocephalus. Variable mental retardation. At least some patients show normal intelligence, suggesting that craniosynostosis repair should be undertaken, when necessary, to allow for normal brain development.

ORTHOPEDIC: Radiohumeral synostosis. Femoral and ulnar bowing. Multiple joint contractures with severely limited range of motion in hands, wrists, hips, knees, and ankles. Arachnodactyly. Slender nails. Camptodactyly. Rocker-bottom feet. May have skeletal fractures as a neonate. Narrow pelvis.

GI/GU: Occasional renal or urogenital defects including vaginal atresia and hypoplastic or fused labia.

ANESTHETIC CONSIDERATIONS

Upper airway obstruction may require immediate intervention at birth. An oral airway or choanal stenting may be helpful. Tracheostomy can be required for definitive treatment of airway obstruction. Choanal atresia precludes placement of a nasal airway, nasal intubation, or placement of a nasogastric tube. A laryngeal mask airway (LMA) has been used successfully intraoperatively.

Meticulous perioperative eye protection is necessary in patients with significant proptosis. Careful perioperative positioning is required secondary to multiple joint contractures, which may limit vascular access. Skeletal fractures have been reported only in the neonatal period.

Bibliography:

1. LeBard SE, Thiemann LJ. Antley-Bixler syndrome: a case report and discussion. *Paediatr Anaesth* 1998;8:89–91.
2. Crisponi G, Porcu C, Piu ME. Antley-Bixler syndrome: case report and review of the literature. *Clin Dysmorphol* 1997;6:61–68.
3. Hassell S, Butler MG. Antley-Bixler syndrome: a report of a patient and review of literature. *Clin Genet* 1994;46:372–376.
4. Escobar LF, Bixler D, Sadove M, et al. Antley-Bixler syndrome from a prognostic perspective: report of a case and review of the literature. *Am J Med Genet* 1988;29:829–836.

Apert Syndrome

SYNONYM: Acrocephalosyndactyly type I

MIM #: 101200

This autosomal dominant disorder is characterized by craniosynostosis and acrocephaly, midfacial hypoplasia, and syndactyly. This syndrome is caused by mutations in the fibroblast growth factor receptor-2 gene (*FGFR2*). Most cases occur sporadically and are thought to be due to a new gene mutation. Two distinct causative mutations have thus far been identified. Different mutations of the same gene cause Crouzon syndrome, Antley-Bixler syndrome, Beare-Stevenson syndrome, and some cases of Pfeiffer syndrome, syndromes that have many phenotypic similarities. The findings in Apert syndrome tend to be more severe and more widespread than those with the other craniosynotosis syndromes.

HEENT/AIRWAY: Acrocephaly, high forehead, flat occiput. Horizontal forehead groove. Irregular craniosynostosis. Large fontanelles. Midfacial hypoplasia. Hypertelorism and shallow orbits. Down-slanting palpebral fissures. Strabismus, myopia. Can have hearing loss. Occasional choanal stenosis or atresia. Small beaked nose and nasopharynx. High, narrow palate. Can have cleft palate. Can have tracheal stenosis or abnormal tracheal cartilage.

Upper airway compromise can occur secondary to the small nasopharynx, choanal stenosis or atresia, tracheal stenosis, or abnormal tracheal cartilage.

CHEST: Narrowed trachea with fused tracheal rings. Rare anomalous tracheal cartilage or pulmonary aplasia, which can result in respiratory compromise. Can have obstructive sleep apnea.

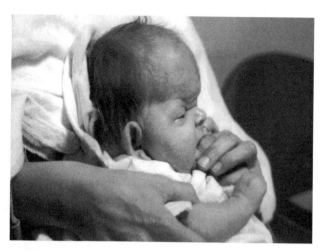

Apert syndrome. FIG. 1. An infant with Apert syndrome scheduled for craniofacial surgery.

CARDIOVASCULAR: Ten percent incidence of congenital cardiac defects, which include pulmonary stenosis, overriding aorta, and ventricular septal defect.

NEUROMUSCULAR: Variable mental retardation. Intelligence can be normal. Can have hydrocephalus or increased intracranial pressure. Craniosynostosis repair should be undertaken, when indicated, to maximize brain development. However, craniosynostosis repair alone does not prevent mental retardation. There is a high incidence of brain malformations, including agenesis of the corpus callosum, anomalies of the septum pellucidum, and gyral and hippocampal abnormalities.

ORTHOPEDIC: Syndactyly—partial or total, osseous or cutaneous—most commonly in digits two through four. Fingers are usually more severely affected than toes. Broad distal phalanx of thumb and great toe. Occasional

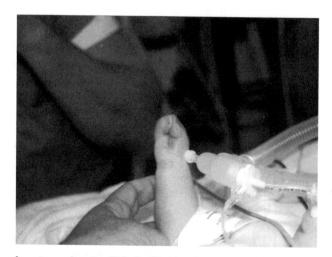

Apert syndrome. FIG. 2. Hands of the patient in Figure 1, showing syndactyly. Establishing adequate venous access in this child was challenging.

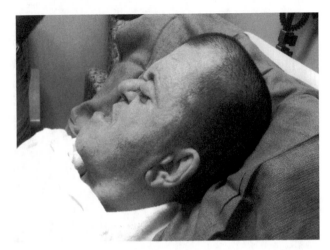

Apert syndrome. FIG. 3. A 47-year-old man with Apert syndrome. He is profoundly retarded and institutionalized. (Courtesy of Dr. William Arnold, Department of Anesthesiology, University of Virginia Health System.)

radiohumeral synostosis. Progressive synostosis can occur at other joints. Fusion of single or multiple cervical vertebrae, C5-6 most commonly.

GI/GU: Ten percent incidence of genitourinary anomalies, including polycystic kidneys, hydronephrosis, bicornuate uterus, vaginal atresia, and cryptorchidism.

OTHER: Growth deceleration in childhood, which becomes more striking after puberty. Severe acne on face and forearms at puberty. Hyperhidrosis.

MISCELLANEOUS: Apert was a French pediatrician, first at Hôpital Saint-Louis and later at Hôpital des Enfants-Malades. "His" syndrome was actually first reported in 1894 by Wheaton. In 1906, Apert summarized nine cases.

ANESTHETIC CONSIDERATIONS

Laryngoscopy and endotracheal intubation may be difficult, particularly if the patient has a small nasopharynx or cervical spine fusion. Because cervical anomalies can complicate an already compromised airway in Apert syndrome, Kreiborg et al. (7) concluded that it is imperative to obtain radiographs of the cervical spine before undertaking anesthesia and surgery in these patients. Placement of a maxillary distraction device can increase the difficulty of tracheal intubation (1), and difficult intubation following midface distraction surgery has been ascribed to temporalis muscle fibrosis (3). Tracheal stenosis or abnormal tracheal cartilage can result in a reduced ability to clear secretions, an increased risk of tracheal injury during suctioning, or respiratory compromise (6). One series reported a high incidence of perioperative wheezing (2). Choanal stenosis or atresia precludes placement of a nasal airway or a nasogastric tube. Preoperative evaluation of renal function should be considered in patients with a history of renal abnormalities which predispose to renal insufficiency. Perioperative antibiotic prophylaxis may be indicated if there is associated congenital heart disease. Patients can have elevated intracranial pressure, in which case precautions should be taken to avoid further elevations in pressure. Excessive premedication and intraoperative hypoventilation may exacerbate preexisting increases in intracranial pressure. Vascular access may be difficult.

Bibliography:

1. Roche J, Frawley G, Heggie A. Difficult tracheal intubation induced by maxillary distraction devices in craniosynostosis syndromes. *Paediatr Anaesth* 2002;12:227–234.
2. Elwood T, Sarathy PV, Geiduschek JM, et al. Respiratory complications during anesthesia in Apert syndrome. *Paediatr Anaesth* 2001;11:701–703.
3. Morris GP, Cooper MG. Difficult tracheal intubation following midface distraction surgery. *Paediatr Anaesth* 2000;10:99–102.
4. Perkins JA, Sie KC, Milczuk El, et al. Airway management in children with craniofacial anomalies. *Cleft Palate Craniofac J* 1997;34:135–140.
5. Reiner D, Arnaud E, Cinalli G, et al. Prognosis for mental function in Apert's syndrome. *J Neurosurg* 1996;85:66–72.
6. Cohen MM, Kreiborg S. Upper and lower airway compromise in the Apert syndrome. *Am J Med Genet* 1992;44:90–93.
7. Kreiborg S, Barr M, Cohen MM. Cervical spine in the Apert syndrome. *Am J Med Genet* 1992;43:704–708.
8. Cohen MM Jr, Kreiborg S. The central nervous system in the Apert syndrome. *Am J Med Genet* 1990;35:36–45.

Aplasia Cutis Congenita

See Adams-Oliver syndrome

Apparent Mineralocorticoid Excess, Syndrome of

See 11β-hydroxysteroid dehydrogenase deficiency

ARC Syndrome

MIM #: 208085

This autosomal recessive syndrome of **A**rthrogryposis, **R**enal dysfunction, and **C**holestasis is due to mutations in the gene *VPS33*, which is involved in the Golgi to lysosomal transfer. Neonatal death is common.

HEENT/AIRWAY: Can have deafness. Can have high-arched palate. Can have redundant nuchal skin.

CARDIOVASCULAR: Can have congenital heart disease.

NEUROMUSCULAR: Rarefaction of the anterior horn of the spinal cord. Developmental delay.

ORTHOPEDIC: Arthrogryposis multiplex congenita (see later) on a neurogenic basis. Proximally placed thumbs.

GI/GU: Cholestatic liver disease. Intrahepatic biliary hypoplasia. Eventual progression to cirrhosis. Diarrhea, probably secondary to fat malabsorption. Nephropathy. Renal tubular acidosis (see Fanconi syndrome). May have nephrogenic diabetes insipidus. May have cryptorchidism.

OTHER: Abnormal platelet morphology and function, similar to gray platelet syndrome (not discussed in this text). Ichthyosis. Recurrent febrile illnesses.

ANESTHETIC CONSIDERATIONS

Severe and fatal hemorrhage has been reported after liver and kidney biopsies. Children may die before renal manifestations become clinically important. Because there is evidence of muscle denervation, succinylcholine should be avoided in these patients. Isosthenuria (fixed specific gravity, neither concentrated nor dilute) or polyuria can complicate perioperative fluid management. Protracted preoperative fasting should be avoided to prevent dehydration. Urine output may be a poor indicator of intravascular fluid status, so central venous pressure monitoring might be appropriate in these patients if surgery will involve major fluid shifts. Chronic renal failure has implications for the choice and dosages of anesthetics and other drugs. Intravenous fluids may be supplemented with bicarbonate or potassium. May require more water in intravenous fluids because of excessive and relatively dilute urine.

Bibliography:
1. Hayes JA, Kahr WHA, Lo B, et al. Liver biopsy complicated by hemorrhage in a patient with ARC syndrome. *Paediatr Anaesth* 2004;14960–14963.
2. Eastham KM, McKiernan PJ, Milford DV, et al. ARC syndrome: an expanding range of phenotypes. *Arch Dis Child* 2001;85:415–420.

Arginase Deficiency

SYNONYM: Argininemia

MIM #: 207800

This autosomal recessive disorder is one of the urea cycle defects and is a potential cause of hyperammonemia. The urea cycle degrades amino acids to urea. Because arginase appears relatively late in the urea cycle, the disease may be less severe than other urea cycle defects. Symptoms can be triggered by stress, such as surgery or infection, or episodes of protein catabolism, such as involution of the postpartum uterus. Unlike the other urea cycle defects, the most common findings with arginase deficiency are neurologic. Liver transplantation is curative.

NEUROMUSCULAR: Spastic tetraplegia is often the presenting feature with arginase deficiency. These children are often originally diagnosed with cerebral palsy, but the progressive nature of the neurologic disease differentiates arginase deficiency from cerebral palsy. The legs are much more severely affected than the arms. Can have psychomotor retardation, hyperactivity, and seizures. Hyperammonemic encephalopathy is clinically similar to hepatic encephalopathy and proceeds through the stages of lethargy and agitation to coma with cerebral edema.

GI/GU: Possible hepatomegaly.

OTHER: Growth failure. Episodes of hyperammonemia are not as severe or as frequent as those with the other urea cycle defects. During episodes of hyperammonemia, ammonia levels are lower than those with the other urea cycle defects.

ANESTHETIC CONSIDERATIONS

Acute metabolic encephalopathy can present after anesthesia. Patients should have high carbohydrate intake (and low protein intake) perioperatively. An orogastric tube or throat packs should be placed if the surgery has the potential to cause oral or intestinal bleeding because blood aspirated into the gastrointestinal tract after oral or nasal surgery might present an excessive protein load and trigger an acute decompensation.

FIGURE: See **Appendix C**

Bibliography:
1. Urea Cycle Disorders Conference group. Consensus statement from a conference for the management of patients with urea cycle disorders. *J Pediatr* 2001;138:S1–5.
2. Schuerle AE, McVie R, Beaudet AL, et al. Arginase deficiency presenting as cerebral palsy. *Pediatrics* 1993;91:995–996.
3. Bernar J, Hanson RA, Kern R, et al. Arginase deficiency in a 12-year-old boy with mild impairment of intellectual function. *J Pediatr* 1986;108:432–435.
4. Brusilow SW, Danney M, Waber LJ, et al. Treatment of episodic hyperammonemia in children with inborn errors of urea synthesis. *N Engl J Med* 1984;310:1630–1634.
5. Snyderman SE, Sansaricq C, Chen WJ, et al. Argininemia. *J Pediatr* 1977;90:563–568.

Argininemia

See Arginase deficiency

Argininosuccinic Acid Lyase Deficiency

SYNONYM: Argininosuccinic aciduria

MIM #: 207900

This autosomal recessive disorder is one of the urea cycle defects and is a potential cause of hyperammonemia. Both early onset (severe) and late-onset (less severe) types have been described. The urea cycle degrades amino acids to urea. Symptoms can be triggered by stress, such as surgery or infection, or episodes of protein catabolism, such as involution of the postpartum uterus. Neonates are treated with dietary arginine. Episodes of hyperammonemia usually resolve with intravenous arginine. Liver transplantation is curative.

The clinical presentations of the urea cycle defects, carbamyl phosphate synthetase, ornithine transcarbamylase, argininosuccinic acid synthetase, and argininosuccinic acid lyase deficiencies, are essentially identical.

NEUROMUSCULAR: Mental retardation, seizures. Hyperammonemic encephalopathy is clinically similar to hepatic encephalopathy and proceeds through the stages of lethargy and agitation to coma with cerebral edema.

GI/GU: Hepatomegaly. Hepatic synthetic function is normal, although there may be elevations in serum transaminase levels, both during and between episodes of hyperammonemia.

OTHER: Particular to this specific urea cycle defect is the presence of brittle hair (which fluoresces red) in approximately half the patients, possibly related to a low-protein diet. Skin on the dorsum of the hands and arms is rough. Episodes of hyperammonemia begin with anorexia and lethargy and can progress through agitation, irritability, and confusion. Vomiting and headaches can be prominent. Untreated, central nervous system deterioration ensues, with worsening encephalopathy, and eventually results in coma with cerebral edema and death.

MISCELLANEOUS: This enzyme has structural and enzymatic activity. It can accumulate in high concentration without precipitating, making it transparent, and is found in particularly high concentration in duck lenses.

ANESTHETIC CONSIDERATIONS
Acute metabolic encephalopathy can present after anesthesia. Patients should have high carbohydrate intake (and low protein intake) perioperatively. An orogastric tube or throat packs should be placed if the surgery has the potential to cause oral or intestinal bleeding because blood aspirated into the gastrointestinal tract after oral or nasal surgery might present an excessive protein load, triggering an acute decompensation. A case of fatality on the first postoperative day of an otherwise stable child with the disease after inguinal herniorrhaphy with enflurane anesthesia has been reported (2).

FIGURE: See **Appendix C**

Bibliography:
1. Urea Cycle Disorders Conference group. Consensus statement from a conference for the management of patients with urea cycle disorders. *J Pediatr* 2001;138:S1–5.
2. Asai K, Ishii S, Ohta S, et al. Fatal hyperammonaemia in argininosuccinic aciduria following enflurane anaesthesia [Letter]. *Eur J Paediatr* 1997;157:169–170.
3. Worthington S, Christodoulou J, Wilcken B, et al. Pregnancy and argininosuccinic aciduria. *J Inherit Metab Dis* 1996;19:621–623.
4. Widhalm K, Koch S, Scheibenreiter S, et al. Long-term follow-up of 12 patients with the late-onset variant of argininosuccinic acid lyase

deficiency: no impairment of intellectual and psychomotor development during therapy. *Pediatrics* 1992;89:1182–1184.
5. Brusilow SW, Danney M, Waber LJ, et al. Treatment of episodic hyperammonemia in children with inborn errors of urea synthesis. *N Engl J Med* 1984;310:1630–1634.
6. Collins FS, Summer GK, Schwartz RP, et al. Neonatal argininosuccinic aciduria-survival after early diagnosis and dietary management. *J Pediatr* 1980;96:429–431.

Argininosuccinic Acid Synthetase Deficiency

SYNONYM: Citrullinuria; Citrullinemia

MIM #: 215700

This autosomal recessive disorder is one of the urea cycle defects and is a potential cause of hyperammonemia. The urea cycle degrades amino acids to urea. Symptoms can be triggered by stress, such as surgery or infection, or episodes of protein catabolism, such as involution of the postpartum uterus. Onset is usually in the neonatal period, but a late-onset form of the disease has been described in Japan. The clinical presentations of the urea cycle defects, carbamyl phosphate synthetase, ornithine transcarbamylase, argininosuccinic acid synthetase, and argininosuccinic acid lyase deficiencies, are essentially identical. Liver transplantation is curative.

NEUROMUSCULAR: Mental retardation, developmental delay. Seizures. Lethargy, episodic coma. Hyperammonemic encephalopathy is clinically similar to hepatic encephalopathy and proceeds through stages of lethargy and agitation to coma with cerebral edema.

GI/GU: Vomiting, diarrhea. Hepatic synthetic function is normal, although there can be elevations in serum transaminase levels, both during and between episodes of hyperammonemia.

OTHER: Episodes of hyperammonemia begin with anorexia and lethargy and can progress through agitation, irritability, and confusion. Vomiting and headaches can be prominent. Untreated, central nervous system deterioration ensues, with worsening encephalopathy, and eventually results in coma with cerebral edema and death.

MISCELLANEOUS: The amino acid citrulline derives its name from its high concentrations in the watermelon, *Citrullis vulgaris.* The disorder has also been reported in a strain of Australian dairy cows.

ANESTHETIC CONSIDERATIONS
Acute metabolic encephalopathy can present after anesthesia. Patients should have high carbohydrate intake (and low protein intake) perioperatively. An orogastric tube or throat packs should be placed if the surgery has the potential to cause oral or intestinal bleeding because blood aspirated into the gastrointestinal tract after oral or nasal surgery might present an excessive protein load, triggering an acute decompensation. Worsening encephalopathy has been reported in patients receiving glycerol for cerebral edema.

FIGURE: See **Appendix C**

Bibliography:

1. Urea Cycle Disorders Conference group. Consensus statement from a conference for the management of patients with urea cycle disorders. *J Pediatr* 2001;138:S1–5.
2. Brusilow SW, Danney M, Waber LJ, et al. Treatment of episodic hyperammonemia in children with inborn errors of urea synthesis. *N Engl J Med* 1984;310:1630–1634.
3. Whelan DT, Brusso T, Spate M. Citrullinemia: phenotypic variations. *Pediatrics* 1976;57:935–941.

Argininosuccinic Aciduria

See Argininosuccinic acid lyase deficiency

Arima Syndrome

SYNONYM: Cerebrooculohepatorenal syndrome

MIM #: 243910

This autosomal recessive syndrome shares phenotypic characteristics with Joubert syndrome (see later). The gene and gene product are not known.

HEENT/AIRWAY: Abnormal eye movements. Leber congenital amaurosis (see later). Chorioretinal coloboma. Abnormal eye movements. Rhythmic tongue protrusion. Large mouth.

CHEST: Episodic hyperventilation.

NEUROMUSCULAR: Aplasia of the cerebellar vermis, ataxia, hypotonia, mental retardation. Can have brainstem malformations including pachygyria.

ORTHOPEDIC: Postaxial polydactyly of hands and feet.

GI/GU: Can have liver disease. Infantile polycystic disease of the kidneys. Renal failure.

ANESTHETIC CONSIDERATIONS
Hepatic and renal dysfunction can affect metabolism of a variety of anesthetic medications. There have been reports of difficult airway management. A laryngeal mask airway (LMA) has been used successfully. A case of intraoperative hyperkalemia has been reported, but the etiology is unclear because the child had renal failure with baseline hyperkalemia.

Bibliography:

1. Koizuka S, Nishikawa K-I, Nemoto H, et al. Intraoperative QRS-interval changes caused by hyperkalaemia in an infant with Arima syndrome. *Paediatr Anaesth* 1998;8:425–428.

Arnold-Chiari Malformation

SYNONYM: Chiari malformation

MIM #: 207950

The Arnold-Chiari malformation is the most common anomaly of the hindbrain and results in caudal displacement of the cerebellum and lower brainstem. The etiology of this malformation appears to be multifactorial. The disorder has been subdivided into three types, depending on the extent of caudal displacement. Patients with type I are usually asymptomatic. Patients with type II may become symptomatic, often before the age of 3 months. Patients with type III are almost always symptomatic before the age of 3 months. The Arnold-Chiari malformation, usually type II, is present in virtually all children with meningomyelocele. Symptoms are a result of the impairment of the lower cranial nerves, brainstem, cerebellum, and, occasionally, cervical spinal cord secondary to caudal displacement and sometimes herniation of parts of the cerebellum and brainstem. Typically, there is herniation of the cerebellar vermis and choroid plexus through the foramen magnum. The most common symptoms are vocal cord paralysis, dysphagia, stridor, apnea, upper extremity weakness, and opisthotonos. In older children and adults, the Arnold-Chiari malformation can be associated with syringomyelia.

HEENT/AIRWAY: Vocal cord paralysis, dysphagia.

CHEST: Stridor, respiratory distress, apnea (central or obstructive). Abnormal swallowing increases the risk of pulmonary aspiration.

CARDIOVASCULAR: Significant brainstem involvement can be reflected in changes in heart rate or rhythm.

NEUROMUSCULAR: Can have cranial nerve VI, VII, IX, X, XI, or XII; brainstem; cerebellar; or cervical cord dysfunction, with various manifestations. Headaches are common. Diminished or absent gag reflex. Central apnea. Ataxia, vertigo, nystagmus. Paresthesias, weakness, or spasticity of an extremity. Opisthotonos. Symptomatic patients may benefit from surgical decompression of the posterior fossa.

Brainstem compression may lead to complete obstruction of the foramina of Luschka and Magendie and to progressive hydrocephalus. Possible increased intracranial pressure. Patients with symptomatic hydrocephalus benefit from placement of a ventriculoperitoneal shunt.

ORTHOPEDIC: May have cervical spondylolysis or other deformities.

MISCELLANEOUS: In 1883 John Cleland described the basilar impression syndrome, now known as the Arnold-Chiari malformation, 8 years before Chiari (1891) and 11 years before Arnold (1894).

ANESTHETIC CONSIDERATIONS

Patients are at increased risk of aspiration secondary to swallowing difficulties with pooling of oral secretions, diminished or absent gag reflex, and vocal cord paralysis. Patients with a history of recurrent aspiration may have chronic lung disease. Patients may also have other cranial nerve defects. Brainstem dysfunction can result in an abnormal response to hypoxia and hypercarbia, or frank apnea. Intraoperative controlled ventilation is necessary in patients with frequent apneic episodes. Significant brainstem compression has been associated with intraoperative refractory hypotension and bigeminy (3). Precautions against elevations in intracranial pressure are indicated in some patients. Spinal and epidural anesthesia for Cesarian section have been reported several times for women with type I lesions. Subarachnoid needle entry is a concern if elevated intracranial pressure is present but has not been reported.

Posterior fossa decompression surgery is usually performed with the patient in the prone position with the neck flexed. Care should be taken in positioning because extreme neck flexion can cause brainstem compression or endobronchial intubation. If prone, the patient's face and eyes should be well padded. There is the potential for the development of an air embolism during posterior fossa surgery.

After posterior fossa decompression, the recovery of neurologic function takes time. Patients with inability to maintain or protect their airway preoperatively (vocal cord paralysis, absent gag reflex) will not have immediate improvement in function and will need to remain intubated until adequate function returns.

Bibliography:

1. Chantigian RC, Koehn MA, Ramin KD, et al. Chiari I malformation in parturients. *J Clin Anesth* 2002;14:201–205.
2. Nel MR, Robson V, Robinson PN. Extradural anaesthesia for caesarean section in a patient with syringomyelia and Chiari type I anomaly. *Br J Anaesth* 1998;80:512–515.
3. Tanaka M, Harukuni I, Naito H. Intraoperative cardiovascular collapse in an infant with Arnold-Chiari malformation. *Paediatr Anaesth* 1997;7:163–166.
4. Semple DA, McClure JH. Arnold-Chiari malformation in pregnancy. *Anaesthesia* 1996;51:580–582.
5. Davidson Ward SL, Nickerson BG, van der Hal A, et al. Absent hypoxic and hypercapneic arousal responses in children with myelomeningocele and apnea. *Pediatrics* 1986;78:44–50.

Aromatic L-Amino Acid Decarboxylase Deficiency

SYNONYM: AADC deficiency

MIM #: 608643

This autosomal recessive disorder, due to mutations in the gene *AADC*, is a disorder of neurotransmitter synthesis. This enzyme decarboxylates L-dopa to dopamine, and 5-hydroxytryptophan to serotonin. There are low levels of multiple catecholamine neurotransmitters, including dopamine, epinephrine, norepinephrine, and serotonin.

Parasympathetic function is intact, leading to an autonomic imbalance with parasympathetic predominance. Diagnosis is made by finding low levels of these neurotransmitters in the spinal fluid or blood. Plasma enzyme activity can also be assayed. Treatment may include ropinirole (a D_2 dopamine receptor agonist), pergolide (a dopamine receptor agonist), pyridoxine (a cofactor of the enzyme), cholinergics, monoamine oxidase inhibitors, and serotoninergic agents.

HEENT/AIRWAY: Ptosis, miosis. Nasal congestion. Drooling.

CARDIOVASCULAR: Impaired heart rate and blood pressure control. Hypotension. Bradycardia.

NEUROMUSCULAR: Severe autonomic dysregulation. Severe mental retardation. Markedly diminished voluntary movements. Truncal hypotonia, limb hyperreflexia, intermittent oculogyric crises, dystonic posturing. Myoclonus. Emotional lability.

GI/GU: Gastroesophageal reflux, constipation, diarrhea.

OTHER: Temperature instability. Hypoglycemia. Diaphoresis.

ANESTHETIC CONSIDERATIONS

The autonomic imbalance produces significant challenges to intraoperative homeostasis. There is decreased ability to respond appropriately to hypovolemia. Prophylactic atropine has been suggested, given the propensity to bradycardia. Patients can develop hypothermia or hyperthermia (not malignant hyperthermia related). Painful stimuli can result in bradycardia and cardiorespiratory arrest due to unopposed vagal tone. Infusion of dopamine at 5 µg/kg/minute resulted in an excessive hypertensive and tachycardic response in one child. Doses of 1 to 2 µg/kg/minute of dopamine were tolerated. It is unclear whether this was due to an abnormal expression of dopaminergic receptors or an interaction with the dopaminergic medications the patient was receiving. Phenylephrine can result in profound reflex bradycardia. Ephedrine will have diminished effect because of its indirect mechanism of action. Arterial catheters should be considered for procedures with possible blood or fluid loss. Blood glucose should be followed perioperatively. Hemodynamic monitoring should be continued into the postoperative period. There can be delayed gastric emptying.

Bibliography:

1. Vutskits L, Menache C, Manzano S, et al. Anesthesia management in a young child with aromatic L-amino acid decarboxylase deficiency. *Paediatr Anaesth* 2006;16:82–84.
2. Swoboda KJ, Saul JP, McKenna CE, et al. Aromatic L-amino acid decarboxylase deficiency: overview of clinical features and outcomes. *Ann Neurol* 2003;54(Suppl 6):S49–S55.

Arrhythmogenic Right Ventricular Dysplasia

See Uhl anomaly

Arteriohepatic Dysplasia

See Alagille syndrome

Arthrodentoosteo Dysplasia

See Hajdu-Cheney syndrome

Arthrogryposis

SYNONYM: Distal arthrogryposis; Arthrogryposis multiplex congenita (AMC), distal

MIM #: 108120, 108130

Arthrogryposis, meaning "curved joints," is a general term that describes multiple joint contractures of prenatal onset. Arthrogryposis can be found associated with a variety of diseases. It can be the result of a fetal myopathy, fetal neuropathy, or severe oligohydramnios resulting in intrauterine constraint.

Distal arthrogryposis is an autosomal dominant form of arthrogryposis in which there is involvement primarily of the distal joints (hands and feet). There is marked variability in expression, and the manifestations in some patients are mild. It is characterized by congenital contractures that primarily affect the distal joints, clenched fists with medially overlapping fingers in the neonate (similar to the hand positioning noted in trisomy 18), ulnar deviation of

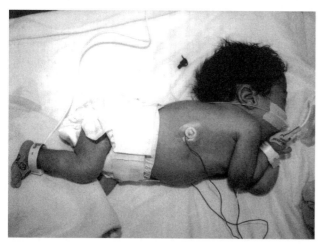

Arthrogryposis. FIG. 1. The neck is in fixed extension in this infant with arthrogryposis.

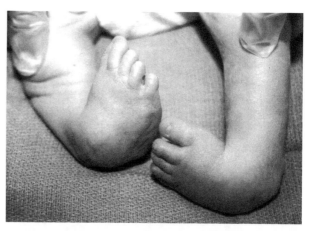

Arthrogryposis. FIG. 2. Fixed foot deformity in arthrogryposis.

the fingers, and clubfeet. Distal arthrogryposis is due to mutations in the gene *TPM2*, which encodes β-tropomyosin.

HEENT/AIRWAY: Patients can have associated ptosis, cleft lip or palate, micrognathia, short neck, trismus.

CHEST: Myopathy, a poor cough, and skeletal deformities can result in alveolar hypoventilation, atelectasis, and restrictive lung disease and may increase the risk of aspiration.

CARDIOVASCULAR: A variety of congenital heart defects have been noted in a small percentage of patients. Severe respiratory disease can result in cor pulmonale.

NEUROMUSCULAR: Intelligence is usually normal. Spinal stenosis has been reported.

ORTHOPEDIC: Multiple joints exhibit fixed flexion or contracture deformities, severely limiting joint mobility. The affected extremities are often atrophic. There can be webbing of overlying skin. Joints often exhibit a good response to physical therapy. Hip involvement is common—congenital dislocation, decreased abduction, and mild flexion contracture deformities. Clubfeet in most cases. Occasional scoliosis. Occasional fusion of cervical vertebrae. Occasional short stature.

Neonates' hands are clenched tightly in a fist, with medially overlapping fingers and thumb. Ulnar deviation of the fingers and camptodactyly occur in adults, after the hands have unclenched.

MISCELLANEOUS: Arthrogryposis can be seen in any circumstance in which there is immobilization of the developing fetal joints. An unusual example is treatment of a mother with curare for tetanus.

ANESTHETIC CONSIDERATIONS
Micrognathia or limited mandibular excursion, a short neck, or fusion of the cervical vertebrae can make laryngoscopy

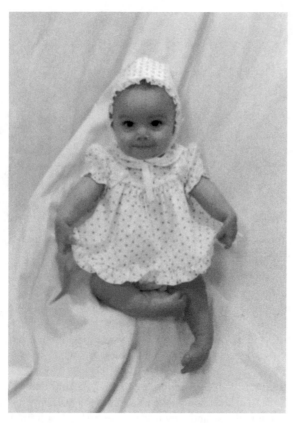

Arthrogryposis. FIG. 3. The fixed wrist, foot and knee deformities are obvious in this girl with arthrogryposis.

and tracheal intubation difficult. Difficult intubations have not been reported in patients with isolated limb findings. Peripheral regional techniques can be appropriate, even in neonates (2). Significant cardiac or pulmonary disease is rare. Intravenous access and appropriate positioning may be difficult because of flexion or contracture deformities, especially of the distal extremities. This disease is not associated with malignant hyperthermia. The hypermetabolism and hyperthermia sometimes seen in association with anesthesia are not believed to represent malignant hyperthermia (5, 7, 9).

Bibliography:

1. Martin S, Tobias JD. Perioperative care of the patient with arthrogryposis. *Paediatr Anaesth* 2006;16:31–37.
2. Ion T, Cook-Sather SD, Finkel RS. Fascia iliaca block for an infant with arthrogryposis multiplex congenital undergoing muscle biopsy. *Anesth Analg* 2005;100:82–84.
3. Nguyen NH, Morvant EM, Mayhew JF. Anesthetic management for patients with arthrogryposis multiplex congenita and severe micrognathia: case reports. *J Clin Anesth* 2000;12:227–230.
4. Ferris PE. Intraoperative convulsions in a child with arthrogryposis. *Anaesth Intensive Care* 1997;25:546–549.
5. Audenaert SM. Arthrogryposis is not a diagnosis [Letter]. *Paediatr Anaesth* 1994;4:201–202.
6. Zamudio IA, Brown TCK. Arthrogryposis multiplex congenita (AMC): a review of 32 years' experience. *Paediatr Anaesth* 1993;3:101–106.
7. Hopkins PM, Ellis FR, Halsall PJ. Hypermetabolism in arthrogryposis multiplex congenita. *Anaesthesia* 1991;46:374–375.
8. Oberoi G, Kaul HL, Gill IS. Anaesthesia in arthrogryposis multiplex congenita: case report. *Can J Anaesth* 1987;34:288–290.
9. Baines DB, Douglas ID, Overton JH. Anaesthesia for patients with arthrogryposis multiplex congenita: what is the risk of malignant hyperthermia? *Anaesth Intensive Care* 1986;14:370–372.
10. Hall JG, Reed SD, Greene D. The distal arthrogryposes. Delineation of new entities: review and nosologic discussion. *Am J Med Genet* 1982;11:185–239.

Arthrogryposis Multiplex Congenita (AMC), Distal

See Arthrogryposis

Asperger Syndrome

Included in Autism

Asphyxiating Thoracic Dystrophy

See Jeune syndrome

Asplenia

SYNONYM: Ivemark syndrome; Heterotaxy syndrome

MIM #: 208530

Asplenia and the related syndrome of polysplenia are often thought of as disorders of laterality: patients with asplenia are bilaterally right sided (right-sided isomerism, i.e., they have two copies of right-sided structures and they lack normal left-sided structures, the spleen being one), and patients who are polysplenic are bilaterally left sided. Therefore, they have neither situs solitus nor situs inversus but are said to have situs ambiguus. Asplenia is often associated with a primitive heart and right-sided obstruction. Sudden death, particularly during the first few years of life, is primarily due to sepsis, complex cardiac disease, or less commonly, arrhythmias. Familial cases have been reported.

CHEST: There are two right lungs [trilobed with the bronchial—arterial relationship of the right lung (pulmonary artery superior to the bronchus)].

CARDIOVASCULAR: There are two right atria and, therefore, two sinoatrial nodes producing a wandering atrial pacemaker from the two foci. A common atrium, a single ventricle with a single atrioventricular canal type valve, or a single ventricle variant with pulmonary stenosis or atresia may occur. Because there is no left atrium for the pulmonary veins to return to, there is usually some type of anomalous pulmonary venous return. Systemic venous anomalies include bilateral superior vena cavae, bilateral hepatic venous connections directly to the ipsilateral atrium, and unroofing of the coronary sinus. The aorta and inferior vena cava run together on the same side of the spine (normally the inferior vena cava is to the right and the aorta to the left).

GI/GU: There is laterality to the "tacking down" of the fetal gastrointestinal tract in normal fetuses (that is why the appendix fairly reliably ends up in the right lower quadrant). In this disease of abnormal laterality, there may be malrotation of the gut, which can present with volvulus. There are two right lobes of the liver, and on radiographs the abnormal liver can be seen interposed between the air-filled stomach and the base of the left lung. The stomach and pancreas can be left sided, right sided, or midline. There is, of course, no spleen. Can have horseshoe kidney.

OTHER: Because of absence of the spleen, patients are immunoincompetent and are susceptible to infection with encapsulated organisms. They should have received the pneumococcal and *Hemophilus* vaccines and probably also the meningococcal vaccine if older than 2 years. Patients are also at increased risk for fatal malaria and severe babesiosis. Red cell inclusions, particularly Howell-Jolly bodies, can be seen in the peripheral blood smear of patients with asplenia.

ANESTHETIC CONSIDERATIONS
Meticulous aseptic technique is imperative in these patients with an immune deficiency, and appropriate antibiotic prophylaxis particularly important. Specific anesthetic management varies with the individual cardiac lesions. Patients with cardiac anomalies require perioperative antibiotic prophylaxis as indicated. Although not reported, it might be expected that a left-sided double-lumen endobronchial tube might occlude the takeoff of the left upper lobe bronchus, which would arise more proximally than usual in this left-sided lung that has the anatomy of a right lung.

Bibliography:
1. Wu MH, Wang JK, Lue HC. Sudden death in patients with right isomerism (asplenism) after palliation. *J Pediatr* 2002;140:93–96.
2. Winer-Muram HT. Adult presentation of heterotaxic syndromes and related complexes. *J Thorac Imag* 1995;10:43–57.
3. Phoon CK, Neill CA. Asplenia syndrome: insight into embryology through an analysis of cardiac and extracardiac anomalies. *Am J Cardiol* 1994;73:581–587.
4. Winer-Muram HT, Tonkin IL. The spectrum of heterotaxic syndromes. *Radiol Clin North Am* 1989;27:1147–1170.

Asymmetric Crying Facies

SYNONYM: Cayler syndrome

MIM #: 125520

This syndrome is due to congenital hypoplasia or absence of the depressor anguli oris muscle, resulting in asymmetry of the mouth during crying or laughing. It is hypothesized to be either an autosomal dominant or a multifactorial trait. It can occur in isolation or in association with defects in other organs, most commonly ventricular septal defects

of the heart. The specific gene and gene product are not known. It is thought that the syndrome might represent another manifestation of the 22q11.2 deletion syndrome (see DiGeorge syndrome).

HEENT/AIRWAY: Variable microcephaly. Asymmetry of the lower lip, seen particularly with crying or laughing.

CARDIOVASCULAR: Ventricular septal defect.

NEUROMUSCULAR: Rare mental retardation.

OTHER: May fail to thrive.

MISCELLANEOUS: Glenn Cayler, who first described this disorder, was a pediatric cardiologist who noted an "epidemic of congenital paresis and heart disease."

ANESTHETIC CONSIDERATIONS
Patients with congenital heart disease need perioperative antibiotic prophylaxis as indicated. The asymmetric facies should be documented preoperatively to avoid miscommunication postoperatively.

Bibliography:
1. Lahat E, Heyman E, Barkay A. Asymmetric crying facies and associated congenital anomalies: prospective study and review of the literature. *J Child Neurol* 2000;15:808–810.
2. Lin DS, Huang FY, Lin SP, et al. Frequency of associated anomalies in congenital hypoplasia of depressor anguli oris muscle: a study of 50 patients. *Am J Med Genet* 1997;71:215–218.
3. Silengo MC, Lopez Bell G, Biagioli M, et al. Asymmetric crying facies with microcephaly and mental retardation: an autosomal dominant syndrome with variable expressivity. *Clin Genet* 1986;30:481–484.

Ataxia—Telangiectasia

SYNONYM: Louis-Bar syndrome

MIM #: 208900

This autosomal recessive disorder involves oculocutaneous telangiectasis, variable immunodeficiency, cerebellar ataxia, and a predisposition to malignancy. The ataxia—telangiectasia gene encoding the ATM (ataxia—telangiectasia mutated) protein encodes phosphatidylinositol-3 kinase, which is a member of a family of proteins that respond to DNA damage by phosphorylating substances involved in DNA repair or cell cycle control. Patients with ataxia—telangiectasia have defective DNA repair after ionizing radiation, and their cells have increased chromosomal breakage. Survival, which used to be uncommon into the teenager years is now often into adulthood in the United States.

HEENT/AIRWAY: Telangiectasis first appears on the conjunctivae, at approximately 3 to 5 years of age. Nystagmus. Oculomotor apraxia (inability to make purposeful movements). Recurrent sinusitis. Dysarthria, drooling.

CHEST: Recurrent pulmonary infections and bronchiectasis. These are with "routine" pathogens and not opportunistic organisms. Thymus remains embryonic.

NEUROMUSCULAR: Progressive cerebellar ataxia. Difficulty in learning to walk is typically the initial presentation, followed by choreoathetosis, myoclonic jerks, and oculomotor abnormalities. Abnormal fetal cerebellar Purkinje cell migration and degeneration. Progressive muscle weakness from degeneration of peripheral nerve Schwann cells. Patients have normal intelligence, but severe short-term memory loss has been reported in older adults. Progressive spinal muscle atrophy may develop in adults.

ORTHOPEDIC: Interosseous muscle atrophy of the hands, in combination with dystonia, leads to a combination of flexion-extension contractures of the hands in adults.

GI/GU: May have elevated liver enzymes associated with fatty infiltration and round cell infiltration of the portal area. There is hypogonadism, more so in female than in male patients. Delayed development of secondary sexual characteristics in girls is associated with absent or hypoplastic ovaries. Can have premature menopause.

OTHER: Telangiectases appear on the skin, particularly on sun-exposed areas and areas of trauma. There are also areas of vitiligo, *café au lait* spots, early loss of subcutaneous fat, and premature graying of the hair. Endocrine abnormalities are common, and most patients have some degree of glucose intolerance. There is an increased incidence of malignancy of a variety of types, often leukemia or lymphoma, and approximately 15% of patients eventually die of malignant disease. A variety of immunologic defects are seen, variable even within the same family. These include immunoglobulin A (IgA) deficiency in most patients (interestingly, all the patients in whom carcinoma of the stomach develops are IgA deficient), IgE deficiency, IgG subtype deficiency, an abnormal IgM (7S monomorphic form rather than the usual 19S pentameric form), anergy to delayed hypersensitivity skin testing, depressed lymphocyte proliferative responses to mitogens or viral pathogens, and abnormalities in helper T-cell function. Despite these abnormalities, systemic viral, bacterial, and fungal infections are uncommon. Premature aging. Can have hypertrichosis.

MISCELLANEOUS: These patients are extremely sensitive to ionizing radiation, and treatment of malignancies with conventional doses of radiation therapy may be fatal. DNA repair mechanisms are abnormal in four other inherited diseases: xeroderma pigmentosum, Fanconi anemia, Bloom syndrome, and Cockayne syndrome.

Louis-Bar is one person (Denise Louis-Bar). She began using the hyphenated surname after she was married.

ANESTHETIC CONSIDERATIONS
Perioperative x-ray studies are indicated only when absolutely necessary. Patients may have glucose intolerance, and the perioperative serum glucose level can be elevated. The likelihood of an immunodeficiency suggests that particularly good aseptic technique is obligatory. Patients may benefit from anticholinergic medication for excessive drooling. Succinylcholine may cause hyperkalemia in patients with significant neuropathy and muscle weakness.

Bibliography:
1. Lavin MF, Shiloh Y. The genetic defect in ataxia-telangiectasia. *Annu Rev Immunol* 1997;15:177–202.
2. Gatti RA. Ataxia-telangiectasia. *Dermatol Clin* 1995;13:1–6.

ATP Synthetase (ATPase) Deficiency

See Complex V deficiency

ATR-X Syndrome

SYNONYM: X-linked alpha thalassemia/mental retardation syndrome

MIM #: 301040

This X-linked recessive disorder of alpha thalassemia, mental retardation, genital abnormalities, and characteristic facies is due to a defect in the gene encoding X-linked helicase-2. Helicases are involved in a wide variety of intracellular functions, including DNA recombination and repair and regulation of transcription, including regulation of alpha-globin expression. The typical facies of patients with this syndrome are similar to that seen with Coffin-Lowry syndrome. Specific mutations in this gene can result in dysmorphic features and mental retardation without thalassemia. A second, less common and more phenotypically variable form of this syndrome is due to a partial deletion of chromosome 16 that involves hemoglobin alpha$_1$ and alpha$_2$ genes.

HEENT/AIRWAY: Microcephaly, midface hypoplasia. Can have absent frontal sinuses. Telecanthus, epicanthal folds. Small or malformed, low-set ears. Small, triangular nose, anteverted nostrils, alae nasi extend below columella and septum, flat nasal bridge. Carp-shaped mouth, large, protuberant tongue, full lips.

CHEST: Missing rib.

CARDIOVASCULAR: Occasional ventricular septal defect.

NEUROMUSCULAR: Severe mental and gross motor retardation, almost absent speech. Hypotonia. Seizures.

ORTHOPEDIC: Clinodactyly. Occasional clubfoot deformity. Occasional growth retardation.

GI/GU: Gastroesophageal reflux is common. Genital anomalies including shawl scrotum, cryptorchidism and hypospadias. Recurrent urinary tract infections. Occasional renal agenesis, hydronephrosis, hydroureter.

OTHER: Alpha thalassemia (see Thalassemia). Cells containing hemoglobin H inclusions are detectable in a peripheral blood smear. Hematologic abnormalities tend to be relatively minor.

ANESTHETIC CONSIDERATIONS

A preoperative hematocrit should be obtained. Severe mental retardation and absent speech may make the induction of anesthesia more challenging. Gastroesophageal reflux is common, increasing the risk of perioperative aspiration. Patients may have renal dysfunction, which has implications for perioperative fluid management and choice of anesthetic drugs. Patients with congenital cardiac defects will require appropriate antibiotic prophylaxis.

Bibliography:

1. Gibbons RJ, Higgs DR. Molecular-clinical spectrum of the ATR-X syndrome. *Am J Med Genet* 2000;97:204–212.
2. Ellis NA. DNA helicases in inherited human disorders. *Curr Opin Genet Dev* 1997;7:354–363.
3. Gibbons RJ, Picketts DJ, Villard L, et al. Mutations in a putative global transcriptional regulator cause X-linked mental retardation with alpha thalassemia (ATR-X syndrome). *Cell* 1995;80:837–845.

Auriculoosteodysplasia

SYNONYM: Beals auriculoosteodysplasia syndrome

MIM #: 109000

This autosomal dominant disorder involves malformation of the external ear and dysplasia of multiple bones. The specific gene and gene products are not known. Note that this is not the same as Beals contractural arachnodactyly syndrome (see later).

HEENT/AIRWAY: Abnormal ear shape—usually elongation of the lobe with an attached, small, slightly posterior lobule.

ORTHOPEDIC: Short stature. Multiple osseous dysplasias, especially radiocapitellar joint dysplasia, radial head dislocation, hip dysplasia.

ANESTHETIC CONSIDERATIONS

Patients must be carefully positioned perioperatively because of the presence of multiple osseous dysplasias. Vascular access might be limited.

Bibliography:

1. Beals RK. Auriculo-osteodysplasia: a syndrome of multiple osseous dysplasia, ear anomaly, and short stature. *J Bone Joint Surg Am* 1967;49:1541–1550.

Autism

SYNONYM: Infantile autism; Autistic disorder; Kanner syndrome. (Includes Asperger syndrome)

MIM #: 608636, 608638

Autism is a pervasive developmental disorder that is characterized by an inability to socialize and form normal relationships, severe limitations in verbal and nonverbal communication skills, and stereotypical repetitive patterns of behavior. Intelligence testing in children with autism usually places them in the normal to functionally retarded range. Occasionally, children with autism display isolated, but remarkable, talents—analogous to that of the adult savant. Autism is apparent by 3 years of age and is typically diagnosable at 18 months of age. Autism is more common in males than in females (3 to 4:1). Autism may be associated with other neurologic disorders, particularly seizure disorders. Autism has also been linked to tuberous sclerosis, fragile X syndrome, and untreated phenylketonuria (see later). There is controversy over whether the incidence of autism is increasing. The cause of autism is multifactorial. There appears to be no association between the use of the measles, mumps, and rubella (MMR) vaccine and autism (8). Family and twin studies have shown that genetic factors play a significant role. The disease is genetically heterogeneous.

Asperger syndrome is a form of childhood autism also exhibiting genetic heterogeneity. Children with Asperger syndrome exhibit impaired social interactions and repetitive behaviors but lack the severe language impairments that characterize autism. Also, unlike autism, intelligence in children with Asperger syndrome is almost always in the normal range. The prevalence of Asperger syndrome is approximately 30 per 10,000 children, and Asperger syndrome may be diagnosed at a later age than autism. There is debate whether Asperger syndrome is a separate disorder or whether it represents the "high-functioning" end of the spectrum of autism.

NEUROMUSCULAR: May have macrocephaly. May have seizure disorder. Studies have demonstrated structural anatomic changes in the brains of patients with autism, none of which are diagnostic for autism. Structural changes may be demonstrable in the hippocampus, the temporal lobe, the cerebellum, the reticular activating system, or the anterior cingulate gyrus, an area of the brain that is associated with processing feelings and thoughts and with decision making. Abnormal neurotransmitter levels have also been implicated in autism, with particular interest focused on the dopamine, catecholamine, and serotonin pathways.

OTHER: Children with higher-functioning autism and those with Asperger syndrome may be at greater risk for having other psychiatric disorders, particularly oppositional-defiant disorder, obsessive-compulsive disorder, and anxiety or mood disorders.

MISCELLANEOUS: Leo Kanner, an Austrian psychiatrist who practiced in the United States, was the first to describe autism. In 1943 he wrote of a disorder in which children showed "an innate inability to form the usual, biologically provided affective contact with people." Kanner noted that in most cases the child's behavior was abnormal from early infancy, which suggested to him that the disorder was genetically based. In 1944, the Austrian pediatrician Hans Asperger described a syndrome in which children exhibited impaired social interaction coupled with seemingly normal intelligence. He dubbed this disorder "autistic psychopathy." Asperger was a prolific writer, who published more than 350 articles in his lifetime and an indefatigable academician, lecturing 6 days before his death at the age of 74 years.

ANESTHETIC CONSIDERATIONS

Children with autism become particularly difficult to manage in the hospital setting because they react poorly to changes in their routine. There is great variability in the severity of autism and in the needs of individuals with autism. Early and comprehensive communication with the patient's family and a willingness to be flexible with the anesthetic plan are imperative. Oral midazolam has been shown to be an effective premedicant for milder cases, and oral ketamine a reliable premedicant for moderate to severe cases (4). It is important to return the patients as quickly as possible to their baseline state. To this end, the intravenous cannula should be removed as soon as is clinically acceptable and the patient should be discharged as quickly as possible (ideally on the same day as surgery).

Bibliography:
1. Arndt TL, Stodgell CJ, Rodier PM. The teratology of autism. *Int J Dev Neurosci* 2005;23:189–199.
2. Khouzam HR, El-Gabalawi F, Pirwani N, et al. Asperger's disorder: a review of its diagnosis and treatment. *Compr Psychiatry* 2004;45:184–191.
3. Muhle R, Trentacoste SV, Rapin I. The genetics of autism. *Pediatrics* 2004;113:e472–e486.
4. van der Walt JH, Moran C. An audit of perioperative management of autistic children. *Paediatr Anaesth* 2001;11:401–408.
5. Tsang RW, Solow HL, Ananthanarayan C, et al. Daily general anaesthesia for radiotherapy in unco-operative patients: ingredients for successful management. *Clin Oncol (R Coll Radiol)* 2001;13:416–421.
6. Institute of Medicine Immunization Safety Reviews. *Measles-Mumps-Rubella Vaccine and Autism*. Washington: National Academy Press, 2001:13–69.
7. Gillberg C. Asperger syndrome and high-functioning autism. *Br J Psychiatry* 1998;172:200–209.
8. Jensen RA. Autism and the use of hypnotic barbiturates in obstetrics and pediatrics [Letter]. *J Autism Dev Disord* 1991;21:254–257.

Autistic Disorder

See Autism

Autonomic Neuropathy with Insensitivity to Pain

See Congenital insensitivity to pain and anhydrosis

Axenfeld Syndrome

SYNONYM: Axenfeld-Rieger syndrome
See also Rieger syndrome

MIM #: 109120

This autosomal dominant disorder is similar to Rieger syndrome (see later) and probably represents a different manifestation of the same genetic defect. The Axenfeld anomaly has findings limited to the peripheral anterior segment of the eye. The Axenfeld syndrome includes the Axenfeld anomaly and other facial and skeletal anomalies. The Rieger anomaly consists of the Axenfeld anomaly and abnormalities of the iris. The Rieger syndrome involves eye abnormalities and other developmental defects (see later). These disorders are sometimes referred to as the **Axenfeld-Rieger anomalies**. Several different cytogenetic abnormalities have been associated with development of the syndrome.

HEENT/AIRWAY: Brachycephaly. Prominent forehead with flat midface. Facial asymmetry. Abnormalities of the anterior chamber, absent eye muscles, proptosis, hypertelorism, glaucoma. Mild sensorineural deafness. Maxillary hypoplasia.

CARDIOVASCULAR: Can be associated with a variety of congenital cardiac defects.

NEUROMUSCULAR: May have communicating hydrocephalus or psychomotor retardation. Hypotonia. Absent corpus callosum.

ORTHOPEDIC: Flat femoral epiphyses. Coxa valga. Hip dislocation. Hypoplastic shoulder. Lax joints. Short stature.

ANESTHETIC CONSIDERATIONS

Care must be taken perioperatively to protect the proptotic eyes from trauma.

Bibliography:
1. Cok OY, Ozkose Z, Atabekoglu S, et al. Intravenous patient-controlled analgesia using remifentanil in a child with Axenfeld-Rieger syndrome. *Paediatr Anaesth* 2005;15:162–166.
2. Chitty LS, McCrimmon R, Temple IK, et al. Dominantly inherited syndrome comprising partially absent eye muscles, hydrocephaly, skeletal abnormalities, and a distinctive facial phenotype. *Am J Med Genet* 1991;40:417–420.

B

Baller-Gerold Syndrome

SYNONYM: Craniosynostosis-radial aplasia syndrome

MIM #: 218600

This autosomal recessive disorder has as its main features craniosynostosis, radial aplasia, and absent or hypoplastic thumbs. Death during infancy is common. There may be overlap with Fanconi anemia and Saethre-Chotzen syndrome (see later), and the question whether Baller-Gerold syndrome represents a distinct entity has been raised.

HEENT/AIRWAY: Craniosynostosis involving single or multiple sutures. Flattened forehead. Down-slanting palpebral fissures, epicanthal folds, hypertelorism. Low-set and posteriorly rotated ears. Prominent nasal bridge. Micrognathia with small mouth. Occasional cleft palate or choanal stenosis.

CARDIOVASCULAR: Twenty-five percent incidence of cardiac anomalies including subaortic valvular hypertrophy, ventricular septal defect, tetralogy of Fallot.

NEUROMUSCULAR: Mental retardation is common. Occasional seizures, hydrocephalus, absent corpus callosum.

ORTHOPEDIC: Growth retardation. Absent or hypoplastic radius. Ulnar hypoplasia and curvature. Absent or hypoplastic thumbs. Malformed or absent carpals. Occasional humeral hypoplasia, vertebral and pelvic defects, fused ribs, scoliosis.

GI/GU: Anal anomalies are common, including anteriorly placed anus and imperforate anus. Renal anomalies are common, including ectopic, hypoplastic, dysplastic, or absent kidneys.

ANESTHETIC CONSIDERATIONS
Patients must be evaluated for congenital cardiac defects. Micrognathia or small mouth may make direct laryngoscopy difficult. Choanal stenosis precludes nasal intubation or placement of a nasogastric tube. Vascular access may be difficult secondary to radial aplasia and humeral hypoplasia. Radial anomalies may also make placement of a radial arterial catheter more difficult. Patients with renal dysfunction require careful titration of perioperative fluids and judicious use of renally excreted drugs. Patients with congenital cardiac defects require appropriate antibiotic prophylaxis.

Bibliography:
1. Cohen MM, Toriello HV. Is there a Baller-Gerold syndrome [Editorial]? *Am J Med Genet* 1996;61:63–64.
2. Farrell SA, Paes BA, Lewis MES. Fanconi anemia in a child previously diagnosed as Baller-Gerold syndrome [Letter]. *Am J Med Genet* 1994;50: 98–99.
3. Ramos Fuentes FJ, Nicholson L, Scott CI. Phenotypic variability in the Baller-Gerold syndrome: report of a mildly affected patient and review of the literature. *Eur J Pediatr* 1994;153:483–487.
4. Lin AE, McPherson E, Nwokoro NA, et al. Further delineation of the Baller-Gerold syndrome. *Am J Med Genet* 1993;45:519–524.

Bannayan-Riley-Ruvalcaba Syndrome

See Riley-Smith syndrome

Bannayan-Zonana Syndrome

See Riley-Smith syndrome

Baraitser-Burn Syndrome

Included in Oral-facial-digital syndrome, type I

Bardet-Biedl Syndrome

MIM #: 209900

This is an autosomal recessive disorder with marked variability of clinical expression. The classic findings are mental retardation, retinal dystrophy, obesity, polydactyly, hypogenitalism, and renal insufficiency. Genetic heterogeneity is likely in this syndrome, with linkage analysis in different families implicating nine loci on different chromosomes. Some require a recessive mutation in one locus plus an additional mutation in a second locus. It has been suggested that the involved proteins attach to the basal body of ciliated cells, making this a ciliary dysfunction disorder. This disorder is similar to, but possibly distinct from, the Laurence-Moon syndrome (see later). Unlike the patients described by Bardet and Biedl, the patients described by Laurence and Moon had spastic paraplegia, and did not have obesity or polydactyly. The two syndromes have sometimes been recognized as distinct, and sometimes not. Thus, the literature contains many references to the Laurence-Moon-Biedl syndrome or the Laurence-Moon-Biedl-Bardet syndrome. Some children were diagnosed as having McKusick-Kaufman syndrome (not discussed in this text) early in life only to be rediagnosed with Bardet-Biedl syndrome later as clinical findings developed.

HEENT/AIRWAY: Occasional macrocephaly. Retinal dystrophy and pigmentation result in problems such as night vision, peripheral vision, color vision, and visual acuity. Most patients are blind by the age of 20 years. Astigmatism, nystagmus, cataracts. Occasional glaucoma. Partial or complete loss of sense of smell. High-arched palate with tooth crowding. Hypodontia with small tooth roots. May have bifid epiglottis.

CARDIOVASCULAR: Hypertension is common, particularly in patients with renal disease. A variety of minor cardiac defects have been described.

NEUROMUSCULAR: Mild to moderate mental retardation. Behavioral problems and flat affect are common. Delayed speech. Ataxia. Poor coordination.

ORTHOPEDIC: Postaxial polydactyly. Syndactyly. Brachydactyly of hands. Short, broad feet.

GI/GU: Hirschsprung disease (see later) has been reported in several patients. Can develop hepatic fibrosis. Hypogenitalism—male patients appear to be sterile, but some affected women have given birth. Multiple renal anomalies have been reported, including abnormal calyces, calyceal diverticulae, abnormal lobulations, renal cysts, cortical loss, and scarring. Most patients exhibit mild renal insufficiency, and renal failure develops in some patients. Nephrogenic diabetes insipidus.

OTHER: Morbid obesity. Occasional diabetes mellitus. Poor wound healing.

MISCELLANEOUS: Biedl was a prominent Hungarian endocrinologist who practiced in Germany. He can be considered the founder of modern endocrinology.

ANESTHETIC CONSIDERATIONS

Behavioral problems may make the smooth induction of anesthesia a challenge. Keep in mind that patients will likely have impaired vision. Venous access and identification of landmarks for regional anesthesia may be difficult secondary to morbid obesity. Obesity may result in desaturation with induction of anesthesia because of increased airway closure and decreased functional residual capacity. Obesity is also a risk factor for perioperative aspiration. Drug doses (on a per kilogram basis) should be reduced in cases of massive obesity. Patients with renal dysfunction need careful titration of perioperative fluids and judicious use of renally excreted drugs.

Bibliography:

1. Beales PL, Warner AM, Hitman GA. et al. Bardet-Biedl syndrome: a molecular and phenotypic study of 18 families. *J Med Genet* 1997;34:92–98.
2. Uçar B, Yakut A, Kural N. Renal involvement in the Laurence-Moon-Bardet-Biedl syndrome: report of five cases. *Pediatr Nephrol* 1997;11:31–35.
3. Elbedour K, Zucker N, Zalzstein E. et al. Cardiac abnormalities in the Bardet-Biedl syndrome: echocardiographic studies of 22 patients. *Am J Med Genet* 1994;52:164–169.
4. Low J, Brown TCK. Bardet-Biedl syndrome: review of anaesthetic problems. *Paediatr Anaesth* 1992;2:245–248.
5. Green JS, Parfrey PS, Harnett JD, et al. The cardinal manifestations of Bardet-Biedl syndrome, a form of Laurence-Moon-Biedl syndrome. *N Engl J Med* 1989;321:1002–1009.

Bare Lymphocyte Syndrome

Included in Severe combined immunodeficiency syndrome

Barth Syndrome

MIM #: 302060

This X-linked recessive disorder of dilated cardiomyopathy, neutropenia, skeletal myopathy, and abnormal mitochondria is due to mutations in the gene *TAZ* (also known as *G4.5*).

The role of the protein product, tafazzin, is unknown, but it is possibly an acyltransferase. The phenotype is widely variable, and the syndrome is suspected to be underdiagnosed. An etiologic role may be played by cardiolipin. There are abnormalities in cardiolipin, a phospholipid structural component of the mitochondrial inner membrane, resulting in leaky mitochondria with abnormal ATP production.

HEENT/AIRWAY: Recurrent mouth ulcers related to neutropenia.

CARDIOVASCULAR: Dilated cardiomyopathy, usually presenting in infancy. Endomyocardial fibroelastosis. Left-ventricular noncompaction. Cardiac function tends to improve in preadolescence, worsen during the teenage years, and then improve yet again. Can develop ventricular arrhythmias.

NEUROMUSCULAR: Myopathy. Hypotonia. Sparing of bulbar and ocular muscles. Weakness, myalgia.

ORTHOPEDIC: Moderate growth retardation. Growth velocity increases during the teenage years.

OTHER: Intermittent lactic acidemia. Neutropenia. Recurrent infections in infancy and early childhood. Structurally abnormal mitochondria. Elevated levels of urinary 3-methylglutaconic acid.

ANESTHETIC CONSIDERATIONS

Because cardiac function can fluctuate, a cardiac evaluation should be performed in proximity to anesthesia and surgery. Cardiac medications should be continued perioperatively. Anesthetic technique may have to be modified in the presence of cardiac dysfunction. Succinylcholine would be contraindicated in this myopathy secondary to the risk of exaggerated hyperkalemia. Patients needing prolonged orotracheal intubation will require good mouth care because of the presence of oral ulcers.

Bibliography:

1. Barth PG, Valianpour F, Bowen VM, et al. X-linked cardioskeletal myopathy and neutropenia (Barth syndrome). *Am J Med Genet A* 2004;126:349–354.

Bartter Syndrome

SYNONYM: Hyperprostaglandin E syndrome. (Includes Gitelman syndrome)

MIM #: 601678, 241200, 607364, 602522

This clinical syndrome of salt-losing renal tubulopathy has various autosomal recessive types, all linked by hyperreninemic hypokalemic metabolic alkalosis. There is inadequate salt reabsorption from the thick ascending loop of Henle. Autosomal recessive antenatal Bartter syndrome type 1 is due to abnormalities in the Na^+-K^+-$2Cl^-$ cotransporter gene *SLC12A1*. It is marked by hypokalemic, hypochloremic metabolic alkalosis, high levels of renin and aldosterone, and the absence of hypertension. The clinically and biochemically indistinguishable antenatal Bartter syndrome type 2 is caused by a mutation in the gene for the ATP-sensitive inwardly-rectifying potassium channel ROMK and is associated with high levels of prostaglandin E. Classic Bartter syndrome (type 3) is caused by defects in the kidney chloride channel B gene (*CLCNKB*). Infantile Bartter syndrome with sensorineural deafness (type 4) is caused by defects in the gene *BSND*, which is present in the inner ear as well as the kidney, or by simultaneous mutations in *CLCNKA* and *CLCNKB*. Neonatal disease presents with antenatal onset. Similar hypokalemic alkalosis in older children and adults but with hypocalciuria is known as **Gitelman syndrome**, and is caused by defects in the thiazide-sensitive sodium chloride cotransporter *SLC12A3*. Gitelman syndrome also has episodes of muscle weakness and tetany with hypokalemia, hypomagnesemia, and hypocalciuria. Unlike the other forms that affect the ascending loop of Henle, the defect in Gitelman syndrome affects the distal tubule.

NEUROMUSCULAR: Mental retardation. Muscular weakness, muscle cramps.

ORTHOPEDIC: Short stature, rickets.

GI/GU: Hypokalemia can result in ileus, delayed gastric emptying, or constipation. The primary renal defect is the diminished chloride reabsorption in the ascending loop of Henle. Excessive sodium delivery (as sodium chloride) to the collecting duct causes excessive potassium secretion, which is enhanced by the hyperaldosteronism. There is increased urinary prostaglandin E_2 (a secondary phenomenon from protracted potassium depletion). There is juxtaglomerular cell hyperplasia. Hypokalemia inhibits renal tubular function, resulting in polyuria and polydipsia. Nephrocalcinosis (not in the classic type). Hypercalciuria.

OTHER: Anorexia, failure to thrive. In addition to the hypokalemic, hypochloremic metabolic alkalosis, there is also hypomagnesemia, hypocalcemia, hypercalciuria, and hyperuricemia. There is hyperaldosteronism and hyperreninemia, but no hypertension. There is an impaired vasopressor response to angiotensin II. There may be platelet dysfunction due to abnormalities in prostaglandins. Type 2 disease can be associated with transient neonatal hyperkalemia.

MISCELLANEOUS: Bartter also described the syndrome of inappropriate antidiuretic hormone (SIADH). Because this less-common syndrome was described first, it retains the eponymous association. It has been speculated that given the lack of severity in Bartter's original patients, they may have actually had Gitelman syndrome.

Bartter was an expert on mushrooms and an authority in the diagnosis and treatment of amanita-type mushroom poisoning.

ANESTHETIC CONSIDERATIONS

Neonates in particular can have severe intravascular volume depletion. Preoperative medications should be continued until surgery and reinstituted as soon as possible thereafter. Medications may include a prostaglandin synthetase inhibitor (such as indomethacin), spironolactone, potassium chloride, ammonium chloride, and sodium chloride, but treatment rarely totally corrects the hypokalemia. A nonkaliuretic diuretic should be chosen, if possible. However, chronic hypokalemia does not carry the same risk of arrhythmia as does acute hypokalemia. Hypovolemia should be avoided and prophylactic volume expansion considered. Prostaglandin synthetase inhibitors can also additionally inhibit platelet function, and the potential for dysfunctional platelets needs to be considered. Patients may be volume contracted at the baseline and the hematocrit may fall with volume expansion.

Decreased gastric motility from hypokalemia may increase aspiration risk. Aggressive ventilation with respiratory alkalosis may worsen a preexisting metabolic alkalosis, and may also further lower serum potassium. The effects of muscle relaxants may be potentiated by the hypotonia. The urinary concentrating defect may make urinary output a poor guide to intravascular volume. Propofol may increase urinary uric acid excretion in normal patients (4), and propofol may therefore be contraindicated for prolonged anesthesia or sedation in patients with Bartter syndrome.

A patient with abnormal baroreceptor responses has been described (8); however, there have been no reported problems with blood pressure control in response to anesthetics. Perioperative changes in plasma renin activity, angiotensin II, and plasma aldosterone responses all mirror changes seen in unaffected patients.

Bibliography:
1. Vetrugno L, Cheli G, Bassi F, et al. Cardiac anesthesia management of a patient with Bartter syndrome. *J Cardiothorac Vasc Anesth* 2005;19:373–376.
2. Bichet DG, Fujiwara TM. Reabsorption of sodium chloride–lessons lessons from the chloride channels. *N Engl J Med* 2004;350: 1281–1283.
3. Scheinman SJ, Guay-Woodford LM, Thakker RV, et al. Genetic disorders of renal electrolyte transport. *N Engl J Med* 1999;340:1177–1187.
4. Miyazawa N, Takeda J, Izawa H. Does propofol change uric acid metabolism? *Anesth Analg* 1998;86:S486.
5. Kannan S, Delph Y, Moseley HSL. Anaesthetic management of a child with Bartter's syndrome. *Can J Anaesth* 1995;42:808–812.
6. Higa K, Ishino H, Sato S, et al. Anesthetic management of a patient with Bartter's syndrome. *J Clin Anesth* 1993;5:321–324.
7. Kataja J, Viinamaki O, Punnonen R, et al. Renin-angiotensin-aldosterone system and plasma vasopressin in surgical patients anesthetized with halothane or isoflurane. *Eur J Anaesthesiol* 1988;5:121–129.
8. Nishikawa T, Dohi S. Baroreflex function in a patient with Bartter's syndrome. *Can Anaesth Soc J* 1985;32:646–650.
9. Abston PA, Priano LL. Bartter's syndrome: anesthetic implications based on pathophysiology and treatment. *Anesth Analg* 1981;60:764–766.

Basal Cell Nevus Syndrome

SYNONYM: Gorlin-Goltz syndrome; Gorlin-Gold syndrome; Gorlin syndrome; Nevoid basal cell carcinoma syndrome

MIM #: 109400

This autosomal dominant disorder results in the development of multiple nevoid basal cell carcinomas, along with characteristic facies, rib anomalies, and mandibular cysts. Penetrance is variable, but seems similar within a family. Many cases represent fresh mutations, and advanced paternal age probably plays a role in these new mutations. The syndrome is caused by a mutation in the gene *PTC*, the human homolog of the *Drosophila* "patched" gene. *PTC*, which is expressed in the developing tissues that are involved in the clinical syndrome, encodes a transmembrane protein and functions as a tumor suppressor gene.

HEENT/AIRWAY: Macrocephaly. Bony bridging of the sella turcica. Frontal bossing and prominent supraorbital ridges, with overlying thick eyebrows. Hypertelorism. Cataracts. Strabismus. Iris coloboma. Broad nasal bridge. May have cleft lip or palate. Abnormally shaped teeth. Dental caries is common. Prognathism. Mandibular cysts, which may enlarge during puberty.

CHEST: Bifid ribs or other rib anomalies. May have pectus excavatum. Congenital lung cysts.

CARDIOVASCULAR: Occasional cardiac fibromas.

NEUROMUSCULAR: May have mental deficiency, hydrocephalus. May have calcification of the falx cerebri, falx cerebelli, petroclinoid ligament, dura, pia, or choroid plexus. Occasional agenesis of the corpus callosum. At risk for medulloblastoma, astrocytoma.

ORTHOPEDIC: Scoliosis. May have cervical vertebral anomalies. Kyphoscoliosis. Sloping, narrow shoulders. Short fourth metacarpals. Occasional polydactyly, arachnodactyly.

GI/GU: Lymphomesenteric cysts. Hamartomatous stomach polyps. Ovarian fibromas—these may contain vasoactive substances. Ovarian sarcomas. Occasional hypogonadism in male patients. Occasional renal anomalies.

OTHER: Multiple (up to several hundred) nevoid basal cell carcinomas, especially over the face, neck, arms, and chest. The nevi are rarely present at birth, but begin to proliferate at puberty. Basal cell carcinomas usually develop between the age of 15 and 35 years, but have appeared as early as age 2 years. Milia. Palmar and plantar pits. Epidermal cysts. Occasional calcification of subcutaneous tissue. Can have a Marfanoid habitus.

Other neoplasms may develop, including medulloblastoma, astrocytoma, meningioma, melanoma, lipoma, fibroma, breast cancer, ovarian cancer, lung cancer, chronic lymphoid leukemia, non-Hodgkin lymphoma.

MISCELLANEOUS: Patients are extremely radiosensitive, and therapeutic doses of ionizing radiation have led to the development of large numbers of basal cell carcinomas. African Americans are less likely to have basal cell carcinomas than whites, even though other components of the syndrome are expressed equivalently. Increased skin pigmentation in African Americans is presumably protective against the effects of ultraviolet radiation in these very radiosensitive patients. The protein product of *PTC* in *Drosophila* is a transmembrane receptor for the ligand Sonic Hedgehog.

Robert Gorlin is a dentist and a leading dysmorphologist. His *Syndromes of the Head and Neck* is a classic reference text.

ANESTHETIC CONSIDERATIONS
Dental abnormalities/dental caries may predispose to dental loss during laryngoscopy. Teeth should be inventoried before laryngoscopy. Patients may require extreme care in positioning and laryngoscopy if cervical vertebral anomalies are present. Patients may have unrecognized hydrocephalus.

Bibliography:
1. Gorlin RJ. Nevoid basal cell carcinoma (Gorlin) syndrome. *Genet Med* 2004;6:530–539.
2. Kimonis VE, Goldstein AM, Pastakia B, et al. Clinical manifestations in 105 persons with nevoid basal cell carcinoma syndrome. *Am J Med Genet* 1997;69:299–308.
3. Wicking C, Shanley S, Smyth I, et al. Most germ-line mutations in the nevoid basal cell carcinoma syndrome lead to a premature termination of the PATCHED protein, and no genotype-phenotype correlations are evident. *Am J Hum Genet* 1997;60:21–26.
4. Shanley S, Ratcliffe J, Hockey A, et al. Nevoid basal cell carcinoma syndrome: review of 118 affected individuals. *Am J Med Genet* 1994;50:282–290.
5. Evans DGR, Ladusans EJ, Rimmer S, et al. Complications of the nevoid basal cell carcinoma syndrome: results of a population based study. *J Med Genet* 1993;30:460–464.
6. Yoshizumi J, Vaughan RS, Jasani B. Pregnancy associated with Gorlin's syndrome. *Anaesthesia* 1990;45:1046–1048.
7. Gorlin RJ. Nevoid basal-cell carcinoma syndrome. *Medicine (Baltimore)* 1987;66:98–113.
8. Southwick GJ, Schwartz RA. The basal cell nevus system: disasters occurring among a series of 36 patients. *Cancer* 1979;44:2294–2305.

Batten Disease

See Spielmeyer-Vogt disease

Beals Auriculoosteodysplasia Syndrome

See Auriculoosteodysplasia
Note: This is distinct from Beals syndrome (see later)

Beals Contractural Arachnodactyly Syndrome

See Beals syndrome

Beals Syndrome

SYNONYM: Beals contractural arachnodactyly syndrome

MIM #: 121050

This autosomal dominant syndrome has as its main features joint contractures, arachnodactyly, and a "crumpled"-appearing ear. The gene responsible is likely fibrillin-2 (*FNB2*). It is somewhat phenotypically similar to Marfan syndrome, caused by abnormalities in the gene fibrillin-1. Note that this is a distinct entity from Beals auriculoosteodysplasia syndrome (see earlier).

HEENT/AIRWAY: May have scaphocephaly, brachycephaly, or dolichocephaly. May have frontal bossing. Occasional iris coloboma. "Crumpled"-appearing ear. Micrognathia. Short neck. High-arched palate.

CHEST: Occasional sternal defects. May have pectus carinatum.

CARDIOVASCULAR: Mitral prolapse with regurgitation. Occasional atrial septal defect, ventricular septal defect, or aortic hypoplasia.

ORTHOPEDIC: Congenital joint contractures, especially of the elbows, hips, and knees. Can also have contractures of the fingers. Joint mobility improves over time. Long, slim limbs with arachnodactyly. Camptodactyly. Ulnar deviation of the fingers. Calf muscle hypoplasia. May have mild clubfoot deformity. Generalized osteopenia. Thoracolumbar kyphoscoliosis—can be congenital and usually progressive over time.

MISCELLANEOUS: Beals and Hecht, who originally described this syndrome in 1971, have suggested that the patient described by Marfan in 1896 actually had contractural arachnodactyly syndrome rather than the syndrome now known as Marfan syndrome. Because the ocular and cardiovascular complications of Marfan syndrome do not occur or are different in contractural arachnodactyly syndrome, the distinction between these two syndromes has clinical significance to the anesthesiologist.

ANESTHETIC CONSIDERATIONS
Relatively short neck and mild micrognathia have not been associated with difficult direct laryngoscopy or intubation. Careful perioperative positioning is required secondary to multiple joint contractures. Thoracolumbar scoliosis may be severe enough to cause restrictive lung disease. Patients may have mitral regurgitation, but significant aortic disease (as with Marfan syndrome) has not been reported. Patients with mitral regurgitation will require antibiotic prophylaxis as indicated.

Bibliography:
1. De Coster PJ, Martens LC, De Paepe A. Orofacial manifestations of congenital fibrillin deficiency: pathogenesis and clinical diagnostics. *Pediatr Dent* 2004;26:535–537.
2. Putnam EA, Zhang H, Ramirez F, et al. Fibrillin-2 (FBN2) mutations result in the Marfan-like disorder, congenital contracture arachnodactyly. *Nat Genet* 1995;11:456–458.
3. Viljoen D. Congenital contracture arachnodactyly (Beals syndrome). *J Med Genet* 1994;31:640–643.

Bean Syndrome

See Blue rubber bleb nevus syndrome

Beare-Stevenson Syndrome

SYNONYM: Cutis gyrata syndrome of Beare-Stevenson

MIM #: 123790

This autosomal dominant disorder has as its primary components craniofacial, skin, and genital abnormalities. The most typical finding is cutis gyrata (widespread heavily corrugated skin folds), particularly of the scalp. The syndrome is associated with increased paternal age. It is due to defects in the gene encoding fibroblast growth factor receptor 2 (*FGFR2*), although the inability to document a defect in this gene in several patients suggests there may be some heterogeneity. Death usually occurs in childhood. Different mutations of this gene cause Apert syndrome, Crouzon syndrome, Antley-Bixler syndrome, and some cases of Pfeiffer syndrome, syndromes that have many phenotypic similarities.

HEENT/AIRWAY: Cloverleaf skull (kleeblattschaedel), craniosynostosis, midface hypoplasia, hypertelorism, proptosis, downward-slanting palpebral fissures, low-set ears, choanal stenosis or atresia, narrow palate. Can have cleft palate.

CHEST: Can have recurrent pulmonary infections. Tracheal stenosis has been reported.

NEUROMUSCULAR: Hydrocephalus. Can have agenesis of the corpus callosum. Arnold-Chiari malformation. Developmental delay. Central sleep apnea requiring nighttime oxygen has been reported in one infant.

ORTHOPEDIC: Can have limited elbow extension.

GI/GU: Prominent umbilical stump. Anteriorly placed anus. Bifid scrotum. Heavily wrinkled labia majora.

OTHER: Cutis gyrata, furrowed palms and soles, acanthosis nigricans.

ANESTHETIC CONSIDERATIONS

Neonates with choanal stenosis or atresia can have airway obstruction with or without apnea. Choanal atresia precludes placement of a nasal airway, nasal intubation, or nasogastric tube. Arnold-Chiari malformation can predispose to apnea and postoperatively patients need to be observed closely. Cervical spine abnormalities have not been reported, but can be seen in other disorders due to *FGFR2* mutations. Proptosis requires close attention to eye protection intraoperatively. Intravenous access may be challenging due to cutis gyrata.

Bibliography:
1. Upmeyer S, Bothwell M, Tobias JD. Perioperative care of a patient with Beare-Stevenson syndrome. *Paediatr Anaesth* 2005;15:1131–1136.

Becker Disease

MIM #: 255700

This disease is a separate entity from Becker muscular dystrophy. It is an autosomal recessive myotonia due to an abnormality in the skeletal muscle chloride channel gene (*CLCN1*). It is sometimes called myotonia congenita, but the autosomal dominant type (Thomsen disease, see later) is more frequently referred to as myotonia congenita. Thomsen disease is caused by mutations in the same gene. Becker disease does not become clinically apparent until 4 to 12 years of age, and sometimes even later in boys.

HEENT/AIRWAY: Lid lag.

NEUROMUSCULAR: Clumsiness, muscle cramping. The hallmark finding, myotonia, refers to delayed relaxation of contracted muscle. Examples include the inability to release a handshake ("action myotonia"), or the sustained contraction with direct tapping or stimulation of a tendon reflex ("percussion myotonia"—best elicited by tapping the thenar eminence or finger extensors). Severe myotonia affects the legs first. It progresses to the arms and finally to the facial and masticatory muscles. Muscle dystrophy may be seen on muscle biopsy. Hypertrophy of lower limb muscles. Asymptomatic heterozygotes may have electromyographic evidence of myotonia.

MISCELLANEOUS: Peter Emil Becker was a German neurologist and geneticist.

ANESTHETIC CONSIDERATIONS

Anesthetic or surgical manipulations can induce myotonic contractions. Even the pain from an intravenous injection of propofol can cause myotonic contractions, as can cold or shivering. These patients can have abnormal drug reactions. Neither regional anesthesia nor muscle relaxants prevent or reverse myotonic contractions. Drugs that have been used to attenuate the contractions are quinine, procainamide, phenytoin, volatile anesthetics, and steroids. When all

else fails, direct infiltration of the muscle with a local anesthetic has been recommended. Succinylcholine can induce sustained contraction of chest wall muscles, making positive-pressure ventilation difficult even in the intubated patient. Because of dystrophic muscle changes, it is possible that in advanced cases succinylcholine might result in an exaggerated hyperkalemic response—another reason to avoid the drug. Responses to nondepolarizing muscle relaxants are normal. Anticholinesterase drugs used to reverse muscle relaxants can precipitate myotonia, and the use of shorter-acting muscle relaxants that do not require reversal has been suggested.

Succinylcholine-induced muscle rigidity without myoglobinuria or hyperthermia, but with a positive halothane contracture test, has been reported in two sisters (3).

FIGURES: See Myotonic dystrophy

Bibliography:
1. Russell SH, Hirsch NP. Anaesthesia and myotonia. *Br J Anaesth* 1994;72:210–216.
2. Koch MC, Steinmeyer K, Lorencz C, et al. The skeletal muscle chloride channel in dominant and recessive human myotonia. *Science* 1992;257:797–800.
3. Heiman-Patterson T, Martino C, Rosenberg H, et al. Malignant hyperthermia in myotonia congenita. *Neurology* 1988;38:810–812.

Becker Muscular Dystrophy

MIM #: 310200

This X-linked muscular dystrophy is similar to Duchenne muscular dystrophy. While patients with Duchenne muscular dystrophy (see later) lack detectable dystrophin in skeletal muscle because of genetic defects that disrupt transcription of the gene, patients with Becker muscular dystrophy have dystrophin of altered size or reduced abundance because the genetic defect allows continued transcription of the gene. Dystrophin is responsible for connecting the sarcolemma to the extracellular matrix. Patients with Becker muscular dystrophy have a more benign disease than those with Duchenne muscular dystrophy. The age at onset is later, and the progression of the disease is slower.

CHEST: Respiratory muscle weakness and swallowing difficulties late in the disease can lead to recurrent respiratory infections.

CARDIOVASCULAR: Patients may have a dilated cardiomyopathy. A full cardiologic evaluation demonstrates that a significant percentage of patients with mild or subclinical skeletal muscle involvement have cardiac involvement, typically beginning in the right ventricle (4).

NEUROMUSCULAR: Myopathy. Pseudohypertrophy of calf muscles. Serum creatine kinase levels are elevated, but not as high as in Duchenne muscular dystrophy. Onset of weakness is delayed compared with Duchenne muscular dystrophy, with loss of ambulation in the third to fifth decade.

ORTHOPEDIC: Pes cavus (high-arched foot).

GI/GU: Increased incidence of infertility.

ANESTHETIC CONSIDERATIONS

Succinylcholine has resulted in fatal rhabdomyolysis with hyperkalemia (6). Massive rhabdomyolysis can occur in the presence of only minimal symptoms. Patients with advanced disease may have swallowing difficulties and are at increased risk for perioperative aspiration. Patients with advanced disease are also at risk for perioperative respiratory complications, secondary to respiratory muscle weakness. A preoperative cardiac evaluation should be done to evaluate for cardiomyopathy. Myocardial depressant agents should be avoided in patients with a significant cardiomyopathy. The association of Becker muscular dystrophy and malignant hyperthermia remains unclear (1). *In vitro* contracture testing may be positive, but it has been suggested that *in vitro* muscle testing may not be accurate with neuromuscular diseases (3).

Bibliography:

1. Kleopa KA, Rosenberg H, Heiman-Patterson T. Malignant hyperthermia-like episode in Becker muscular dystrophy. *Anesthesiology* 2000;93: 1535–1537.
2. Beggs AH. Dystrophinopathy, the expanding phenotype. *Circulation* 1997;95:2344–2347.
3. Wappler F, Scholz J, von Richthofen V, et al. Association of neuromuscular diseases with malignant hyperthermia [Abstract]. *Anesthesiology* 1997;87:861.
4. Melacini P, Fanin M, Danieli GA. et al. Myocardial involvement is very frequent among patients affected with subclinical Becker's muscular dystrophy. *Circulation* 1996;94:3168–3175.
5. Farrell PT. Anaesthesia-induced rhabdomyolysis causing cardiac arrest: case report and review of anaesthesia and the dystrophinopathies. *Anaesth Intensive Care* 1994;22:597–601.
6. Bush A, Dubowitz V. Fatal rhabdomyolysis complicating general anaesthesia in a child with Becker muscular dystrophy. *Neuromuscul Disord* 1991;1:201–204.

Beckwith-Wiedemann Syndrome

MIM #: 130650

The main features of this syndrome are macrosomia, visceromegaly, macroglossia, omphalocele, and earlobe creases. Although Beckwith-Wiedemann syndrome is likely inherited in an autosomal dominant manner, there may be incomplete penetrance, or there may be other genetic factors that influence the clinical manifestations of this syndrome. Most cases occur sporadically. Defects in the region 11p15.5 have been documented in patients with Beckwith-Wiedemann syndrome. Underexpression of the p57 gene (*KIP2*), which encodes a protein that is a negative regulator of cell proliferation, and overexpression of the insulin-like growth factor 2 gene (*IGF2*) probably play an important role in cellular and tissue overgrowth in this

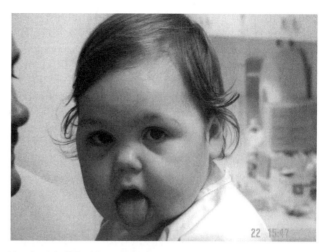

Beckwith-Wiedemann syndrome. The macroglossia in this young infant with Beckwith-Wiedemann syndrome is apparent. (Courtesy of Dr. Michel Sommer, Department of Anesthesiology, University of Maastricht, The Netherlands.)

syndrome. It may be that the disease is caused by inheriting two paternal copies of the gene.

HEENT/AIRWAY: Metopic ridge, large fontanelles, prominent occiput. Microcephaly can develop in later childhood. Capillary hemangioma on central forehead and eyelids. Relative exophthalmos. Linear earlobe creases or indentations of the external helix. Macroglossia—often severe enough to cause upper airway obstruction or feeding problems. Malocclusion. Prognathism.

CARDIOVASCULAR: Cor pulmonale from chronic airway obstruction. A variety of congenital defects have been described. Cardiomegaly, asymptomatic and resolving by 6 months of age, can be part of the visceromegaly.

NEUROMUSCULAR: May have mild to moderate mental deficiency. Problems with extrauterine transition have occurred, resulting in apnea or seizures.

ORTHOPEDIC: Increased muscle mass and subcutaneous tissue (macrosomia). Accelerated osseous maturation leads to advanced bone age during childhood.

GI/GU: Visceromegaly—may involve kidneys, pancreas, adrenals, liver, and gonads. Omphalocele or other umbilical abnormality. Overgrowth of the external genitalia. Dysplasia of the renal medulla. Increased risk of intraabdominal tumors, such as Wilms tumor, hepatoblastoma, adrenocortical carcinoma, neuroblastoma, rhabdomyosarcoma, nephroblastoma, or gonadoblastoma.

OTHER: Occasional hemihypertrophy. Premature birth is common. Large for gestational age. May have neonatal polycythemia. High incidence of neonatal hypoglycemia, potentially very severe, secondary to hyperinsulinism from pancreatic islet cell hyperplasia or nesidioblastosis. Hypoglycemia usually subsides by 4 months of age, and is usually responsive to therapy with corticosteroids, but may require a central venous infusion of glucose or a partial pancreatectomy. Gigantism may develop later in childhood. Occasional immunodeficiency. Increased incidence (7.5% to 10%) of early childhood cancer, especially Wilms tumor.

MISCELLANEOUS: Wiedemann, a professor of pediatrics at Kiel (Germany), was one of the first to bring attention to the thalidomide disaster.

ANESTHETIC CONSIDERATIONS

Macroglossia can cause upper airway obstruction, which may worsen with the induction of anesthesia. Airway obstruction is also a risk in a lethargic patient after extubation. Placing the patient face down or on his/her side may help relieve the obstruction. As the child grows, there is relatively more room for the oversized tongue. However, partial glossectomy is sometimes necessary. Macroglossia may make visualization of the vocal cords difficult during direct laryngoscopy. A laryngeal mask airway has been used successfully. Intravenous access may be difficult.

There is a significant risk of death in infants with Beckwith-Wiedemann syndrome (up to 20% mortality rate in the first year of life). There is a high incidence of neonatal hypoglycemia, which may be severe. Serum glucose must be closely monitored in these patients, and neonates and young infants may require perioperative glucose infusions. Infants treated with steroids may require perioperative stress doses. Care may be complicated by concurrent diseases and conditions of prematurity.

Bibliography:

1. Celiker V, Basgul E, Karagoz AH. Anesthesia in Beckwith-Wiedemann syndrome. *Paediatr Anaesth* 2004;14:778–780.
2. Goldman LJ, Nodal C, Jimenez E. Successful airway control with the laryngeal mask in an infant with Beckwith-Wiedemann syndrome and hepatoblastoma for central line catheterization. *Paediatr Anaesth* 2000;10:445–448.
3. Suan C, Ojeda R, Garcia-Perla JL, et al. Anaesthesia and the Beckwith-Wiedemann syndrome. *Paediatr Anaesth* 1996;6:231–233.
4. Hatada I, Ohashi H, Fukushima Y, et al. An imprinted gene p57(KIP2) is mutated in Beckwith-Wiedemann syndrome. *Nat Genet* 1996;14:171–173.
5. Weng EY, Moeschler JB, Graham JM. Longitudinal observations on 15 children with Wiedemann-Beckwith syndrome. *Am J Med Genet* 1995;56:366–373.
6. Elliott M, Bayly R, Cole T, et al. Clinical features and natural history of Beckwith-Wiedemann syndrome: presentation of 74 new cases. *Clin Genet* 1994;46:168–174.
7. Tobias JD, Lowe S, Holcomb GW. Anesthetic considerations of an infant with Beckwith-Wiedemann syndrome. *J Clin Anesth* 1992;4:484–486.
8. Gurkowski MA, Rasch DK. Anesthetic considerations for Beckwith-Wiedemann syndrome. *Anesthesiology* 1989;70:711–712.

Berardinelli Lipodystrophy

See Lipodystrophy

Bernard-Soulier Syndrome

MIM #: 231200

This autosomal recessive disorder of platelets results in variable degrees of mucocutaneous bleeding, and is due to deficiencies in one of three genes encoding platelet surface glycoproteins. Most patients have episodes that are severe enough to require transfusion. Platelet aggregation remains normal in response to adenosine diphosphate, collagen, and epinephrine, but abnormal in response to plasma or ristocetin. These platelets are deficient in all the platelet surface glycoprotein Ib members: Ib alpha and Ib beta, V and IX, and lack binding sites for the von Willebrand factor (glycoprotein Ib).

HEENT/AIRWAY: Epistaxis.

GI/GU: Gastrointestinal bleeding. Menorrhagia.

OTHER: Purpuric skin lesions. The platelet count is normal or moderately decreased. Platelets are large, but otherwise morphologically normal. Bone marrow megakaryocytes are normal or increased. The bleeding dyscrasia can worsen during adolescence and adulthood.

MISCELLANEOUS: In platelet abnormalities, total platelet mass, rather than platelet number or concentration, tends to be preserved. Thus, perhaps, the low platelet concentration that is found in this disorder with large platelets.

During the German occupation of France during World War II, Bernard was a member of the French resistance. He was arrested and during his imprisonment he composed poetry, which was later published.

ANESTHETIC CONSIDERATIONS

Preparations should be made for surgical bleeding, which is expected to be excessive. Nasal intubation should be avoided if possible. 1-Deamino-8-D-arginine vasopressin (DDAVP) may improve, but not normalize, the platelet function. Platelet transfusions control bleeding. Aspirin, nonsteroidal drugs, and other inhibitors of platelet function should be avoided. Neuraxial techniques are probably contraindicated. Patients may have developed antiplatelet antibodies from prior platelet transfusions, thereby complicating therapy.

Bibliography:

1. Kostopanagiotou G, Siafaka I, Sikiotis G, et al. Anesthetic and perioperative management of a patient with Bernard-Soulier syndrome. *J Clin Anesth* 2004;16:458–460.
2. Lopez JA, Andrews RK, Afshar-Kharghan V, et al. Bernard-Soulier syndrome. *Blood* 1998;91:4397–4418.
3. Caen JP, Rosa JP. Platelet-vessel wall interaction: from the bedside to molecules. *Thromb Haemost* 1995;74:18–24.

Bernheimer-Seitelberger Disease

Included in Tay-Sachs disease

Beta-Glucuronidase Deficiency

See Sly syndrome

Beta-Ketothiolase Deficiency

SYNONYM: Acetyl-CoA acetyltransferase-1 deficiency, 2-methylacetoacetyl-CoA thiolase deficiency; 3-oxothiolase deficiency; ketothiolase deficiency

MIM #: 203750

This autosomal recessive disorder of branched-chain amino acid metabolism is due to deficiencies in the enzyme acetyl-CoA acetyltransferase-1 (also known as methylacetoacetyl-CoA thiolase, beta-ketothiolase or 3-oxothiolase), which is responsible for the penultimate step in isoleucine catabolism, the conversion of 2-methylacetoacetyl-CoA into acetyl CoA and propionyl CoA. Symptomatic presentation is variable, but typically involves intermittent metabolic acidosis and ketosis with vomiting, worsened by increased protein intake. With appropriate management of acute episodes, long-term prognosis is good.

CARDIOVASCULAR: One patient who died of congestive cardiomyopathy has been reported.

NEUROMUSCULAR: Coma can accompany severe episodes after upper respiratory or gastrointestinal infections, or increased protein intake. Headaches and ataxia have been reported as chronic problems in older children.

GI/GU: Vomiting with acidotic episodes. Diarrhea, often bloody.

OTHER: Intermittent severe metabolic acidosis and ketosis.

MISCELLANEOUS: One method of salicylate measurement gives a false-positive salicylate reaction because of the high levels of acetoacetic acid present. Salicylate toxicity is also a cause of metabolic acidosis in the age-group 1 to 2 years, the age when most of these patients first show the effects of this disorder.

ANESTHETIC CONSIDERATIONS

Treatment of acute episodes is with bicarbonate and glucose, and by restriction of protein. Infections can precipitate acute acidotic episodes. It is not known if they can be precipitated by the stress of surgery. An orogastric tube or throat packs should be placed if the surgery has the potential to cause oral or intestinal bleeding because blood aspirated into the gastrointestinal tract after oral or nasal surgery might present an excessive protein load, triggering decompensation.

FIGURE: See **Appendix D**

Bibliography:
1. Sabetta G, Bachmann C, Giardini O, et al. Beta-ketothiolase deficiency with favourable evolution. *J Inherit Metab Dis* 1987;10:405–406.

Biotinidase Deficiency

SYNONYM: Multiple carboxylase deficiency

MIM #: 253260, 253270

This autosomal recessive disease is a form of multiple carboxylase deficiency, and affects the metabolism of valine and isoleucine. The primary defect is the inability to cleave biocytin, a proteolytic degradation product of the carboxylase enzymes, liberating biotin (a water-soluble vitamin), resulting in biotin deficiency and functional deficiency of the four carboxylases, propionyl CoA carboxylase, 3-methylcrotonyl CoA carboxylase, pyruvate carboxylase, and acetyl CoA carboxylase. Disease severity can be similar to the organic acidemias, with potentially fatal episodes of ketoacidosis early in life, or the disease may be less severe. Treatment with biotin should correct all symptoms (unless fixed, such as optic atrophy). A neonatal form is due to defects in the gene encoding holocarboxylase synthetase (see later, Holocarboxylase synthetase deficiency). There is considerable interpatient variability, even within a family.

HEENT/AIRWAY: Conjunctivitis, optic atrophy, myopia, abnormal retinal pigment. Auditory nerve atrophy with hearing loss is common and variable. Laryngeal stridor.

CHEST: Hyperventilation, apnea.

NEUROMUSCULAR: Mental retardation, developmental delay, hypotonia, ataxia, myoclonic and other seizures, lethargy, coma, basal ganglia calcifications. Spastic paraparesis. Cerebral and cerebellar atrophy.

OTHER: Lactic acidosis with ketosis. Mild hyperammonemia. Seborrheic dermatitis, alopecia, acrodermatitis enteropathica. Abnormal cellular immunity. Recurrent fungal infections.

ANESTHETIC CONSIDERATIONS

Laryngeal stridor may be the presenting finding (3). Abnormal cellular immunity suggests that careful aseptic technique is essential. Long-term use of anticonvulsant medications may alter the metabolism of some anesthetic drugs. Patients should receive appropriate biotin if they are to be on prolonged intravenous fluids.

Bibliography:
1. Grunewald S, Champion MP, Leonard JV, et al. Biotinidase deficiency: a treatable leukoencephalopathy. *Neuropediatrics* 2004;35:211–216.
2. Wolf B, Heard GS. Biotinidase deficiency. *Adv Pediatr* 1991;38:1–21.
3. Dionisi-Vici C, Bachmann C, Graziani MC, et al. Laryngeal stridor as a leading symptom in a biotinidase-deficient patient. *J Inherit Metab Dis* 1988;11:312–313.

4. Sweetman L, Nyhan WL. Inheritable biotin-treatable disorders and associated phenomena. *Annu Rev Nutr* 1986;6:317–343.

Blackfan-Diamond Syndrome

SYNONYM: Diamond-Blackfan syndrome; Aase-Smith syndrome II

MIM #: 105650

This disease of congenital red blood cell hypoplasia appears to have multiple etiologies. Many cases are sporadic. Approximately 25% are due to defects in the gene encoding ribosomal protein S19. A second locus has been mapped to chromosome 8. It can be autosomal dominant or recessive.

HEENT/AIRWAY: Hypertelorism. Snub nose. Thick upper lip.

ORTHOPEDIC: Short stature. May have triphalangeal thumbs or other hand anomalies.

GI/GU: Hepatosplenomegaly.

OTHER: Congenital red blood cell hypoplasia. This may be steroid responsive, and may require long-term transfusions. There is an increased risk of leukemia. Fetal anemia can present with hydrops fetalis.

MISCELLANEOUS: Dr. Blackfan was the first (with Dandy) to describe Dandy-Walker malformation. He was offered the deanship of the Harvard Medical School, which he refused in order to remain active clinically. Dr. Louis Diamond was responsible for introducing exchange transfusion as a successful treatment for hemolytic disease of the newborn (Rh sensitization). He is also the Diamond of Shwachman-Diamond syndrome.

ANESTHETIC CONSIDERATIONS
The patient's hematocrit should be obtained before undertaking any procedure that has the potential for significant blood loss. Patients who are on long-term steroid therapy need perioperative stress doses of steroids. Long-term transfusion can potentially result in iron overload, with cardiomyopathy.

Bibliography:
1. Orfali KA, Ohene-Abuakwa Y, Ball SE. Diamond-Blackfan anaemia in the UK; clinical and genetic heterogeneity. *Br J Haematol* 2004;125:243–252.
2. Krijanovski OI, Sieff CA. Diamond-Blackfan anemia. *Hematol Oncol Clin North Am* 1997;11:1061–1077.
3. Ball SE, McGuckin CP, Jenkins G, et al. Diamond-Blackfan anaemia in the U.K.: analysis of 80 cases from a 20-year birth cohort. *Br J Haematol* 1996;94:645–653.

Bland-White-Garland Syndrome

See Anomalous origin, left coronary artery

Blepharophimosis Syndrome

SYNONYM: Blepharophimosis, ptosis, and epicanthus inversus syndrome (BPES syndrome)

MIM #: 110100

This autosomal dominant disorder predominantly affects the eyelids and is characterized by blepharophimosis, ptosis, and epicanthus inversus. There are two types of blepharophimosis syndrome, with type I additionally involving infertility in women from premature ovarian failure. The infertility is inherited as an autosomal dominant sex-limited trait, as occurs in the Stein-Leventhal syndrome. Both types of blepharophimosis syndrome are due to defects in the gene *FOXL2* (forkhead transcription factor). This is a nuclear protein expressed in the clinically involved tissues. Plastic surgery is often required to preserve ocular function.

HEENT/AIRWAY: Blepharophimosis—short palpebral fissures secondary to lateral displacement of the inner canthi. Ptosis. Epicanthus inversus (a fold of skin curving in the mediolateral direction, inferior to the inner canthus). Arched eyebrows. Hypoplasia of the levator palpebrae muscle. Strabismus. Amblyopia is very common. Occasional ocular abnormalities, including microphthalmia, optic nerve hypoplasia, and nystagmus. Simple ears, with cupping. Flat nasal bridge. One patient has been reported with a small larynx. High-arched palate.

CARDIOVASCULAR: Occasional cardiac defects.

NEUROMUSCULAR: May exhibit hypotonia in infancy. Rare mental deficiency.

GI/GU: Menstrual irregularity leading to amenorrhea and infertility in women with type I blepharophimosis syndrome. Scant pubic and axillary hair in females. One patient has been reported with severe, chronic feeding difficulties.

ANESTHETIC CONSIDERATIONS
Patients must receive meticulous perioperative eye care to prevent corneal injuries.

Bibliography:
1. Chandler KE, de Die-Smulders CEM. Severe feeding problems and congenital laryngostenosis in a patient with 3q23 deletion. *Eur J Pediatr* 1997;156:636–638.
2. Oley C, Baraitser M. Blepharophimosis, ptosis, epicanthus inversus syndrome (BPES syndrome). *J Med Genet* 1988;25:47–51.
3. Zlotogora J, Sagi M, Cohen T. The blepharophimosis, ptosis and epicanthus inversus syndrome: delineation of two types. *Am J Hum Genet* 1983;35:1020–1027.

Blepharophimosis, Ptosis, and Epicanthus Inversus Syndrome (BPES Syndrome)

See Blepharophimosis syndrome

Bloch-Sulzberger Syndrome

See Incontinentia pigmenti

Bloom Syndrome

MIM #: 210900

This autosomal recessive disorder is marked by short stature, malar hypoplasia, facial telangiectasis, and a predisposition to malignancy. Many affected people are of Ashkenazic Jewish ancestry. This syndrome is due to mutations in the gene encoding DNA helicase RecQ protein-like-3.

HEENT/AIRWAY: Mild microcephaly with dolichocephaly. Malar hypoplasia. Recurrent otitis. May have small nose. Facial, sun-sensitive telangiectasis and chronic erythema involving the butterfly midface region, exacerbated by sunlight. The rash is rarely present at birth, becomes noticeable during the first year, and improves with age. Occasional absence of upper lateral incisors. Occasional high-pitched voice.

CHEST: May have bronchiectasis or pulmonary fibrosis after repeated lung infections.

NEUROMUSCULAR: Occasional mild mental retardation. Occasional attention deficit disorder or learning disabilities.

ORTHOPEDIC: Proportionately very short stature.

GI/GU: Can have episodes of diarrhea and vomiting in infancy leading to dehydration. Infertility in males from failure of spermatogenesis, and decreased fertility in female patients; however, pregnancy can occur, and premature delivery may be common.

OTHER: Predisposition to malignancy—usually solid tumors or leukemia. Hypersensitivity to sunlight. Patchy areas of hypopigmentation or hyperpigmentation. May have immunoglobulin deficiency, with increased susceptibility to infection, which appears to resolve with age. May acquire non–insulin-dependent diabetes. Growth retardation and wasting, prenatal onset with low birth weights. Decreased subcutaneous fatty tissue.

MISCELLANEOUS: There is evidence of multiple chromosomal breaks and sister chromatid exchanges, which probably account for the predisposition to malignancy. A high ratio of diagnosed male to female patients is probably secondary to underdiagnosis of this disorder in women, in whom the skin lesion tends to be milder. DNA repair mechanisms are abnormal in four other inherited diseases: ataxia-telangiectasia, Fanconi anemia, xeroderma pigmentosum, and Cockayne syndrome.

ANESTHETIC CONSIDERATIONS
Patients should be addressed in a manner appropriate to their chronologic and developmental age, not their "height age."

Bibliography:
1. Keller C, Keller KR, Shew SB, et al. Growth deficiency and malnutrition in Bloom syndrome. *J Pediatr* 1999;134:472–479.
2. Ellis NA, German J. Molecular genetics of Bloom's syndrome. *Hum Mol Genet* 1996;5:1457–1463.
3. German J, Passarge E. Bloom's syndrome. XIII. Report from the Registry for 1987. *Clin Genet* 1989;35:57–69.
4. Van Kerckhove CW, Ceuppens JL, Vanderschueren-Lodeweyckx M, et al. Bloom's syndrome: clinical features and immunologic abnormalities of four patients. *Am J Dis Child* 1988;142:1089–1093.

Blount Disease

MIM #: 259200

This disease, which is essentially tibia vara, has been ascribed to both autosomal and multifactorial causes. It is due to disordered growth of the proximal medial physis and metaphysis resulting in a localized tibia vara deformity, and is often associated with tibial torsion. The incidence of tibia vara is higher in African Americans and increased in association with obesity, where the deformity is thought to be due to mechanical stress converting physiologic (and transient) bowlegs to a fixed tibia vara. Treatment is by bracing, and then surgical osteotomy if unsuccessful.

ORTHOPEDIC: Genu varum (bowlegs).

MISCELLANEOUS: Walter Blount was a leading American pediatric orthopedic surgeon.

ANESTHETIC CONSIDERATIONS
There are no anesthetic implications of Blount disease; however, a good number of patients are obese, with attendant aspiration risk and possible difficulty with venous access.

Bibliography:
1. Myers TG, Fishman MK, McCarthy JJ, et al. Incidence of distal femoral and distal tibial deformities in infantile and adolescent blount disease. *J Pediatr Orthop* 2005;25:215–218.
2. Cheema JI, Grissom LE, Harcke HT. Radiographic characteristics of lower-extremity bowing in children. *Radiographics* 2003;23:871–880.
3. Bathfield CA, Beighton PH. Blount disease: a review of etiological factors in 110 patients. *Clin Orthop* 1978;135:29–33.

Blue Diaper Syndrome

MIM #: 211000

This is a defect in intestinal tryptophan transport. Bacterial degradation of the excessive tryptophan results in increased indole production, and eventually in the production of indigo blue, which stains the diapers (hence the name of the syndrome). The disease is probably inherited as autosomal recessive, although X-linkage cannot be excluded.

HEENT/AIRWAY: Microconia, hypoplastic optic disks, and abnormal eye movements have been described in one patient.

GI/GU: Nephrocalcinosis.

OTHER: Hypercalcemia.

MISCELLANEOUS: A false-positive diagnosis has been ascribed to the presence of blue pigments of *Pseudomonas* in the stool, also coloring the diapers blue.

ANESTHETIC CONSIDERATIONS
It is important to provide adequate intravenous fluid perioperatively to maintain reasonable diuresis in the face of hypercalcemia. The role of calciuretic diuretics in potentiating nephrocalcinosis is unknown.

Bibliography:
1. Chen Y, Wu L, Xiong Q. The ocular abnormalities of blue diaper syndrome. *Metab Pediatr Syst Ophthalmol* 1991;14:73–75.

Blue Rubber Bleb Nevus Syndrome

SYNONYM: Bean syndrome

MIM #: 112200

This syndrome of large venous malformations has been reported both within families and sporadically. These lesions are congenital malformations and are not neoplastic. Bleeding from hemangiomas is a major concern. A similar syndrome related to abnormalities in the *TEK* gene (tyrosine kinase receptor, epithelial-specific) has been reported, and may be the same or very similar.

HEENT/AIRWAY: Can involve the oropharynx. Can involve the orbit with visual impairment.

CHEST: Endobronchial involvement has been reported.

CARDIOVASCULAR: May have thromboembolic pulmonary hypertension.

NEUROMUSCULAR: May develop cerebellar medulloblastoma. Can have central nervous system involvement with seizures or intracerebral hemorrhage.

ORTHOPEDIC: A patient with angiomatous gigantism of an affected arm requiring amputation has been reported.

GI/GU: Bleeding hemangiomas are distributed throughout the gastrointestinal tract, from the oropharynx to the anus, and can lead to acute and chronic bleeding. Has been the leading point for intussusception. Can have hepatic hemangiomas.

OTHER: The hemangiomas are found particularly on the trunk and upper arms. They are large, rubbery, and promptly refill following compression. Disseminated intravascular coagulation from a consumption coagulopathy has been reported.

ANESTHETIC CONSIDERATIONS
Patients can have chronic and/or acute anemia. Clotting status could be abnormal, contraindicating regional techniques. Particular care must be exercised during laryngoscopy when there is oropharyngeal involvement. Because of the diffuse distribution of these lesions throughout the length of the gastrointestinal system they cannot all be addressed by either upper or lower endoscopy. A technique combining endoscopy with endoscopic examination through open laparotomy and enterotomy has been described. A case of venous air embolism during distension of the bowel lumen with air, during endoscopic visualization has been reported (1). In a single case, disseminated intravascular coagulation has been treated successfully with interferon beta.

Bibliography:
1. Holzman RS, Yoo L, Fox VL, et al. Air embolism during intraoperative endoscopic localization and surgical resection for blue rubber bleb nevus syndrome. *Anesthesiology* 2005;102:1279–1280.
2. Ertem D, Acar Y, Kotiloglu E, et al. Blue rubber bleb nevus syndrome. *Pediatrics* 2001;107:418–421.

BOFS

See Branchiooculofacial syndrome

BOR Syndrome

See Melnick-Fraser syndrome

Börjeson Syndrome

See Börjeson-Forssman-Lehmann syndrome

Börjeson-Forssman-Lehmann Syndrome

SYNONYM: Börjeson syndrome

MIM #: 301900

This syndrome involves severe mental retardation, seizures, large ears, hypogonadism, and obesity. The syndrome is inherited in an X-linked recessive manner. An abnormality of neuronal migration leads to the central nervous system manifestations. The gene responsible for this disorder is *PHF6*. This gene, active in the embryonic central nervous system, probably has a role in transcription. Female carriers of the gene defect may show some characteristics of the syndrome.

HEENT/AIRWAY: Microcephaly. Coarse facies. Prominent supraorbital ridges and deep-set eyes. Nystagmus, ptosis, narrow palpebral fissures, and decreased vision. Retinal or optic nerve abnormalities. Large ears. Subcutaneous tissue of the face is swollen.

CHEST: Two patients died of bronchopneumonia, but there is no apparent increased susceptibility to respiratory infections.

NEUROMUSCULAR: Severe mental retardation. Hypotonia. Significant motor and speech delay. Abnormal electroencephalogram—seizures are common. Narrow cervical spinal canal. It has been suggested that there might be abnormalities of midline neurodevelopment, including the hypothalamic-pituitary axis.

ORTHOPEDIC: Short stature. Vertebral osteochondrosis. Mild scoliosis or kyphosis. Hypoplasia of the distal and middle phalanges. Fingers are tapered. Short, widely spaced and flexed toes. Subcutaneous tissue of the hands is swollen.

GI/GU: Hypogonadotropic hypogonadism. Cryptorchidism. Small penis.

OTHER: Obesity. Postpubertal gynecomastia.

ANESTHETIC CONSIDERATIONS
Severe mental retardation may complicate preoperative management. Intravenous access may be difficult secondary to obesity and swelling of the subcutaneous tissue of the hands. Patients who are obese are at increased risk for aspiration, and may warrant a rapid-sequence induction of anesthesia. Obesity may result in desaturation with induction of anesthesia because of increased airway closure and decreased functional residual capacity. Obese patients require lower than expected drug doses on a per kilogram basis. Long-term use of anticonvulsant medications may alter the metabolism of some anesthetic drugs. The narrowed cervical spinal canal has not been associated with spinal cord abnormalities.

Bibliography:
1. Visootsak J, Rosner B, Dykens E, et al. Clinical and behavioral features of patients with Borjeson-Forssman-Lehman syndrome with mutations in *PHF6. J Pediatr* 2004;145:819–825.
2. Petridou M, Kimiskidis V, Deligiannis K, et al. Borjeson-Forssman-Lehmann syndrome: two severely handicapped females in a family. *Clin Neurol Neurosurg* 1997;99:148–150.
3. Turner G, Gedeon A, Mulley J, et al. Borjeson-Forssman-Lehmann syndrome: clinical manifestations and gene localization to Xq26-27. *Am J Med Genet* 1989;34:463–469.

Brachmann-de Lange Syndrome

See Cornelia de Lange syndrome

Brachydactyly Syndrome, Type E

MIM #: 113300

This autosomal dominant disorder is characterized by short stature and short fingers. There are several other types of brachydactyly syndrome, similarly identified by a letter type. This type, and brachydactyly type D, can be caused by defects in the gene *HOXD13*.

HEENT/AIRWAY: Round facies. Multiple impacted teeth.

CARDIOVASCULAR: May have atrial septal defect.

NEUROMUSCULAR: Normal intelligence.

ORTHOPEDIC: Moderate short stature. Brachydactyly, short metacarpals, short metatarsals (variable). Short, straight clavicles. Radiologically, this syndrome is indistinguishable from pseudohypoparathyroidism and pseudopseudohypoparathyroidism (see later).

OTHER: Normal parathyroid function.

ANESTHETIC CONSIDERATIONS
The short, straight clavicle may make placement of a subclavian venous catheter more difficult.

Bibliography:
1. Czeizel A, Goblyos P. Familial combination of brachydactyly, type E and atrial septal defect, type II. *Eur J Pediatr* 1989;149:117–119.
2. Cartwright JD, Rosin M, Robertson C. Brachydactyly type E: a report of a family. *S Afr Med J* 1980;58:255–257.

Brancher Deficiency

SYNONYM: Glycogen storage disease type IV; Andersen disease; Alpha-1,4-glucan:alpha-1,4-glucan-6-alpha-glucosyltransferase deficiency

MIM #: 232500

This relatively uncommon form of glycogen storage disease is an autosomal recessive disease that is due to abnormalities in brancher enzyme, which results in insufficient branching of glycogen when it is synthesized. Glucose release from this abnormal glycogen is abnormal. This type of glycogen storage disease is differentiated from the other forms by early development of hepatic failure with cirrhosis. Liver transplantation is the only successful therapy. It resolves the cirrhosis (obviously) and may decrease amylopectin storage in the heart; however, progressive cardiac failure after liver transplantation has been reported. A neuromuscular presentation also exists.

CARDIOVASCULAR: Congestive heart failure is rare and is due to amylopectin storage in the heart.

NEUROMUSCULAR: Hypotonia, muscle atrophy, delayed milestones. An adult patient who had symptoms of limb-girdle muscular dystrophy with hyperlordotic posture, waddling gait, and proximal limb weakness has been described.

ORTHOPEDIC: Growth retardation.

GI/GU: Hepatomegaly, hepatic failure with cirrhosis, ascites, portal hypertension with splenomegaly. Esophageal varices. In some, liver disease may not be progressive.

OTHER: Fasting hypoglycemia may occur. Failure to thrive.

ANESTHETIC CONSIDERATIONS
Although congestive heart failure is rare, a thorough preoperative cardiac examination is indicated. Early hepatic failure may lead to abnormal coagulation and may affect protein binding of some anesthetic drugs. Esophageal probes and catheters should be placed with caution, as varices can be present. Fasting hypoglycemia may occur. Serum glucose levels should be monitored perioperatively, and perioperative glucose-containing intravenous fluids would seem appropriate. Succinylcholine should be used with caution in patients with muscle atrophy because of the risk of exaggerated hyperkalemia.

FIGURE: See **Appendix E**

Bibliography:
1. Bruno C, van Diggelen OP, Cassandrini D, et al. Clinical and genetic heterogeneity of branching enzyme deficiency (glycogenosis type IV). *Neurology* 2004;63:1053–1058.
2. Talente GM, Coleman RA, Alter C, et al. Glycogen storage disease in adults. *Ann Intern Med* 1994;120:218–226.
3. Howell RR. Continuing lessons from glycogen storage diseases. *N Engl J Med* 1991;324:55–56.
4. Selby R, Starzl TE, Yunis E, et al. Liver transplantation for type IV glycogen storage disease. *N Engl J Med* 1991;324:39–42.
5. Servidei S, Riepe R, Langston C, et al. Severe cardiopathy in branching enzyme deficiency. *J Pediatr* 1987;111:51–56.

Branchiooculofacial Syndrome

SYNONYM: BOFS

MIM #: 113620

This autosomal dominant disorder involves defects of the branchial arch, eyes, and face. The most consistent abnormalities are branchial cleft sinuses, nasolacrimal duct obstruction, and pseudocleft lip (looks like a surgically repaired cleft lip). The specific gene and gene product are not known.

HEENT/AIRWAY: Subcutaneous scalp cysts. Nasolacrimal duct obstruction, strabismus, coloboma, microphthalmia, cataracts, hemangiomatous cysts of the orbit. Malformed ears, ear pits, postauricular linear skin lesions, conductive hearing loss. Mastoid hypoplasia. Fusion of ear ossicles. Broad nasal bridge, flat nasal tip, broad philtrum. Pseudocleft lip, high-arched palate, cleft lip or palate, carp-shaped mouth, lip pits, dental anomalies, mild micrognathia. Nasal speech. Branchial cleft sinuses (of the neck).

CHEST: Supernumerary nipples.

NEUROMUSCULAR: Most have normal intelligence. Rare mild mental retardation.

ORTHOPEDIC: Retarded growth. Polydactyly, clinodactyly. Hypoplastic fingernails.

GI/GU: Renal anomalies, including agenesis and cysts. Hydronephrosis.

OTHER: Low birth weight, premature graying. Ectopic thymus.

ANESTHETIC CONSIDERATIONS
In the absence of renal involvement, there are no specific anesthetic considerations.

Bibliography:
1. Lin AE, Gorlin RJ, Lurie IW, et al. Further delineation of the branchiooculo-facial syndrome. *Am J Med Genet* 1995;56:42–59.
2. McCool M, Weaver DD. Branchio-oculo-facial syndrome: broadening the spectrum. *Am J Med Genet* 1994;49:414–421.
3. Fujimoto A, Lipson M, Lacro RV, et al. New autosomal dominant branchio-oculo-facial syndrome. *Am J Med Genet* 1987;27:943–951.

Branchiootorenal Syndrome

See Melnick-Fraser syndrome

C

C Syndrome

MIM #: 211750

The prominent features of this autosomal recessive disorder are trigonocephaly, unusual facies, polydactyly, cardiac abnormalities, and cryptorchidism. When viewed from above, the widened biparietal diameter and narrow forehead give the appearance of a triangular cranium (trigonocephaly). Trigonocephaly may be found in other disorders also.

HEENT/AIRWAY: Abnormal skull with trigonocephaly, synostosis of the metopic suture, narrow pointed forehead, and biparietal widening. Up-slanting palpebral fissures, strabismus. Low-set ears with abnormal helix. Hypoplastic nasal root. Deeply furrowed palate. Short neck. Micrognathia with large mouth.

CHEST: Pectus deformities. Anomalous ribs.

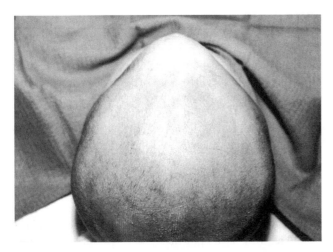

C syndrome. Trigonocephaly, viewed from above. (Courtesy of K. Lin, MD and the Craniofacial Anomalies Clinic, University of Virginia Health System.)

CARDIOVASCULAR: Congenital heart defects of a variety of types.

NEUROMUSCULAR: Mental retardation, hypotonia.

ORTHOPEDIC: Polydactyly, syndactyly. Ulnar deviation of the fingers. Syndactyly. Flexion deformities of the elbows, wrists and fingers. Short stature. Dislocated hips.

GI/GU: Omphalocele. Hepatomegaly. Cryptorchidism, prominent labia majora and clitoris.

OTHER: Loose skin.

MISCELLANEOUS: The term "C syndrome" comes from Opitz's use of a patient's initials to refer to this syndrome.

ANESTHETIC CONSIDERATIONS
Direct laryngoscopy and tracheal intubation may be more difficult secondary to the short neck. Flexion deformities may make correct positioning difficult. Patients with congenital heart disease require perioperative antibiotic prophylaxis as indicated.

Bibliography:
1. Haaf T, Hofmann R, Schmid M. Opitz trigonocephaly syndrome. *Am J Med Genet* 1991;40:444–446.

C1 Esterase Inhibitor Deficiency

See Hereditary angioedema

Caffey Disease

SYNONYM: Infantile cortical hyperostosis

MIM #: 114000

This probably autosomal dominant disease involves apparent inflammatory swelling of a variety of bones. It is due to mutations in the collagen gene *COL1A1*. Oddly for a genetic disorder, signs and symptoms are not present at birth; they appear and then regress. It usually does not present until about 5 months of age and is gone by age 2 years, although a case with recurrences through adolescence has been reported. A severe phenotype with prenatal onset has also been reported.

HEENT/AIRWAY: The mandible is the most commonly affected bone, and may be very tender, warm, and swollen.

ORTHOPEDIC: Inflammatory changes in bone and periosteum, which eventually resolve. Bones are tender, warm, and swollen. The mandible, ribs, and scapulae are most commonly affected. There is infiltration of the periosteum by round cells with periosteal thickening. There is cortical hyperostosis and cortical irregularity.

OTHER: Fever.

MISCELLANEOUS: John Caffey was the dean of American pediatric radiologists. He worked until the day of his death at age 83. Caffey played a critical role in the recognition of the battered baby syndrome of child abuse.

ANESTHETIC CONSIDERATIONS
There are no specific anesthetic considerations, although mandibular tenderness is an indication for extreme gentleness during physical examination of the airway, and gentle positioning would seem appropriate.

Bibliography:
1. Emmery L, Timmermans J, Christens J, et al. Familial infantile cortical hyperostosis. *Eur J Pediatr* 1983;141:56–58.

Campomelic Dwarfism

See Campomelic dysplasia

Campomelic Dysplasia

SYNONYM: Campomelic dwarfism

MIM #: 114290

This disorder is distinguished by short stature, flat facies, hypoplastic scapulae, and bowed limbs. It was once thought to be autosomal recessive, but is now thought to be autosomal dominant with lethality in most cases. Campomelic dysplasia is due to mutations of the *SOX9* gene. This gene is involved in cartilage formation, testicular development, and sex determination. Most patients with campomelic dysplasia die in early infancy secondary to respiratory insufficiency or critical airway narrowing.

HEENT/AIRWAY: Macrocephaly, large anterior fontanelle. Flat facies, high forehead. Hypertelorism, short palpebral fissures. Abnormal or low-set ears. May have hearing loss. Low nasal bridge. Cleft palate. Micrognathia. Short neck.

CHEST: Small thorax and thoracic kyphoscoliosis may lead to restrictive lung disease. Missing or hypoplastic ribs. May have tracheobronchomalacia with intrathoracic airway obstruction. Small thoracic cage. Eleven pairs of ribs.

CARDIOVASCULAR: Rare cardiac defects.

NEUROMUSCULAR: Gross abnormalities may be found in the cerebral cortex, thalamus, and caudate nucleus. Significant central nervous system abnormalities, including apnea. Hydrocephalus. Hypoplastic olfactory tracts. Hypotonia.

ORTHOPEDIC: Short stature. Short-limbed dwarfism. Abnormal vertebrae, particularly in the cervical region. Hypoplastic scapulae. Bowed limbs, especially the tibiae, with pretibial skin dimpling. Short fibulae. Abnormal hand positioning. Clubfoot deformity. Hip dislocation. Delayed osseous maturation.

GI/GU: May have hydronephrosis. Many XY individuals have sex reversal (patients have male gonadal dysgenesis and develop normal female external genitalia).

MISCELLANEOUS: "Camptomelique" was introduced in the French literature to describe this syndrome. The name derives from the Greek *camptos* ("bent") and *melos* ("limb").

ANESTHETIC CONSIDERATIONS
Direct laryngoscopy and tracheal intubation may be difficult secondary to micrognathia and short neck. Patients might require a smaller-than-expected endotracheal tube if sized for age. Patients may have significant cervical vertebral abnormalities and may have an unstable cervical spine. Respiratory insufficiency is common, and patients are at risk for postoperative respiratory complications. Patients with tracheobronchomalacia often have airway obstruction, which may require a tracheostomy. Patients are at risk for perioperative apnea. Consider preoperative evaluation of renal function in patients with a history of renal abnormalities which predispose to renal insufficiency.

Bibliography:
1. Bell DM, Leung KK, Wheatley SC, et al. *SOX9* directly regulates the type-II collagen gene. *Nat Genet* 1997;16:174–178.
2. Mansour S, Hall CM, Pembrey ME. A clinical and genetic study of campomelic dysplasia. *J Med Genet* 1995;32:415–420.
3. Berkowitz I, Raja S, Bender K, et al. Dwarfs: pathophysiology and anesthetic implications. *Anesthesiology* 1990;73:739–759.

Camurati-Engelmann Syndrome

SYNONYM: Progressive diaphyseal dysplasia

MIM #: 131300

This autosomal dominant syndrome is marked by diaphyseal dysplasia with leg pain and weakness. There is wide variability in expression, and some patients may manifest only radiographic evidence of the disease. Microscopically, osteoblastic hyperactivity has been demonstrated in the diaphyseal portions of most long bones. This disorder is progressive through adolescence, then stabilizes during adulthood. The disorder is due to specific mutations in the gene encoding transforming growth factor $\beta 1$. A second type of the disease, Camurati-Engelmann syndrome type II, is not associated with defects in this gene.

HEENT/AIRWAY: Occasional sclerosis of the cranium, mandible. May have optic nerve compression secondary to hyperostosis of the skull. Exophthalmos. May have hearing loss from nerve compression.

NEUROMUSCULAR: May have cranial nerve compression secondary to hyperostosis of the skull. Muscle weakness, particularly of the pelvic girdle.

ORTHOPEDIC: Progressive diaphyseal dysplasia, including diaphyseal widening with cortical thickening and irregularity. The diaphyseal dysplasia is bilateral and symmetric. The femur and tibia are most affected. The medullary canal is narrowed, even though overall the bone is widened. Waddling gait. Leg pain and weakness. Occasional scoliosis. Over years, the disease may also affect the upper extremities and the spine.

GI/GU: Hepatosplenomegaly. Hypogonadism. Delayed puberty.

OTHER: Patients are typically tall, thin, and "malnourished" appearing. May be anemic, leukopenic.

MISCELLANEOUS: Mario Camurati was an Italian orthopedic surgeon. Engelmann practiced orthopedics primarily in Vienna. Camurati published his discussion several years before Engelmann. Cockayne actually probably published the first case report of this syndrome, and considered syphilitic osteitis in the differential.

ANESTHETIC CONSIDERATIONS
Patients are often taking steroids for symptomatic relief of bone pain and clinical improvement of their bone disease. These patients require perioperative stress doses of steroids. There may be excessive perioperative heat loss in these very thin patients.

Bibliography:
1. Ramanan AV, Hall MJ, Baildam EM, et al. Camurati-Engelmann disease— a case report and literature review [Letter]. *Rheumatology* 2005;44:1069–1072.
2. Grey AC, Wallace R, Crone M. Engelmann's disease: a 45-year follow-up. *J Bone Joint Surg Br* 1996;78:488–1491.

Canavan Disease

SYNONYM: Acetylaspartic aciduria

MIM #: 271900

This autosomal recessive leukodystrophy is due to a defect in the gene for aspartoacylase, with accumulation of *N*-acetylaspartic acid. The disease affects myelin formation. It is a leukodystrophy, and patients' brains show spongy degeneration, a nonspecific finding. Congenital, infantile (the most common), and juvenile forms have been described. Its features are similar to those of Alexander disease (see earlier). Onset is typically in the first 2 months of life with death in the first decade.

HEENT/AIRWAY: Macrocephaly. Delayed closure of the anterior fontanelle. Absence of blinking to visual threat. Optic atrophy. Blindness. Deafness. Copious oral secretions.

NEUROMUSCULAR: Hypotonia early in life, followed by hypertonicity and decerebrate or decorticate posturing. Arrested developmental milestones. Seizures, spastic diplegia or quadriplegia, choreoathetosis, opisthotonic posturing.

GI/GU: Increased incidence of gastroesophageal reflux. Poor nutrition.

MISCELLANEOUS: One of the leukodystrophies, the others of which are adrenoleukodystrophy, metachromatic leukodystrophy, Krabbe disease, Pelizaeus-Merzbacher disease, and Alexander disease. Leukodystrophies involve defective formation of myelin.

ANESTHETIC CONSIDERATIONS

Macrocephaly may be severe enough to require elevation of the rest of the body to obtain the "sniffing" position. Patients are at risk for perioperative aspiration because of airway hypotonia, gastroesophageal reflux, and copious oral secretions. Consideration should be given to anticholinergic premedication to dry oral secretions. Care must be taken around the patient's eyes perioperatively because their blink reflex is impaired. Careful intraoperative positioning and padding is important in these patients with poor nutrition. Phenothiazines, butyrophenones, metoclopramide, and other dopaminergic blockers may exacerbate movement disorders. Ondansetron should be safe to use as an antiemetic because it does not have antidopaminergic effects. Anticonvulsant medications must be continued (or a parenteral form substituted) perioperatively, and chronic use of anticonvulsant medications may alter the metabolism of some anesthetic drugs. Postoperative respiratory observation is particularly important because of airway hypotonia. Increased risk from succinylcholine has not been demonstrated, but it seems reasonable to avoid it if appropriate because of the potential for hyperkalemia.

Bibliography:

1. Matalon R, Michals K, Kaul R. Canavan disease: from spongy degeneration to molecular analysis. *J Pediatr* 1995;127:511–517.
2. Aicardi J. The inherited leukodystrophies: a clinical overview. *J Inherit Metab Dis* 1993;16:733–743.
3. Tobias JD. Anaesthetic considerations for the child with leukodystrophy. *Can J Anaesth* 1992;39:394–397.

Cantrell's Pentalogy

See Pentalogy of Cantrell

Carbamoyl Phosphate Synthetase Deficiency

See Carbamyl phosphate synthetase deficiency

Carbamyl Phosphate Synthetase deficiency

SYNONYM: Carbamoyl phosphate synthetase deficiency

MIM #: 237300

This autosomal recessive disorder is one of the urea cycle defects, and is a potential cause of hyperammonemia. These disorders are marked by hyperammonemia, encephalopathy and respiratory alkalosis. The urea cycle degrades amino acids to urea. The involved enzyme is mitochondrial carbamyl phosphate synthetase. Symptoms similar to those of hepatic encephalopathy can be triggered by stress such as surgery or infection, or episodes of protein catabolism such as involution of the postpartum uterus. Patients may self-select a low protein diet. There are two types of the disease: a lethal neonatal type and a less severe type with delayed onset. The clinical presentations of the urea cycle defects carbamyl phosphate synthetase, ornithine transcarbamylase, argininosuccinic acid synthetase, and argininosuccinic acid lyase deficiencies are essentially identical. Liver transplantation is curative.

CHEST: Neonatal respiratory distress.

NEUROMUSCULAR: Muscle weakness with acute episodes. Seizures, ataxia. Developmental delay. May have strokelike episodes. Untreated hyperammonemic encephalopathy is clinically similar to hepatic encephalopathy and proceeds through stages of lethargy and agitation, to coma with cerebral edema.

GI/GU: Vomiting and mild abdominal pain with exacerbations. Hepatic synthetic function is normal, although there may be elevations in serum transaminases, both during and between episodes of hyperammonemia.

OTHER: Episodes of hyperammonemia begin with anorexia and lethargy, and may progress through agitation, irritability, and confusion. Vomiting and headaches may be prominent.

MISCELLANEOUS: Carbamyl phosphate synthetase is a large protein that constitutes 15% to 30% of mitochondrial protein.

ANESTHETIC CONSIDERATIONS

Acute metabolic encephalopathy can present after anesthesia. Patients should have high carbohydrate intake (and low protein intake) perioperatively. An orogastric tube or throat packs should be placed if the surgery has the potential to cause oral or intestinal bleeding because blood aspirated into the gastrointestinal tract after oral or nasal surgery might present an excessive protein load.

FIGURE: See **Appendix C**

Bibliography:
1. Urea Cycle Disorder Conference group. Consensus statement from a conference for the management of patients with urea cycle disorders. *J Pediatr* 2001;138:S1–5.
2. Brusilow SW, Danney M, Waber LJ, et al. Treatment of episodic hyperammonemia in children with inborn errors of urea synthesis. *N Engl J Med* 1984;310:1630–1634.

Cardiac-Limb Syndrome

See Holt-Oram syndrome

Cardiofaciocutaneous Syndrome

SYNONYM: CFC syndrome

MIM #: 115150

This sporadically occurring syndrome includes congenital cardiac defects, frontal bossing, ectodermal defects, neurologic abnormalities, and growth failure. It is thought to be possibly related to Noonan syndrome, as there is phenotypic overlap and in some families some individuals have been diagnosed with Noonan syndrome, and others with cardiofaciocutaneous syndrome. The syndrome might be due to deletions on chromosome 12.

HEENT/AIRWAY: Macrocephaly, bitemporal narrowing, frontal bossing. Shallow orbital ridges, hypoplastic supraorbital ridges, hypertelorism, down-slanting palpebral fissures, exophthalmos, ptosis, strabismus, nystagmus. Absent eyebrows and eyelashes. Abnormal external ears, which are posteriorly rotated. May have hearing loss. Depressed nasal bridge, short, upturned nose. Wide, long philtrum. May have submucous cleft palate. Micrognathia.

CHEST: Pectus carinatum or excavatum.

CARDIOVASCULAR: Atrial septal defect and pulmonic stenosis are the most common of the congenital cardiac defects.

NEUROMUSCULAR: Mental retardation. Developmental delay. Hypotonia. Cortical atrophy, brainstem atrophy, mild hydrocephalus. Seizures may develop.

ORTHOPEDIC: Growth retardation, short stature. Thin nails. Hyperextensible fingers. Multiple palmar creases.

OTHER: Abnormalities of the skin, including atopic dermatitis, hyperkeratosis, ichthyosis. Sparse, friable, slow-growing hair. Decreased sweating (hypohidrosis).

ANESTHETIC CONSIDERATIONS

Patients with congenital cardiac defects require antibiotic prophylaxis as indicated. Chronic use of anticonvulsant medications may alter the metabolism of some anesthetic drugs. Patients may have heat intolerance secondary to sweat gland dysfunction.

Bibliography:
1. Kavamura MI, Peres CA, Alchorne MM, et al. CFC index for the diagnosis of cardiofaciocutaneous syndrome. *Am J Med Genet* 2002;112: 12–16.
2. Wieczorek D, Majewski F, Gillessen-Kaesbach G. Cardio-facio-cutaneous (CFC) syndrome—a distinct entity? Report of three patients demonstrating the diagnostic difficulties in delineation of CFC syndrome. *Clin Genet* 1997;52:37–46.
3. Krajewska-Walasek M, Chrzanowska K, Jastrzbska M. The cardio-facio-cutaneous (CFC) syndrome: two possible new cases and review of the literature. *Clin Dysmorphol* 1996;5:65–72.

Carney Complex

MIM #: 160980, 605244

This autosomal dominant multiple neoplasia syndrome is due to mutations in the gene *PRKAR1A*, a cyclic AMP-dependent protein kinase A regulatory gene which is a tumor suppressing gene. A second form, type 2, is linked to chromosome 2. The disease is marked by spotty skin pigmentation, cardiac and other myxomas, endocrine tumors, and melanotic schwannomas. Carney complex is somewhat heterogeneous, and has also been described in concert with Dutch-Kentucky syndrome (see later), in which case it was due to a mutation in the gene *MYH8*.

HEENT/AIRWAY: Spotty pigmentation on the lips and face. Scleral and conjunctival pigmentation. Eyelid myxoma.

CARDIOVASCULAR: Atrial and ventricular myxomas.

OTHER: Profuse ephelides, or freckles and lentigines, and other pigmented skin lesions and nevi. Blue nevi. Cushing disease, acromegaly. Red hair. A variety of thyroid gland abnormalities. Neoplasias include myxoid cutaneous tumors, adrenocortical nodular hyperplasia, Sertoli cell tumor of testes, pituitary adenoma, mammary ductal fibroadenoma, schwannoma, and pheochromocytoma.

MISCELLANEOUS: In 1995, Carney published an account of his search for Harvey Cushing's patient Minnie G, who was reported in Cushing's 1912 monograph on the pituitary and its disorders. Carney believed that this patient might have had 'his' syndrome. Carney succeeded in identifying her, locating her death certificate, and finding her family. However, the cause of her Cushing syndrome remains unknown.

ANESTHETIC CONSIDERATIONS

Patients should be screened preoperatively for the presence of cardiac myxomas. Luckily, these are relatively easily diagnosed by echocardiography. These tumors are often pedunculated and can obstruct valve orifices with changes in body position. They can also directly affect valve function, and in rare cases they can embolize. Patients can present with the biochemical abnormalities of Cushing disease, with hypertension, hyperglycemia, weakness, and obesity. If acromegaly has developed, there is concern about difficult laryngoscopy and intubation, as well as obstructive sleep apnea and cardiomyopathy. Although schwannomas can develop, there is inadequate information currently to contraindicate regional techniques.

Bibliography:

1. Veugelers M, Bressan M, McDermott DA, et al. Mutation of perinatal myosin heavy chain associated with a Carney complex variant. *N Engl J Med* 2004;351:460–469.
2. Szokol JW, Franklin M, Murphy GS, et al. Left ventricular mass in a patient with Carney's complex. *Anesth Analg* 2002;95:874–875.
3. Stratakis CA, Kirschner LS, Carney JA. Clinical and molecular features of the carney complex: diagnostic criteria and recommendations for patient evaluation. *J Clin Endocrinol Metab* 2001;86:4041–4046.

Carnitine Palmitoyltransferase Deficiency

MIM #: 255120, 255110, 608836, 600649

This disorder is due to two distinct and separate autosomal recessive mutations. There are two carnitine palmitoyltransferase (CPT) enzymes. Both are involved in the transfer of fatty acids into the mitochondria. To cross the mitochondrial membrane, fatty acids are first activated by coenzyme A (CoA), and are then reversibly conjugated with L-carnitine. CPT I converts fatty acyl-CoA into a fatty acylcarnitine, which is required for transport through the mitochondrial membrane. CPT II, on the inner aspect of the membrane, liberates carnitine, and in association with several other enzymes, makes the fatty acyl-CoA available for beta-oxidation.

CPT I deficiency is marked by hypoketotic hypoglycemia, and potentially with seizures and coma. Attacks are precipitated by fasting, exercise, cold exposure, infection, stress, or a high-fat and low-carbohydrate diet. It usually presents at 8–18 months of age.

CPT II is found in a variety of tissues, but the clinical manifestations are restricted to muscle. This represents the most common inherited disorder of long-chain fatty acid oxidation. It usually presents in young adults, but there is also a neonatal-onset type that is severe and presents with (potentially fatal) cardiomyopathy, weakness, and coma. The milder adult form has muscle weakness and episodes of rhabdomyolysis triggered by exercise, prolonged fasting, cold, or by conditions of stress that are associated with increased supply of energy as lipid to muscle.

Medium-chain triglycerides bypass the CPT-mediated transfer process.

CHEST

CPT I: Acute respiratory failure.

CARDIOVASCULAR

CPT I: Cardiomyopathy.

CPT II (neonatal form): Arrhythmia, cardiomyopathy.

NEUROMUSCULAR

CPT I: Muscle aching and stiffness, rhabdomyolysis. This form does not have muscle weakness. Episodes similar to hepatic encephalopathy progressing eventually to coma.

CPT II: Episodes of rhabdomyolysis and myoglobinuria are associated with aching muscle pain and elevations in creatine phosphokinase. Muscle weakness following exercise.

GI/GU

CPT I: Hepatomegaly with fatty infiltration. After acute episodes, there are major abnormalities in liver function tests and serum bilirubin that remain abnormal for several weeks. There may also be transient renal tubular acidosis because fatty acids are an energy source for the kidney.

CPT II: Episodic pancreatitis, even without myoglobinuria. Episodes of rhabdomyolysis and myoglobinuria may lead to renal dysfunction.

OTHER

CPT I: Hypoketotic hypoglycemia, hyperammonemia, Reye syndrome-like episodes.

CPT II (neonatal form): Hypoketotic hypoglycemia.

MISCELLANEOUS: Mothers carrying fetuses with CPT I can develop acute fatty liver of pregnancy or HELLP syndrome. This is also the case with other acyl-CoA dehydrogenase deficiencies, such as long-chain acyl-CoA dehydrogenase deficiency (see later). Presumably abnormal fetal metabolites overwhelm the ability of the heterozygote mother's mitochondria to oxidize them.

ANESTHETIC CONSIDERATIONS

Protracted perioperative fasting must be avoided because it may lead to hypoketotic hypoglycemia. Perioperative intravenous fluids should include glucose. In patients who are hypoglycemic, 5% dextrose may be inadequate. The limitations of caloric intake as supplied by intravenous lipids are unclear. Medium chain triglycerides are fully metabolized and are an appropriate energy source. Hepatic function should be evaluated. Anesthesia and/or surgical stress can precipitate an attack of rhabdomyolysis (3–5) or hepatic coma (1). The consequences of succinylcholine use in the presence of this myopathy are not known.

Bibliography:

1. Neuvonen PT, van den Berg AA. Postoperative coma in a child with carnitine palmitoyltransferase I deficiency. *Anesth Analg* 2001;92:646–647.
2. Keyes MA, Van de Wiele B, Stead SW. Mitochondrial myopathies: an unusual cause of hypotonia in infants and children. *Paediatr Anaesth* 1996;6:329–335.
3. Zierz S, Schmitt U. Inhibition of carnitine palmitoyltransferase by malonyl-CoA in human muscle is influenced by anesthesia [Letter]. *Anesthesiology* 1989;70:373.
4. Katsuya H, Misumi M, Ohtani Y, et al. Postanesthetic acute renal failure due to carnitine palmitoyltransferase deficiency. *Anesthesiology* 1988;68:945–948.
5. Schaer H, Steinmann B, Jerusalem S, et al. Rhabdomyolysis induced by anaesthesia with intraoperative cardiac arrest. *Br J Anaesth* 1977;49:495–499.

Carpenter Syndrome

SYNONYM: Acrocephalosyndactyly type II. (Includes Summitt syndrome)

MIM #: 201000

This autosomal recessive disorder is characterized by craniosynostosis, acrocephaly, lateral displacement of the inner canthi, syndactyly, and polydactyly of the feet. A variant, known as **Summitt syndrome,** has been described with the findings of Carpenter syndrome with obesity and normal intelligence.

HEENT/AIRWAY: Craniosynostosis (coronal, sagittal and lambdoid). Acrocephaly, brachycephaly, or Kleeblattschaedel deformity (see later). Hypoplastic supraorbital ridges. Flat midface. Lateral displacement of the inner canthi, may have inner canthal folds. Microcornea, cataracts. Low-set, malformed ears. May have conductive or sensorineural hearing loss. Flat nasal bridge. High-arched palate. Abnormal dentition, including missing teeth, delayed loss of deciduous teeth and delayed emergence of teeth. Hypoplastic mandible. May have short neck.

CARDIOVASCULAR: Congenital cardiac defects occur in approximately half, and include atrial septal defect, ventricular septal defect, patent ductus arteriosus, tetralogy of Fallot, and transposition of the great vessels.

NEUROMUSCULAR: Variable mental retardation, from none to severe. May have speech delay. May have elevated intracranial pressure if craniosynostosis is severe.

ORTHOPEDIC: Growth retardation. Hands show syndactyly, brachydactyly, clinodactyly, camptodactyly. Single palmar crease. Feet show preaxial polydactyly, partial syndactyly. Hypoplastic or missing middle phalanges of fingers and toes.

Coxa valga. Angulation deformities at the knees. Metatarsus varus.

GI/GU: Umbilical hernia, omphalocele. Cryptorchidism, hypogonadism. May have hydronephrosis or hydroureter.

OTHER: Obesity. Precocious puberty.

MISCELLANEOUS: George Carpenter described a patient with "his" syndrome thus: "When looked at from the front, the face and skull form an ace of diamonds shaped figure, the eyes protruding frog-like, the eyeballs being kept in position merely by their lids, so that it is possible to readily dislocate the globes and permit the organs to hang suspended by their muscular and nerve attachments."

ANESTHETIC CONSIDERATIONS
The hypoplastic mandible may make direct laryngoscopy and tracheal intubation difficult. Patients may have elevated intracranial pressure, in which case precautions should be taken to avoid further elevations in pressure. Consider preoperative evaluation of renal function in patients with a history of renal abnormalities which predispose to renal insufficiency. Patients with congenital heart disease need antibiotic prophylaxis as indicated.

Bibliography:

1. Richieri-Costa A, Pirolo Junior L, Cohen MM. Carpenter syndrome with normal intelligence: Brazilian girl born to consanguineous parents. *Am J Med Genet* 1993;47:281–283.
2. Gershoni-Baruch R. Carpenter syndrome: marked variability of expression to include the Summitt and Goodman syndromes. *Am J Med Genet* 1990;35:236–240.
3. Robinson LK, James HE, Mubarak SJ, et al. Carpenter syndrome: natural history and clinical spectrum. *Am J Med Genet* 1985;20:461–469.

Cartilage-Hair Hypoplasia Syndrome

SYNONYM: Metaphyseal chondrodysplasia, McKusick type; Metaphyseal dysplasia, McKusick type

MIM #: 250250

There are many types of metaphyseal chondrodysplasia—see also Jansen, Pyle, Schmid, Shwachman, and Spahr type [Spahr type not included in this text (*MIM #* 250400)]. This autosomal recessive form of metaphyseal chondrodysplasia is characterized by flared and irregular metaphyses, mild bowing of the legs, and fine, sparse hair. The hematologic and immunologic abnormalities that can be seen with this syndrome are similar to those seen in Shwachman syndrome. The gene responsible for this disorder, *RMRP*, is interesting. The product of this gene, mitochondrial RNA-processing endoribonuclease, cleaves mitochondrial RNA. The enzyme is a ribonucleoprotein whose RNA component is produced by a nuclear gene and imported into the mitochondria. The *RNRP* gene is untranslated—it encodes an RNA, not a protein.

HEENT/AIRWAY: May have abnormal dentition and dental caries.

CHEST: Prominent sternum. Mild flaring of the ribs at the costochondral junction.

ORTHOPEDIC: Growth deficiency and short stature with short limbs and long trunk. Mild bowing of the legs. Long fibula distally relative to the tibia. Incomplete extension of the elbow. Flared and irregular metaphyses, with epiphyses essentially normal. Short hands. Lax joints in the hands. Flat feet. Small pelvic inlet. Genu varum. Scoliosis, lumbar lordosis.

GI/GU: May have esophageal atresia, intestinal malabsorption, Hirschsprung disease (see later), anal stenosis. May have impaired spermatogenesis.

OTHER: Fine, sparse, hypopigmented hair. Abnormal cellular immune function and neutropenia lead to significantly increased risk of serious infection, with a noted susceptibility to varicella infection (chicken pox). Humeral immune deficiency of a variety of immunoglobulin types and subtypes. Mild macrocytic anemia. Rare congenital hypoplastic anemia which is usually transient, but occasionally persistent. May have thrombocytosis. Malignancy, particularly non-Hodgkin lymphoma and basal cell carcinoma may develop, presumably due to the immunologic defect. May develop obesity.

MISCELLANEOUS: Particularly common in Old Order Amish and in Finland.

ANESTHETIC CONSIDERATIONS
A baseline hematocrit should be obtained. Carious teeth can be dislodged during laryngoscopy. Attention to good aseptic technique is indicated because patients may have a significant immunologic abnormality. Patients must be carefully positioned secondary to orthopedic abnormalities. Patients with concomitant Hirschsprung disease are at increased risk for postoperative morbidity and mortality.

Bibliography:
1. Makitie O, Heikkinen M, Kaitila I, et al. Hirschsprung's disease in cartilage-hair hypoplasia has poor prognosis. *J Pediatr Surg* 2002;37: 1585–1588.
2. Clayton DA. Molecular biology: a big development for a small RNA. *Nature* 2001;410:29–31.
3. Makitie O, Sulisalo T, de la Chapelle A, et al. Cartilage-hair hypoplasia. *J Med Genet* 1995;32:39–43.
4. Sulisalo T, van der Burgt I, Rimoin D, et al. Genetic homogeneity of cartilage-hair hypoplasia. *Hum Genet* 1995;95:157–160.

Cat Eye Syndrome

MIM #: 115470

This syndrome classically involves colobomas of the iris and anal atresia. However, there are many patients with

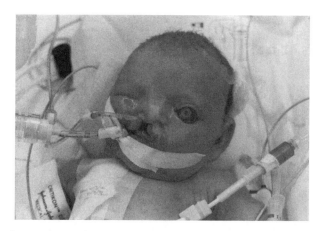

Cat eye syndrome. In addition to the expected ocular findings, this 5 day old infant with cat eye syndrome has complex cyanotic congenital heart disease, anal atresia, cleft lip and palate, and brainstem hypoplasia.

this syndrome who exhibit only one of the characteristic features. Genetic studies (fluorescent *in situ* hybridization, FISH) have been able to confirm atypical cases in which only one of the classic features is present. This syndrome is due to the presence of a partial extra chromosome or a duplication of the 22q11 region, including the centromere. Patients may have mosaicism.

HEENT/AIRWAY: Mild hypertelorism, down-slanting palpebral fissures. Inferior coloboma of the iris, giving the appearance of a cat's eye. May have colobomas of the choroid or optic nerve. Inner epicanthal folds, microphthalmia, strabismus. May have abnormal external ear, atresia of the external auditory canal, preauricular tags/pits. Flat nasal bridge. May have choanal atresia. May have cleft palate. Mild micrognathia.

CHEST: Absence or synostosis of ribs.

CARDIOVASCULAR: Congenital cardiac defects, including persistence of the left superior vena cava, tetralogy of Fallot and total anomalous pulmonary venous return.

NEUROMUSCULAR: Intelligence is normal or near normal.

ORTHOPEDIC: May have growth retardation. May have radial aplasia, duplication of the hallux.

GI/GU: Anal atresia with a fistula from the rectum to the bladder, vagina, urethra, or peritoneum. May have inguinal hernias, malrotation of the gut, Meckel diverticulum, Hirschsprung disease (see later), biliary atresia. Renal abnormalities include hypoplasia, unilateral or bilateral agenesis, hydronephrosis, supernumerary kidneys.

MISCELLANEOUS: The association of coloboma of the iris and anal atresia was first reported by Haab in 1879.

ANESTHETIC CONSIDERATIONS

Patients invariably need surgical correction of anal atresia. Difficult intubation has been reported, with successful use of a laryngeal mask airway or awake nasal fiberoptic intubation. Renal abnormalities are common, and renal insufficiency has implications for perioperative fluid management and the choice of anesthetic drugs. Radial anomalies may make placement of a radial arterial catheter more difficult. Patients with congenital cardiac disease require prophylactic antibiotics as indicated. Choanal atresia, although uncommon, precludes placement of a nasal airway, nasal intubation, or placement of a nasogastric tube.

Bibliography:

1. Devavaram P, Seefelder C, Lillehei CW. Anaesthetic management of cat eye syndrome [Letter]. *Paediatr Anaesth* 2001;11:746–748.
2. Bellinghieri G, Triolo O, Stella NC, et al. Renal function evaluation in an adult female with cat-eye syndrome. *Am J Nephrol* 1994;14:76–79.

CATCH-22 Syndrome

MIM #: None

Deletions of the long arm of chromosome 22 in the region of 22q11.2 can present with a variety of phenotypes, including DiGeorge syndrome (see later), Shprintzen syndrome (velocardiofacial syndrome, see later), conotruncal anomaly face syndrome (Takao syndrome, not discussed in this text), or isolated conotruncal cardiac defects (tetralogy of Fallot, truncus arteriosus, or interrupted aortic arch).

This somewhat whimsical designation has been proposed as a catch-all acronym to include these various presentations: **C**ardiac, **A**bnormal facies, **T**-cell deficit from thymic hypoplasia, **C**left palate, **H**ypocalcemia from hypoparathyroidism. This term, though cute, is no longer in routine use.

See DiGeorge syndrome later for a complete discussion.

Catel-Manzke Syndrome

MIM #: 302380

This sporadic, possibly X-linked recessive disorder is characterized by severe micrognathia, cleft palate, and anomalies of the index finger. The responsible gene and gene product are not known.

HEENT/AIRWAY: May have hypertelorism. Abnormal or posteriorly rotated external ears. Cleft palate, may have cleft lip. Large tongue. Severe micrognathia. Pierre-Robin. Short neck.

CHEST: May have pectus excavatum or carinatum.

CARDIOVASCULAR: Cardiac defects are common, and include atrial septal defects, ventricular septal defects, overriding aorta, coarctation of the aortic, dextrocardia.

NEUROMUSCULAR: Intelligence is normal. Occasional developmental delay, seizures. May have facial paresis.

ORTHOPEDIC: Prenatal and postnatal growth failure. Accessory bone at the base of the index finger, with resultant ulnar deviation (bilateral duplication of the proximal phalanges of the index fingers). Hypoplasia of the associated metacarpal. Over time the accessory bone fuses to the proximal phalangeal epiphysis. Clinodactyly. Single palmar crease. May have radial defects. Dislocatable knees. Camptodactyly. Clubfoot.

GI/GU: May have umbilical and inguinal hernias. Cryptorchidism.

OTHER: Failure to thrive secondary to respiratory problems or cardiac anomalies.

ANESTHETIC CONSIDERATIONS

Endotracheal intubation may be extremely difficult or impossible secondary to severe micrognathia. Alternatives to direct laryngoscopy, such as fiberoptic intubation, retrograde intubation, blind nasal intubation, and the laryngeal mask airway, must be considered. Patients may have significant upper airway obstruction even without the induction of anesthesia. Placing the patient prone so that the tongue does not fall posteriorly into the pharynx may improve spontaneous ventilation. Radial anomalies may make placement of a radial arterial catheter more difficult. Patients must be closely observed after surgery for evidence of airway obstruction. Patients with congenital cardiac defects need prophylactic antibiotics as indicated.

Bibliography:

1. Puri RD, Phadke SR. Catel-Manzke syndrome without cleft palate: a case report. *Clin Dysmorphol* 2003;12:279–281.
2. Wilson GN, King TE, Brookshire GS. Index finger hyperphalangy and multiple anomalies: Catel-Manzke syndrome? *Am J Med Genet* 1993;46:176–179.
3. Dignan PS, Martin LW, Zenni EJ. Pierre Robin anomaly with an accessory metacarpal of the index fingers: the Catel-Manzke syndrome. *Clin Genet* 1986;29:168–173.

Caudal Regression Syndrome

SYNONYM: Sacral agenesis

MIM #: None

This syndrome involves a spectrum of abnormalities of the sacrum and lower extremities (the caudal region). There is no discernible Mendelian inheritance pattern. The syndrome is probably secondary to a defect in neural plate and neural tube development or fetal vascular supply. Infants of diabetic mothers are at increased risk for development of this syndrome. The most severely affected patients have complete sacral agenesis, and their prognosis is poor.

HEENT/AIRWAY: May have cleft lip or palate.

CARDIOVASCULAR: Rare congenital heart disease.

NEUROMUSCULAR: Disruption of the distal spinal cord secondary to sacral or lumbar defects may lead to neurogenic bladder, fecal incontinence, lower extremity paralysis. May have microcephaly, meningomyelocele.

ORTHOPEDIC: Varying degrees of sacral and lower extremity hypoplasia. The buttocks are shortened and flattened. May have hypoplasia of the lumbar vertebrae. May have hypoplasia of the femur, defects of the tibiae/fibulae. The most extreme cases have sacral agenesis, flexion and abduction deformities of the lower extremities, popliteal webs, or fusion of the lower extremities. Clubfoot deformity is common.

GI/GU: May have imperforate anus. May have renal anomalies.

ANESTHETIC CONSIDERATIONS
Baseline renal function should be evaluated if neurogenic bladder is present. Self-catheterization for neurogenic bladder is a major risk factor for the development of latex allergy. Lower lumbar and caudal anesthesia/analgesia are technically difficult or impossible with the complete absence of those structures. The patient's lower extremities may need to be carefully positioned secondary to contracture deformities.

Bibliography:
1. Yegin A, Sanli S, Hadimioglu N, et al. Anesthesia in caudal regression syndrome [Letter]. *Paediatr Anaesth* 2005;15:174–175.
2. Adra A, Cordero D, Mejides A, et al. Caudal regression syndrome: etiopathogenesis, prenatal diagnosis, and perinatal management. *Obstet Gynecol Surv* 1994;49:508–516.
3. Goto MP, Goldman AS. Diabetic embryopathy. *Curr Opin Pediatr* 1994;6:486–491.

Cayler Syndrome

See Asymmetric crying facies

Central Core Disease

MIM #: 117000
This autosomal dominant congenital myopathy is characterized by nonprogressive, primarily proximal muscle weakness. The name is derived from the fact that there is decreased stain uptake in the central areas (cores) of muscle fibers on histologic examination. This is a result of quantitative and qualitative abnormalities of mitochondria, sarcoplasmic reticulum, and glycogen in these areas. This disorder is due to one of several reported defects in the ryanodine receptor-1 gene (*RYR1*), a calcium channel gene that has been mapped to the long arm of chromosome 19. Less calcium is taken up by the sarcoplasmic reticulum in the cores, which leads to an elevated calcium concentration in the muscle fiber. The abnormality appears to be limited to type 1 muscle fibers.

The other congenital myopathies are mini-core myopathy (not covered in this text), myotubular myopathy (see later) and nemaline rod myopathy (see later).

HEENT/AIRWAY: Mandibular hypoplasia and a short neck may occur secondary to congenital muscle weakness.

NEUROMUSCULAR: Proximal or, more rarely, diffuse, nonprogressive myopathy. Hypotonia in infancy. Intelligence is normal. Cranial nerve function is normal. Delayed motor development.

ORTHOPEDIC: May have kyphoscoliosis, dislocated hips, pes cavus, joint contractures.

ANESTHETIC CONSIDERATIONS
Central core disease is one of the few diseases where patients are clearly susceptible to the development of malignant hyperthermia (see later). Patients with central core disease must always receive a nontriggering anesthetic. Interestingly, both central core disease and malignant hyperthermia susceptibility are due to mutations in *RYR1*. However, malignant hyperthermia susceptibility does not always correlate with central core disease and central core disease does not always cosegregate with the identified region on chromosome 19 (3).

Although statin drugs have been associated with rhabdomyolysis and myopathy, there is an isolated report of uncomplicated use in a patient for coronary bypass surgery (2).

Bibliography:
1. Avila G. Intracellular Ca^{2+} dynamics in malignant hyperthermia and central core disease: established concepts, new cellular mechanisms involved. *Cell Calcium* 2005;37:121–127.
2. Johi RR, Mills R, Halsall PJ, et al. Anaesthetic management of coronary artery bypass grafting in a patient with central core disease and susceptibility to malignant hyperthermia on statin therapy. *Br J Anaesth* 2003;91:744–747.
3. Curran JL, Hall WJ, Halsall PJ, et al. Segregation of malignant hyperthermia, central core disease and chromosome 19 markers. *Br J Anaesth* 1999;83:217–222.

Central Hypoventilation Syndrome

See Ondine's curse

Centronuclear Myopathy

See Myotubular myopathy

Cerebral Gigantism

See Sotos syndrome

Cerebrocostomandibular Syndrome

MIM #: 117650

This possibly autosomal recessive disorder consists of mental retardation, rib gap defects, and severe micrognathia. Patients have a very small thoracic cage, and usually die during early childhood of respiratory insufficiency. The responsible gene and gene product are not known.

HEENT/AIRWAY: May have microcephaly. Severe micrognathia, large tongue. May have hearing loss. Cleft palate. Dental anomalies. May have abnormal cartilaginous tracheal rings.

CHEST: Defects (gaps) in ribs between the posterior incompletely ossified ribs and the anterior cartilaginous ribs, with resultant small, bell-shaped thoracic cage. The defects become pseudoarthroses over time. Ribs may be aberrantly attached to the vertebrae posteriorly. Sternum and clavicles may be hypoplastic. Rib defects may cause flail chest.

CARDIOVASCULAR: May have ventricular septal defect.

NEUROMUSCULAR: Mental retardation. Porencephaly. Speech delay. May have meningomyelocele.
Orthopedic. Growth retardation. Vertebral defects. May have sacral fusion, congenital hip dislocation, clubfoot deformity. May have hypoplastic humerus.

GI/GU: May have cystic renal disease.

ANESTHETIC CONSIDERATIONS
Endotracheal intubation can be extremely difficult or impossible secondary to severe micrognathia. Alternatives to direct laryngoscopy, such as fiberoptic intubation, retrograde intubation, blind nasal intubation, and the laryngeal mask airway should be considered. Patients have severe restrictive lung disease secondary to thoracic cage defects. These patients are at increased risk for perioperative respiratory complications. Clavicular anomalies may make placement of a subclavian venous catheter more difficult. Renal disease is rare, but when present, has implications for perioperative fluid management and the choice of anesthetic drugs. Patients with congenital cardiac defects require prophylactic antibiotics as indicated.

Bibliography:
1. Plotz FB, van Essen AJ, Bosschaart AN, et al. Cerebro-costo-mandibular syndrome. *Am J Med Genet* 1996;62:286–292.
2. Drossou-Agakidou V, Andreou A, Soubassi-Griva V, et al. Cerebrocostomandibular syndrome in four sibs, two pairs of twins. *J Med Genet* 1991;28:704–707.

Cerebrohepatorenal Syndrome

See Zellweger syndrome

Cerebrooculofacioskeletal Syndrome

SYNONYM: COFS syndrome; Pena-Shokeir syndrome, type II

MIM #: 214150

This autosomal recessive syndrome consists of microcephaly, microphthalmia, arthrogryposis, and failure to thrive. It is a progressive disorder involving degeneration of the brain and spinal cord. Evidence of the degenerative process is usually present at birth. Most patients die in early childhood. The disorder is due to mutations in the gene *ERCC6*, which is involved in DNA repair. Defects in this gene are also responsible for the late-onset type of Cockayne syndrome (see later).

HEENT/AIRWAY: Microcephaly. Microphthalmia, blepharophimosis, cataracts, nystagmus. Large ears. Can have decreased hearing, and abnormal inner ear pathology has been described. Broad nasal root. Mild micrognathia. Overhanging upper lip.

CHEST: Pulmonary infections are common, particularly as malnutrition progresses. Widely spaced nipples.

NEUROMUSCULAR: Degeneration of white matter. Cerebellar degeneration. Mental retardation. Hypotonia, hyporeflexia. May have seizures, infantile spasms. Focal gliosis of the third ventricle, focal microgyria, hypoplastic optic tracts and chiasm, agenesis of the corpus callosum, intracranial calcifications.

ORTHOPEDIC: Severe growth deficiency. Arthrogryposis, particularly of elbows and knees. Camptodactyly. Coxa valga. Rocker-bottom feet. Kyphoscoliosis. Osteoporosis.

GI/GU: May have renal abnormalities.

OTHER: Severe failure to thrive with progressive malnutrition. Hirsutism.

ANESTHETIC CONSIDERATIONS
Patients exhibit progressive neurologic degeneration, and may be at risk for hyperkalemia with the administration of succinylcholine. Chronic use of anticonvulsant medications may affect the metabolism of some anesthetic drugs. Micrognathia is usually mild, and should not interfere with ease of intubation. Pulmonary infections are common. Patients must be carefully positioned secondary to joint contractures and osteoporosis.

Bibliography:
1. Del Bigio MR, Greenberg CR, Rorke LB, et al. Neuropathological findings in eight children with cerebro-oculo-facio-skeletal (COFS) syndrome. *J Neuropathol Exp Neurol* 1997;56:1147–1157.
2. Gershoni-Baruch R, Ludatscher RM, Lichtig C, et al. Cerebro-oculofacio-skeletal syndrome: further delineation. *Am J Med Genet* 1991;41:74–77.

Cerebrooculohepatorenal Syndrome

See Arima syndrome

Cerebroside Lipidosis

See Krabbe disease

Ceroid Lipofuscinosis

See Jansky-Bielschowsky disease and Spielmeyer-Vogt disease

Cervicooculoacoustic Syndrome

See Wildervanck syndrome

CFC Syndrome

See Cardiofaciocutaneous syndrome

Charcot-Marie-Tooth Syndrome

MIM #: 118200, 118210, 118220, 302800

This hereditary peripheral neuropathy is the most common form of peripheral neuropathy in children, but is genetically and clinically heterogeneous. Patients exhibit distal motor and sensory nerve dysfunction, with the primary manifestation being peroneal muscle atrophy. The sympathetic postganglionic fibers may also be involved, leading to autonomic dysfunction. Symptoms are usually evident by the midteen years, and are slowly progressive with periods of remission and exacerbation. Life expectancy is unaffected. Exacerbations of symptoms can occur during pregnancy.

A relatively common autosomal dominant form of Charcot-Marie-Tooth syndrome (CMT type 1) is a peripheral demyelinating disease with bilaterally slowed motor nerve conduction velocities. It presents in the second or third decade of life with progressive disease. Overexpression of the *PMP22* gene results in CMT type 1A. CMT type 1B is caused by mutations in the gene *MPZ*, and is related clinically and genetically to Dejerine-Sottas syndrome (see later). Both the *PMP22* and *MPZ* genes encode a peripheral myelin protein. There are many other subtypes of CMT type 1 that have been associated with defects in a variety of other genes. Another dominant form, CMT type 2, is caused by mutations in the gene *K1F1B* (whose gene product transports mitochondria along microtubules) or the gene *MFN2* (which regulates mitochondrial fusion). CMT type 2 presents later in life than CMT type 1. An X-linked form is due to mutations in the gene *GJB1*, which encodes connexin-32, a gap junction protein.

HEENT/AIRWAY: May have vocal cord paresis.

CHEST: Severe disease can result in respiratory insufficiency in adults secondary to respiratory muscle involvement. The presence of proximal arm weakness may be a marker for respiratory muscle involvement.

NEUROMUSCULAR: Slowly progressive neuropathy with muscle wasting and early loss of deep tendon reflexes. Muscle weakness begins in the feet and legs. Peroneal muscle atrophy is a hallmark finding, with foot drop. Involvement of the sympathetic postganglionic fibers impairs autonomic function. Weakness and wasting of intrinsic muscles of the hands in severe disease. Difficulty manipulating thumb for tasks that require thumb opposition or fine motor movements. Thickened ulnar and peroneal nerves. Tremor.

ORTHOPEDIC: High-arched feet (pes cavus), clubfoot deformity, hammer toe deformity. Foot deformities may precede muscle atrophy by many years.

OTHER: Temperature regulation by sweating may be impaired secondary to autonomic dysfunction. The neuropathy may be exacerbated by pregnancy. Symptoms often, but not always, return to baseline after delivery. Some patients may have new or exacerbated symptoms postpartum. Alcohol can exacerbate symptoms in CMT 1 disease, and all patients are very sensitive to vincristine.

MISCELLANEOUS: Described separately by Charcot and Marie in France and Tooth in England. Charcot and Marie thought it to be a primary muscular disease, but Tooth correctly identified it as a peripheral neuropathy.

ANESTHETIC CONSIDERATIONS

Both depolarizing and nondepolarizing muscle relaxants have been used uneventfully in these patients (1, 4, 5, 7, 8). Hypersensitivity did occur in a patient with advanced disease (9). It has been suggested that succinylcholine be avoided, particularly during acute exacerbations, because of the risk of hyperkalemia secondary to denervation muscle atrophy. Succinylcholine has been used during stable disease without symptomatic problems (8). Temperature regulation by sweating may be impaired secondary to autonomic dysfunction, leading to thermal lability and mottled cyanosis. Spinal and epidural anesthesia have been used successfully in these patients (3, 6). Vocal cord paresis is well-tolerated in adults but has resulted in tracheostomies in children. Pregnancies have resulted in a higher incidence of emergency and instrumented deliveries. There is no association between CMT and malignant hyperthermia.

Bibliography:

1. Schmitt HJ, Wick S, Münster T. Onset and duration of mivacurium-induced neuromuscular blockade in children with Charcot-Marie-Tooth disease. A case series with five children. *Paediatr Anaesth* 2006;16: 182–187.

2. Hoff JM, Gilhus NE, Daltveit AK. Pregnancies and deliveries in patients with Charcot-Marie-Tooth disease. *Neurology* 2005;64:459–462.
3. Schmitt HJ, Muenster T, Schmidt J, et al. Central neural blockade in Charcot-Marie-Tooth disease [Letter]. *Can J Anaesth* 2004;51: 1049–1050.
4. Naguib M, Samarkandi AH. Response to atracurium and mivacurium in a patient with Charcot-Marie-Tooth disease. *Can J Anaesth* 1998; 45:56–59.
5. Baraka AS. Vecuronium neuromuscular block in a patient with Charcot-Marie-Tooth syndrome. *Anesth Analg* 1997;84:927–928.
6. Scull T, Weeks S. Epidural analgesia for labour in a patient with Charcot-Marie-Tooth disease. *Can J Anaesth* 1996;43:1150–1152.
7. Greenberg RS, Parker SD. Anesthetic management for the child with Charcot-Marie-Tooth disease. *Anesth Analg* 1992;74:305–307.
8. Antognini JF. Anaesthesia for Charcot-Marie-Tooth disease: a review of 86 cases. *Can J Anaesth* 1992;39:398–400.
9. Brian JE Jr, Boyles GD, Quirk JG Jr, et al. Anesthetic management for cesarean section of a patient with Charcot-Marie-Tooth disease. *Anesthesiology* 1987;66:410–412.
10. Roelofse JA, Shipton EA. Anaesthesia for abdominal hysterectomy in Charcot-Marie-Tooth disease. *S Afr Med J* 1985;67:605–606.

CHARGE Association

MIM #: 214800

The acronym CHARGE stands for **C**olobomas of the eye, **H**eart disease, **A**tresia of the choanae, **R**etarded growth or central nervous system anomalies, **G**enital anomalies or hypogonadism, and **E**ar anomalies or deafness. These anomalies are frequently seen in nonrandom association, and at least four must be present to make the diagnosis. All of the organ systems involved are at a critical stage of development during the second month of gestation, and it has been hypothesized that a midline developmental abnormality during the second month of gestation is responsible for the variety of defects seen with the CHARGE association. The association is due to abnormalities in one of two genes, *CHD7* (chromodomain helicase DNA-binding protein 7) or *SEMA3E* (semaphorin 3E). *SEMA3E* is involved in embryonic endothelial and vasculature development.

HEENT/AIRWAY: Microcephaly. Colobomas of the eye (iris, choroid, retina, disc or optic nerve). May have morning glory syndrome (see later, Papillorenal syndrome). Upslanting palpebral fissures. May have anophthalmia. External ear abnormalities, sensorineural or conductive hearing loss. Choanal atresia or stenosis. Cleft lip or palate. Velopharyngeal incompetence. May have single maxillary central incisor. Micrognathia, which may be severe. Short neck. Laryngomalacia. Subglottic stenosis. May have esophageal atresia, tracheoesophageal fistula.

CHEST: May have rib anomalies, pectus carinatum, respiratory insufficiency.

CARDIOVASCULAR: Congenital heart disease, including tetralogy of Fallot (most commonly), patent ductus arteriosus, atrial septal defect, ventricular septal defect, double-outlet right ventricle with an atrioventricular canal, right-sided aortic arch.

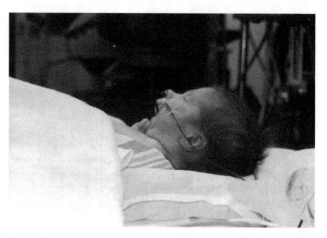

CHARGE association. This neonate presented for choanal atresia repair. The micrognathia is obvious. She was extubated without difficulty, but when she required additional surgery 2 weeks later neither the anesthesiologist nor the otolaryngologist could visualize the vocal cords, and the trachea was intubated through a laryngeal mask airway.

NEUROMUSCULAR: Variable mental retardation. Developmental delay. Cranial nerve abnormalities may result in facial nerve palsy, abnormal gag reflex, sensorineural hearing loss. Severe cases may manifest arhinencephaly, holoprosencephaly.

ORTHOPEDIC: Growth retardation. May have syndactyly, nail hypoplasia.

GI/GU: Gastroesophageal reflux. May have omphalocele, anal atresia or stenosis. Genital anomalies or hypogonadism. Renal anomalies.

OTHER: Failure to thrive. May have parathyroid hypoplasia.

ANESTHETIC CONSIDERATIONS

Consider having an interpreter present before surgery to ease communication with those patients who are deaf. In addition, many patients have visual defects. Gastroesophageal reflux is common, and some patients also have an impaired gag reflex. Patients are at increased risk for perioperative aspiration. Patients with congenital heart disease require perioperative antibiotic prophylaxis as indicated.

Micrognathia can make direct laryngoscopy and tracheal intubation difficult. Intubation can become more difficult with increasing age. Patients with laryngomalacia may have trouble maintaining an airway while ventilating through a mask or a laryngeal mask airway without additional positive end-expiratory pressure. They may do better in the lateral position. Patients with subglottic stenosis require a smaller-than-expected endotracheal tube. Choanal atresia may cause severe respiratory distress in the newborn, and precludes the use of a nasal airway or nasogastric tube.

Bibliography:

1. Blake KD, Davenport SL, Hall BD, et al. CHARGE association: an update and review for the primary pediatrician. *Clin Pediatr* 1998;37: 159–173.
2. Perkins JA, Sie KC, Milczuk H, et al. Airway management in children with craniofacial anomalies. *Cleft Palate Craniofac J* 1997;34:135–140.
3. Van Meter TD, Weaver DD. Oculo-auriculo-vertebral spectrum and the CHARGE association: clinical evidence for a common pathogenetic mechanism. *Clin Dysmorphol* 1996;5:187–196.
4. Stack CG, Wyse RK. Incidence and management of airway problems in CHARGE association. *Anaesthesia* 1991;46:582–585.
5. Lin AE, Siebert JR, Graham JM. Central nervous system malformations in the CHARGE association. *Am J Med Genet* 1990;37:304–310.
6. Cyran SE, Martinez R, Daniels S, et al. Spectrum of congenital heart disease in CHARGE association. *J Pediatr* 1987;110:576–580.

Chediak-Higashi Syndrome

MIM #: 214500

This autosomal recessive disorder involves granular cells. It is characterized by the presence of large intracellular inclusions, best seen in neutrophils, monocytes, and lymphocytes, but present in a variety of other granular cells, such as renal tubular epithelium, gastric mucosa, Schwann cells and melanocytes. Death is usually secondary to infection or a lymphoreticular malignancy occurring during an accelerated phase of the disease. The disorder is due to mutations in the gene *LYST*, a lysosomal trafficking regulator gene, which is likely responsible for sorting lysosomal proteins.

During an accelerated phase patients can develop anemia, thrombocytopenia and qualitative platelet defects.

HEENT/AIRWAY: Partial oculocutaneous albinism with abnormal pigmentation of the eyes. Photophobia and nystagmus, particularly in patients with light-colored eyes. Decreased retinal pigmentation. Abnormal electroretinogram and auditory and visual evoked responses, suggesting abnormal neural routing. Epistaxis. Gingivitis.

CHEST: Recurrent upper and lower respiratory tract infections.

NEUROMUSCULAR: Cranial nerve abnormalities. Peripheral neuropathy (late, perhaps due to invasion by lymphohistiocytic cells). Abnormal electroencephalogram, electromyogram, and nerve conduction velocity. Peripheral neuropathy. May have disorders of muscle function secondary to neuropathy. May have seizures. Diffuse brain and spinal cord atrophy.

GI/GU: Hepatosplenomegaly. Gastrointestinal tract bleeding. Abnormal liver function as a late finding during the accelerated phase.

OTHER: Partial albinism. Hair has an abnormal metallic, frosted-gray sheen, and has been described as ashen or silvery-blond. Even darker hair has a silvery appearance. Skin color varies from light to slate gray, and burns easily on exposure to sunlight. Pigmented and papillary skin lesions are common. Easy bruising. Patients are highly susceptible to bacterial infections, usually staphylococcal or streptococcal, and to infection with Epstein-Barr virus. Infections are related to both quantitative and qualitative neutrophil, monocyte, and natural killer cell defects. May have lymphoma-like lymphoproliferative disease. Quantitative and qualitative abnormalities of platelet function. In late stages can have lymphohistiocytic infiltrates and erythrophagocytosis.

MISCELLANEOUS: Chediak-Higashi syndrome is a disease of Aleutian mink, Hereford cattle, killer whales, cats, beige mice, and humans.

ANESTHETIC CONSIDERATIONS

Patients are highly susceptible to bacterial infections, and good perioperative aseptic technique is imperative. Patients often have photophobia, and may be sensitive to the bright operating room lights. Bleeding dyscrasia is a contraindication to neuraxial anesthesia. Excessive operative blood loss may occur secondary to quantitative or qualitative defects in platelet function. Succinylcholine may be relatively contraindicated in patients with a significant neuropathy because of the risk of hyperkalemia. Patients taking steroids to ameliorate the symptoms of the accelerated phase should receive perioperative stress dose steroids.

Bibliography:

1. Demirkiran O, Utku T, Urkmez S, et al. Chediak-Higashi syndrome in the intensive care unit. *Paediatr Anaesth* 2004;14:685–688.
2. Huizing M, Anikster Y, Gahl WA. Hermansky-Pudlak syndrome and Chediak-Higashi syndrome: disorders of vesicle formation and trafficking. *Thromb Haemost* 2001;86:233–245.
3. Asian Y, Erduran E, Gedik Y, et al. The role of high dose methylprednisolone and splenectomy in the accelerated phase of Chediak-Higashi syndrome. *Acta Haematol* 1996;96:105–107.
4. Ulsoy H, Erciyes N, Ovali E. Anesthesia in Chediak-Higashi syndrome: case report. *Middle East J Anesthesiol* 1995;13:101–105.
5. Stolz W, Graubner U, Gerstmeier J. Chediak-Higashi syndrome: approaches in diagnosis and treatment. *Curr Probl Dermatol* 1989;18: 93–100.

Chiari Malformation

See Arnold-Chiari malformation

CHILD Syndrome

MIM #: 308050

CHILD is an acronym for **C**ongenital **H**emidysplasia with **I**chthyosiform erythroderma and **L**imb **D**efects. Congenital cardiac defects are also common. Most cases have been female, suggesting X-linked dominant inheritance with lethality in boys. The disorder is due to mutations in the gene *NSDHL* (NAD[P]H steroid-dehydrogenase-like protein), which may be involved in cholesterol synthesis. Interestingly, the right side of the body is more often affected

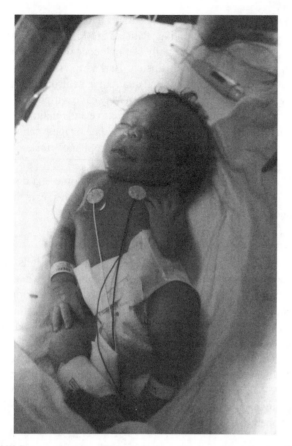

CHILD syndrome. This 2.3 kg 16-day-old infant with complex congenital heart disease has CHILD syndrome. Note that her left humerus is shorter than the right and her left forearm is also shortened. Her left femur is shorter than her right, and she has bilateral clubfoot and four fingers on her left hand.

than the left. Left-sided disease is associated with cardiac defects. A variety of organs can be asymmetrically hypoplastic, ipsilateral to the side of ichthyosis and limb malformations.

HEENT/AIRWAY: May have hearing loss. May have cleft lip. May have unilateral mandibular hypoplasia.

CHEST: May have unilateral pulmonary hypoplasia. May have unilateral clavicular, scapular or rib hypoplasia.

CARDIOVASCULAR: Congenital cardiac defects, especially atrial septal defects, ventricular septal defects, single coronary ostium, single ventricle.

NEUROMUSCULAR: May have mild mental retardation. May have unilateral cortical, cranial nerve, brainstem, or spinal cord hypoplasia. Rare meningomyelocele.

ORTHOPEDIC: Unilateral hypomelia, varying from phalangeal hypoplasia to complete absence of a limb. Ipsilateral nail dysplasia. May have hypoplastic mandible, clavicle, scapula, ribs, or vertebrae ipsilateral to the affected limb.

Joint contractures, webbing at the elbows and knees. May have scoliosis. May have unilateral pelvic hypoplasia.

GI/GU: May have umbilical hernia. Unilateral renal agenesis. Unilateral ovarian hypoplasia or fallopian tube hypoplasia.

OTHER: Congenital unilateral ichthyosiform erythroderma–erythematous, scaling skin, present at birth or soon thereafter. There is a sharp demarcation in the midline between normal and abnormal skin. Unilateral alopecia, hyperkeratosis. The face is usually spared. May have unilateral thyroid or adrenal hypoplasia.

MISCELLANEOUS: Although the snappy acronym has been followed for many decades, the first description was by Otto Sachs in 1903.

ANESTHETIC CONSIDERATIONS
Peripheral intravenous access is limited in patients with significant limb defects. Clavicular anomalies may make placement of a subclavian venous catheter more difficult. Renal insufficiency affects intraoperative fluid management and the kinetics of some anesthetic drugs. Patients with congenital cardiac defects require antibiotic prophylaxis as indicated. Difficult laryngoscopy secondary to mandibular hypoplasia has not yet been reported. Patients with pulmonary hypoplasia may require additional attention to ventilator settings.

Bibliography:
1. Happle R, Effendy I, Megahed M, et al. CHILD syndrome in a boy. *Am J Med Genet* 1996;62:192–194.
2. Emami S, Rizzo WB, Hanley KP, et al. Peroxisomal abnormality in fibroblasts from involved skin of CHILD syndrome: case study and review of peroxisomal disorders in relation to skin disease. *Arch Dermatol* 1992;128:213–222.

Cholesterol Ester Storage Disease

Included in Wolman disease

Chondrodysplasia Punctata–Autosomal Recessive Type

SYNONYM: Rhizomelic chondrodysplasia punctata

MIM #: 215100

This autosomal recessive type of chondrodysplasia punctata is characterized by rhizomelic limb shortening, vertebral clefting, and punctate epiphyseal calcifications.

Patients usually die in infancy or early childhood. This disorder is due to a mutation in the *PEX7* gene, which encodes the peroxisomal type 2 targeting signal receptor, leading to quantitative or qualitative defects in peroxisomes. There are also X-linked dominant, autosomal dominant, and X-linked recessive types of chondrodysplasia punctata (see following). Fetal warfarin syndrome (see later) is phenotypically similar to chondrodysplasia punctata.

HEENT/AIRWAY: May have microcephaly. Frontal bossing. Flat facies. Bilateral cataracts. May have upward-slanting palpebral fissures. Flat nasal bridge with small nares. May have micrognathia. May have cleft palate.

CHEST: Neonates are prone to respiratory insufficiency.

NEUROMUSCULAR: Severe mental retardation. May exhibit spasticity. Cortical atrophy. Severely delayed myelination. Seizures.

ORTHOPEDIC: Dwarfism. Rhizomelic limb shortening (proximal limb shortening). Hypoplastic distal phalanges. Coronal clefting of the vertebrae. Vertebrae may be dysplastic. Punctate epiphyseal calcifications and irregularity. Metaphyseal splaying. Joint contractures.

OTHER: Ichthyosis, which develops postnatally. May have alopecia.

MISCELLANEOUS: Chondrodysplasia punctata has also been described in beagles.

ANESTHETIC CONSIDERATIONS

Neonates are prone to respiratory insufficiency. Patients must be carefully positioned perioperatively secondary to joint contractures. Patients with ichthyosis may be using topical agents with an oily base that prevents adhesives from sticking to their skin. Tubes and catheters may need to be sewn or tied into place perioperatively. In patients with severe ichthyosis, temperature regulation may be impaired. Small nares may impede passage of nasal or nasogastric tubes.

Bibliography:
1. Agamanolis DP, Novak RW. Rhizomelic chondrodysplasia punctata: report of a case with review of the literature and correlation with other peroxisomal disorders. *Pediatr Pathol Lab Med* 1995;15:503–513.
2. Heikoop JC, Wanders RJ, Strijland A, et al. Genetic and biochemical heterogeneity in patients with the rhizomelic form of chondrodysplasia punctata: a complementation study. *Hum Genet* 1992;89:439–444.
3. Wardinsky TD, Pagon RA, Powell BR, et al. Rhizomelic chondrodysplasia punctata and survival beyond one year: a review of the literature and five case reports. *Clin Genet* 1990;38:84–93.

Chondrodysplasia Punctata–Autosomal Dominant and X-linked Dominant Types

SYNONYM: Conradi-Hunermann syndrome

MIM #: 118650, 302960

Also known as Conradi-Hunermann syndrome, this autosomal dominant type of chondrodysplasia punctata is

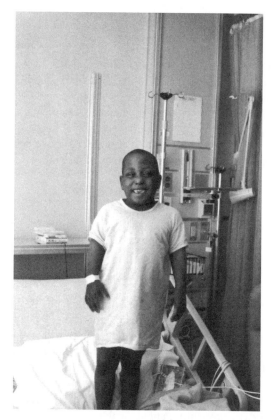

Chondrodysplasia punctata–autosomal recessive type. This young boy with autosomal recessive chondrodysplasia punctata has obvious rhizomelic asymmetry of his arms. He is hyperactive with developmental delay.

characterized by asymmetric limb shortening and punctate epiphyseal calcifications that usually improve in the first year of life. The long-term prognosis is good because intelligence is usually normal and the epiphyseal abnormalities usually improve with age. The specific gene and gene product are unknown. The X-linked dominant form is also referred to, perhaps inappropriately, as Conradi-Hunermann syndrome. It is due to defects in the gene coding for delta(8)-delta(7) sterol isomerase emopamil-binding protein. There is an X-linked recessive form (*MIM #* 302950) which is due to defects in the gene encoding arylsulfatase E. There is also an autosomal recessive type of chondrodysplasia punctata (see preceding). The fetal warfarin syndrome (see later) is phenotypically similar to chondrodysplasia punctata.

HEENT/AIRWAY: Frontal bossing. Flat facies. Down-slanting palpebral fissures. May have cataracts. May have abnormal external ears. May have hearing loss. May have microphthalmia, glaucoma. Low nasal bridge. Micrognathia. Short neck. Laryngeal and tracheal calcifications with associated tracheal stenosis. Laryngomalacia.

CARDIOVASCULAR: May have congenital cardiac defects, including patent ductus arteriosus, atrial septal defects, ventricular septal defects, pulmonary artery stenosis.

NEUROMUSCULAR: May have mental retardation.

ORTHOPEDIC: May have mild to moderate growth deficiency. Asymmetric limb shortening related to areas of punctate epiphyseal calcification, but limb length not as profoundly shortened as in the autosomal recessive type. Scoliosis, related to areas of punctate calcification. May have joint contractures. May have vertebral anomalies, including hypoplasia, aplasia, clefting. May have odontoid hypoplasia or agenesis with atlantoaxial instability.

GI/GU: May have renal anomalies.

OTHER: Congenital ichthyosis. Large skin pores. Coarse, sparse hair. May have alopecia. May have failure to thrive in infancy.

ANESTHETIC CONSIDERATIONS
Direct laryngoscopy and tracheal intubation may be difficult secondary to the short neck and micrognathia. Patients who have laryngeal and tracheal calcifications with associated tracheal stenosis may need a smaller-than-expected endotracheal tube. Laryngomalacia may cause perioperative upper airway obstruction, which is usually responsive to positive pressure (positive end-expiratory pressure, continuous positive airway pressure). Patients with odontoid hypoplasia or agenesis may have atlantoaxial instability and an unstable cervical spine.

Patients with ichthyosis may be using topical agents on their skin. The oily base in these agents prevents adhesives from sticking to the skin. Perioperatively, tubes and catheters may need to be sewn or tied into place. In patients with severe ichthyosis, temperature regulation may be impaired.

Patients must be carefully positioned perioperatively secondary to asymmetric limb shortening and joint contractures. Patients with congenital heart disease need antibiotic prophylaxis as indicated.

Bibliography:
1. Hascalik M, Togal T, Doganay S, et al. Anaesthetic management of an infant with Conradi's syndrome. *Paediatr Anaesth* 2003;13:841–842.
2. Karoutsos S, Lansade A, Terrier G, et al. Chondrodysplasia punctata and subglottic stenosis. *Anesth Analg* 1999;89:1322–1323.
3. Garcia Miguel FJ, Galindo S, Palencia J, et al. Anaesthetic management of a girl with chondrodysplasia punctata [Letter]. *Paediatr Anaesth* 1997;7:355.
4. Fourie DT. Chondrodysplasia punctata: case report and literature review of patients with heart lesions. *Pediatr Cardiol* 1995;16:247–250.

Chondrodystrophica Myotonia

See Schwartz-Jampel syndrome

Chondroectodermal Dysplasia

See Ellis-van Creveld syndrome

Christmas Disease

See Hemophilia B

Chronic Granulomatous Disease

MIM #: 306400

Chronic granulomatous disease describes a genetically heterogeneous group of disorders in which neutrophils are unable to deliver activated oxygen to the phagocytic vacuole. Thus, neutrophils can phagocytize but cannot kill fungi or catalase negative bacteria, resulting in severe fungal or bacterial infections in a variety of organs and tissues. Chronic infections can lead to the formation of noncaseating granulomas. Most defects are X-linked and due to abnormalities of each of the four polypeptides required for nicotinamide adenine dinucleotide phosphate (NADPH) oxidase activity. Rare forms are autosomal recessive. One X-linked disease is due to defects in the gene *CYBB*, encoding p91-phox. Cytochrome $b(-245)$ is a component of phagocytic NADPH oxidase, which generates large amounts of superoxide and other oxidants upon activation by a variety of inflammatory stimuli. Cytochrome $b(-245)$ is a heterodimer of p91-phox beta polypeptide and a smaller phox (for phagocytic oxidase) alpha peptide. Very rarely, cases of this disease present for the first time in previously healthy older adults.

HEENT/AIRWAY: Ulcerative stomatitis and gingivitis.

CHEST: There may be sequelae of chronic pulmonary infections with granulomatous infiltration or fibrosis.

ORTHOPEDIC: Osteomyelitis.

GI/GU: There may be granulomas throughout the gastrointestinal tract leading to local complications. Esophageal strictures. There may be splenic infections and perirectal and perianal abscesses and fistulae. There may be granulomatous ureteral strictures, or bladder involvement with urinary obstruction. Tubo-ovarian abscesses may develop in female patients.

OTHER: May have cutaneous granulomas, lymphadenitis, lymphadenopathy. Discoid lupus in carriers or in adults with mild disease. Large deletions may also affect the Kell red blood cell blood group system, which lies adjacent on the X chromosome.

MISCELLANEOUS: The disease has been treated with gamma-interferon and bone marrow transplantation.

ANESTHETIC CONSIDERATIONS
Good aseptic technique is of particular importance. Chronic use of aminoglycosides or amphotericin may affect renal function. Potential sites of infection (e.g., wound, catheter)

must be monitored carefully postoperatively. Double-lumen endobronchial tubes may be of use in thoracic surgery to minimize spillage of infectious materials from one lung to the other. Granulomatous lesions of the gastrointestinal tract may involve the gastroesophageal sphincter or may delay gastric emptying. For this reason, rapid sequence induction of anesthesia has been recommended (2). A small number of patients may have abnormalities in the Kell red blood cell blood group system. This could delay the availability of blood or limit the amount of blood that can be made available.

Bibliography:

1. Segal BH, Leto TL, Gallin JI, et al. Genetic, biochemical, and clinical features of chronic granulomatous disease. *Medicine (Baltimore)* 2000;79:170–200.
2. Wall RT, Buzzanell CA, Epstein TA, et al. Anesthetic considerations in patients with chronic granulomatous disease. *J Clin Anesth* 1993;2: 306–311.
3. Babior BM, Woodman RC. Chronic granulomatous disease. *Semin Hematol* 1991;27:247–259.

Citrullinemia

See Argininosuccinic acid synthetase deficiency

Citrullinuria

See Argininosuccinic acid synthetase deficiency

Cleidocranial Dysostosis

SYNONYM: Cleidocranial dysplasia

MIM #: 119600

This autosomal dominant disorder is characterized by dysplasia of osseous and dental tissue. The most frequent defects are seen in the clavicle and the cranium, hence the name "cleidocranial." There is wide variability in the clinical expression of this syndrome. The gene responsible for this disorder encodes transcription factor CBFA1, and the gene is also known as *Runx2. Runx2* (homologous to the "runt domain") is an osteoblast-specific transcription factor. It is the osteogenic "master switch" and is a regulator of osteoblast differentiation. One third of patients represent a new mutation.

HEENT/AIRWAY: Brachycephaly, thick calvarium, Delayed and poor calcification of cranial sutures, wormian bones. Frontal, parietal and occipital bossing. Very delayed closure of the fontanelles, may be open in adults. Midfacial hypoplasia. Hypoplastic sinuses and mastoid air cells. Hypertelorism. May have hearing loss. Low nasal bridge. High-arched palate, may have cleft palate. Dental abnormalities, including delayed eruption, enamel hypoplasia, root abnormalities, dental caries. May have micrognathia. May have abnormality of temporomandibular joint. Hypoplastic hyoid bone.

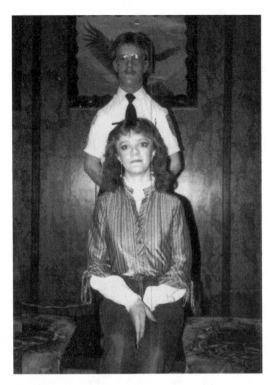

Cleidocranial dysostosis. FIG. 1. This brother and sister have cleidocranial dysostosis. Note the narrow upper chest and sloping shoulders.

CHEST: Small, narrow thoracic cage with short ribs. Cervical ribs. Aplastic or hypoplastic clavicles. Neonatal respiratory distress.

CARDIOVASCULAR: May have subclavian artery damage from the clavicular anomaly.

NEUROMUSCULAR: Intelligence is usually normal. Syringomyelia. Large foramen magnum.

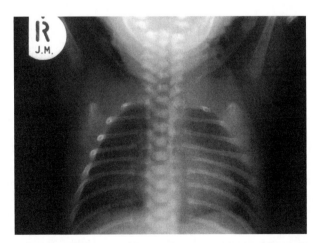

Cleidocranial dysostosis. FIG. 2. Chest radiograph of a child with cleidocranial dysostosis. Note the absent clavicles. (Courtesy of Dr. Philip A. Henning, Neonatal Service, Tygerberg Children's Hospital, Cape Town, South Africa.)

ORTHOPEDIC: Short stature. Hypoplastic or aplastic clavicles. May have hypoplastic phalanges. Delayed calcification of pubic bone with wide symphysis pubis. Hypoplastic iliac bones, narrow pelvis. May have coxa vara. Vertebral abnormalities, scoliosis, kyphosis, spondylosis, spondylolisthesis. Bones susceptible to fracture.

MISCELLANEOUS: A Neanderthal skull with features of cleidocranial dysostosis has been described (4). It has also been postulated that Thersites, a character in the *Iliad*, had this disorder (1).

ANESTHETIC CONSIDERATIONS
Hypoplasia or aplasia of the clavicles alters the landmarks for insertion of a subclavian intravenous catheter. Dental abnormalities should be documented preoperatively. Root abnormalities or severe dental caries predispose the teeth to loss during direct laryngoscopy. A single patient with limited mouth opening secondary to temporomandibular joint deformity has been reported. Patients should be carefully positioned and padded because bones are fragile and susceptible to fracture. Given the single reported case of an adult with arm ischemia from impingement of the subclavian artery, documentation of arm pulses after positioning is encouraged. A narrow thoracic cage can lead to respiratory distress in early infancy.

Bibliography:
1. Altschuler EL. Cleidocranial dysostosis and the unity of Homeric epics: an essay. *Clin Orthop Relat Res* 2001;(383):286–289.
2. Chitayat D, Hodgkinson KA, Azouz EM. Intrafamilial variability in cleidocranial dysplasia: a three generation family. *Am J Med Genet* 1992;42:298–303.
3. Dore DD, MacEwen GD, Boulos MI. Cleidocranial dysostosis and syringomyelia: review of the literature and case report. *Clin Orthop* 1987;214:229–234.
4. Grieg DM. Neanderthal skull presenting features of cleidocranial dysostosis and other peculiarities. *Edinburgh Med J* 1933;40:407.

Cleidocranial Dysplasia

See Cleidocranial dysostosis

Clouston Syndrome

MIM #: 129500

This autosomal dominant hidrotic ectodermal dysplasia consists of nail dysplasia, palmar and plantar dyskeratosis, and alopecia. At least one form of hidrotic ectodermal dysplasia is due to mutations in the gene *GJB6* (gap junction protein, beta-6) which encodes a connexin. Connexins are the protein subunits for gap junctions. Unlike forms of hypohidrotic ectodermal dysplasia, patients with hidrotic ectodermal dysplasia have normal sweat and sebaceous gland function.

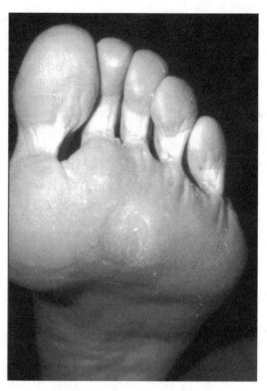

Clouston syndrome. Dyskeratosis on the sole in Clouston syndrome. (Courtesy of Dr. Neil Prose, Department of Dermatology, Duke University.)

HEENT/AIRWAY: Thick skull. Hypoplastic or absent eyebrows and eyelashes, strabismus. May have cataracts or photophobia. Teeth are normal.

NEUROMUSCULAR: May have mental retardation.

ORTHOPEDIC: May have short stature. Nail dysplasia. May have clubbing of the fingers.

OTHER: Thickened palmar and plantar dyskeratosis. Hair hypoplasia. Alopecia or fine, brittle hair. Alopecia may be more total in females. Hyperpigmentation over joints and intertriginous areas. Sweat production is normal. Severe nail changes with onychodystrophy, onycholysis, nail hypoplasia and thick, discolored nails.

ANESTHETIC CONSIDERATIONS
Dental abnormalities, typical of other ectodermal dysplasias, are not seen in Clouston syndrome. Sweat production is normal, so perioperative thermoregulation is maintained. Patients with photophobia may be sensitive to bright operating room lights.

Bibliography:
1. Tan E, Tan YK. What syndrome is this? Hidrotic ectodermal dysplasia (Clouston syndrome). *Pediatr Dermatol* 2000;17:65–67.
2. Hassed SJ, Kincannon JM, Arnold GL. Clouston syndrome: an ectodermal dysplasia without significant dental findings. *Am J Med Genet* 1996;61:274–276.

Cloverleaf Skull

See Kleeblattschaedel

Cobalamin (A–G) Deficiency

MIM #: 236270, 250940, 251100, 251110, 277380, 277400, 277410

There are seven distinct autosomal recessive abnormalities that result in defective intracellular metabolism of cobalamin. The cobalamins (Cbl) are cobalt-containing organometallic substances. The basic structure of the cobalamins is vitamin B_{12}. Once absorbed from the gastrointestinal tract and transported to the cells [complexed with transcobalamin II (see later, Transcobalamin II deficiency)], cells endocytose the complexes, dissociate the transcobalamin II, and either methylate cobalamin in the cytoplasm (forming Me Cbl, required for the enzyme methylmalonyl CoA mutase) or adenosylate it in the mitochondria (forming Ado Cbl, required for N-5-methyltetrahydrofolate methyltransferase). Cobalamin A and B defects lead to abnormal adenosylcobalamin synthesis and result in methylmalonic acidemia (see later). Treatment with cobalamin (cyanocobalamin or hydroxocobalamin) results in improvement for most cobalamin A patients and some cobalamin B patients. Cobalamin E and G abnormalities affect only Me Cbl, and produce homocystinuria with hypomethioninemia (see later). Treatment with cobalamin corrects the clinical problem. Cobalamin C, D, and F abnormalities affect the synthesis of both Me Cbl and Ado Cbl. Patients with cobalamin C and D mutations have methylmalonic aciduria and homocystinuria. Patients with cobalamin C defects tend to be more severely affected. Cobalamin F defects result in mild methylmalonic acidemia.

OTHER: In general, disorders affecting only Ado Cbl produce metabolic ketoacidosis in young infants. Me Cbl defects present as failure to thrive and megaloblastic changes. Disorders affecting both forms result in a variable combination of the two phenotypes.

MISCELLANEOUS: Cobalamin was first described as "extrinsic factor," the complement to "intrinsic factor," which is the transport factor necessary for the absorption of vitamin B_{12} in the distal ileum. The discovery of this factor won a Nobel prize.

ANESTHETIC CONSIDERATIONS
See under the specific type of amino acid disorder caused, methylmalonic acidemia or homocystinuria.

Bibliography:
1. Rosenblatt DS, Whitehead VM. Cobalamin and folate deficiency: acquired and hereditary disorders in children. *Semin Hematol* 1999;36: 19–34.
2. Kano Y, Sakamoto S, Miura Y, et al. Disorders of cobalamin metabolism. *Clin Rev Oncol Hematol* 1985;3:1–34.
3. Matthews DM, Linnell JC. Cobalamin deficiency and related disorders in infancy and childhood. *Eur J Pediatr* 1982;138:6–16.

Cocaine

See Fetal cocaine effect

Cockayne Syndrome

MIM #: 216400

This autosomal recessive disease has multisystem findings, including precocious senile-like changes, growth failure, mental retardation, accelerated atherosclerosis, retinal degeneration, optic atrophy, sensorineural hearing loss, and photosensitivity dermatitis. Cockayne syndrome has been divided into an early-onset form (congenital) and a late-onset form (with onset in early childhood). The pathogenesis of both forms appears to be similar. There is decreased ability to repair ultraviolet light-induced damage to DNA strands. The two types of the disorder are due to mutations in the DNA repair genes *ERCC8* or *ERCC6*. Patients with the early-onset form of Cockayne syndrome usually die in childhood, those with the late-onset form die in their early teens. DNA repair mechanisms are abnormal in four other inherited diseases: ataxia-telangiectasia, Fanconi anemia, Bloom syndrome, and xeroderma pigmentosum.

HEENT/AIRWAY: Microcephaly, thick calvarium. Gaunt face (lacking subcutaneous fat) with a long, slender nose. Retinal degeneration, cataracts, optic atrophy, nystagmus, miotic pupils. Decreased lacrimation. Sensorineural hearing loss. Dental abnormalities include delayed eruption, missing teeth, hypoplastic teeth, dental caries, malocclusion. Small mandible.

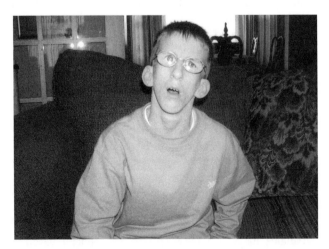

Cockayne syndrome. Typical facies in a young man with Cockayne syndrome.

CHEST: Pneumonia is common, and often is a contributing cause of death.

CARDIOVASCULAR: Premature hypertension, coronary atherosclerosis and peripheral vascular disease. May have cardiac arrhythmias.

NEUROMUSCULAR: Progressive mental retardation. Intracranial calcifications, especially in the basal ganglia, resulting in unsteady gait, ataxia, tremor, incoordination, dysarthric speech. Muscle atrophy. May have increased ventricular size, cerebral atrophy, demyelination of subcortical white matter, peripheral neuropathy. Seizures may develop. May have accelerated cerebral atherosclerosis.

ORTHOPEDIC: Growth failure. Relatively short trunk such that the limbs appear inappropriately long. Limited joint mobility with formation of flexion contractures. Vertebral abnormalities, kyphosis. Osteoporosis may develop.

GI/GU: Gastroesophageal reflux. Progressive renal disease in some. May have hepatomegaly, splenomegaly.

OTHER: Photosensitivity dermatitis. Thin, dry skin. Thin, dry, prematurely gray hair. Absence of subcutaneous fat. Impaired sweat production. Cool hands and feet, which sometimes appear cyanotic. Rare basal cell carcinomas.

MISCELLANEOUS: Edward Cockayne, of the Great Ormond Street Hospital, London, was a pioneer in the study of genetic diseases and the skin. As a hobby, he developed a very large collection of butterflies and moths and was in fact awarded the Order of the British Empire for his services to entomology.

ANESTHETIC CONSIDERATIONS

A small mandible and normal (for age) sized teeth has made direct laryngoscopy difficult (5, 7). Fiberoptic intubation using a laryngeal mask has been successful (5). The trachea may be smaller than expected and may require a smaller-than-expected endotracheal tube (4, 7). Gastroesophageal reflux is common, and patients may be at increased risk for perioperative aspiration. However, mask inductions and laryngeal mask airways have been used successfully (4, 5). Dental abnormalities should be documented before surgery. Decreased lacrimation increases the risk of corneal abrasion, and the eyes should be adequately protected. Note that the pupils may be miotic at baseline. Impaired sweat production may lead to perioperative hyperthermia. The hands may be cool and cyanotic-appearing, even when there is no arterial desaturation. Patients must be carefully positioned secondary to contractures. Contractures may make vascular access more challenging.

Patients may have hypertension or peripheral vascular disease. Accelerated coronary atherosclerosis and cardiac arrhythmias are of particular concern. Consideration should be given to evaluating for ischemic cardiac disease. A report suggested that nifedipine-induced hypotension may have caused transient cerebral ischemia, possibly related to cerebral atherosclerotic disease (3).

Patients with significant renal disease need careful titration of intraoperative fluids and consideration of the mode of metabolism in choosing anesthetic drugs. Chronic use of anticonvulsant medication alters the metabolism of some anesthetic drugs. Succinylcholine induced hyperkalemia has not been reported, but is a potential concern in patients with muscle atrophy or advanced renal disease.

Bibliography:

1. Gozal Y, Gozal D, Galili D, et al. Cockayne syndrome with premature aging: anesthetic implications. *Am J Anesth* 2000;27:149–150.
2. Rapin I, Lindenbaum Y, Dickson DW, et al. Cockayne syndrome and xeroderma pigmentosum. *Neurology* 2000;55:1442–1449.
3. Sasaki R, Hirota K, Masuda A. Nifedipine-induced transient cerebral ischaemia in a child with Cockayne syndrome [Letter]. *Anaesthesia* 1997;52:1236.
4. Woolridge WJ, Dearlove OR, Khan AA. Anaesthesia for Cockayne syndrome: three case reports. *Anaesthesia* 1996;51:478–481.
5. Woolridge WJ, Dearlove OR. Anaesthesia for Cockayne's syndrome: contemporary solutions to an old problem. *Anaesthesia* 1994;4:191–195.
6. Nance MA, Berry SA. Cockayne syndrome: review of 140 cases. *Am J Med Genet* 1992;42:68–84.
7. Cook S. Cockayne syndrome: another cause of difficult intubation. *Anaesthesia* 1982;37:1104–1107.

Coenzyme Q-cytochrome *c* Reductase Deficiency

See Complex III deficiency

Coffin-Lowry Syndrome

MIM #: 303600

This X-linked dominant disorder is characterized by mental retardation, short stature, coarse facies, down-slanting palpebral fissures, a bulbous nose, and puffy hands with tapering fingers. This disorder is caused by mutations in the *RSK2* (ribosomal S6 kinase-2) gene. The RSK genes encode growth factor-regulated serine-threonine kinases. Female heterozygotes have more mild manifestations.

HEENT/AIRWAY: May have microcephaly, thick calvarium, delayed closure of anterior fontanelle. Hypoplastic sinuses. Coarse facies, which worsen with age. Midfacial hypoplasia. Down-slanting palpebral fissures, hypertelorism. Heavy arched eyebrows. Large, protuberant ears. May have sensorineural hearing loss. Short, broad, bulbous nose, anteverted nares. Wide mouth, thick lower lip. Dental abnormalities including hypoplastic teeth, malocclusion, premature loss, and large medial incisors.

CHEST: Short bifid sternum. Pectus carinatum or excavatum.

CARDIOVASCULAR: May have mitral regurgitation. May have cardiomyopathy.

NEUROMUSCULAR: Severe mental retardation. Severe speech delay—may never acquire speech. Hypotonia. May have dilated lateral ventricles, seizures. May have calcification of the ligamentum flavum, with resultant narrowing of the spinal canal and subsequent radiculopathy. Can have nonepileptic drop attacks, with features of cataplexy and hyperekplexia.

ORTHOPEDIC: Short stature. Puffy hands with tapering fingers. Small fingernails. "Drumstick" terminal phalanges. May have simian creases. Flat feet. Hypermobile joints. Vertebral dysplasia. Cervical lordosis. Thoracolumbar kyphoscoliosis. Characteristic stooped posture.

GI/GU: Inguinal hernia. Rectal or uterine prolapse.

OTHER: Cutis marmorata. Dependent acrocyanosis.

MISCELLANEOUS: This syndrome was described by Coffin et al. in 1966, and then by Lowry et al. in 1971. These were later recognized as the same syndrome.

ANESTHETIC CONSIDERATIONS
Dental abnormalities should be documented preoperatively. Patients are prone to premature tooth loss. Patients must be carefully positioned secondary to hypermobile joints. Chronic use of anticonvulsant medications may alter the metabolism of some anesthetic drugs. Patients with mitral regurgitation need perioperative antibiotic prophylaxis as indicated.

Calcification of the ligamentum flavum has been reported, with resultant narrowing of the spinal canal and subsequent radiculopathy. It may be wise to avoid regional anesthesia if there is evidence of a radiculopathy. If regional anesthesia is undertaken, note that there may be technical difficulties finding the epidural or subarachnoid space, and that a decreased amount of drug may be needed in the narrowed subarachnoid space.

Bibliography:

1. Hanauer A, Young ID. Coffin-Lowry syndrome: clinical and molecular features. *J Med Genet* 2002;39:705–713.
2. Hunter AG. Coffin-Lowry syndrome: a 20-year follow-up and review of long-term outcomes. *Am J Med Genet* 2002;111:345–355.
3. Gilgenkrautz S, Mujica P, Gruet P, et al. Coffin-Lowry syndrome: a multicenter study. *Clin Genet* 1988;34:230–245.

Coffin-Siris Syndrome

MIM #: 135900

This possibly autosomal recessive syndrome is characterized by mental retardation, coarse facies, hypoplastic to absent fifth fingers, and hypoplastic toenails. Most affected individuals are females. Similar nail changes have been observed in the fetal hydantoin syndrome.

HEENT/AIRWAY: Microcephaly. Coarse facies. Thick eyebrows, long eyelashes. May have hypotelorism, ptosis, strabismus, nystagmus. May have hearing loss. Preauricular skin tag. Depressed nasal bridge, broad nose, anteverted nares. Long philtrum. Wide mouth, thick lips, macroglossia. May have choanal atresia, cleft palate. Delayed dentition. Short neck.

CHEST: Recurrent upper and lower respiratory tract infections are common. May have diaphragmatic hernia.

CARDIOVASCULAR: May have a congenital cardiac defect, including patent ductus arteriosus, atrial septal defect, ventricular septal defect, tetralogy of Fallot.

NEUROMUSCULAR: Mental retardation. Speech delay. May exhibit aggressive behavior. Hypotonia. May have agenesis of the corpus callosum, Dandy-Walker malformation. Seizures.

ORTHOPEDIC: Short stature. Hypoplastic or absent digits, especially the fifth finger and fifth toe. Hypoplastic toenails. Clinodactyly. Hypermobility of joints. Radial dislocation at the elbow. Coxa valga. May have vertebral abnormalities. Sacral dimple.

GI/GU: May have inguinal or umbilical hernias, intussusception, malrotation of the gut, gastric outlet obstruction. May have renal anomalies including hydronephrosis, ureteral stenosis, microureter, ectopic kidney. Cryptorchidism, absent uterus.

OTHER: Sparse scalp hair with generalized hirsutism. Cutis marmorata. One patient has been reported in whom recurrent hypoglycemia developed.

ANESTHETIC CONSIDERATIONS
A smooth induction of anesthesia may be difficult in patients with aggressive behavioral characteristics. It has been suggested that the difficulty of endotracheal intubation increases with age. Dysmorphic features are said to worsen with aging, and a patient has been reported who underwent uncomplicated anesthesia as a child but whose trachea could not be successfully intubated as a 45-year-old (3). Upper and lower respiratory tract infections are common in these patients. Acutely, this may lead to cancellation of an anesthetic. Chronically, this may indicate the presence of residual lung disease in patients, with subsequent increased risk of postoperative pulmonary complications. Choanal atresia, if present, precludes the use of a nasal airway or a nasogastric tube. Patients must be carefully positioned secondary to hypermobility of the joints. Consider preoperative evaluation of renal function in patients with a history of renal abnormalities which predispose to

renal insufficiency. Patients with congenital cardiac disease require perioperative antibiotic prophylaxis as indicated.

One patient has been reported who had recurrent hypoglycemia. The cause of the hypoglycemia is unknown. The possibility of perioperative hypoglycemia should be kept in mind, particularly during a general anesthetic.

Bibliography:
1. Shirakami G, Tazuke-Nishimura M, Hirakata H, et al. Anesthesia for a pediatric patient with Coffin-Siris syndrome [Japanese]. *Masui* 2005;54:42–45.
2. Silvani P, Camporesi A, Zoia E, et al. Anesthetic management of a child with Coffin-Siris syndrome [Letter]. *Paediatr Anaesth* 2004;14:698–699.
3. Dimaculangan DP, Lokhandwala BS, Wlody DJ, et al. Difficult airway in a patient with Coffin-Siris syndrome. *Anesth Analg* 2001;92:554–555.
4. Imaizumi K, Nakamura M, Masuno M, et al. Hypoglycemia in Coffin-Siris syndrome. *Am J Med Genet* 1995;59:49–50.
5. Swillen A, Glorieux N, Peeters M, et al. The Coffin-Siris syndrome: data on mental development, language, behavior and social skills in children. *Clin Genet* 1995;48:177–182.
6. deJong G, Nelson MM. Choanal atresia in two unrelated patients with the Coffin-Siris syndrome. *Clin Genet* 1992;42:320–322.
7. Levy P, Baraitser M. Coffin-Siris syndrome. *J Med Genet* 1991;28: 338–341.

COFS Syndrome

See Cerebrooculofacioskeletal syndrome

Cohen Syndrome

MIM #: 216550

This autosomal recessive disorder is distinguished by mental retardation, hypotonia, muscle weakness, obesity, and prominent upper central incisors. The disorder is due to abnormalities in the gene *COH1*. The exact role of the large, complex protein product of this gene is unknown, but it may have to do with intracellular protein transport.

HEENT/AIRWAY: Microcephaly. Malar hypoplasia, down-slanting palpebral fissures. Poor vision, retinal anomalies, strabismus. May have microphthalmia, coloboma. Large ears. High nasal bridge. Short philtrum. Prominent upper central incisors, open mouth. High-arched palate. Mild micrognathia. May have increased susceptibility to oral cavity infections.

CARDIOVASCULAR: May have a cardiac anomaly, especially mitral valve prolapse.

NEUROMUSCULAR: Mental retardation, hypotonia and muscle weakness. Motor delay. Cheerful disposition. May have seizures. Autistic-like behavioral problems.

ORTHOPEDIC: May have short stature. Narrow hands and feet, long fingers and toes. Simian creases. Joint hypermobility. Genu valgus, cubitus valgus. Lumbar lordosis, scoliosis. Narrow feet.

GI/GU: May have hiatal hernia with gastroesophageal reflux. May have periureteral obstruction.

OTHER: Central obesity starting in childhood. May have intermittent neutropenia. Delayed puberty.

ANESTHETIC CONSIDERATIONS
The prominent upper central incisors must be carefully avoided during laryngoscopy. Difficult laryngoscopy and intubation has been reported in an adult (1). Venous access and identification of landmarks for regional anesthesia may be difficult secondary to obesity. Obesity may result in desaturation with induction of anesthesia because of increased airway closure and decreased functional residual capacity. Obesity is also a risk factor for perioperative aspiration. Patients must be carefully positioned intraoperatively secondary to hyperextensibility of the joints. Chronic use of anticonvulsant medications may affect the metabolism of some anesthetic drugs. Patients with hypotonia and muscle weakness might be at risk for hyperkalemia after the administration of succinylcholine. Although patients may have intermittent neutropenia, they do not appear to have an increased risk of infection. Patients with cardiac anomalies should receive perioperative prophylactic antibiotics as indicated.

Bibliography:
1. Meng L, Quinlan JJ, Sullivan E. The anesthetic management of a patient with Cohen syndrome. *Anesth Analg* 2004;99:697–698.
2. Orbach-Zinger S, Kaufman E, Donchin Y, et al. Between Scylla and Charybdis: a bleomycin-exposed patient with Cohen syndrome. *Acta Anaesthesiol Scand* 2003;47:1047–1049.
3. Kivitie-Kallio S, Norio R. Cohen syndrome: essential features, natural history, and heterogeneity. *Am J Med Genet* 2001;102:125–135.

Collodion Membranes

Included in Ichthyosis

Complex I Deficiency

SYNONYM: NADH-coenzyme Q reductase deficiency; NADH-ubiquinone oxidoreductase deficiency

MIM #: 252010

There are a total of five protein complexes that make up the mitochondrial electron transport chain. Complex I has at least 36 polypeptide subunits that are encoded by nuclear DNA and 7 that are encoded by mitochondrial DNA. Thus, both nuclear and mitochondrial gene defects can lead to defects in complex I. Electrons are transferred independently by complexes I and II to coenzyme Q, and then sequentially to complexes III and IV. Complex V converts adenosine diphosphate (ADP) to ATP. Complex I is capable of utilizing both pyruvate (when complexed to malate) and glutamate as carbon sources. Complex II can only utilize succinate. Complex I deficiency is the most common oxidative-phosphorylation enzymatic defect. The phenotype is variable.

HEENT: Leber hereditary optic atrophy (see later).

CHEST: Neonatal respiratory distress.

CARDIOVASCULAR: Cardiomyopathy, biventricular hypertrophy.

NEUROMUSCULAR: Encephalopathy, seizures. Myopathy, with generalized muscle weakness and muscle wasting. Fatigue to exercise, fasting, and ethanol. Mitochondria in muscles have abnormal morphology with inner and outer membranes arranged in whirls.

GI/GU: Hypospadias, micropenis.

OTHER: Hypoglycemia. Lactic acidemia, worse with exercise. Leigh disease (see later).

ANESTHETIC CONSIDERATIONS

Patients are at risk for perioperative respiratory failure and must be monitored closely both during and after surgery for signs of respiratory insufficiency. There is a report of three patients with Leigh disease (which may occur in complex I deficiency) in whom respiratory failure was precipitated by general anesthesia, leading to death. All three patients had preoperative respiratory abnormalities. Patients with complex I deficiency can have a cardiomyopathy, so cardiac function should be evaluated preoperatively. Patients should not undergo a protracted perioperative fast without concomitantly receiving an intravenous glucose-containing solution. Perioperative serum glucose levels should be monitored closely. Succinylcholine should be used with caution in patients with evidence of a myopathy because of the risk of hyperkalemia. Chronic use of anticonvulsant medications may alter the metabolism of some anesthetic drugs.

Although there are no clinical reports, it is reasonable to avoid the use of nitroprusside because cyanide can inhibit the electron transport chain. Although barbiturates, propofol and volatile anesthetics can inhibit mitochondrial respiration, anesthesia with each of these drugs has been used without any complications in patients with mitochondrial defects. Patients with Complex I deficiency have been shown to be very sensitive to sevoflurane (1, 3), but sevoflurane has been used successfully. Propofol has been used successfully as the primary anesthetic (4), although some would avoid it in these patients.

Bibliography:

1. Lee TB, Sedensky MM, Morgan PG. Intraoperative and complications in patients with mitochondrial disease [Abstract]. *Anesthesiology* 2005;103: A1359.
2. Kuhnick H, Wunder C, Roewer N. Anaesthetic considerations for a 2-month-old infant with suspected complex I respiratory chain disease. *Paediatr Anaesth* 2003;13:83–85.
3. Morgan PG, Hoppel CL, Sedensky MM. Mitochondrial defects and anesthetic sensitivity. *Anesthesiology* 2002;96:1268–1270.
4. Cheam EWS, Cheam LAH. Anesthesia for a child with complex I respiratory chain enzyme deficiency. *J Clin Anesth* 1998;10:524–527.
5. Keyes MA, Van de Wiele B, Stead SW. Mitochondrial myopathies: an unusual cause of hypotonia in infants and children. *Paediatr Anaesth* 1996;6:329–335.

Complex II Deficiency

SYNONYM: Succinate-coenzyme Q reductase deficiency

MIM #: 252011

This autosomal recessive disorder involves one of the five protein complexes that make up the mitochondrial electron transport chain. Unlike the other four, this enzyme is coded for solely by nuclear (and not a combination of nuclear and mitochondrial) DNA. Four nuclear-encoded proteins form the complex. Electrons are transferred independently by complexes I and II to coenzyme Q, and then sequentially to complexes III and IV. Complex V converts adenosine diphosphate (ADP) to ATP. Complex I is capable of utilizing both pyruvate (when complexed to malate) and glutamate as carbon sources. Complex II can only utilize succinate.

CARDIOVASCULAR: May have isolated hypertrophic cardiomyopathy.

NEUROMUSCULAR: Progressive encephalopathy with dementia. Myoclonic seizures.

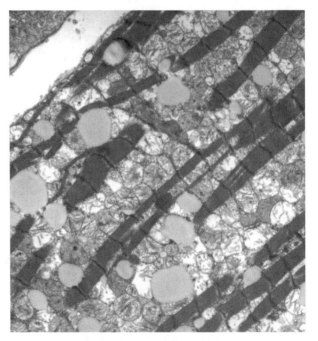

Complex II deficiency. Cardiac pathology from a 2-year-old girl with Complex II deficiency who died while awaiting a heart transplantation. This electron micrograph shows a proliferation of large abnormal mitochondria with simplified architecture of the cristae.

ORTHOPEDIC: Small stature.

GI/GU: Hepatic cirrhosis has been reported in a patient with complex II/III deficiency.

OTHER: Kearns-Sayre syndrome (see later).

ANESTHETIC CONSIDERATIONS

Patients with complex II deficiency can have a hypertrophic cardiomyopathy, so cardiac function should be evaluated preoperatively. Patients should not undergo a protracted perioperative fast without concomitantly receiving an intravenous glucose-containing solution. Perioperative serum glucose levels should be monitored closely. Succinylcholine should be used with caution in patients with evidence of a myopathy because of the risk of hyperkalemia. Chronic use of anticonvulsant medications may alter the metabolism of some anesthetic drugs.

Although there are no clinical reports, it is reasonable to avoid the use of nitroprusside because cyanide can inhibit the electron transport chain. Although barbiturates, propofol and volatile anesthetics can inhibit mitochondrial respiration, anesthesia with each of these drugs has been used without any complications in patients with mitochondrial defects. However, complex II deficiency has been implicated in the case of a child who developed metabolic acidosis from the propofol infusion syndrome (1). Hepatic disease can affect the binding and metabolism of some anesthetic drugs.

Bibliography:
1. Wolf A, Weir P, Segar P, et al. Impaired fatty acid oxidation in propofol infusion syndrome. *Lancet* 2001;357:606–607.
2. Sewell AC, Sperl W, Herwig J, et al. Cirrhosis in a child with deficiency of mitochondrial respiratory-chain succinate-cytochrome c-oxidoreductase [Letter]. *J Pediatr* 1997;131:166–167.
3. Keyes MA, Van de Wiele B, Stead SW. Mitochondrial myopathies: an unusual cause of hypotonia in infants and children. *Paediatr Anaesth* 1996;6:329–335.
4. Arpa J, Campos Y, Gutierrez-Molina M, et al. Benign mitochondrial myopathy with decreased succinate cytochrome C reductase activity. *Acta Neurol Scand* 1994;90:281–284.

Complex III Deficiency

SYNONYM: Coenzyme Q-cytochrome *c* reductase deficiency; Ubiquinone-cytochrome *c* oxidoreductase deficiency

MIM #: 516020

Complex III includes mitochondrial cytochrome *b*, and is one of five protein complexes that make up the mitochondrial electron transport chain. This is the second enzyme in the sequence, and catalyzes the transfer of electrons from reduced coenzyme Q10 to cytochrome *c*. The energy generated is used to translocate protons from the inside to the outside of the mitochondrial inner membrane. This disorder may be inherited as a mitochondrial gene defect, and thus it can be maternally transmitted. Onset of symptoms is in the second and third decades.

HEENT/AIRWAY: External ophthalmoplegia or other ocular myopathy, ptosis, sudden swollen optic disc, Leber hereditary optic atrophy (see later) with sudden central field defect.

CARDIOVASCULAR: Cardiomyopathy with evidence of abnormal accumulations of mitochondria.

NEUROMUSCULAR: Headaches. Myopathy, easy fatigability, areflexia, dementia.

GI/GU: Dysphagia. Hepatic cirrhosis has been reported in a patient with complex II/III deficiency.

ANESTHETIC CONSIDERATIONS

Patients with complex III deficiency can have a cardiomyopathy, so cardiac function should be evaluated preoperatively. Patients should not undergo a protracted perioperative fast without concomitantly receiving an intravenous glucose-containing solution. Perioperative serum glucose levels should be monitored closely. Patients with significant dysphagia are at increased risk for perioperative aspiration. Succinylcholine should be used with caution in patients with evidence of a myopathy because of the risk of hyperkalemic arrest.

Although there are no clinical reports, it is reasonable to avoid the use of nitroprusside because cyanide can inhibit the electron transport chain. Although barbiturates, propofol and volatile anesthetics can inhibit mitochondrial respiration, anesthesia with each of these drugs has been used without any complications in patients with mitochondrial defects. Hepatic disease can affect the binding and metabolism of some anesthetic drugs.

Bibliography:
1. Wallace JJ, Perndt H, Skinner M. Anaesthesia and mitochondrial disease. *Paediatr Anaesth* 1998;8:249–254.
2. Sewell AC, Sperl W, Herwig J, et al. Cirrhosis in a child with deficiency of mitochondrial respiratory-chain succinate-cytochrome c-oxidoreductase [Letter]. *J Pediatr* 1997;131:166–167.
3. Keyes MA, Van de Wiele B, Stead SW. Mitochondrial myopathies: an unusual cause of hypotonia in infants and children. *Paediatr Anaesth* 1996;6:329–335.

Complex IV Deficiency

SYNONYM: Cytochrome *c* oxidase deficiency

MIM #: 220110

Complex IV is one of five protein complexes that make up the mitochondrial electron transport chain. Electrons are transferred independently by complexes I and II to coenzyme Q, and then sequentially to complexes III and IV. Complex IV collects electrons from cytochrome *c* and transfers them to oxygen to produce water. Complex V converts adenosine diphosphate (ADP) to ATP. There are said to be up to nine distinct clinical presentations of this disorder; thus, the clinical findings given here are inclusive, and will not all be seen in every patient. This complex is encoded by both nuclear and mitochondrial DNA, and therefore some cases are inherited as a mitochondrial gene defect (i.e., they are maternally transmitted). Most cases, however, are due to nuclear gene mutations. In addition, complex IV deficiency can occur secondarily in diseases such as Menkes kinky hair syndrome (see later). It can present in the neonate as Fanconi syndrome, Leber hereditary optic atrophy, or Leigh disease (see later for each).

HEENT/AIRWAY: Leber hereditary optic atrophy (see later) with sudden central visual loss, swollen optic disc. Sensorineural hearing loss.

CHEST: Respiratory failure due to muscle weakness.

CARDIOVASCULAR: Hypertrophic cardiomyopathy (*COX10* mitochondrial gene defect only).

NEUROMUSCULAR: Headaches. Fatal neonatal myopathy, hypotonia, hyporeflexia. Ataxia. Delayed development. Seizures. Abnormal mitochondria in muscles.

GI/GU: Early and fatal liver dysfunction has been reported. Neonatal renal dysfunction. Fanconi syndrome (see later).

OTHER: Lactic acidosis. Failure to thrive. Anemia (*COX10* mitochondrial gene defect only). Leigh disease.

ANESTHETIC CONSIDERATIONS
Patients are at risk for perioperative respiratory failure and must be monitored closely both during and after surgery for signs of respiratory insufficiency. There is a report of three patients with Leigh disease (which may occur in complex IV deficiency) in whom respiratory failure was precipitated by general anesthesia, leading to death. All three patients had preoperative respiratory abnormalities. Patients with the *COX10* mitochondrial gene defect can have a cardiomyopathy, so cardiac function should be evaluated preoperatively. Patients should not undergo a protracted perioperative fast without concomitantly receiving an intravenous glucose-containing solution. Perioperative serum glucose levels should be monitored closely. Succinylcholine should be used with caution in patients with evidence of a myopathy because of the risk of hyperkalemia.

Although there are no clinical reports, it is reasonable to avoid the use of nitroprusside because cyanide can inhibit the electron transport chain. Although barbiturates, propofol and volatile anesthetics can inhibit mitochondrial respiration, anesthesia with each of these drugs has been used without any complications in patients with mitochondrial defects. Hepatic disease can affect the binding and metabolism of some anesthetic drugs. Careful attention must be paid to intravascular volume, electrolyte, and acid–base status in patients with Fanconi syndrome.

Bibliography:
1. Wallace JJ, Perndt H, Skinner M. Anaesthesia and mitochondrial disease. *Paediatr Anaesth* 1998;8:249–254.
2. Keyes MA, Van de Wiele B, Stead SW. Mitochondrial myopathies: an unusual cause of hypotonia in infants and children. *Paediatr Anaesth* 1996;6:329–335.

Complex V Deficiency

SYNONYM: ATP synthetase deficiency

MIM #: 516060

There are a total of five protein complexes that make up the mitochondrial electron transport chain. Electrons are transferred independently by complexes I and II to coenzyme Q, and then sequentially to complexes III, and IV. Complex V converts adenosine diphosphate (ADP) to ATP. Complex V has 10–16 polypeptide subunits encoded by nuclear DNA and 2 polypeptide subunits encoded by mitochondrial DNA. Mitochondrial, autosomal recessive, and X-linked forms have been described. Specific mutations can present as Leber hereditary optic atrophy, NARP syndrome, or Leigh disease (see later for each).

HEENT/AIRWAY: Retinitis pigmentosa, nystagmus and other abnormalities in eye movements, Leber hereditary optic atrophy (see later) with sudden central field defect, sluggish pupils, blindness.

CHEST: Hyperventilation, dyspnea, Cheyne-Stokes respirations, respiratory failure.

CARDIOVASCULAR: Hypertrophic cardiomyopathy.

NEUROMUSCULAR: Mental retardation. Seizures, apnea, ataxia, hypotonia, tremor, areflexia, spastic quadriplegia, chorea. Neurodegenerative disease of brainstem and basal ganglia, intermittent coma.

GI/GU: Dysphagia.

OTHER: Intermittent lactic acidosis. Leigh disease.

MISCELLANEOUS: Accumulation of a subunit of ATP synthase has been found very early in the development of neurofibrillatory degeneration in Alzheimer disease.

ANESTHETIC CONSIDERATIONS
Patients are at risk for perioperative respiratory failure and must be monitored closely both during and after surgery for signs of respiratory insufficiency. There is a report of three patients with Leigh disease (which may occur in complex V deficiency) in whom respiratory failure was precipitated by general anesthesia, leading to death. All three patients had preoperative respiratory abnormalities.

Also, acute respiratory compromise has been reported in two children who received chloral hydrate for a radiologic procedure. Both had a history of apnea and gagging. Patients with complex V deficiency can have a hypertrophic cardiomyopathy, so cardiac function should be evaluated preoperatively.

Patients should not undergo a protracted perioperative fast without concomitantly receiving an intravenous glucose-containing solution. Perioperative serum glucose levels should be monitored closely. Patients with significant dysphagia are at increased risk for perioperative aspiration. Succinylcholine should be used with caution in patients with evidence of a myopathy because of the risk of hyperkalemia. Although there are no clinical reports, it is reasonable to avoid the use of nitroprusside because cyanide can inhibit the electron transport chain. Although barbiturates, propofol and volatile anesthetics can inhibit mitochondrial respiration, anesthesia with each of these drugs has been used without any complications in patients with mitochondrial defects.

Bibliography:

1. Keyes MA, Van de Wiele B, Stead SW. Mitochondrial myopathies: an unusual cause of hypotonia in infants and children. *Paediatr Anaesth* 1996;6:329–335.
2. Ciafaloni E, Santorelli FM, Shanske S, et al. Maternally inherited Leigh syndrome. *J Pediatr* 1993;122:419–422.

Congenital Adrenal Hyperplasia

SYNONYM: Adrenogenital syndrome. (Includes 21-hydroxylase deficiency; 11β-hydroxylase deficiency; 17α-hydroxylase deficiency; 3β-hydroxysteroid dehydrogenase deficiency)

MIM #: 201910

Congenital adrenal hyperplasia is an autosomal recessive disease resulting from a defect in one of the enzymes of cortisol biosynthesis. In approximately 95% of cases it is due to **21-hydroxylase deficiency** in the adrenal cortex. Because of the defect in cortisol synthesis, adrenocorticotropic hormone levels rise, resulting in overproduction of cortisol precursors, particularly 17-OH progesterone, which causes excessive androgen production, and results in fetal virilization. There are four clinical types: salt-wasting, simple virilizing, nonclassic, and late onset (also called attenuated, or acquired). The different types are due to different allelic mutations in the 21-hydroxylase gene.

This clinical disease can also be secondary to abnormal function of the gene for **11β-hydroxylase**, which is also an autosomal recessive defect. 11β-Hydroxylase is the final step in aldosterone synthesis. There is accumulation of 11-deoxycorticosterone, a potent salt retainer, with consequent hypertension, which differentiates it clinically from congenital adrenal hyperplasia due to 21-hydroxylase deficiency. Patients respond well to supplemental mineralocorticoids.

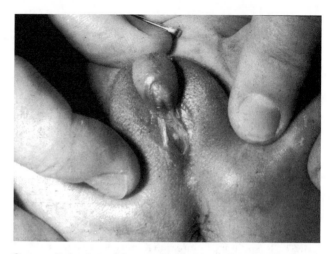

Congenital adrenal hyperplasia. Masculinized female external genitalia in a newborn girl with congenital adrenal hyperplasia. (Courtesy of Dr. Kenneth E. Greer, Department of Dermatology, University of Virginia Health System.)

An alternative cause of this syndrome is **17α-hydroxylase deficiency**. Excessive production of corticosterone and deoxycorticosterone results in hypokalemic alkalosis. There is almost complete absence of aldosterone synthesis. There is estrogen deficiency, resulting in primary amenorrhea and absent sexual maturation in girls. Although deficient 17,20-desmolase (see earlier) and 17α-hydroxylase activities can occur separately, and these were thought to represent two distinct enzymes, they are now known to reside in a single protein. The gene for this protein has been localized to chromosome 10, and at least 16 distinct mutations have been described.

Congenital adrenal hyperplasia can also be due to a deficiency of the enzyme **3β-hydroxysteroid dehydrogenase**. This variant of the disease has much less marked virilization, suggesting that the gene product has testicular as well as adrenal activity. Boys with this type can have hypospadias or even pseudohermaphroditism, and salt wasting may be severe, even fatal.

CARDIOVASCULAR: Hypertension, depending on the defect. Cortisol deficiency can contribute to poor cardiac function and diminished vascular response to catecholamines. When combined with hypovolemia this can result in shock.

ORTHOPEDIC: Untreated, it can cause early rapid growth in children, with early epiphyseal closure and eventual short stature.

GI/GU: Newborn girls have masculinization of the external genitalia, but the degree of masculinization depends on the specific enzyme deficiency. Girls have normal female internal genitalia. Boys have normal male external and internal genitalia. Untreated, it can cause penile or clitoral enlargement in boys and girls. There is also precocious adrenarche and centrally mediated precocious puberty.

OTHER: Approximately half of all patients with 21-hydroxylase deficiency have an additional defect in aldosterone synthesis (conversion of progesterone to 11-deoxycorticosterone). Some 21-hydroxylase precursors can act as mineralocorticoid antagonists, worsening the effects of aldosterone deficiency. If left untreated, this can cause severe salt wasting and death (analogous to Addisonian crisis). Adrenal medullary development is partially dependent on glucocorticoids, so patients with salt-wasting 21-hydroxylase deficiency can also be catecholamine deficient, potentially exacerbating the shock. Patients can also have hypoglycemia. A mild form can present in adults with hirsutism as the only manifestation. Patients may be hyperkalemic, which can be symptomatic. Girls are reported to have boy-like behavior in childhood, but their adult gender and sexual identity is as females.

Patients with 17α-hydroxylase deficiency have hypertension and hypokalemic alkalosis. They can also have non–life-threatening, mild symptoms of glucocorticoid deficiency.

Patients with 3β-hydroxysteroid dehydrogenase deficiency can have severe and fatal salt wasting, which may not respond to apparently appropriate adrenal replacement therapy.

MISCELLANEOUS: The Yupik Eskimos of Alaska have the highest prevalence of 21-hydroxylase deficiency in the world.

ANESTHETIC CONSIDERATIONS

Serum electrolytes, hydration status, and glucose should be followed closely perioperatively. Steroid therapy must be continued perioperatively, and patients should receive perioperative stress doses of steroids as indicated. Parenteral corticosteroids may need to be substituted for the usual oral preparations. Stress-dose hydrocortisone is 2 mg/kg every 6 hours. The acute treatment of salt-losing crises includes the administration of salt-containing intravenous fluids, intravenous mineralocorticoid (such as fludrocortisone), and intravenous cortisol. Pregnancy is possible for many women, but delivery is often via Caesarean section. A certain amount of sensitivity is required when speaking with patients or families whose children have intersex disorders.

FIGURE: See **Appendix A**

Bibliography:
1. Merke DP, Bornstein SR. Congenital adrenal hyperplasia. *Lancet* 2005;365:2125–2136.
2. Speiser PW, White PC. Congenital adrenal hyperplasia. *N Engl J Med* 2003;349:776–788.
3. Okamoto T, Minami K. Anesthesia for a girl with severe hypertension due to 11β-hydroxylase deficiency [Letter]. *Anaesth Int Care* 2003;31:596.
4. MacLean HE, Warne GL, Zajac JD. Intersex disorders: shedding light on male sexual differentiation beyond SRY. *Clin Endocrinol* 1997;46:101–108.
5. Cutler GB Jr, Laue L, Congenital adrenal hyperplasia due to 21-hydroxylase deficiency. *N Engl J Med* 1990;323:1806–1813.
6. Holler W, Scholz S, Knorr D, et al. Genetic differences between the salt-wasting, simple virilizing, and nonclassical types of congenital adrenal hyperplasia. *J Clin Endocrinol Metab* 1985;60:757–763.
7. Kuttenn F, Couillin P, Girard F, et al. Late-onset adrenal hyperplasia in hirsutism. *N Engl J Med* 1985;313:224–231.

Congenital Cutis Laxa

See Cutis laxa

Congenital Insensitivity to Pain and Anhydrosis

SYNONYM: Familial dysautonomia, type II; Hereditary sensory and autonomic neuropathy (HSAN IV); Autonomic neuropathy with insensitivity to pain

MIM #: 256800

This autosomal recessive disease is caused by mutations in the gene *NTRK1*, which encodes a tyrosine kinase receptor of nerve growth factor. Peripheral unmyelinated nerve fibers and small myelinated fibers are markedly diminished in number, or even absent. There are at least five genetically distinct sensory and autonomic neuropathies. This type, and type III (Familial dysautonomia, see later) are the most common types. As suggested, the disease is marked by insensitivity to pain (and temperature) and anhydrosis, despite anatomically normal sweat glands. Insensitivity to pain includes visceral pain. Tactile sensation is intact. Patients can have self-mutilation of the mouth and hands. Death in infants and young children from hyperpyrexia can occur in approximately 20%.

HEENT/AIRWAY: Hypotrichosis of the scalp. Can have absent corneal sensation with secondary corneal opacities, abrasions and scarring. Poor corneal healing. Normal lacrimation. Accidental oral trauma from decreased sensation. Self-mutilation of the lips and tongue.

CARDIOVASCULAR: Postural hypotension with reflex tachycardia, though not as marked as in familial dysautonomia. Absent innervation of vessel walls, although in one report baroreceptor function was intact.

NEUROMUSCULAR: Developmental delay, mental retardation. Hyperactivity. Rage attacks. Diffuse autonomic dysfunction. Insensitivity to pain, including visceral pain. Absent or diminished deep tendon reflexes. Temperature insensitivity. Episodic fever, sometimes severe [109°F (42.8°C)] has been reported. Decreased small unmyelinated and myelinated fibers. Loss of sympathetic innervation of eccrine sweat glands.

ORTHOPEDIC: Neuropathic arthropathy. Distal ulceration and osteomyelitis of fingers and toes leading to autoamputation. Fractures.

OTHER: Anhydrosis or markedly diminished sweating, thick calloused skin and palms. Skin ulcers. Dystrophic nails. Delayed wound healing. Absent flare response to injection of subcutaneous histamine.

MISCELLANEOUS: This disease has a particularly high incidence in a group of Israeli Bedouins.

ANESTHETIC CONSIDERATIONS
Despite congenital analgesia, anesthesia is required to maintain hemodynamic stability, and anesthetics are generally uneventful. Most surgeries are orthopedic procedures for injury-induced osteomyelitis. No atypical responses to anesthetic agents have been reported. Atropine use has not resulted in excessive temperature elevations. Intraoperative temperature can usually be controlled by the customary means. Operating room temperature should be controlled and forced air warmers and cooling mattresses used as necessary. Adequate preoperative sedation will ameliorate fever caused by excitement. Postoperative hyperthermia can develop. Nonsteroidal anti-inflammatory drugs are ineffective in lowering temperature. Patients will not feel pain and may be susceptible to additional orthopedic trauma from excessive postoperative movement. Sedation might be required.

Bibliography:
1. Axelrod FB, Hilz MJ. Inherited autonomic neuropathies. *Semin Neurol* 2003;23:381–390.
2. Tomioka T, Awaya Y, Nihei K, et al. Anesthesia for patients with congenital insensitivity to pain and anhydrosis: a questionnaire study in Japan. *Anesth Analg* 2002;94:271–274.
3. Okuda K, Arai T, Miwa T, et al. Anaesthetic management of children with congenital insensitivity to pain with anhydrosis. *Paediatr Anaesth* 2000;10:545–548.
4. Rosemberg S, Nagahashi Marie SK, Kliemann S. Congenital insensitivity to pain with anhydrosis (hereditary sensory and autonomic neuropathy type IV). *Pediatr Neurol* 1994;11:50–56.
5. Mitaka C, Tsunoda Y, Hikawa Y, et al. Anesthetic management of congenital insensitivity to pain with anhydrosis. *Anesthesiology* 1985;63:328–329.

Congenital Methemoglobinemia

See Methemoglobinemia

Congenital Microgastria-Limb Reduction Complex

SYNONYM: Microgastria-limb reduction complex

MIM #: 156810

This syndrome of unknown etiology is characterized by microgastria, limb reduction defects, and splenic anomalies. There is no evidence of a Mendelian inheritance pattern; however, a severe form with hydrocephalus and agenesis of the corpus callosum has recurred in a consanguinous family, suggesting that at least some cases might be inherited.

CHEST: Rare anomalies of lung lobation.

CARDIOVASCULAR: May have congenital cardiac defects, in particular atrial septal defect or truncus arteriosus.

NEUROMUSCULAR: May have arhinencephaly, microphthalmia, polymicrogyria, agenesis of the corpus callosum, or porencephalic cyst.

ORTHOPEDIC: Limb reduction defects include absent thumbs, oligodactyly, radial hypoplasia, ulnar hypoplasia, transverse defects of the humerus, and phocomelia.

GI/GU: Microgastria, resulting in failure to thrive. A surgically created gastric reservoir is usually beneficial. Intestinal malrotation, congenital megacolon. Splenic anomalies include asplenia, splenic hypoplasia, splenogonadal fusion. Renal anomalies include pelvic kidney, horseshoe kidney, unilateral renal agenesis, renal dysplasia.

MISCELLANEOUS: This association was first noted by Roberts in 1842.

ANESTHETIC CONSIDERATIONS
Patients with microgastria usually have significant gastroesophageal reflux, and are at increased risk for perioperative aspiration. Nasogastric tubes should be advanced cautiously. Limb reduction defects may make peripheral vascular access more difficult to obtain. Radial anomalies may make placement of a radial arterial catheter more difficult. Limb reduction defects may make fixation of an appropriately sized blood pressure cuff difficult, and falsely high pressures might be displayed by noninvasive monitors. An appropriate blood pressure cuff should cover two-thirds of the upper arm length. Patients with congenital cardiac disease should receive perioperative prophylactic antibiotics as indicated.

Bibliography:
1. Cunniff C, Williamson-Kruse L, Olney AH. Congenital microgastria and limb reduction defects. *Pediatrics* 1993;91:1192–1194.
2. Meinecke P, Bonnemann CG, Laas R. Microgastria-hypoplastic upper limb association: a severe expression including microphthalmia, single nostril and arhinencephaly. *Clin Dysmorphol* 1992;1:43–46.

Congenital Myotonic Dystrophy

Included in Myotonic dystrophy

Congenital Rubella Syndrome

See Fetal rubella syndrome

Congenital Spherocytosis

See Hereditary spherocytosis

Conradi-Hunermann Syndrome

See Chondrodysplasia punctata–autosomal dominant and X-linked dominant types

Cooley Anemia

Included in Thalassemia

Cori Disease

See Debrancher deficiency

Cornelia de Lange Syndrome

SYNONYM: de Lange syndrome; Brachmann-de Lange syndrome

MIM #: 122470

This syndrome is characterized by small stature, severe mental retardation, eyebrow fusion, a thin upper lip with a long philtrum, down-turned angles of the mouth, and micromelia. The disorder can be due to defects in the human homolog of the Drosophila gene *Nipped-B*. The protein product of this gene has acquired the name delangin. Inheritance is thought to be autosomal dominant.

HEENT/AIRWAY: Microbrachycephaly. Low anterior and posterior hairlines. Bushy eyebrows that fuse in the midline (synophrys). Long eyelashes. Myopia, ptosis, nystagmus. Low-set ears. Hearing loss. Depressed nasal bridge, upturned nasal tip, anteverted nares. Thin upper lip with long philtrum, down-turned angles of the mouth. High-arched palate.

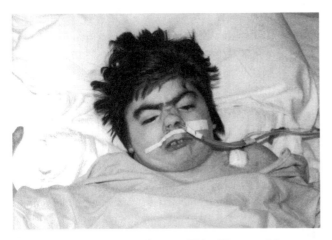

Cornelia de Lange syndrome. This 30-year-old woman with Cornelia de Lange syndrome was hospitalized for cecal volvulus. She is only slightly over 90 cm (3 feet) tall and weighs 20 kg. She is unable to talk or walk.

Occasional choanal atresia, cleft palate. Teeth erupt late and are widely spaced. Micrognathia. Short neck.

CHEST: Short sternum. Thirteen ribs. May contract lung disease secondary to repeated aspiration.

CARDIOVASCULAR: Occasional ventricular septal defect.

NEUROMUSCULAR: Severe mental and motor retardation. Hypertonia. May have seizures. Risk of apnea in infancy. Delayed speech is sometimes secondary to hearing loss. May exhibit autistic, stereotypical, self-destructive, or antisocial behavior. Broad-based gait.

ORTHOPEDIC: Prenatal and postnatal growth deficiency. Micromelia of the upper extremities. Simian crease. Proximal origination of the thumbs. Clinodactyly. Flexion contractures at the elbows. Dislocated or hypoplastic radial head. Syndactyly of the second and third toes. Delayed osseous maturation.

GI/GU: Gastroesophageal reflux. Bowel anomalies, including duplication of the gut, malrotation with volvulus, pyloric stenosis. Occasional hiatal hernia, diaphragmatic hernia, inguinal hernia. Hypospadias. Cryptorchidism.

OTHER: Characteristic weak, low-pitched, growling cry in infancy. Cutis marmorata (transient skin mottling). Perioral cyanosis without arterial desaturation. Hirsutism. Occasional thrombocytopenia.

MISCELLANEOUS: Cornelia de Lange qualified as a physician in 1897, very much in discord with the expected gender roles of her time. She went on to become a leading Dutch pediatrician, and originally reported this syndrome in 1933. Brachmann had described a child with similar features at autopsy in 1916, and this syndrome is sometimes known as the Brachmann-de Lange syndrome. It was Opitz, in 1963, who discovered Brachmann's description of the syndrome, when a volume of the journal *Jahrbuch fur Kinderheilkunde* was brought to his attention because it had been damaged by water such that it opened only in one place. He was then "startled to find out that here was an article on the Cornelia de Lange syndrome written 17 years before de Lange's first paper of 1933. The author, Dr. W. Brachmann, was then a young physician in training, who apologized that his study of this remarkable case was interrupted by sudden orders to report for active duty (in the German Army)" (9). Brachmann was killed in World War I, and his portrait and most of his academic papers were destroyed in World War II.

ANESTHETIC CONSIDERATIONS
Severe mental retardation and behavioral characteristics make smooth induction of anesthesia a challenge. Patients with Cornelia de Lange syndrome may have decreased

anesthetic requirements (8). Infants are at risk for perioperative apnea. Micrognathia and short neck may make direct laryngoscopy difficult. Choanal atresia, if present, precludes the use of a nasal airway or a nasogastric tube. Because of the high incidence of gastroesophageal reflux, these patients are at significant risk for pulmonary aspiration. Cutis marmorata (transient skin mottling) and perioral cyanosis without arterial desaturation can be misleading perioperatively. Peripheral vascular access can be difficult secondary to micromelia, and the shortened arm may require use of a narrower-than-usual blood pressure cuff. The short neck may make central venous access more difficult. Chronic use of anticonvulsant medications affects the kinetics of some anesthetic drugs. Patients with a congenital cardiac defect need perioperative antibiotic prophylaxis as indicated.

Bibliography:

1. Munoz Corsini L, De Stefano G, Porras MC, et al. Anaesthetic implications of Cornelia de Lange syndrome. *Paediatr Anaesth* 1998;8: 159–161.
2. Allanson JE, Hennekam RC, Ireland M. de Lange syndrome: subjective and objective comparison of the classical and mild phenotypes. *J Med Genet* 1997;34:645–650.
3. Tsukazaki Y, Tachibana C, Satoh K, et al. A patient with Cornelia de Lange syndrome with difficulty in orotracheal intubation [Japanese]. *Masui* 1996;45:991–993.
4. Veall GR. An unusual complication of Cornelia de Lange syndrome. *Anaesthesia* 1994;49:409–410.
5. Jackson L, Kline AD, Barr MA, et al. de Lange syndrome: a clinical review of 310 individuals. *Am J Med Genet* 1993;47:940–946.
6. Ireland M, Donnai D, Burn J. Brachmann-de Lange syndrome: delineation of the clinical phenotype. *Am J Med Genet* 1993;47:959–964.
7. Rosenbach Y, Zahavi I, Dinari G. Gastroesophageal dysfunction in Brachmann-de Lange syndrome. *Am J Med Genet* 1992;42:379–380.
8. Sargent WW. Anesthetic management of a patient with Cornelia de Lange syndrome. *Anesthesiology* 1991;74:1162–1163.
9. Opitz JM. The Brachmann-de Lange syndrome. *Am J Med Genet* 1985;22:89–102.

Corticosterone Methyl Oxidase I Deficiency

See 18-hydroxylase deficiency

Costello Syndrome

MIM #: 218040

This likely autosomal dominant disorder is characterized by mental retardation, coarse facies, hypertrophic cardiomyopathy, and perioral, nasal, and anal papillomas. The defect can be caused by mutations in the gene *HRAS*. *HRAS* is homologous to a retroviral oncogene. There is an association with older paternal age, suggesting a possible autosomal dominant inheritance with germline mosaicism.

HEENT/AIRWAY: Macrocephaly. Coarse and characteristic facies that worsen with age. Epicanthal folds, strabismus, downslanting palpebral fissures. Low-set ears with thick lobes. Flat nasal bridge with upturned nose. May have

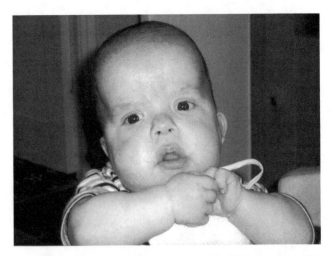

Costello syndrome. FIG. 1. 15-month-old boy with difficulty swallowing and gastroesophageal reflux. He required a Nissen fundoplication and a gastrostomy tube, and later developed a rapidly progressive fatal lung tumor.

choanal atresia. Thick lips. Macroglossia. May have high-arched palate. Short neck. Hypertrophied supraglottic tissue. Hoarse voice. Perioral and nasal papillomas with onset during childhood. Rare laryngeal papillomas. The papillomas may become malignant. The craniofacial phenotype resembles that of the lysosomal storage diseases.

CHEST: Barrel chest. May have copious tracheobronchial secretions. Pulmonary deposits of abnormal collagen and elastic fibers have been reported.

CARDIOVASCULAR: Hypertrophic cardiomyopathy, which can be associated with fatal dysrhythmias. Supraventricular tachyarrhythmias have also been reported, primarily during infancy. Cardiomyocytes contain accumulations of chondroitin-6-sulfate. May have ventricular septal defect, mitral valve prolapse, pulmonic stenosis.

NEUROMUSCULAR: Moderate to severe mental retardation. Speech delay. Hypotonia. Cheerful personality. Cerebral atrophy. May have seizures.

ORTHOPEDIC: Short stature. Decreased mobility at the elbow. Hyperextensible fingers. Deep palmar and plantar creases. Brittle nails. May have dislocated hips. Short Achilles tendon. Clubfoot deformity. Unsteady gait.

GI/GU: Swallowing difficulties. Gastroesophageal reflux. May have hepatosplenomegaly. May have inguinal hernias. Undescended testes. Perianal papillomas. The papillomas can become malignant.

OTHER: Polyhydramnios. Fetal macrosomia. Feeding problems and failure to thrive in infancy. Obesity in childhood.

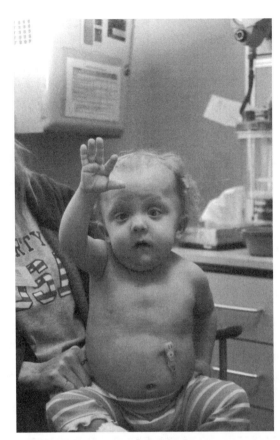

Costello syndrome. FIG. 2. A 3-year-old with congenital heart disease and cardiomyopathy, developmental delay and strabismus. A severe gag reflex required feeding via a gastric tube.

Cutis laxa, particularly of the neck, hands, and feet. Hyperkeratotic palms and soles. Darkly pigmented skin. Sparse, curly hair. Acanthosis nigricans. Can have deficiency of growth hormone. Can have abnormal glucose metabolism, with fasting hypoglycemia and postprandial hyperglycemia. May be associated with malignancies, particularly rhabdomyosarcoma, neuroblastoma and bladder cancer. Sudden death.

ANESTHETIC CONSIDERATIONS
Swallowing difficulties and gastroesophageal reflux are common, and patients are at increased risk for perioperative aspiration. Macroglossia and short neck may impact airway management. Thickened aryepiglottic folds have complicated laryngoscopy and tracheal intubation (7). Laryngeal papillomas and a tracheal web have also been described. Nasal papillomatosis may be a contraindication to nasotracheal intubation. Alternatively, patients may have choanal atresia preventing nasal intubation.

Patients often have hypertrophic cardiomyopathy, and are at risk for fatal dysrhythmias. It has been suggested that all children with Costello syndrome receive an electrocardiogram, a 24-hour Holter monitor and an echocardiogram (6). If not already done, it would seem prudent to complete these studies prior to elective surgery. Patients with congenital cardiac defects require perioperative antibiotic prophylaxis as indicated. In at least one instance, Costello syndrome has been associated with fasting hypoglycemia.

Bibliography:
1. White SM, Graham JM Jr, Kerr B, et al. The adult phenotype in Costello syndrome. *Am J Med Genet A*. 2005;136:128–135.
2. Katcher K, Bothwell M, Tobias JD. Anaesthetic implications of Costello syndrome. *Paediatr Anaesth* 2003;13:257–262.
3. Benni F, Leoni T, Iacobucci T, et al. Anaesthesiological considerations in Costello syndrome [Letter]. *Paediatr Anaesth* 2002;12:376–377.
4. van Eeghen AM, van Gelderen I, Hennekam RCM. Costello syndrome: report and review. *Am J Med Genet* 1999;82:187–193.
5. Johnson JP, Golabi M, Norton ME, et al. Costello syndrome: phenotype, natural history, differential diagnosis, and possible cause. *J Pediatr* 1998;133:441–448.
6. Siwik ES, Wiesner GL. Cardiac disease in Costello syndrome. *Pediatrics* 1998;101:706–709.
7. Dearlove O, Harper N. Costello syndrome [Letter]. *Paediatr Anaesth* 1997;7:476–477.
8. Costello JM. Costello syndrome: update on the original cases and commentary. *Am J Med Genet* 1996;62:199–201.

Coumarin

See Fetal warfarin syndrome

Cowden Disease

MIM #: 158350

This autosomal dominant disease is a disease of multiple hamartomas and a variety of benign and malignant tumors. It is caused by a germline mutation in the gene *PTEN* (phosphatase and tensin homolog gene). *PTEN* is a tumor suppressor gene. Cowden disease has been only poorly described in young children, and it has been suggested that the defect is allelic with Riley-Smith syndrome (Bannayan-Riley-Ruvalcaba syndrome), with which it has overlapping clinical features (see later). Malignant transformation has not been found in Riley-Smith syndrome, unlike in Cowden syndrome. There is a high incidence of breast cancer in affected women, and also a significant risk of malignant thyroid cancer, although the majority of tumors of those organs will be benign.

HEENT/AIRWAY: Progressive macrocephaly, "birdlike facies," multiple facial papules, cataracts, myopia, angioid streaks, hearing loss, hypoplastic mandible and maxilla, microstomia, high-arched palate, scrotal tongue, oral papules and papillomas.

CHEST: Pectus excavatum, gynecomastia in boys, breast fibrocystic disease, breast cancer.

NEUROMUSCULAR: Seizures, intention tremor, mild to moderate retardation and psychomotor delay, cerebellar dysplastic gangliocytoma (Lhermitte-Duclos disease).

ORTHOPEDIC: Kyphosis, scoliosis.

GI/GU: Hamartomatous polyps, colonic diverticulae. Polyps and adenomas can involve esophagus and stomach. Hydrocele, varicocele. Ovarian cysts, uterine leiomyomas.

OTHER: Multiple skin tags and palmoplantar keratoses. Subcutaneous lipomas. Trichilemmomas (hamartomas of the hair follicle). Cutaneous hemangiomas. Endocrinopathies include goiter, thyroid adenoma and follicular cell cancer, hyperthyroidism and thyroiditis. Other neoplasias include ovarian carcinoma, cervical carcinoma, uterine adenocarcinoma, transitional cell cancer of the bladder, adenocarcinoma of the colon, and meningioma.

MISCELLANEOUS: The first major report was that of Weary et al. from the University of Virginia. The disease is named after the first reported case, Ms. Cowden.

ANESTHETIC CONSIDERATIONS

Oropharyngeal papillomas can make laryngoscopy and intubation difficult (2). These can be friable. Chronic use of anticonvulsant medications can affect the kinetics of some anesthetic drugs.

Bibliography:

1. Corredor J, Wambach J, Barnard J. Gastrointestinal polyps in children: advances in molecular genetics, diagnosis and management. *J Pediatr* 2001;138:621–628.
2. Omote K, Kawamata T, Imaizumi H, et al. A case of Cowden's disease that caused airway obstruction during induction of anesthesia. *Anesthesiology* 1999;91:1537–1540.
3. Smid L, Zargi M. Cowden's disease: its importance for otolaryngologists. *J Laryngol Otol* 1993;107:1063–1065.

Craniocarpotarsal Dysplasia

See Whistling face syndrome

Craniodiaphyseal Dysplasia

MIM #: 218300, 122860

This metabolic bone disease leads to massive hyperostosis (progressive thickening) and sclerosis of multiple bones, particularly the craniofacial bones and the long tubular bones. It is an autosomal recessive disorder, although a single family with apparent autosomal dominant transmission has been reported. Impingement on cranial foramina can result in a variety of problems.

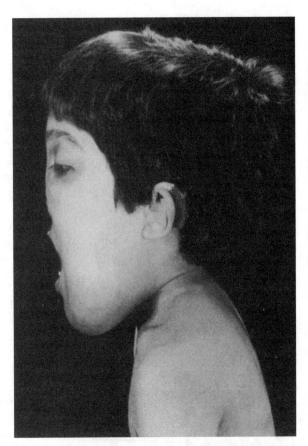 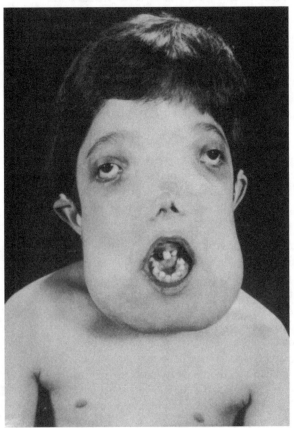

Craniodiaphyseal dysplasia. A young boy with craniodiaphyseal dysplasia. (From Appleby JN, Bingham RM. Craniodiaphyseal dysplasia: another cause of difficult intubation. *Paediatr Anaesth* 1996;6:225–229, with permission.)

HEENT/AIRWAY: Bony overgrowth of the skull, mandible, and maxilla. Calvarial thickness of 4 cm has been reported. Hypertelorism. May have vision loss. Hearing loss. Choanal stenosis. Respiratory distress can occur secondary to narrowing of the nasal passages, and patients eventually become obligate mouth breathers. Obliterated sinuses. Limited mouth opening.

CHEST: Thickening of the ribs and clavicles.

CARDIOVASCULAR: Bony overgrowth can impede jugular venous drainage.

NEUROMUSCULAR: May have mental retardation. Encroachment of the foramina may cause compression and impairment of cranial nerves IX and X. Stenosis of the cervical canal has led to quadraparesis in an adult.

ORTHOPEDIC: Restricted cervical spine and atlantoaxial mobility. Hyperostosis and sclerosis of the diaphyses, with diaphyseal widening. No metaphyseal flaring. Pelvic bones can also be involved. Bone pain.

ANESTHETIC CONSIDERATIONS
Direct laryngoscopy and visualization of the larynx may be extremely difficult. Fiberoptic intubation through a laryngeal mask airway has been successful (1). The large mandible, bulky occiput and limited cervical spine mobility may severely limit the ability to flex the neck. Massive mandibular overgrowth may prevent placement of a tracheostomy because the jaw can extend down to the level of the manubrium. Choanal stenosis may preclude placement of a nasal airway, nasal intubation, or placement of a nasogastric tube. Bone reduction surgery can result in significant blood loss.

Bibliography:
1. Appleby JN, Bingham RM. Craniodiaphyseal dysplasia: another cause of difficult intubation. *Paediatr Anaesth* 1996;6:225–229.
2. Brueton LA, Winter RM. Craniodiaphyseal dysplasia. *J Med Genet* 1990;27:701–706.
3. Schaefer B, Stein S, Oshman D, et al. Dominantly inherited craniodiaphyseal dysplasia: a new craniotubular dysplasia. *Clin Genet* 1986;30:381–391.

Craniofacial Dysostosis

See Crouzon syndrome

Craniofrontonasal Dysplasia

MIM #: 304110

This likely X-linked dominant disorder is characterized by brachycephaly, hypertelorism, down-slanting palpebral fissures, cleft nasal tip, and digital anomalies. Curiously, unlike other X-linked disorders, girls are far more severely affected than are boys. The gene responsible for this disorder is *EFNB1*, although there may be additional etiologies. *EFNB1* is a receptor for a protein-tyrosine kinase.

HEENT/AIRWAY: Coronal synostosis with brachycephaly in females. Low posterior hairline. Facial asymmetry. Frontal bossing, down-slanting palpebral fissures, nystagmus, all in females. Hypertelorism in males. Broad nasal root, cleft nasal tip. High-arched palate. May have cleft lip or palate. May have webbed neck.

CHEST: Pectus excavatum in males. Clavicular pseudoarthrosis in males. Sprengel deformity (winged scapula) in females. May have diaphragmatic hernia. Unilateral breast hypoplasia.

NEUROMUSCULAR: May have mental retardation.

ORTHOPEDIC: Short stature. Asymmetric lower limb shortness. Digital anomalies, including syndactyly (females), brachydactyly (males), clinodactyly, broad toes. Longitudinally grooved fingernails. May have limited forearm pronation, limited hip and shoulder abduction. Joint laxity.

GI/GU: Hypospadias. Shawl scrotum.

OTHER: Thick, wiry hair (females). Widow's peak.

ANESTHETIC CONSIDERATIONS
May require frontal advancement surgery. There are no specific anesthetic implications with this syndrome, although limited hip, shoulder, and arm mobility may occasionally affect positioning.

Bibliography:
1. Orr DJ, Slaney S, Ashworth GJ, et al. Craniofrontonasal dysplasia. *Br J Plast Surg* 1997;50:153–161.
2. Saavedra D, Richieri-Costa A, Guion-Almeida ML, et al. Craniofrontonasal syndrome: study of 41 patients. *Am J Med Genet* 1996;61:147–151.
3. Devriendt K, Van Mol C, Fryns JR. Craniofrontonasal dysplasia: more severe expression in the mother than in her son. *Genet Couns* 1995;6:361–364.

Craniometaphyseal Dysplasia

MIM #: 123000, 218400

This syndrome is similar to Pyle metaphyseal dysplasia (see later), but involves greater craniofacial hyperostosis and less metaphyseal splaying than is seen with Pyle disease. Craniometaphyseal dysplasia can be inherited in an autosomal dominant or an autosomal recessive fashion. The autosomal dominant form is due to mutations in the gene *ANKH*, the homolog of the mouse progressive ankylosis gene. The autosomal recessive type is more rare and more severe. Specifically, it is more likely to result in hearing loss, facial paralysis, and loss of vision.

HEENT/AIRWAY: Macrocephaly. Thick calvarium and skull base. Hypertelorism, proptosis. The recessive form can have optic atrophy. May have conductive hearing loss. Bony wedge over the bridge of the nose. Progressive flattening of the nose. Narrow nasal passages, chronic rhinitis. Prognathism. Malaligned teeth. Delayed eruption of permanent teeth in the recessive form.

NEUROMUSCULAR: Intelligence is usually normal. Hyperostosis can lead to obstructive hydrocephalus, cranial nerve compression and headaches. Cranial nerve compression can result in hearing loss (cranial nerve VIII), facial paralysis (cranial nerve VII), and loss of vision (cranial nerve II). Stenosis of the foramen magnum can occur—cerebellomedullary compression has been reported.

ORTHOPEDIC: Mild metaphyseal splaying. "Erlenmeyer flask" deformity of distal femur in childhood, club-shaped distal femur in adulthood. Diaphyseal sclerosis.

ANESTHETIC CONSIDERATIONS

Patients with proptosis or facial paralysis may not be able to close their eyelids fully over their eyes. Meticulous perioperative eye care is necessary to prevent corneal abrasions. Patients may have extremely narrow nasal passages or have nasal obstruction. In either case, it may be impossible to place a nasal airway, a nasotracheal tube, or a nasogastric tube. Patients may have obstructive sleep apnea.

Bibliography:
1. Sheppard WM, Shprintzen RJ, Tatum SA, et al. Craniometaphyseal dysplasia: a case report and review of medical and surgical management. *Int J Pediatr Otorhinolaryngol* 2003;67:687–693.
2. Beighton P. Craniometaphyseal dysplasia (CMD), autosomal dominant form. *J Med Genet* 1995;32:370–374.
3. Cole DE, Cohen MM. A new look at craniometaphyseal dysplasia. *J Pediatr* 1988;112:577–579.

Cranioorofacial Digital Syndrome

See Otopalatodigital syndrome, type II

Craniosynostosis-Radial Aplasia Syndrome

See Baller-Gerold syndrome

Cri du Chat Syndrome

SYNONYM: 5p- syndrome

MIM #: 123450

This chromosomal disorder is due to a partial deletion of the short arm of chromosome 5. It is thought that many of the phenotypic changes are specifically due to the loss of the gene *TERT*, the telomerase reverse transcriptase gene. Cri du chat is one of the most common chromosomal deletion syndromes, and is characterized by microcephaly, mental retardation, downward-slanting palpebral fissures, and a distinctive cat-like cry in infancy. The abnormal cry is caused by laryngeal deformity. The larynx normalizes with aging, and the distinctive cry diminishes. Most cases are the result of new deletions. Most patients die in early childhood.

HEENT/AIRWAY: Microcephaly, round face, facial asymmetry. Downward-slanting palpebral fissures, hypertelorism, epicanthal folds, strabismus. Abnormal, low-set ears. May have cleft lip or palate. May have dental abnormalities, including delayed eruption, malocclusion. Micrognathia. Long, floppy epiglottis. Laryngeal deformity, consisting of diamond-shaped vocal cords on inspiration with a large air space in the area of the posterior commissure. May have short neck.

CHEST: May have recurrent aspiration.

CARDIOVASCULAR: Congenital heart disease in one-third, predominantly patent ductus arteriosus, atrial septal defect, ventricular septal defect and/or pulmonic stenosis.

NEUROMUSCULAR: Severe mental retardation. Hypotonia.

ORTHOPEDIC: Growth retardation. Scoliosis. Simian crease. May have hemivertebrae. May have flat feet.

GI/GU: May have inguinal hernia.

MISCELLANEOUS: The name "cri du chat" ("cat cry") comes from the plaintive, high-pitched cry reminiscent of the mewing of a cat.

ANESTHETIC CONSIDERATIONS

Direct laryngoscopy and tracheal intubation may be difficult secondary to micrognathia, a short neck, a long, floppy epiglottis, and a small, narrow larynx. A variety of alternative laryngoscope blades and intubation techniques should be available. A laryngeal mask airway has been used during a thoracotomy in a young child who could not be otherwise successfully intubated (4).

Patients are at risk for perioperative aspiration. Those patients who have a history of recurrent aspiration may have chronic lung disease. Hypotonia can include the pharyngeal muscles, and patients should be observed closely perioperatively for airway obstruction. It has been suggested that intraoperative maintenance of body temperature is particularly difficult in these patients. There is no known association with malignant hyperthermia or succinylcholine-induced rhabdomyolysis. Patients with congenital heart disease need perioperative antibiotic prophylaxis as indicated.

Bibliography:
1. Cornish K, Bramble D. Cri du chat syndrome: genotype-phenotype correlations and recommendations for clinical management. *Dev Med Child Neurol* 2002;44:494–497.

2. Cornish KM, Pigram J. Developmental and behavioural characteristics of cri du chat syndrome. *Arch Dis Child* 1996;75:448–450.
3. Brislin RP, Stayer SA, Schwartz RE. Anaesthetic considerations for the patient with cri du chat syndrome. *Paediatr Anaesth* 1995;5:139–141.
4. Castresana MR, Stefansson S, Cancel AR, et al. Use of the laryngeal mask airway during thoracotomy in a pediatric patient with cri-du-chat syndrome [Letter]. *Anesth Analg* 1994;78:817.
5. Yamashita M, Tanioka F, Taniguchi K, et at. Anesthetic considerations in cri du chat syndrome: a report of three cases. *Anesthesiology* 1985;63:201–202.
6. Miyake K, Kobayashi H, Nakazawa K, et al. Experience of general anesthesia in dental treatment for a patient with 5p- syndrome (cat cry syndrome). *J Jpn Dent Anes Soc* 1983;11:80–85.

Crigler-Najjar Syndrome

MIM #: 218800

This usually autosomal recessive disease is due to a defect in the enzyme uridine diphosphate glucuronyltransferase (UDP-glucuronyltransferase) resulting in unconjugated hyperbilirubinemia. In type I disease there is absent enzyme activity. In type II disease there is markedly diminished activity, and both autosomal dominant inheritance with incomplete penetrance and autosomal recessive inheritance have been suggested. Type I disease can be treated with phototherapy, often for many hours a day, which converts bilirubin to more polar compounds that can be excreted without conjugation. Phototherapy usually becomes less effective at around the time of puberty due to skin changes and a decreased surface-to-mass ratio. Type II disease is often less severe and is responsive to therapy with barbiturates, which induces microsomal enzymes.

Acute exacerbations of the disease can occur with trauma or other stresses such as surgery or infection, and have been treated with plasmapheresis and plasma exchange. Without treatment death occurs from kernicterus, often in young childhood, but as late as adolescence in some.

Liver transplantation is curative. A single patient has been treated successfully with transplantation of isolated hepatocytes.

Gilbert disease (see later) is also due to a defect in the enzyme UDP-glucuronyltransferase, and the two syndromes are likely allelic. Other diseases of hepatic bilirubin metabolism include the Dubin-Johnson and Rotor syndromes (see later).

NEUROMUSCULAR: Kernicterus, if not treated. Late bilirubin encephalopathy can develop in older patients who were otherwise doing well with the exception of jaundice. Acute stress can raise bilirubin levels, even in type II, with the development of new neurologic manifestations.

GI/GU: Congenital nonhemolytic unconjugated hyperbilirubinemia with otherwise normal hepatic function and histology, although canalicular and biliary duct cholestasis has been described, probably from excretion of unconjugated bilirubin with phototherapy. There is essentially no conjugated bilirubin. Although the bile is pale, stool color is normal because of normal fecal urobilinogen. Jaundice appears within the first days of life.

MISCELLANEOUS: Phototherapy for hyperbilirubinemia was first appreciated by a nurse in an English nursery who noticed that infants near the windows were less likely to have jaundice. Indeed, the bilirubin levels of these patients can go down during the summertime.

The family of one of the first reported cases was fairly inbred, and also harbored other recessive diseases including Morquio syndrome, homocystinuria, metachromatic leukodystrophy and Seckel syndrome.

ANESTHETIC CONSIDERATIONS
Phototherapy should be continued as long as possible perioperatively, and has even been used intraoperatively (3). Fasting increases bilirubin levels. The stress of surgery or a perioperative infection can exacerbate the hyperbilirubinemia.

Some drugs, the most common being rifampin, cause enzyme inhibition with increased serum bilirubin levels and jaundice. Although sulfonamides, some cephalosporins, and intravenous contrast agents can increase free bilirubin levels by displacement of bilirubin from albumin, no currently used anesthetic agents are known to displace bilirubin significantly enough to contraindicate their use. Phenobarbital has been used in an effort to decrease bilirubin levels in type II, although it is likely of little benefit acutely. Some patients may be on long-term phenobarbital therapy, which can affect the metabolism of some anesthetic drugs. Morphine is metabolized by a different glucuronyltransferase system, and can be used in these patients.

Bibliography:
1. Bosma PJ. Inherited disorders of bilirubin metabolism. *J Hepatol* 2003;38:107–117.
2. Hamada T, Miyamoto M, Oda S, et al. Anesthetic and postoperative care of a patient with Crigler-Najjar syndrome type II [Japanese]. *Masui* 1996;45:345–347.
3. Prager MC, Johnson KL, Ascher NL. Anesthetic care of patients with Crigler-Najjar syndrome. *Anesth Analg* 1992;74:162–164.

Cross Syndrome

SYNONYM: Oculocerebral hypopigmentation syndrome

MIM #: 257800

This autosomal recessive disorder consists of ocular, cerebral, and cutaneous abnormalities. The gene and gene product are not known.

HEENT/AIRWAY: Ocular abnormalities, including hypopigmentation, cloudy corneas, cataracts, iris atrophy. May have hearing loss. May have dental defects.

CARDIOVASCULAR: May have interventricular septal hypertrophy.

NEUROMUSCULAR: Mental retardation, motor delay, spastic tetraplegia, athetosis, Dandy-Walker cyst, encephalopathy.

GI/GU: May have inguinal hernias. May have urinary tract anomalies.

OTHER: Growth retardation. Hypopigmented skin, silver-gray hair.

ANESTHETIC CONSIDERATIONS

There are no specific anesthetic implications with this syndrome.

Bibliography:

1. Tezcan I, Demir E, Asan E, et al. A new case of oculocerebral hypopigmentation syndrome (Cross syndrome) with additional findings. *Clin Genet* 1997;51:118–121.
2. Lerone M, Pessagno A, Taccone A, et al. Oculocerebral syndrome with hypopigmentation (Cross syndrome): report of a new case. *Clin Genet* 1992;41:87–89.

Crouzon Syndrome

SYNONYM: Craniofacial dysostosis

MIM #: 123500

This craniofacial dysmorphic syndrome is inherited in an autosomal dominant fashion, but there is wide variability in expression. Anomalies are confined to the craniofacial region, and include craniosynostosis, hypertelorism, shallow orbits, and a parrot-like beaked nose. Craniofacial surgery is undertaken to correct elevated intracranial pressure and to allow for normal brain development, or strictly for cosmetic reasons.

Crouzon syndrome results from mutations in the fibroblast growth factor receptor-2 gene (*FGFR2*). About half of all cases are new mutations with a suggestion of advanced paternal age. Different mutations of the same gene cause Apert syndrome, Antley-Bixler syndrome, Beare-Stevenson syndrome and some cases of Pfeiffer syndrome. Crouzon

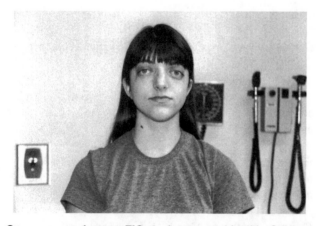

Crouzon syndrome. FIG. 1. A young girl with Crouzon syndrome.

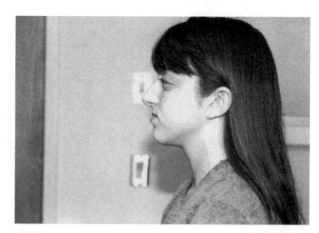

Crouzon syndrome. FIG. 2. Lateral view of the girl in Figure 1.

syndrome with acanthosis nigricans results from a mutation in the fibroblast growth factor receptor-3 gene (*FGFR3, MIM #* 134934.0011).

HEENT/AIRWAY: Craniosynostosis, especially of coronal, lambdoid, and sagittal sutures. Frontal bossing. Hypertelorism, shallow orbits with ocular proptosis. Exposure keratitis or conjunctivitis is common. May have strabismus, nystagmus, optic atrophy. Mild to moderate conductive hearing loss. May have external auditory canal atresia. Hypoplastic maxilla. Parrot-like beaked nose. Choanal atresia has been described in Crouzon syndrome with acanthosis nigricans. Short philtrum. High-arched palate, occasional cleft lip or palate. Dental crowding. Relative prognathism. Crouzon syndrome with acanthosis nigricans may be associated with cementomas of the jaw.

Upper airway obstruction is common—many patients become obligate mouth breathers, but acute respiratory distress develops only rarely. May develop sleep apnea.

NEUROMUSCULAR: Intelligence is normal. Rarely, may have mental deficiency, hydrocephalus, or increased intracranial pressure secondary to abnormal suture closure. May have seizures, agenesis of the corpus callosum.

ORTHOPEDIC: May have dislocation of the radial head. Cervical spine fusion, typically C2-3. Scoliosis and spinal stenosis may occur in Crouzon syndrome with acanthosis nigricans.

OTHER: May have acanthosis nigricans involving skin of the head and neck.

MISCELLANEOUS: Octave Crouzon was a leading French neurologist during the first part of the 20th century.

ANESTHETIC CONSIDERATIONS

Tracheal intubation may be difficult secondary to the craniofacial anomalies. Placement of a maxillary distraction device may increase the difficulty of tracheal intubation (1). Ocular proptosis often leads to exposure keratitis or conjunctivitis. Meticulous intraoperative eye care is indicated. Patients may have elevated intracranial pressure, in which case precautions should be taken to avoid further elevations in pressure. Airway anomalies are less common than in the related Apert and Pfeiffer syndromes.

Bibliography:

1. Roche J, Frawley G, Heggie A. Difficult tracheal intubation induced by maxillary distraction devices in craniosynostosis syndromes. *Paediatr Anaesth* 2002;12:227–234.
2. Payne JF, Cranston AJ. Postoperative airway problems in a child with Crouzon's disease. *Paediatr Anaesth* 1995;5:331–333.
3. Cinalli G, Renier D, Sebag G, et al. Chronic tonsillar herniation in Crouzon's and Apert's syndromes: the role of premature synostosis of the lambdoid suture. *J Neurosurg* 1995;83:575–582.
4. Reardon W, Winter RM, Rutland P, et al. Mutations in the fibroblast growth factor receptor 2 gene cause Crouzon syndrome. *Nat Genet* 1994;8:98–103.

Cryptophthalmos Syndrome

See Fraser syndrome

Cryptophthalmos-Syndactyly Syndrome

See Fraser syndrome

Cutis Gyrata Syndrome of Beare-Stevenson

See Beare-Stevenson syndrome

Cutis Laxa

SYNONYM: Congenital cutis laxa

MIM #: 123700, 219100, 219200

Cutis laxa is a rare congenital disorder of elastin synthesis, affecting both skin and internal organs. Inheritance may be autosomal recessive or autosomal dominant. The recessive and some of the dominant forms are due to abnormalities in the fibulin gene *FBLN5*. It has been suggested that *FBLN5* is a vascular ligand for integrin receptors and is involved in vascular development and remodeling. The dominant form is less severe, and lacks pulmonary manifestations, although there is a single case report of emphysema (2). It can be due to mutations in the gene encoding elastin. There is also an acquired form of cutis laxa, called generalized elastolysis. Skin biopsy specimens show deficient and disorganized elastin fibers in the dermis and vascular walls. An X-linked form of cutis laxa is also referred to as Ehlers-Danlos syndrome, type IX (see later).

HEENT/AIRWAY: Delayed closure of fontanelles. May have hoarse cry from vocal cord laxity.

CHEST: Diaphragmatic atony, diaphragmatic hernia, emphysema, pulmonary hypertension in recessive form.

CARDIOVASCULAR: Aneurysmal aortic dilatation or aortic and arterial tortuousity, peripheral pulmonary artery stenosis, valvular insufficiency. Cor pulmonale may develop in patients with significant pulmonary hypertension. Acquired form may have severe coronary artery disease. Renal artery dysplasia.

ORTHOPEDIC: Less joint hypermobility than in the clinically similar Ehlers-Danlos syndrome. Generalized osteoporosis.

GI/GU: Umbilical, inguinal hernias. GI and GU diverticulae, including esophageal and bladder diverticulae. Rectal prolapse in recessive form.

OTHER: Skin hangs on the body in loose, pendulous folds like an ill-fitting suit. Child may look prematurely wrinkled and aged. Skin does not bruise easily and it heals normally (unlike skin in Ehlers-Danlos syndrome).

ANESTHETIC CONSIDERATIONS
Abnormal skin may make vascular access more difficult. Patients may have significant pulmonary disease, aortic or coronary artery disease. Nasogastric tubes should be placed with care because of possible esophageal diverticula. Patients who are receiving chronic steroid treatment require perioperative stress doses of steroids.

Bibliography:

1. Ringpfeil F. Selected disorders of connective tissue: pseudoxanthoma elasticum, cutis laxa, and lipoid proteinosis. *Clin Dermatol* 2005;23:41–46.
2. Corbett E, Glaisyer H, Chan C, et al. Congenital cutis laxa with a dominant inheritance and early onset emphysema. *Thorax* 1994;49:836–837.
3. Thomas WO, Moses MH, Craver RD, et al. Congenital cutis laxa: a case report and review of loose skin syndromes. *Ann Plast Surg* 1993;30:252–256.

Cyclic Neutropenia

MIM #: 162800

This autosomal dominant disease is characterized by regular cyclic variations in neutrophils, monocytes, eosinophils, lymphocytes, platelets, and reticulocytes. Cycles among individuals vary from approximately 15 to 35 days. It is due to mutations in the gene encoding neutrophil elastase. Patients may be treated with granulocyte colony-stimulating factor (G-CSF).

HEENT/AIRWAY: Recurring mucosal ulcers.

OTHER: Recurrent fever and malaise. There may be serious skin and other infections during periods of neutropenia.

MISCELLANEOUS: A very similar disease occurs in gray collie dogs.

ANESTHETIC CONSIDERATIONS
Careful aseptic technique is required, particularly during periods of neutropenia. Patients with mucosal ulcers will require extra care during laryngoscopy and intubation.

Bibliography:
1. Dale DC, Bolyard AA, Aprikyan A. Cyclic neutropenia. *Semin Hematol* 2002;39:89–94.
2. Wright DG, Dale DC, Fauci AS, et al. Human cyclic neutropenia: clinical review and long-term follow-up of patients. *Medicine (Baltimore)* 1981;60:1–13.

Cystathionase Deficiency

See Cystathioninuria

Cystathioninuria

SYNONYM: Cystathionase deficiency

MIM #: 219500

This autosomal recessive defect is due to decreased activity of gamma-cystathionase, with urinary excretion and accumulation in tissues of large amounts of cystathionine and other metabolites. Gamma-cystathionase catalyzes the conversion of cystathionine, derived from methionine, to cysteine plus alpha-ketobutyrate. There appears to be significant genetic heterogeneity. Many patients are responsive to pyridoxine.

Cystathioninuria may also be caused by a number of other abnormalities, including overproduction of cystathionine secondary to other enzymatic defects, excessive transport of cystathionine into the urine secondary to renal defects, pyridoxine deficiency, liver disease, and several tumor types. Neonates may have transient cystathioninuria because the activity of gamma-cystathionase is normally low in the newborn.

Although we have listed several associated clinical findings, it has been suggested that these findings merely reflect ascertainment bias, because the earliest patients first came to medical attention for other, probably unrelated, medical problems. Cystathioninuria is considered to be biochemically benign.

HEENT/AIRWAY: Ear defects.

NEUROMUSCULAR: Mental retardation, seizures.

ORTHOPEDIC: Clubfoot.

GI/GU: Urinary calculi.

OTHER: Thrombocytopenia.

ANESTHETIC CONSIDERATIONS
It is likely that these purported clinical findings are related to ascertainment bias rather than the metabolic defect. There are no apparent deleterious effects in pregnant mothers or neonates. Thus, there are no specific anesthetic considerations.

Bibliography:
1. Endres W, Wuttge B. Occurrence of secondary cystathioninuria in children with inherited metabolic disorders, liver diseases, neoplasms, cystic fibrosis and celiac disease. *Eur J Pediatr* 1978;129:29–35.
2. Pascal TA, Gaull GE, Beratis NG, et al. Cystathionase deficiency: evidence for genetic heterogeneity in primary cystathioninuria. *Pediatr Res* 1978;12:125–133.

Cystic Fibrosis

SYNONYM: Mucoviscidosis

MIM #: 219700

Cystic fibrosis (CF) is an autosomal recessive disorder characterized by copious viscid mucous production that affects multiple organ systems, particularly the lungs and the exocrine pancreas. This disorder is due to a defect in the CF transmembrane conductance regulator gene (*CFTR*). The protein product of the gene appears to function as a chloride ion channel, the only ion channel of its type that is currently recognized. Since the discovery of the CF gene, more than 1300 *CFTR* gene mutations that lead to the disease

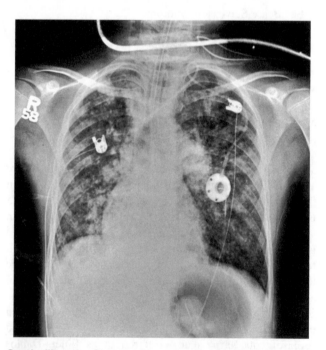

Cystic fibrosis. Chest radiograph of a 15-year-old boy with end-stage cystic fibrosis. This film was taken shortly after tracheal intubation. His arterial PCO_2 before intubation was 104 mm Hg. The following day he underwent bilateral, living unrelated donor pulmonary lobe transplantation.

have been identified. Genetic defects are varied, and can be single nucleotide-polymorphisms or large deletions, and can affect channel synthesis, maturation, regulation, conductance or stability. The mutation that accounts for approximately 70% of defective *CFTR* alleles and 90% of CF cases in the United States is known as the ΔF508 mutation. This mutation causes a deletion of phenylalanine at position 508 in the protein product of the gene. The abnormal protein is recognized as misfolded and is rapidly degraded before it can reach its site of action at the cell membrane.

CF most often occurs in people of European descent, where the incidence is 1:2,000 to 1:5,000, making it the most common autosomal recessive disease in that population. The *CFTR* gene has been constructed *in vitro*, and work is ongoing to determine a viral or nonviral vector that is capable of delivering and inserting the normal gene into a patient's cells to correct the genetic defect. It has been proposed that polymorphisms, or minor variations, in other genes, specifically in *TGFβ*1 (the gene encoding transforming growth factor β1) or a nearby upstream region can modify the clinical severity of lung disease.

HEENT/AIRWAY: Chronic sinusitis. Nasal polyps occur in older children and adults, and are usually asymptomatic but may cause nasal obstruction or epistaxis. With advanced disease, the trachea may enlarge and become flaccid.

CHEST: Recurrent or persistent chest infections are the rule. Electrolyte abnormalities and mucous gland and goblet cell hypertrophy lead to viscid mucous. Viscid mucous is hard to clear, leading to mucous plugging and patchy atelectasis. The lungs become colonized with bacteria, typically *Pseudomonas* or *Staphylococcus* species. Colonization and intermittent infection contribute to lung damage through inflammation and destruction of lung tissue. Bronchopulmonary aspergillosis may also develop. Bronchial hyperreactivity causes additional gas trapping and hyperinflation. In addition, there is decreased ciliary clearance. The incidence of spontaneous pneumothorax increases with age, and has a high recurrence rate without pleurodesis. Minor hemoptysis is common; major hemoptysis requiring bronchial artery embolization is rare.

CARDIOVASCULAR: Chronic respiratory disease and hypoxemia may result in cor pulmonale. Left ventricular dysfunction has also been reported.

GI/GU: The neonate may present with meconium ileus (secondary to abnormally viscid meconium).

Eighty-five percent of patients have pancreatic exocrine insufficiency secondary to viscid secretions, which causes ductal obstruction. Pancreatic exocrine insufficiency leads to steatorrhea and malabsorption. Malabsorption is usually successfully treated with oral pancreatic enzymes and fat-soluble vitamin supplements. Adults may have intermittent small bowel obstruction, only rarely requiring surgery, but exclusion of other surgical diseases may be difficult. There is an increased incidence of rectal prolapse in children, often recurrent. There is an increased incidence of gastroesophageal reflux.

Pancreatic insufficiency disrupts the enterohepatic circulation of bile acids, and there is an increased incidence of cholelithiasis. Biliary cirrhosis leading to portal hypertension can occur. Hepatic cirrhosis may develop.

Frequent aminoglycoside use has caused renal insufficiency.

Men are infertile; women have decreased fertility.

OTHER: Malnutrition. Anemia of chronic disease. Vitamin K deficiency and prolonged prothrombin time only in severe malabsorption. Progressive pancreatic damage can result in glucose intolerance or even frank diabetes in teenagers and adults. Oral hypoglycemics are rarely useful, and insulin may be needed. High sweat electrolyte losses (the basis of the diagnostic sweat test) can cause heat prostration, particularly with exertion in hot weather.

MISCELLANEOUS: CF has been recognized in European folklore since the 1600s. References such as "the child will soon die whose forehead tastes salty when kissed" have appeared in songs and stories from northern Europe for centuries. Curcumin, a major component of the spice turmeric, can correct ΔF508 processing and has prolonged life in mice homozygous for this gene. Heterozygotes are relatively immune to typhoid, which requires a normal *CFTR* gene to enter cells.

ANESTHETIC CONSIDERATIONS

In the early part of the last century, CF was uniformly fatal in infancy or early childhood. Today, most patients reach adulthood, with a mean survival age of 30 to 35 years. Anesthesiologists are therefore more likely to see CF patients in the operating room, either for surgery related to their disease (nasal polypectomy, lung transplant) or for unrelated surgeries.

Over 90% of CF patients die from respiratory complications. Patients uniformly have some obstructive disease (secondary to mucous plugging and hyperreactivity), but many also have restrictive disease (secondary to chronic lung destruction). Approximately 40% of patients will respond to bronchodilators. Pulmonary infections are common, and should be resolved before elective surgery is undertaken. Clinical evaluation and sputum culture can be misleading—a preoperative chest radiograph may be helpful. Preoperative blood gas and pulmonary function testing may be useful in assessing the severity of the lung disease. Elevated $PaCO_2$ is an indication of severe disease. Patients are likely to have a prolonged forced expiratory volume in 1 second (FEV_1) secondary to obstructive disease, and increased residual volume secondary to gas trapping. Ventilation-perfusion mismatching may lead to hypoxemia. Decreased $PaCO_2$ may be associated with cor pulmonale.

Pulmonary disease may prolong induction of anesthesia by volatile agents. Nasal polyposis is a contraindication to nasal intubation, and may complicate nasogastric tube placement. Some patients depend on hypoxic respiratory drive, and may hypoventilate with supplemental oxygen. Intraoperative assisted or controlled ventilation is recommended. High airway pressures should be avoided if possible, particularly in the presence of known bullae. The anesthesiologist should maintain a high index of suspicion for pneumothorax. Consideration should be given to avoiding the use of nitrous oxide. Perioperative intubation is rarely contraindicated, but prolonged intubation carries the risk of infection and barotrauma. Regional anesthesia or analgesia should be strongly considered when it has the potential to improve postoperative respiratory function.

Perioperative treatment of secretions is usually the anesthesiologist's greatest challenge. Good perioperative chest percussion therapy is critically important. This may be an indication for delaying the patient's procedure until mid-morning to maximize clearance of secretions. Inspired gases should be humidified. Anticholinergic medications decrease the volume of secretions but will not thicken them. Ketamine may increase bronchial secretions, and should be avoided. Intubation is usually necessary for pulmonary toilet in all but the shortest cases. Most patients require frequent suctioning of the airway. Nebulized saline, mucolytic agents (N-acetylcysteine), or recombinant human DNase (which degrades neutrophil DNA and decreases the viscosity of secretions) may be helpful.

Perioperative bronchial hyperreactivity may also be challenging. Coughing and laryngospasm are common. Unfortunately, bronchodilators do not reliably improve air flow, and in some patients they may even exacerbate airway obstruction by causing airway instability during expiration secondary to smooth muscle relaxation.

Patients should receive a cardiac evaluation and a preoperative echocardiogram if cor pulmonale is suspected. Gastroesophageal reflux is common, and patients are at increased risk for perioperative aspiration. Aminoglycosides can prolong the action of nondepolarizing muscle relaxants. Patients with a history of frequent aminoglycoside use may have renal insufficiency.

Patients with pulmonary aspergillosis may be taking steroids, and require perioperative stress doses of steroids.

Venous access may be difficult in patients who require frequent intravenous lines for antibiotic administration. Preoperative laboratory assessment may reveal hyponatremia, anemia, or elevated blood glucose. Some patients will have glucose intolerance or diabetes, and will require appropriate perioperative glucose management.

High-dose ibuprofen, when taken chronically, has been shown to slow the progression of mild pulmonary disease in some patients with CF, presumably through its anti-inflammatory effects. There is no evidence that acute ingestion of nonsteroidal inflammatory drugs has any beneficial effect.

Bibliography:

1. Rowe SM, Miller S, Sorscher EJ. Cystic fibrosis. *N Engl J Med* 2005;352:1992–2001.
2. Bose D, Yentis SM, Fauvel NJ. Caesarean section in a parturient with respiratory failure caused by cystic fibrosis. *Anaesthesia* 1997;52:578–582.
3. Stern RC. The diagnosis of cystic fibrosis. *N Engl J Med* 1997;336:487–491.
4. Walsh TS, Young CH. Anaesthesia and cystic fibrosis. *Anaesthesia* 1995;50:614–622.
5. Weeks AM, Buckland MR. Anaesthesia for adults with cystic fibrosis. *Anaesth Intensive Care* 1995;23:332–338.
6. Webb AK, David TJ. Clinical management of children and adults with cystic fibrosis. *BMJ* 1994;308:459–462.
7. Lamberty KM, Rubin BK. The management of anaesthesia for patients with cystic fibrosis. *Anaesthesia* 1985;40:448–459.
8. Robinson DA, Branthwaite MA. Pleural surgery in patients with cystic fibrosis. *Anaesthesia* 1984;39:655–659.
9. Richardson VF, Robertson CF, Mowat AP, et al. Deterioration in lung function after general anaesthesia in patients with cystic fibrosis. *Acta Paediatr Scand* 1984;73:75–79.

Cystinosis

MIM #: 219750, 219800, 219900

Note: This syndrome is distinct from cystinuria.

This autosomal recessive inborn error of amino acid metabolism consists of three types, an infantile (nephrotic) form, an adolescent form, and an adult form. All three types are due to mutations in the gene *CTNS*, encoding cystinosin, a membrane protein, probably lysosomal, and putative cystine transporter. Multiple specific mutations have been described. There is accumulation of intracellular cystine in a wide variety of organs, but the primary clinical manifestations involve alterations in renal function. In the adolescent form eye findings present early with renal findings presenting with a generally milder course during or after the second decade. The adult form has only eye manifestations. Treatment is with cysteamine, which combines with cystine in the lysosome. The mixed disulfide leaves the lysosome via the lysine transport system. Early treatment with cysteamine has improved the outcome significantly.

HEENT/AIRWAY: Deposition of cystine crystals in the cornea and conjunctivae may cause photophobia or recurrent corneal erosions. Patchy depigmentation of the retina. Decreased visual acuity with aging. Recurrent epistaxis has been described in dialyzed patients. May have choking and gagging due to myopathy.

CARDIOVASCULAR: Hypertension secondary to renal failure.

NEUROMUSCULAR: Poor school performance, seizures, impaired visual memory, and cerebral atrophy may develop with aging. Severely affected patients may have hypotonia, swallowing and speech difficulties, pyramidal and cerebellar signs, and strokes. Ischemic strokes have been seen only in adults. Pseudotumor cerebri has been reported. A myopathy of both proximal and distal muscles, with particular involvement of the interossei and muscles of the thenar eminence has been described. Some myopathy is due to cystine deposits in muscles, but some may be due to excessive carnitine losses in the urine.

ORTHOPEDIC: Severe rickets with the infantile form, if inadequately treated. Short stature.

GI/GU: Involvement of the liver can result in cirrhosis with portal hypertension and esophageal varices. Hepatic enlargement can be due in part to large Kupffer cells that contain cystine crystals and become large foam cells. There can be hypersplenism. Can have pancreatic exocrine dysfunction. Males may have hypogonadism. Cysteamine, used to treat cystinosis, carries a high incidence of gastrointestinal symptoms, which are often acid-mediated.

The infantile form presents with progressive renal failure, beginning with the Fanconi syndrome (see later) with polyuria, followed by glomerular and renal failure requiring dialysis or transplantation. In addition to multiple amino acid and electrolyte losses in the urine, patients also lose vitamin D and carnitine, which need to be replaced. The urine is pale and cloudy with a particular odor, probably due to the aminoaciduria. The adolescent form presents with renal dysfunction in the second decade of life, whereas the adult form has normal renal function. Bartter syndrome (see earlier) can develop in some children. Progression of the renal failure can result in a regression of Fanconi syndrome secondary to decreased glomerular filtrate being presented to the proximal tubules. Dialysis and renal transplantation are routine. Fanconi syndrome does not recur in transplanted kidneys, even though cystine crystals are present, because they are located within macrophages or leukocytes.

Male patients may have an abnormal pituitary-testicular axis with incomplete maturation and infertility. Female patients have normal gonadal function.

OTHER: Pancreatic involvement by cystine deposition can result in diabetes mellitus, and thyroid involvement can result in hypothyroidism. Thyroid dysfunction is common, particularly in adulthood. Pancreatic exocrine function is normal. Decreased sweating may result in heat intolerance, hyperthermia, and flushing with exercise. May have anemia from renal failure. Caucasian patients will have skin and hair pigmentation lighter than their siblings. May have thrombocytosis.

MISCELLANEOUS: Many children crave the four P's of salt-rich (and child-friendly) foods: pizza, pickles, pretzels, and potato chips (2).

ANESTHETIC CONSIDERATIONS

Because of possible Fanconi or Bartter syndromes involving renal electrolyte losses, preoperative measurement of serum electrolytes, calcium, phosphorus, and magnesium is appropriate. The patient's usual doses of electrolytes can be given

orally before surgery, if tolerated. If oral medications are inappropriate, alternative parenteral dosing is necessary. These might include supplemental calcium, bicarbonate, carnitine and cysteamine, which depletes lysosomal cystine.

Isosthenuria (fixed specific gravity, neither concentrated nor dilute) or polyuria may complicate perioperative fluid management. Protracted preoperative fasting should be avoided to prevent dehydration. Urine output may be a poor indicator of intravascular fluid status, so central venous pressure monitoring might be appropriate in these patients if surgery will involve major fluid shifts. Indomethacin significantly diminishes urinary water and electrolyte losses. Chronic renal failure has implications for the choice and dosages of anesthetic and other drugs. Intravenous fluids may be supplemented with bicarbonate or potassium. Because of excessive relatively dilute urine, patients may require more free water in intravenous fluids. Thirst and salt-sensing mechanisms are intact, and if otherwise appropriate, patients should have free access to water and salt.

When clinically indicated, patients should have thyroid and hepatic function evaluated preoperatively. Patients may have esophageal varices. If diabetes mellitus is suspected, the serum glucose should be measured. Preoperative blood counts should be obtained in patients with hypersplenism. Nasal tubes should be avoided in patients with recurrent epistaxis. Patients with photophobia may be bothered by bright operating room lights. Patients may have recurrent corneal erosions, and perioperative eye care is particularly important. If poorly nourished, these patients may have difficulty maintaining their intraoperative body temperature. Poor nutrition is an indication for careful positioning and padding of pressure points. Decreased sweating may result in perioperative hyperthermia. A child with intraoperative hyperthermia, thought not to be related to malignant hyperthermia, has been reported (3). Succinylcholine should presumably be avoided in patients with myopathy due to the potential of an exaggerated hyperkalemic response.

Bibliography:

1. Ray TL, Tobias JD. Perioperative care of the patient with nephrotic syndrome. *Paediatr Anaesth* 2004;14:878–883.
2. Gahl WA, Thoene JG, Schneider JA. Cystinosis. *N Engl J Med* 2002;347: 111–121.
3. Purday JP, Montgomery CJ, Blackstock D. Intraoperative hyperthermia in a paediatric patient with cystinosis. *Paediatr Anaesth* 1995;5:389–392.
4. Schneider JA, Clark KF, Greene AA. Recent advances in the treatment of cystinosis. *J Inherit Metab Dis* 1995;18:387–397.
5. Tobias JD. Anaesthetic implications of cystinosis. *Can J Anaesth* 1993; 40:518–520.

Cystinuria

MIM #: 220100

Note: This syndrome is distinct from cystinosis.

Cystinuria is due to a mutation in the renal amino acid transporter gene. This transporter is involved in the renal and gastrointestinal epithelial transport of cystine, lysine, arginine, and ornithine. Cystinuria is inherited in an autosomal recessive fashion, and there are three clinical phenotypes. Type I disease is due to defects in the gene *SLC3A*, which encodes the heavy subunit of the protein. Types II and III are due to mutations in the gene *SLC7A9*, which encodes the light subunit. The main clinical manifestation in all three types is the formation of cystine renal stones. Patients with type I disease excrete large amounts of cystine, lysine, arginine, and ornithine in the urine. Heterozygotes with type I disease have no abnormal aminoaciduria. Patients with type II disease excrete excessive amounts of cystine and lysine in the urine. Heterozygotes with type II disease also have excessive excretion of cystine and lysine. Patients with type III disease excrete slightly increased amounts of cystine in the urine. Because of the particularly low solubility of cystine, all three types can form cystine stones. Although compliance is an issue, excretion of cystine is diminished with a diet limiting protein and salt.

NEUROMUSCULAR: May have mental retardation.

GI/GU: Radiopaque nephrolithiasis. May develop renal insufficiency secondary to high chronic stone burden. Renal transplantation is curative.

MISCELLANEOUS: An abnormal renal stone was first identified by Wollaston in 1810. It was an odd stone and he named the substance cystic oxide, because it came from the bladder. It turns out he was incorrect on both accounts—it was not restricted to the bladder (stones also occur in the kidney) and it is an amine, not an oxide. Later analysis showed it was a sulfur-containing amino acid, and so this stone eventually was responsible for the names of the amino acids cystine and cysteine. This was one of the four inborn errors of metabolism (the others being albinism, alcaptonuria, and pentosuria) discussed by Garrod in his famous series of lectures in 1902 (3). Cystinuric patients also excrete large amounts of cadaverine and putrescine.

ANESTHETIC CONSIDERATIONS
Children may well have had multiple urologic interventions. Urine output should be maintained. Perioperative hydration to maintain a diuresis should be continued. Cystine solubility is low at acidic urine pH, but does not significantly increase until the urine pH is over 7.5. Cystine stones are not as easily destroyed by extracorporeal lithotripsy as other types of stones, and percutaneous lithotripsy is more effective, although extracorporeal lithotripsy may be more effective in children.

Bibliography:
1. Knoll T, Zollner A, Wendt-Nordahl G, et al. Cystinuria in childhood and adolescence: recommendations for diagnosis, treatment, and follow-up. *Pediatr Nephrol* 2005;20:19–24.
2. Sakhaeee K. Pathogenesis and medical management of cystinuria. *Semin Nephrol* 1996;156:1907–1912.
3. Garrod AE. The incidence of alkaptonuria: a study in individuality. *Lancet* 1902;2:1616–1620.

Cytochrome *c* Oxidase Deficiency

See Complex IV deficiency

D

Dandy-Walker Malformation

MIM #: 220200

Dandy-Walker malformation is characterized by cerebellar hypoplasia and cystic dilation of the fourth ventricle. Inheritance of this malformation is heterogeneous and unlikely Mendelian. Approximately half of the patients have other associated congenital anomalies.

HEENT/AIRWAY: Hypertelorism, cleft lip, microglossia, and micrognathia have been associated in some patients, but are not primary manifestations.

CHEST: Central respiratory failure with periodic breathing or apnea.

NEUROMUSCULAR: Cerebellar hypoplasia (agenesis of the cerebellar vermis) and dilation of the fourth ventricle, often with a posterior fossa cyst, which enlarges the posterior fossa. Obstructive hydrocephalus with enlargement of the third and lateral ventricles is common. There may be associated agenesis of the corpus callosum, poor intellectual development, or interference with medullary control of respiration with apnea and respiratory failure. Most patients require shunting to relieve intracranial pressure, but there can be asymptomatic adults (2). There may be posterior fossa signs such as cranial nerve palsies, nystagmus, and truncal ataxia.

ORTHOPEDIC: Syndactyly, polydactyly, and limb and vertebral anomalies have been described in some patients.

MISCELLANEOUS: This syndrome was first described by Dandy and Blackfan, who incorrectly ascribed it to atresia of the foramina of Luschka and Magendie. Dandy was a surgeon and Blackfan was a pediatrician and the most outstanding pediatric hematologist of his generation (see Blackfan-Diamond syndrome). Taggart and Walker described it almost 30 years later, and 40 years after the original description the current name was suggested.

In 1913, at the age of 27 years, Dandy published a masterly description of the pathogenesis and management of hydrocephalus. His mentor Halsted commented that "Dandy will never do anything equal to this again. Few men make more than one great contribution to medicine." Halsted was wrong.

ANESTHETIC CONSIDERATIONS
Associated micrognathia is rare, but may complicate laryngoscopy and tracheal intubation (1). Obstructive hydrocephalus may increase intracranial pressure. Precautions

should be taken in patients with increased intracranial pressure to avoid further perioperative increases in pressure. Laryngeal incompetence and vocal cord paralysis with postextubation upper airway obstruction have been reported, presumably due to brainstem compression after surgical drainage (4). Patients should be closely observed postoperatively to ensure adequate control of ventilation.

Bibliography:
1. Selim M, Mowafi H, Al-Ghambdi A, et al. Intubation via LMA in pediatric patients with difficult airways. *Can J Anaesth* 1999;46:891–893.
2. Cone AM. Head injury in an adult with previously undiagnosed Dandy-Walker syndrome: a review of the condition and discussion of its anesthetic implications. *Anaesth Intensive Care* 1995;23:613–615.
3. Ewart MC, Oh TE. The Dandy-Walker syndrome. *Anaesthesia* 1990;45:646–648.
4. Mayhew JF, Miner ME, Denneny J. Upper airway obstruction following cyst-to-peritoneal shunt in a child with a Dandy-Walker cyst. *Anesthesiology* 1985;62:183–184.

Debrancher Deficiency

SYNONYM: Glycogen storage disease type III; Amylo-1,6-glucosidase deficiency; Cori disease; Forbes disease

MIM #: 232400

This autosomal recessive glycogen storage disease may involve liver or muscle. The enzyme defect does not allow full degradation of glycogen, which results in hypoglycemia and storage of a polysaccharide with short branches in all tissues. Unlike von Gierke disease, hypoglycemia can be partially ameliorated by gluconeogenesis and ketogenesis. Gluconeogenesis, however, may rob muscles of protein. Most patients have involvement of both liver and muscle (type IIIa), but some only have hepatic involvement (type IIIb). Patients with liver involvement and myopathy lack enzyme activity in both liver and muscle. Patients with liver involvement lack only hepatic but not muscle enzyme. There is marked clinical variability, and in infancy it may be indistinguishable clinically from von Gierke disease (glycogen storage disease type I). Clinical symptoms and hepatomegaly often improve after puberty. There is a report of a patient who developed respiratory failure at 47 years of age after a period of fasting.

HEENT/AIRWAY: Doll-like facies. Macroglossia.

CARDIOVASCULAR: Cardiomyopathy, often subclinical, but may be progressive in adults.

NEUROMUSCULAR: Muscle weakness and wasting. The myopathy can be mild in childhood but becomes more pronounced in adulthood with muscle wasting. Muscle wasting is both myopathic and neuropathic.

ORTHOPEDIC: Growth retardation.

GI/GU: Hepatomegaly, which may be massive. Periportal fibrosis and nodular cirrhosis are rare and may not be progressive. Progressive liver failure is particularly common in Japanese patients. Hepatic adenomas, without malignant transformation. Liver manifestations, including hepatomegaly, usually improve with age and may disappear completely after puberty. Renal tubular acidosis is very rare. Polycystic ovary with normal fertility.

OTHER: Hypoglycemia. Ketoacidosis with stress. Elevated cholesterol and beta-lipoprotein. Truncal obesity. Hypoglycemia risk decreases with aging.

MISCELLANEOUS: Glycogen storage disease type III was the first glycogen storage disease to be described (by van Creveld), a year before von Gierke and 4 years before Pompe described their now eponymous diseases. The disease also occurs in dogs, where it is much more severe.

ANESTHETIC CONSIDERATIONS
Because of the risk of cardiomyopathy, a careful preoperative cardiac examination should be done. A protracted preoperative fast without supplemental glucose must be avoided. Serum glucose should be monitored perioperatively, and perioperative intravenous fluids should contain glucose. Young children can be obese, which can increase the perioperative aspiration risk and make vascular access more challenging. Succinylcholine should be used cautiously, if at all, in patients with myopathy and muscle wasting because of the risk of an exaggerated hyperkalemic response.

FIGURE: See **Appendix E**

Bibliography:
1. Mohart D, Russo P, Tobias JD. Perioperative management of a child with glycogen storage disease type III undergoing cardiopulmonary bypass and repair of an atrial septal defect. *Paediatr Anaesth* 2002;12:649–654.
2. Kiechl S, Kohlendorfer U, Thaler C, et al. Different clinical aspects of debrancher deficiency myopathy. *J Neurol Neurosurg Psychiatr* 1999;67:364–368.
3. Talente GM, Coleman RA, Alter C, et al. Glycogen storage disease in adults. *Ann Intern Med* 1994;120:218–226.
4. Coleman RA, Winter HS, Wolf B, et al. Glycogen debranching enzyme deficiency: long-term study of serum enzyme activities and clinical features. *J Inherit Metab Dis* 1992;15:869–881.

Degos Disease

See Malignant atrophic papulosis

Dejerine-Sottas Syndrome

MIM #: 145900

There are both autosomal dominant and recessive forms of this motor and sensory neuropathy that is characterized by enlarged nerves with slow conduction, nystagmus, hearing loss, and ataxia. Symptoms first occur in infancy and the course is progressive, although marked by acute exacerbations and remissions. This disorder can be due to mutations in the genes *MPZ, PMP22, PRX* or *ERG2. MPZ, PMP22* and *PRX* encode structural proteins in peripheral myelin. *ERG2* induces these three other genes. Different mutations in some of these genes can also cause Charcot-Marie-Tooth syndrome (see earlier), but Dejerine-Sottas syndrome is more clinically severe.

HEENT/AIRWAY: Nystagmus. Hearing loss.

NEUROMUSCULAR: Enlarged nerves secondary to hypertrophic interstitial neuropathy. Demyelination and slow nerve conduction. Muscle weakness and atrophy begins distally and spreads proximally. Lower limbs are affected before upper limbs. Muscle weakness eventually involves the bulbar muscles. Ataxia. Delayed motor development. Loss of deep tendon reflexes. Foot drop. Sensory deficits accompany the motor deficits. May also have autonomic deficits with thermal lability and mottled cyanosis. Eventual muscle atrophy. Normal intelligence.

ORTHOPEDIC: Kyphoscoliosis. Pes cavus. Hammer toes. Clubfoot deformity.

MISCELLANEOUS: Joseph Dejerine was a French neuropathologist. Jules Sottas was his student.

ANESTHETIC CONSIDERATIONS
Patients may be at risk for an exaggerated hyperkalemic response after the administration of succinylcholine secondary to denervation muscle atrophy. Temperature regulation by sweating may be impaired secondary to autonomic dysfunction, leading to thermal lability and mottled cyanosis. Epidural anesthesia has been used successfully. There is no association between Dejerine-Sottas syndrome and malignant hyperthermia.

Bibliography:
1. Gabreels-Festen A. Dejerine-Sottas syndrome grown to maturity: overview of genetic and morphological heterogeneity and follow-up of 25 patients. *J Anat* 2002;200:341–356.
2. Huang J, Soliman I. Anaesthetic management for a patient with Dejerine-Sottas disease and asthma. *Paediatr Anaesth* 2001;11:225–227.

de Lange Syndrome

See Cornelia de Lange syndrome

Delleman Syndrome

SYNONYM: Oculocerebrocutaneous syndrome

MIM #: 164180

This is a sporadically occurring disease whose primary manifestations are central nervous system cysts or hydrocephalus, orbital cysts or microphthalmia, and focal skin defects. It has been suggested that it may be a consequence of the disruption of the anterior neuroectodermal plate. Another possibility is an autosomal dominant lethal mutation, survivable only in mosaics. Males are more commonly affected, and the left side is more commonly involved than the right.

HEENT/AIRWAY: Periorbital skin appendages, orbital cysts, unilateral anophthalmia or microphthalmia. May have bilateral anophthalmia. Colobomas. Punched out lesions over the alae nasi.

NEUROMUSCULAR: A variety of cerebral malformations including intracranial cysts and agenesis of the corpus callosum. Psychomotor developmental delay and seizures, which can be neonatal in onset.

OTHER: Focal dermal hypoplasia or aplasia.

ANESTHETIC CONSIDERATIONS
Neonatal seizures can be difficult to appreciate and aspiration risk can be increased with seizures and feeding problems. Chronic use of anticonvulsant medications can affect the kinetics of some anesthetic drugs.

Bibliography:
1. Jamieson BD, Kuczkowski KM. Delleman syndrome: anesthetic considerations (French, web-based English translation available). *Ann Fr Anesth Reanim* 2005;24:830.
2. Sadhasivam S, Subramaniam R. Delleman syndrome: anesthetic implications. *Anesth Analg* 1998;87:553–555.
3. Moog U, de Die-Smulders C, Systermans JMJ, et al. Oculocerebrocutaneous syndrome: report of three additional cases and aetiological considerations. *Clin Genet* 1997;52:219–225.

Denys-Drash Syndrome

See Drash syndrome

de Sanctis-Cacchione Syndrome

MIM #: 278800

This autosomal recessive disorder is a form of xeroderma pigmentosum (see later) involving xeroderma pigmentosum, neurologic abnormalities, growth deficiency, and hypogonadism. There is slow somatic growth and variable progressive neurologic dysfunction. Skin deterioration begins in infancy and is progressive thereafter, exacerbated by sun exposure. Life span is shortened secondary to neurologic deterioration or malignancy. As with other forms of xeroderma pigmentosum, there is a defect in DNA repair after ultraviolet radiation-induced damage. Patients with de Sanctis-Cacchione syndrome are most often in xeroderma pigmentosum complementation group A. The disorder can be due to mutations in the gene *ERCC6*. This gene is part of the nuclear excision repair network, which eliminates damaged DNA. Mutations in this gene can also result in a type of Cockayne syndrome (see earlier).

HEENT/AIRWAY: Microcephaly. Photophobia. Keratitis. Occasional sensorineural hearing loss.

NEUROMUSCULAR: Progressive neurologic dysfunction—choreoathetosis, ataxia, hypo- or areflexia, spasticity, seizures, peripheral neuropathy. Cerebral and olivoponto-cerebellar atrophy.

ORTHOPEDIC: Growth deficiency.

GI/GU: Hypogonadotropic hypogonadism.

OTHER: Xeroderma pigmentosum. Telangiectasis. Keratoses. Angiomas. Extreme sunlight sensitivity, with progressive skin deterioration. Eventually basal cell carcinomas, squamous cell carcinomas or melanomas develop. Internal malignancies can develop, including solid organ tumors and leukemia. May exhibit immune dysfunction and frequent infections.

MISCELLANEOUS: de Sanctis and Cacchione originally proposed (in Italian) a somewhat less sensitive synonym: xerodermic idiocy. Needless to say, this synonym is no longer routinely used.

ANESTHETIC CONSIDERATIONS
Neurologic dysfunction may make the smooth induction of general anesthesia challenging. Chronic use of anticonvulsant medications can affect the kinetics of some anesthetic drugs. Care must be taken in positioning and padding the patient secondary to atrophic skin changes and the potential for injury to the skin. Patients with photophobia may be sensitive to bright operating room lights.

Bibliography:
1. Kraemer KH, Lee MM, Scotto J. Xeroderma pigmentosa: cutaneous, ocular, and neurologic abnormalities in 830 published cases. *Arch Dermatol* 1987;123:241–250.
2. Roytta M, Anttinen A. Xeroderma pigmentosum with neurological abnormalities: a clinical and neuropathological study. *Acta Neurol Scand* 1986;73:191–199.

Desmolase Deficiency

See 17,20-Desmolase deficiency

de Toni-Debre-Fanconi Syndrome

See Fanconi syndrome

Diamond-Blackfan Syndrome

See Blackfan-Diamond syndrome

Diaphyseal Aclasis

See Multiple exostoses syndrome

Diastrophic Dysplasia

SYNONYM: Diastrophic nanism

MIM #: 222600

This autosomal recessive, short-limbed dwarfism is further characterized by generalized joint dysplasia, decreased joint mobility, clubfeet, and hypertrophic auricular cartilage. There is a significant amount of phenotypic variability with this syndrome. The gene for this disorder, *SLC26A2 (DTDST)*, is a sulfate transporter gene. The gene appears to encode a novel sulfate transporter. Mutations in the *DTDST* gene also cause achondrogenesis type IB (see earlier) and multiple epiphyseal dysplasia (see later); therefore, these

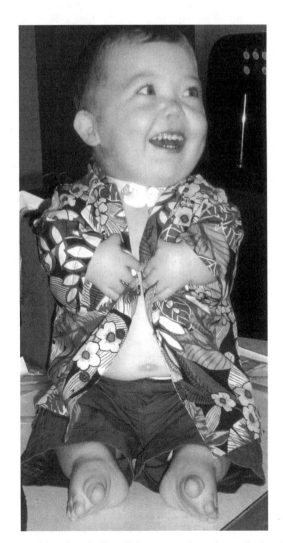

Diastrophic dysplasia. This young boy has diastrophic dysplasia.

disorders are allelic. It is also allelic with atelosteogenesis, type II (not discussed in this text).

HEENT/AIRWAY: Hypertrophic auricular cartilage—may eventually become ossified. Conductive hearing loss. Micrognathia. Malocclusion and occasional hypodontia. Cleft palate. Laryngomalacia, tracheomalacia, and/or bronchomalacia; laryngotracheal stenosis—may cause airway obstruction. Hoarse voice.

CHEST: Premature calcification of the costal cartilages. Accessory manubrial ossification center. Severe kyphoscoliosis leads to restrictive lung disease in some. Small rib cage and tracheal instability can lead to serious neonatal respiratory compromise.

NEUROMUSCULAR: Intelligence is normal. Spinal cord compression can occur as a consequence of severe kyphoscoliosis. Occasional intracranial calcifications.

ORTHOPEDIC: Progressive and marked short stature from lack of pubertal growth spurt. Short limbs. Cervical vertebral hypoplasia or kyphosis with occasional subluxation of C2-3, which may resolve by adulthood. May have odontoid hypoplasia. Broadening of the cervical spine. Cervical lordosis and degenerative changes in adults. Scoliosis. Marked lumbar lordosis and thoracic kyphoscoliosis. Spina bifida occulta in midcervical to upper thoracic vertebrae. Interpeduncular narrowing of L1-5. Generalized joint dysplasia with decreased joint mobility, especially at the elbows, hips, and knees. Early hip degeneration. May have joint webbing. Patellar subluxation. Abduction of the thumbs (hitchhiker thumbs) and great toes. Clubfeet which are particularly difficult to correct surgically.

MISCELLANEOUS: "Diastrophic" is from the Greek, meaning tortuous or crooked, referring to the kyphoscoliosis. It was appropriated from geology, where diastrophism is the process of bending the earth's crust. The disorder is particularly prevalent in Finns.

The location of the *DTDST* gene was found fortuitously by a group mapping the gene for Treacher Collins syndrome.

ANESTHETIC CONSIDERATIONS
Patients may have airway obstruction secondary to laryngotracheobronchomalacia or laryngotracheal stenosis. Up to 25% of infants die of airway complications. Airway complications may be exacerbated by general anesthesia. Patients with laryngotracheal stenosis may require a smaller-than-predicted endotracheal tube. Micrognathia can further complicate laryngoscopy and tracheal intubation.

These patients are at risk for subluxation at C2-3, in addition to baseline cord compression. The head must be carefully positioned during laryngoscopy to avoid hyperextension. Patients must be carefully positioned for the procedure because of limited joint mobility.

Because of their relatively short limbs, these patients may require a smaller than normal blood pressure cuff. An appropriately sized cuff should cover two-thirds of the length of the upper arm.

Bibliography:
1. Makitie O, Kaitila I. Growth in diastrophic dysplasia. *J Pediatr* 1996;130: 641–646.
2. Hall BD. Diastrophic dysplasia: extreme variability within a sibship. *Am J Med Genet* 1996;63:28–33.
3. Poussa M, Merikanto J, Ryoppy S, et al. The spine in diastrophic dysplasia. *Spine* 1991;16:881–887.
4. Berkowitz I, Raja S, Bender K, et al. Dwarfs: pathophysiology and anesthetic implications. *Anesthesiology* 1990;73:739–759.

Diastrophic Nanism

See Diastrophic dysplasia

Dibasic Amino Aciduria Type 2

See Lysinuric protein intolerance

DIDMOAD Syndrome

SYNONYM: Wolfram syndrome

MIM #: 222300

Diabetes **I**nsipidus, **D**iabetes **M**ellitus, **O**ptic **A**trophy, and **D**eafness is likely an autosomal recessive disorder. Only insulin-dependent diabetes mellitus and optic atrophy are required to make the diagnosis. Diabetes mellitus is usually the presenting problem. This autosomal recessive disorder is due to mutations in the gene *WFS1*, which encodes the protein wolframin, an endoplasmic reticulum membrane glycoprotein, but has also been associated with abnormalities at a different locus on chromosome 4. The syndrome is clinically variable.

HEENT/AIRWAY: Optic atrophy, ptosis, nystagmus. Sensorineural hearing loss and deafness.

CARDIOVASCULAR: One adult patient was reported with glycogen deposits in the myocardium.

NEUROMUSCULAR: Autonomic dysfunction, mental retardation, dementia, seizures. Ataxia, tremor, peripheral neuropathy. Dysphagia, dysarthria. Magnetic resonance imaging scans show widespread atrophic brain changes. Psychiatric illness. Patients may be compulsive or physically aggressive. There is an increased risk of suicide.

GI/GU: Hydronephrosis, hydroureter, and distended bladder without vesicoureteral reflux. May have testicular atrophy.

OTHER: Insulin-dependent diabetes mellitus, central diabetes insipidus. Megaloblastic anemia (thiamine responsive) has been reported. May have hypothyroidism.

ANESTHETIC CONSIDERATIONS
Psychiatric illness may make preanesthetic management more difficult. When meeting the patients before surgery, be sensitive to the possibility that they have hearing or visual loss. Glucose control (insulin-dependent diabetes mellitus) and water control (central diabetes insipidus) are critical. Chronic use of anticonvulsant medications may alter the metabolism of some anesthetic drugs.

Bibliography:
1. Barrett TG, Bundey SE. Wolfram (DIDMOAD) syndrome. *J Med Genet* 1997;34:838–841.
2. Peden NR, Gay JD, Jung RT, et al. Wolfram (DIDMOAD) syndrome: a complex long-term problem in management. *Q J Med* 1986;58:167–180.

Diencephalic Syndrome

MIM #: None
This syndrome, which primarily involves abnormal growth and energy metabolism, is secondary to tumors, usually astrocytomas of the anterior third ventricle, or optic gliomas that extend to involve the hypothalamus. Children are typically 18 months to $3\frac{1}{2}$ years of age at diagnosis, but rare cases have been reported in adults. Diencephalic syndrome is probably due to abnormal hypothalamic metabolic control, and the metabolic rate is increased above normal. Patients usually exhibit profound loss of subcutaneous tissue.

HEENT/AIRWAY: Pale, elfin-like facies from loss of subcutaneous fat. Nystagmus, optic atrophy secondary to underlying tumor.

NEUROMUSCULAR: Exceptional alertness or euphoria. Intracranial pressure is normal until late in the progression of the tumor. Peripheral neurologic findings are also late.

ORTHOPEDIC: Accelerated long bone growth.

GI/GU: Vomiting, diarrhea.

OTHER: Normal development initially, with the development of profound inanition and loss of subcutaneous tissue. There may be hypoglycemia. Appetite may be normal, decreased, or excessive, even in the face of continued weight loss. Heat intolerance or abnormal temperature control.

ANESTHETIC CONSIDERATIONS
An adequate perioperative glucose source should be ensured. These very thin patients may have excessive intraoperative heat loss, but may also have abnormal hypothalamic control of body temperature. Patients need careful intraoperative positioning because of thin habitus and lack of subcutaneous cushioning. Precautions must be taken in patients with elevated intracranial pressure to avoid further elevations in pressure.

Bibliography:
1. Carmel PW. Surgical syndromes of the hypothalamus. *Clin Neurosurg* 1980;27:133–159.

DiGeorge Syndrome

SYNONYM: 22q11.2 Deletion syndrome

MIM #: 188400
This well known syndrome has been shown in most cases to be due to microdeletions of chromosome 22 (22q11.2). Mutations in the gene *TBX1*, located in the middle of the microdeletion region, is thought to be involved in producing some of the features. This gene, a transcription factor, is involved in developmental processes. The phenotypic presentation can vary, and the same deletion(s) can result in CATCH-22 syndrome (see earlier), Shprintzen syndrome (velocardiofacial syndrome, see later), conotruncal anomaly face syndrome (Takao syndrome, not discussed in this text), and isolated conotruncal cardiac defects (truncus arteriosus, tetralogy of Fallot, or interrupted aortic arch). Identical twins have had the same genotype, but a different phenotypic presentation. DiGeorge syndrome has also been associated with prenatal exposure to alcohol and to isotretinoin (Accutane).

Approximately 75% of affected people will have cardiac manifestations, and 50% otolaryngologic manifestations. Up to 60% will have at least transient hypocalcemia, but only 2% will have major immunologic deficiencies.

Most features can be traced back to abnormalities of the third and fourth pharyngeal pouches and fourth branchial arch *in utero,* and include defects in the development of the thymus, parathyroids, and great vessels. Neonatal morbidity and mortality are associated with the cardiac defects, sequelae of T-cell immunodeficiency, and seizures related to hypocalcemia.

HEENT/AIRWAY: Telecanthus/lateral displacement of inner canthi and short palpebral fissures with either an upward or downward slant. Low-set ears with lower-than-usual vertical dimension and abnormal folding of the pinna. Bulbous nose. Choanal atresia with velopharyngeal incompetence. The philtrum is short and the mouth small. Overt or submucous cleft palate. Micrognathia in infancy. Trachea may be short.

CARDIOVASCULAR: A variety of conotruncal cardiac defects, namely truncus arteriosus, tetralogy of Fallot, and interrupted aortic arch. Truncus arteriosus and tetralogy of Fallot are often associated with a right aortic arch.

NEUROMUSCULAR: Hypocalcemic tetany or seizures in neonates. Occasional mental deficiency of mild or moderate degree. About 20% of adults carry a psychiatric diagnosis, particularly bipolar disease.

GI/GU: Occasional esophageal atresia, imperforate anus, diaphragmatic hernia. It has been suggested that there is an increase in feeding difficulties due to pharyngeal and esophageal dysmotility.

OTHER: Neonatal hypocalcemia (and subsequent seizures), which can be intermittent, secondary to hypoplastic or absent parathyroid glands. The hypocalcemia typically resolves in early childhood. Abnormal parathyroid function observed in up to 70% cases, but abnormal parathyroid function can only be documented in some children and in adults with provocative tests. Cell-mediated immune deficiency from a T-cell deficiency secondary to a hypoplastic or aplastic thymus gland may result in severe infections. May have short stature, and growth hormone deficiency has recently been documented in some patients.

MISCELLANEOUS: Microdeletions of chromosomal region 22q11 are diagnosed by fluorescence *in situ* hybridization (FISH) testing. In past years, the absence of some features of the syndrome in any particular patient led to the diagnosis of a "forme-fruste" of the syndrome. Approximately one in eight children with tetralogy of Fallot, and one in five with truncus arteriosus, will have DiGeorge syndrome.

ANESTHETIC CONSIDERATIONS

Micrognathia, if present, may make direct laryngoscopy and tracheal intubation difficult. A short trachea can result in inadvertent endobronchial intubation (7). Choanal atresia precludes placement of a nasal airway, nasal intubation, or placement of a nasogastric tube. Neonates should have their serum calcium level evaluated preoperatively. Hyperventilation may worsen hypocalcemia, as may infusions of citrated blood products. Blood products should be irradiated to prevent graft-versus-host disease. Careful aseptic technique is indicated. Patients with cardiac disease should receive antibiotic prophylaxis as indicated. This region of chromosome 22 also includes the gene encoding catechol-O-methyltransferase (*COMT*), responsible for degrading catecholamines. A patient has been reported with unexpected tachycardia from epinephrine containing local analgesic given during dental surgery, possibly from being hemizygous for *COMT* (1).

Bibliography:

1. Passariello M, Perkins R. Unexpected postoperative tachycardia in a patient with 22q11 deletion syndrome after multiple dental extractions [Letter]. *Paediatr Anaesth* 2005;15:1145–1151.
2. Ryan AK, Goodship JA, Wilson DI, et al. Spectrum of clinical features associated with interstitial chromosome 22q11 deletions: a European collaborative study. *J Med Genet* 1997;34:798–804.
3. Johnson MC, Hing A, Wood MK, et al. Chromosome abnormalities in congenital heart disease. *Am J Med Genet* 1997;70:292–298.
4. Thomas JA, Graham JM. Chromosome 22q11 deletion syndrome: an update and review for the primary pediatrician. *Clin Pediatr* 1997;36: 253–266.
5. Wilson DI, Burn J, Scambler P, et al. DiGeorge syndrome, part of CATCH 22. *J Med Genet* 1993;30:852–856.
6. Stevens CA, Carey JC, Shigeoka AO. DiGeorge anomaly and velocardiofacial syndrome. *Pediatrics* 1990;85:526–530.
7. Wells AL, Wells TR, Landing BH, et al. Short trachea, a hazard in tracheal intubation of neonates and infants: syndromal associations. *Anesthesiology* 1989;71:367–373.
8. Flashburg MH, Dunbar BS, August G, et al. Anaesthesia for surgery in an infant with DiGeorge syndrome. *Anesthesiology* 1983;58:479–480.

Dilantin

See Fetal hydantoin syndrome

Disseminated Lipogranulomatosis

See Farber disease

Distal Arthrogryposis

See Arthrogryposis

Distichiasis-Lymphedema Syndrome

MIM #: 153400

This autosomal dominant syndrome is characterized by an extra row of eyelashes and lymphedema. There is marked variability of expression with this syndrome. The syndrome is due to abnormalities in the forkhead family transcription factor gene, *MFH1 (FOXC2)*. This gene is a regulator of adipocyte metabolism. There are several other allelic syndromes with lymphedema being a common factor. It has been suggested that the defect is due to aberrant lymphatic vessel valve formation and an abnormal interaction between the lymphatic endothelial cells and pericytes.

HEENT/AIRWAY: Distichiasis—a double row of eyelashes. Usually at least one row of eyelashes is turned inward, causing corneal irritation. Absence of meibomian glands. Occasional ptosis, microphthalmia, strabismus, epicanthal folds. May have photophobia. Occasional cleft palate, bifid uvula, micrognathia. Webbed neck.

CARDIOVASCULAR: May have a variety of congenital cardiac defects, including defects of the conduction system.

NEUROMUSCULAR: Epidural cysts are common.

ORTHOPEDIC: Vertebral anomalies. Occasional scoliosis/ kyphosis or short stature.

OTHER: Lymphedema, most pronounced in the lower extremities, is usually apparent by the end of puberty. Varicose veins. One family has been reported in which affected members also had renal disease and diabetes.

ANESTHETIC CONSIDERATIONS
Micrognathia, if present, may make laryngoscopy and tracheal intubation more difficult. Peripheral intravenous access may be difficult secondary to lymphedema. Epidural cysts may cause secondary neurologic impairment, which should be well documented before undertaking neuraxial anesthesia/analgesia. Patients with cardiac defects require perioperative antibiotic prophylaxis as indicated.

Bibliography:
1. Brice G, Mansour S, Bell R, et al. Analysis of the phenotypic abnormalities in lymphoedema-distichiasis syndrome in 74 patients with FOXC2 mutations or linkage to 16q24. *J Med Genet* 2002;39:478–483.
2. Temple IK, Collin JRO. Distichiasis-lymphoedema syndrome: a family report. *Clin Dysmorphol* 1994;3:139–142.
3. Corbett CRR, Dale RF, Coltart DJ, et al. Congenital heart disease in patients with primary lymphoedemas. *Lymphology* 1982;15:85–90.
4. Schwartz IF, O'Brien MS, Hoffman JC. Hereditary spinal arachnoid cysts, distichiasis, and lymphedema. *Ann Neurol* 1980;7:340–343.

DK-Phocomelia Syndrome

SYNONYM: von Voss-Cherstvoy syndrome

MIM #: 223340

This possibly autosomal disorder is characterized by phocomelia, thrombocytopenia, encephalocele and urogenital anomalies. The responsible gene and gene product are not known.

HEENT/AIRWAY: Facial asymmetry (particularly in patients with encephalocele). May have cleft palate.

CARDIOVASCULAR: May have valvular defects. May have abnormal branching of coronary arteries.

CHEST: May have abnormal lung lobation. May have agenesis of the diaphragm.

NEUROMUSCULAR: Occipital or parietooccipital encephalocele. May have seizures.

ORTHOPEDIC: Phocomelia. May have congenitally dislocated hips.

GI/GU: Renal anomalies—including horseshoe kidney, renal aplasia. Genital anomalies, including ambiguous genitalia. May have omphalocele, anal atresia, accessory spleens.

OTHER: Thrombocytopenia.

MISCELLANEOUS: The "DK" in the synonym DK-phocomelia comes from the surnames of the two original patients.

ANESTHETIC CONSIDERATIONS
A platelet count should be obtained preoperatively. Phocomelia may make fixation of an appropriate-sized blood pressure cuff difficult, and falsely high pressures may be displayed by noninvasive monitors. An appropriately sized blood pressure cuff should cover two-thirds of the upper arm length. Renal anomalies, if they affect renal function, have implications for perioperative fluid management and the choice of anesthetic drugs.

Bibliography:
1. Brunetti-Pierri N, Mendoza-Londono R, Shah MR, et al. von Voss-Cherstvoy syndrome with transient thrombocytopenia and normal psychomotor development. *Am J Med Genet A* 2004;126:299–302.
2. Bamforth JS, Lin CC. DK phocomelia phenotype (von Voss-Cherstvoy syndrome) caused by somatic mosaicism for del(13q). *Am J Med Genet* 1997;73:408–411.

Donohue Syndrome

See Leprechaunism

Down Syndrome

SYNONYM: Trisomy 21

MIM #: 190685

Trisomy 21 is almost certainly the most widely appreciated chromosomal disease among nongeneticists. Besides the distinctive facies, there are significant airway and cardiac findings, and there is variable mental retardation.

HEENT/AIRWAY: Brachycephaly. Upslanting palpebral fissures. Brushfield spots are seen on the iris. Strabismus is sometimes present. Small external ear canals. Narrowed nasopharynx. Flat nasal bridge. Furrowed tongue. Macroglossia and pharyngeal muscle hypotonia tend to cause upper airway obstruction. High-arched palate, tonsillar and adenoidal hypertrophy. Micrognathia. Teeth may be small or fused. Short, broad neck. Trachea may be small, even in adults without congenital heart disease.

CHEST: May have chronic upper airway obstruction with hypoventilation and obstructive sleep apnea. Recurrent pulmonary infections may develop.

CARDIOVASCULAR: Approximately one half have congenital heart disease. Of those, approximately one half have endocardial cushion defects (including complete atrioventricular canal), and the other half have a variety of defects, typically atrial septal defect, ventricular septal defect or patent ductus arteriosus. Tetralogy of Fallot can also be seen. Children with congenital heart disease with left-to-right shunting are thought to acquire pulmonary hypertension and pulmonary vascular disease at an earlier stage compared to children with a similar cardiac lesion without Down

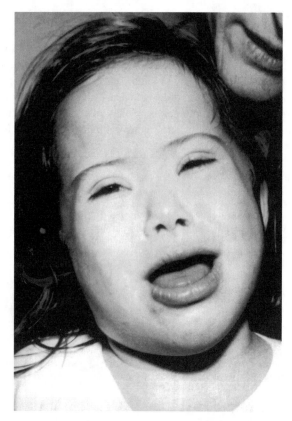

Down syndrome. FIG. 1. A young girl with typical Down syndrome facies. The macroglossia is apparent. (Courtesy of Dr. Jack H. Rubinstein, Cincinnati Center for Developmental Disorders, Cincinnati Children's Hospital Medical Center.)

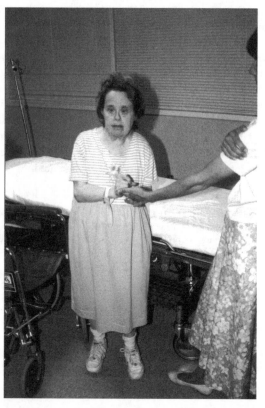

Down syndrome. FIG. 2. A 66-year-old woman with Down syndrome. Other than recurrent pulmonary infections and hypothyroidism, she has been healthy. Her only surgery was a cholecystectomy. Like other adults with Down syndrome, her facial features have lost some of the classic features of children with Down syndrome.

syndrome. This is clouded by upper airway obstruction and hypoventilation that many of these patients have, which can also increase pulmonary arterial pressure.

NEUROMUSCULAR: Hypotonia and variable mental retardation. Children raised at home typically do better than those raised in institutions, which is uncommon today. These children are often very friendly. Dementia and parkinsonism in older adults. Intellectual decline with aging to middle age and older.

ORTHOPEDIC: Height (and weight) below those of normal children. Growth charts for Down syndrome children are available. Joint laxity. Lax cervical ligaments can result in atlantooccipital or atlantoaxial instability and dislocation. Bony abnormalities such as flattening of the occipital condyles can also increase the risk of atlantooccipital instability. There can also be C2 and odontoid abnormalities which can increase the risk of cervical instability. Atlantoaxial instability can be demonstrated in 7% to 36% of children radiographically. The incidence of atlantooccipital instability is approximately 8.5%. Lax ligaments can affect any joint. Patients have clinodactyly of the fifth finger, short, stubby hands, and simian creases (horizontal palmar creases that cross the palm in a single crease).

GI/GU: There is a well known association with congenital duodenal atresia or stenosis. Increased incidence of Hirschsprung disease (see later). Males are infertile. Females have decreased fertility.

OTHER: Patients may have high white blood cell counts in response to infection (leukemoid reaction). The incidence of true leukemia is also high. There is an increased incidence of congenital hypothyroidism and the development of antithyroid antibodies.

MISCELLANEOUS: John Langdon Down was very progressive for his time, and publicly challenged the popular belief that women who sought higher educational degrees were more likely to bear children who would be mentally deficient.

In his original report (1866) on what would become known as Down syndrome, Down tried to differentiate these patients from infants with hypothyroidism ("cretins"). Waardenburg first observed that the disorder might be due to a chromosomal abnormality, which was confirmed by Lejeune in 1959.

Simian creases can be found as normal variants in non-Down patients. One of the authors once knew a genetics fellow with bilateral simian creases.

ANESTHETIC CONSIDERATIONS

Although atlantoaxial instability can occur after approximately 4 years of age, many thousands of children have had laryngoscopy and intubation without untoward incident. However, there are case reports of subluxation after intubation (6,9,13,14). The diagnosis of instability is difficult (1) and involves flexion–extension views. Laryngoscopy should be done with care to minimize flexion or extension of the neck. Recommendations by some practitioners for routine preoperative flexion, neutral, and extension lateral radiographs of the neck seem excessive to most other practitioners. Currently, only a small percentage would obtain radiographs in asymptomatic patients (4), and x-ray criteria are not predictive of a tendency to dislocate. In addition, dislocations are typically preceded by signs or symptoms (11). Rotary cervical dislocations can be related to surgical positioning, often for otolaryngologic surgery. If possible, the patient and table should be rotated as a unit with rotation of the head kept to a minimum. Since dislocations are often preceded by symptoms, the preoperative history should include questions addressing recent changes in gross and fine motor function, or head or neck pain.

Approximately one-fourth of children require an endotracheal tube one to two sizes smaller than that predicted (18), although at least some of this may be due to the generally smaller size of these patients. Adults can also have relatively small tracheas. Postoperative stridor and respiratory complications are more common than in the general population. Macroglossia and pharyngeal muscle hypotonia may lead to upper airway obstruction, and patients must be observed closely in the postanesthesia care unit. Difficult laryngoscopy due to lingual tonsillar hypertrophy has been reported (3).

A significant number of these patients have congenital heart disease. Some patients also have some degree of pulmonary hypertension, due either to heart disease or chronic upper airway obstruction, or a combination of both. A quick screen for endocardial cushion defects (present in approximately 25%) is a superior QRS axis. An increased incidence of intraoperative bradycardia has been reported (2). Patients with congenital heart disease require perioperative antibiotic prophylaxis as clinically indicated.

These patients are more sensitive to the mydriatic and chronotropic effects of atropine (because of altered sensitivity of cholinergic receptors, an imbalance of cholinergic and adrenergic receptors, or altered distribution of the drug), but no ill effects have been seen with normal doses of atropine. Hypothyroidism, when present, could result in delayed gastric emptying, alterations in drug metabolism and impaired temperature regulation.

These patients can be relatively difficult to sedate for cases requiring monitored anesthesia care, without causing hypoventilation.

Bibliography:
1. Hata T, Todd MM. Cervical spine considerations when anesthetizing patients with Down syndrome. *Anesthesiology* 2005;102:680–685.
2. Borland LM, Colligan J, Brandom BW. Frequency of anesthesia-related complications in children with Down syndrome under general anesthesia for noncardiac procedures. *Paediatr Anaesth* 2004;14:733–738.
3. Nakazawa K, Ikeda D, Ishikawa S, et al. A case of difficult airway due to lingual tonsillar hypertrophy in a patient with Down's syndrome. *Anesth Analg* 2003;97:704–705.
4. Litman RS, Zerngast BA, Perkins FM. Preoperative evaluation of the cervical spine in children with trisomy-21: results of a questionnaire study. *Paediatr Anaesth* 1995;5:355–361.
5. Mitchell V, Howard R, Facer E. Down's syndrome and anaesthesia. *Paediatr Anaesth* 1995;5:379–384.
6. Litman RS, Perkins FM. Atlantoaxial subluxation after tympanomastoidectomy in a child with trisomy 21. *Otolaryngol Head Neck Surg* 1994;110:584–586.
7. Rautiainen P, Meretoja OA. Intravenous sedation for children with Down's syndrome undergoing cardiac catheterization. *Paediatr Anaesth* 1994;4:21–26.
8. Hansen DD, Haberkern CM, Jonas RA, et al. Case 1–1991: tracheal stenosis in an infant with Down's syndrome and complex congenital heart disease. *J Cardiothorac Vasc Anesth* 1991;5:8105.
9. Powell JF, Woodcock T, Elliscombe FE. Atlanto-axial subluxation in Down's syndrome. *Anaesthesia* 1990;45:1049–1051.
10. Msall ME, Reese ME, DiGaudio K, et al. Symptomatic atlantoaxial instability associated with medical and rehabilitative procedures in children with Down syndrome. *Pediatrics* 1990;85:447–449.
11. Davidson RG. Atlanto-axial instability in Down's Syndrome: a fresh look at the evidence. *Pediatrics* 1988;81:857–865.
12. Beilin B, Kadari A, Shapira Y, et al. Anaesthetic considerations in facial reconstruction for Down's Syndrome. *J R Soc Med* 1988;81:23–26.
13. Williams JP, Somerville GM, Miner ME, et al. Atlanto-axial subluxation and trisomy-21: another perioperative complication. *Anesthesiology* 1987;67:253–254.
14. Moore RA, McNichols KW, Warran SP. Atlantoaxial subluxation with symptomatic spinal cord compression in a child with Down's syndrome. *Anesth Analg* 1987;66:89–90.
15. Morray JP, MacGillivray R, Duker G. Increased perioperative risk following repair of congenital heart disease in Down's syndrome. *Anesthesiology* 1986;65:220–221.
16. Sherry KM. Post-extubation stridor in Down's syndrome. *Br J Anaesth* 1983;55:53–55.
17. Wark HJ, Overton JH, Marian P. The safety of atropine premedication in children with Down's syndrome. *Anaesthesia* 1983;8:871–879.
18. Kobel M, Creighton RE, Steward DJ. Anaesthetic considerations in Down's syndrome: experience with 100 patients and a review of the literature. *Can Anaesth Soc J* 1982;29:593–598.

Drash Syndrome

SYNONYM: Denys-Drash syndrome

MIM #: 194080

This autosomal dominant syndrome is characterized by pseudohermaphroditism, Wilms tumor, hypertension, and degenerative renal disease. The disorder is due to an abnormality of the Wilms tumor suppressor gene (*WT1*). This gene is a transcription activator or repressor and is required for normal formation of the genitourinary system and mesothelial tissues. There is symptomatic overlap with aniridia-Wilms tumor association (see earlier) and Frasier syndrome (see later), which is also due to abnormalities of *WT1*.

CARDIOVASCULAR: Hypertension secondary to renal failure.

GI/GU: Wilms tumor, usually bilateral. Male pseudohermaphroditism. Ambiguous female genitalia with gonadal dysgenesis, both testicular and ovarian tissue present. Renal failure with mesangial sclerosis presenting as proteinuria and often nephrotic syndrome, and progressing to end-stage renal failure in young childhood. Gonadoblastoma. Primary amenorrhea.

ANESTHETIC CONSIDERATIONS

Renal dysfunction has implications for titration of perioperative fluids and choice of anesthetic drugs. Electrolytes and hematocrit should be evaluated preoperatively in patients with chronic renal failure. A certain amount of sensitivity is required when speaking with patients or families whose children have intersex disorders.

Bibliography:

1. Vila R, Miguel E, Martinez V, et al. Anesthesia for pheochromocytoma in a surgically anephric child. *Anesth Analg* 1997;85:1042–1044.
2. Mueller RF. The Denys-Drash syndrome. *J Med Genet* 1994;31:471–477.
3. Jensen JC, Ehrlich RM, Hanna MK, et al. A report of four patients with the Drash syndrome and a review of the literature. *J Urol* 1989;141:1174–1176.

Dubin-Johnson Syndrome

MIM #: 237500

This is an autosomal recessive disease of hyperbilirubinemia, mostly conjugated. Most patients are asymptomatic. There is a defect in hepatocellular secretion of bilirubin glucuronide and other organic ions. Hepatic cells are stained with a black pigment. The disorder is due to abnormalities in the gene *CMOAT* (canalicular multispecific organic anion transporter), first described in rats. It is also known as *MRP2*, a multidrug resistance protein, which is related to resistance to some chemotherapeutic drugs. Clinically, this syndrome is similar to Rotor syndrome (see later). Other diseases of hepatic bilirubin metabolism include Crigler-Najjar and Gilbert syndromes.

GI/GU: Hyperbilirubinemia without pruritus. Serum bilirubin is typically between 2 to 5 mg/dL, but may be as high as 25 mg/dL. Occasional hepatomegaly, abdominal pain, or splenomegaly. The degree of hyperbilirubinemia can be markedly increased by intercurrent stress, illness, pregnancy, or birth control pills. Black liver. Cholestasis.

MISCELLANEOUS: This disease is particularly common among Iranian Jews, where it is also associated with factor VII deficiency.

Nathan Dubin, chair of pathology at the Medical College of Pennsylvania, often published humorous verse and limericks under a pseudonym. Frank Johnson became curator of the Armed Forces Medical Museum.

ANESTHETIC CONSIDERATIONS

These patients are asymptomatic and there are no specific anesthetic considerations. Some drugs, the most common being rifampin, cause enzyme inhibition with increased serum bilirubin levels and jaundice. Although sulfonamides, some cephalosporins, and intravenous contrast agents can increase free bilirubin levels by displacing bilirubin from albumin, no currently used anesthetic agents are known to displace bilirubin to a degree that would contraindicate their use. The stress of surgery or a perioperative infection can exacerbate the hyperbilirubinemia.

Bibliography:

1. Nowicki MJ, Poley JR. The hereditary hyperbilirubinaemias. *Baillieres Clin Gastroenterol* 1998;12:355–367.
2. Paulusma CC. Oude Elferink RR The canalicular multispecific organic anion transporter and conjugated hyperbilirubinemia in rat and man. *J Mol Med* 1997;75:420–428.
3. Zimniak P. Dubin-Johnson and Rotor syndromes: molecular basis and pathogenesis. *Semin Liver Dis* 1993;13:248–260.
4. Miyakawa H, Matsumoto K, Matsumoto S, et al. Anesthetic and postoperative management of a patient with Gilbert's syndrome and another with Dubin-Johnson syndrome [Japanese]. *Masui* 1991;40:119–123.

Dubowitz Syndrome

MIM #: 223370

This likely autosomal recessive disorder is distinguished by characteristic facies, infantile eczema and growth deficiency. The facies have been likened to those of the fetal alcohol syndrome (see later). The responsible gene and gene product are not known.

HEENT/AIRWAY: Microcephaly. Characteristic small facies with indistinct supraorbital ridge. Facial asymmetry. Short palpebral fissures with telecanthus and apparent hypertelorism. May have ptosis, epicanthal folds, blepharophimosis, strabismus, microphthalmia, hypoplasia of the iris, or colobomas. Malformed ears. Broad nasal tip. Dental abnormalities, including late eruption, caries, and missing teeth. Micrognathia. Occasional submucosal cleft palate, velopharyngeal insufficiency.

CARDIOVASCULAR: Occasional cardiac defect. Occlusion of the internal carotid artery and an aberrant right subclavian artery have been documented in two patients.

NEUROMUSCULAR: Variable degree of mental deficiency. High-pitched, hoarse cry in infancy. Delayed speech. Hyperactivity or attention deficit in most. Other behavioral problems. Cervical vertebral anomalies have been described.

ORTHOPEDIC: Growth deficiency. Delayed osseous maturation. Brachyclinodactyly of fifth fingers. Syndactyly of second and third toes.

GI/GU: Frequent vomiting. Chronic diarrhea. Gastroesophageal reflux. Inguinal hernia. Cryptorchidism. Pilonidal dimple. May have hypospadias.

OTHER: Intrauterine growth retardation. Eczema, noted on face and flexural areas of infants, usually clears by age 2 to

4 years, with occasional flare-ups. Sparse scalp and eyebrow hair. Occasional bone marrow hypoplasia or aplastic anemia. Occasional immunoglobulin deficiency with recurrent respiratory and gastrointestinal infections. Occasional malignancy, including neuroblastoma, lymphoma, and leukemia.

ANESTHETIC CONSIDERATIONS

Behavioral problems may affect the choice of technique for the induction of anesthesia. Missing or loose teeth should be documented before the induction of anesthesia. Patients with cardiac defects should receive perioperative antibiotic prophylaxis as indicated. Micrognathia could potentially result in difficulty with laryngoscopy and intubation, and submental intubation has been reported in a single patient in the Dutch literature.

Bibliography:

1. Tsukahara M, Opitz JM. Dubowitz syndrome: review of 141 cases including 36 previously unreported patients. *Am J Med Genet* 1996;63: 277–289.
2. Hansen KE, Kirkpatrick SJ, Laxova R. Dubowitz syndrome: long-term follow-up of an original patient. *Am J Med Genet* 1995;55:161–164.

Duchenne Muscular Dystrophy

MIM #: 310200

This X-linked muscular dystrophy is biochemically closely related to both Becker muscular dystrophy (see earlier) and X-linked dilated cardiomyopathy (not discussed in this text). Female carriers can have mild clinical manifestations. Patients with Duchenne muscular dystrophy have deletion mutations in the dystrophin gene that prevent any expression of dystrophin in skeletal muscles (frame shifts or stop codons). Patients with Becker muscular dystrophy have dystrophin of altered size or reduced abundance because of deletion mutations that maintain the reading frame during gene transcription. Patients with X-linked cardiomyopathy have defects in a cardiac-specific promotor region or have altered messenger ribonucleic acid (mRNA) splicing, such that only the cardiac but not the striated muscle dystrophin is affected (14).

Dystrophin is a very large protein (accounting for the relatively large number of spontaneous mutations) that resides immediately adjacent to the cell membrane and serves to help anchor the contractile apparatus. Dystrophin is responsible for connecting the sarcolemma to the extracellular matrix. It is found in striated muscle, smooth muscle, and cardiac muscle.

Very large deletions in the dystrophin gene can also affect two nearby genes, leading to hyperglycerolemia (see later) and congenital adrenal hypoplasia (*not* hyperplasia).

HEENT/AIRWAY: Large tongue.

CHEST: Respiratory muscle weakness and swallowing difficulties can lead to recurrent respiratory infections. Abdominal muscle weakness results in early expiratory muscle weakness. Early diaphragmatic preservation preserves

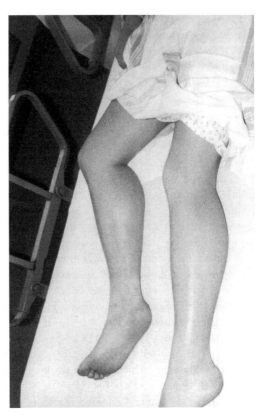

Duchenne muscular dystrophy. Calf pseudohypertrophy in a 12-year-old girl with Duchenne muscular dystrophy. She has mild to moderate muscle weakness, pes cavus, a mild learning disability and hypothyroidism.

inspiratory function through the first decade. Scoliosis may cause restrictive lung disease. Most patients eventually die a respiratory death.

CARDIOVASCULAR: Ninety percent have a typical abnormal electrocardiogram with tall R waves in the right precordium, deep Q waves in the left precordial leads, biventricular hypertrophy, and sinus tachycardia at rest. Heart block or arrhythmias can develop from fibrosis of the conduction system. Heart failure occurs in adolescence. Patients may be relatively asymptomatic for the degree of myocardial dysfunction because they have limited activity. The severity of the cardiomyopathy does not mirror the severity of the peripheral muscular disease. Female carriers also can have a cardiomyopathy, which develops in adulthood.

NEUROMUSCULAR: Generalized myopathy. A classic finding is pseudohypertrophy of the calf muscles. Resting elevations in creatine kinase. Some patients may have mild mental retardation.

GI/GU: There may be gastric hypomotility with delayed gastric emptying. In the extreme, there may be gastric dilatation with the risk of aspiration, or abdominal distention from small bowel ileus. Constipation.

OTHER: The dystrophin gene is closely linked to the gene for glycerol kinase, and patients with Duchenne muscular dystrophy can also have hyperglycerolemia (see later). Typically, those patients with mild mental retardation are also most likely to have hyperglycerolemia and congenital adrenal hypoplasia.

MISCELLANEOUS: Unexpected rhabdomyolysis with hyperkalemic arrest after succinylcholine in boys with undiagnosed Duchenne muscular dystrophy was the primary reason behind the change in the package labeling in the United States for succinylcholine several years ago, cautioning against its use in children.

As a consequence of muscle regeneration (not specifically of dystrophic muscle) there is postsynaptic expression of both fetal and mature nicotinic acetylcholine receptors. Mice have a similar genetic defect but do not become dystrophic. It is thought that a related protein, eutrophin, somehow substitutes function for the missing dystrophin. The gene for eutrophin is active in mouse muscle. It is present but inactive in human muscle.

Separated from his only child after his wife's death, Duchenne led a lonely existence in Paris working primarily in charity clinics. He pursued his clinical neurological studies outside of mainstream Parisian medicine, and was never given any official recognition by the *Académie de Médecine* or the *Institut de France*, although he was made an honorary member of the medical academies in Rome, Madrid, Stockholm, St. Petersburg, Geneva, and Leipzig.

ANESTHETIC CONSIDERATIONS

Although a normal response to succinylcholine has been reported, hyperkalemic cardiac arrest secondary to rhabdomyolysis does occur, and succinylcholine is contraindicated in these patients. Although mild increases in sensitivity to nondepolarizing muscle relaxants have been reported, these are not generally significant (13, 18). Response (in a single patient) to mivacurium was normal (11), however prolonged onset time and duration has been reported with rocuronium (6), and prolonged recovery from mivacurium in an additional study (3).

A patient has been reported who repeatedly had tracheal occlusion when placed prone because of impingement of the trachea between the sternum and a lordotic thoracic spine (17). Postoperative respiratory complications are common secondary to the combination of scoliosis, poor cough, and muscle weakness. Patients may have gastric hypomotility with delayed gastric emptying, and are at increased risk for perioperative aspiration. An intraoperative nasogastric tube may be indicated. Delayed muscle weakness with onset 5 to 36 hours after surgery and leading to respiratory failure has been reported after general anesthesia (all had received succinylcholine) (28).

Heart block or arrhythmias can develop from fibrosis of the conduction system. Heart failure can develop in adolescence, and acute onset of heart failure intraoperatively in a previously (cardiac) asymptomatic patient with a normal preoperative resting echocardiogram has been reported. Anesthetic agents at levels that further depress cardiac function should be avoided. Female carriers of the abnormal gene can also have a cardiomyopathy, but usually not until adulthood.

Epidural anesthesia has been used with success using normal dosing (24), although it could be difficult to perform due to kyphoscoliosis.

An association between Duchenne muscular dystrophy and malignant hyperthermia has been discussed in the past but is unlikely (26, 30, 31). *In vitro* contracture testing can be positive, but it has been suggested that *in vitro* muscle testing may not be accurate in patients with neuromuscular diseases. Halothane has been used without incidence of rhabdomyolysis (34), but cases have been reported of patients experiencing rhabdomyolysis after halothane (22), isoflurane (5,20), enflurane, or sevoflurane (5,6,8,10)—without the concurrent use of succinylcholine. Hyperkalemic arrests, sometimes fatal, have occurred on or shortly following emergence, and not necessarily intraoperatively. Electrocardiographic changes and myoglobinuria can be observed postoperatively. It has been suggested that volatile anesthetics be avoided in patients with known Duchenne dystrophy (1). Halothane is probably of most concern because it is a more potent myocardial depressant than the other volatile agents, and causes additional abnormalities in the sarcoplasmic reticulum's handling of calcium. Cardiac arrest has also been reported after total intravenous anesthesia (12).

Patients who also have congenital adrenal hypoplasia will be on chronic maintenance glucocorticoid and mineralocorticoid replacement therapy and will need perioperative stress doses. Prednisone and anabolic steroids have also been used to improve symptomatology of the myopathy.

Bibliography:

1. Yemen TA, McClain C. Muscular dystrophy, anesthesia and the safety of inhalational agents revisited, again. *Paediatr Anaesth* 2006;16: 105–108.
2. Girshin M, Mukherjee J, Clowney R, et al. The postoperative cardiovascular arrest of a 5-year-old male: an initial presentation of Duchenne's muscular dystrophy. *Paediatr Anaesth* 2006;16: 170–173.
3. Schmidt J, Muenster T, Wick S. Onset and duration of mivacurium-induced neuromuscular block in patients with Duchenne muscular dystrophy. *Br J Anaesth* 2005;95:769–772.
4. Ames WA, Hayes JA, Crawford MW. The role of corticosteroids in Duchenne muscular dystrophy: a review for the anesthetist. *Paediatr Anaesth* 2005;15:3–8.
5. Nathan A, Ganesh A, Godinez RI, et al. Hyperkalemic cardiac arrest after cardiopulmonary bypass in a child with unsuspected Duchenne muscular dystrophy. *Anesth Analg* 2005;100:672–674.
6. Wick S, Muenster T, Schmidt J, et al. Onset and duration of rocuronium-induced neuromuscular blockade in patients with Duchenne muscular dystrophy. *Anesthesiology* 2005;102:915–919.
7. Schmidt GN, Burmeister M-A, Lilje C, et al. Acute heart failure during spinal surgery in a boy with Duchenne muscular dystrophy. *Br J Anaesth* 2003;90:800–804.
8. Takahashi H, Shimokawa M, Sha K, et al. Sevoflurane can induce rhabdomyolysis in Duchenne's muscular dystrophy [Japanese]. *Masui* 2002;51:190–192.
9. Goresky GV, Cox RG. Inhalation anesthetics and Duchenne's muscular dystrophy [editorial]. *Can J Anaesth* 1999;46:525–526.

10. Obata R, Yasumi Y, Suzuki A. Rhabdomyolysis in association with Duchenne's muscular dystrophy. *Can J Anaesth* 1999;46:564–566.
11. Uslu M, Mellinghoff H, Diefenbach C. Mivacurium for muscle relaxation in a child with Duchenne's muscular dystrophy. *Anesth Analg* 1999;89:340–341.
12. Irwin MG, Henderson M. Cardiac arrest during major spinal scoliosis surgery in a patient with Duchenne's muscular dystrophy undergoing intravenous anaesthesia. *Anaesth Int Care* 1995;23:626–629.
13. Ririe DG, Shapiro F, Sethna NF. The response of patients with Duchenne's muscular dystrophy to neuromuscular blockade with vecuronium. *Anesthesiology* 1998;88:351–354.
14. Beggs AH. Dystrophinopathy, the expanding phenotype. *Circulation* 1997;95:2344–2347.
15. Morris P. Duchenne muscular dystrophy: a challenge for the anaesthetist. *Paediatr Anaesth* 1997;7:1–4.
16. Pash MP. Anaesthetic management of a patient with severe muscular dystrophy, lumbar lordosis, and a difficult airway. *Can J Anaesth* 1996;43:959–964.
17. Rittoo DB, Morris P. Tracheal occlusion in the prone position in an intubated patient with Duchenne muscular dystrophy. *Anaesthesia* 1995;50:719–721.
18. Tobias JD, Atwood R. Mivacurium in children with Duchenne muscular dystrophy. *Paediatr Anaesth* 1994;4:57–60.
19. Farrell PT. Anaesthesia-induced rhabdomyolysis causing cardiac arrest: case report and review of anaesthesia and the dystrophinopathies. *Anaesth Intensive Care* 1994;22:597–601.
20. Chalkiadis GA, Branch KG. Cardiac arrest after isoflurane anaesthesia in a patient with Duchenne's muscular dystrophy. *Anaesthesia* 1990;45: 22–25.
21. Larsen UT, Hein-Sorensen O. Complications during anaesthesia in patients with Duchenne's muscular dystrophy [a retrospective study]. *Can J Anaesth* 1989;36:418–422.
22. Sethna NF, Rockoff MA, Worthen HM, et al. Anesthesia-related complications in children with Duchenne muscular dystrophy. *Anesthesiology* 1988;68:462–465.
23. Buzello W, Huttarsch H. Muscle relaxation in patients with Duchenne's muscular dystrophy. *Br J Anaesth* 1988;60:228–231.
24. Murat I, Esteve C, Montay G, et al. Pharmacokinetics and cardiovascular effects of bupivacaine during epidural anesthesia in children with Duchenne muscular dystrophy. *Anesthesiology* 1987;67:249–252.
25. Rubiano R, Chang JL, Carroll J, et al. Acute rhabdomyolysis following halothane anesthesia without succinylcholine. *Anesthesiology* 1987;67:856–857.
26. Wang JM, Stanley TH. Duchenne muscular dystrophy and malignant hyperthermia: two case reports. *Can Anaesth Soc J* 1986;33: 492–497.
27. Sethna NF, Rockoff MA. Cardiac arrest following inhalation induction of anaesthesia in a child with Duchenne's muscular dystrophy. *Can Anaesth Soc J* 1986;33:799–802.
28. Smith CL, Bush GH. Anaesthesia and progressive muscular dystrophy. *Br J Anaesth* 1985;57:1113–1118.
29. Henderson WAV. Succinylcholine-induced cardiac arrest in unsuspected Duchenne muscular dystrophy. *Can Anaesth Soc J* 1984;31: 444–446.
30. Keifer HM, Singer WD, Reynolds RN. Malignant hyperthermia in a child with Duchenne muscular dystrophy. *Pediatrics* 1983;71:118–119.
31. Brownell AKW, Paasuke RT, Elash A, et al. Malignant hyperthermia in Duchenne muscular dystrophy. *Anesthesiology* 1983;58:180–182.
32. McKishnie JD, Muir JM, Girvan DP. Anaesthesia induced rhabdomyolysis: a case report. *Can Anaesth Soc J* 1983;30:295–298.
33. Miller ED, Sanders DB, Rowlingson JC, et al. Anesthesia-induced rhabdomyolysis in a patient with Duchenne's muscular dystrophy. *Anesthesiology* 1978;48:146–148.
34. Richards WC. Anaesthesia and serum creatinine phosphokinase levels in patients with Duchenne's pseudohypertrophic muscular dystrophy. *Anaesth Intensive Care* 1972;1:150–153.

Dutch-Kentucky Syndrome

SYNONYM: Trismus-pseudocamptodactyly syndrome; Hecht Beals syndrome; Hecht syndrome

MIM #: 158300

This autosomal dominant disease is characterized by limited mouth opening and deformities of the extremities. The disease is due to mutations in the gene *MYH8*, which encodes myosin heavy chain 8, which is a perinatal myosin that is active during early skeletal muscle development. This syndrome has also been described in association with the findings of Carney complex (see earlier).

HEENT/AIRWAY: Severely limited mouth opening. The limitation may be due to an enlarged coronoid process of the mandible or to an abnormal ligament from the maxilla to the mandible, anterior to the masseter muscles. Limitation in mouth opening may be so severe as to preclude solid foods. Malformed ears.

CARDIOVASCULAR: May have mitral valve prolapse, aortic root dilatation.

ORTHOPEDIC: Extremity deformities are secondary to short flexor muscles and tendons, which lead to flexion deformities. Pseudocamptodactyly—a flexion deformity of the fingers that occurs with wrist extension. May also have flexion deformities of the feet such as down-turned toes, metatarsus adductus, clubfoot deformity. May have short stature, kyphoscoliosis. Hands are clenched at birth but loosen during infancy.

MISCELLANEOUS: Although doctors Hecht (a pediatrician and medical geneticist) and Beals (an orthopedic surgeon) were in different fields they were assigned to share an office because of a shortage of space. Because of their physical proximity they collaborated on a number of academic projects. The name of this syndrome was suggested after the evaluation of an extensive pedigree of a family in Kentucky was traced back as far as a Dutch girl who migrated to the United States in 1780 and who was described as having "crooked hands and a small mouth."

ANESTHETIC CONSIDERATIONS

Mask ventilation has not been reported to be difficult; however, tracheal intubation may be extremely difficult. The marked limitation in mouth opening necessitates fiberoptic intubation in many children, and a retrograde guidewire-assisted nasal fiberoptic intubation has been required (1). The limitation in mouth opening is anatomic, and will not resolve with muscle relaxants. Successful fiberoptic nasal intubation after unsuccessful blind nasal attempts has been reported in a child (5), and successful blind nasal intubation has been reported in an adult (8). Use of the laryngeal mask has not been reported but might be useful since the anatomy of the glottis and upper airway are normal. However, introduction of an adequate sized device might be difficult or impossible with the very restricted mouth opening. It may be advisable to have a person present for induction who is skilled in obtaining a surgical airway. Patients who have mitral valve prolapse with mitral insufficiency need perioperative antibiotic prophylaxis as indicated.

Bibliography:

1. Seavello J, Hammer GB. Tracheal intubation in a child with trismus pseudocamptodactyly [Hecht] syndrome. *J Clin Anesth* 1999;11:254–256.
2. Nagata O, Tateoka A, Shiro R, et al. Anaesthetic management of two paediatric patients with Hecht-Beals syndrome. *Paediatr Anaesth* 1999;9:444–447.
3. Geva D, Ezri T, Szmuk P, et al. Anaesthesia for the Hecht Beals syndrome [Letter]. *Paediatr Anaesth* 1997;7:178–179.
4. Vaghadia H, Blackstocki D. Anaesthetic implications in Trismus Pseudocamptodactyly [Dutch-Kentucky or Hecht Beals] syndrome. *Can J Anaesth* 1988;35:80–85.
5. Browder FH, Lew D, Shahbazian TS. Anesthetic management of a patient with Dutch-Kentucky syndrome. *Anesthesiology* 1986;65:218–219.
6. Markus AF. Limited mouth opening and shortened flexor muscle-tendon units: 'trismus-pseudocamptodactyly'. *Br J Oral Maxillofac Surg* 1986;24:137–142.
7. Tsukahara M, Shinozaki F, Kajii T. Trismus-pseudocamptodactyly syndrome in a Japanese family. *Clin Genet* 1985;28:247–250.
8. Mercuri LG. The Hecht, Beals and Wilson syndrome. *J Oral Surg* 1981;39:53–56.

Dyggve-Melchior-Clausen Syndrome

MIM #: 223800, 304950

This syndrome, marked by short-trunk dwarfism, characteristic skeletal changes, limited joint mobility, and mental deficiency, is usually inherited in an autosomal recessive fashion. However, a family with X-linked transmission has been described. Superficially, patients resemble those with Hurler and Morquio syndromes. There are some patients who manifest the characteristic skeletal changes (particularly the radiographic and pathologic changes of the iliac crests) but who are not mentally retarded. The autosomal recessive disorder is due to abnormalities in the gene *DYM*, which encodes dymeclin, a ubiquitous transmembrane protein of unknown function. Mutations in this same gene are responsible for Smith-McCort dysplasia (not discussed in this text). Patients with Smith-McCort dysplasia do not have mental retardation.

HEENT/AIRWAY: Microcephaly. Thickened calvarium. Deformed sella turcica. Coarse facies. Relatively large facial bones, prognathism. Odontoid hypoplasia. Very short neck.

CHEST: Barrel chest. Wide costochondral junctions.

NEUROMUSCULAR: Psychomotor retardation varies from moderate to severe. Atlantoaxial instability secondary to odontoid hypoplasia can lead to spinal cord compression.

ORTHOPEDIC: Short trunk dwarfism. Multiple skeletal changes involving the limbs, vertebrae, and pelvis. Rhizomelic limb shortening. Broad hands and feet. Multiple proximal ossification centers of the humerus and femur. Limited joint mobility, especially of elbows, hips, and knees. Flattened vertebrae with ossification defects. Scoliosis, kyphosis, lordosis. Irregularly calcified iliac crests.

Dysplastic acetabulae. Laterally displaced capital femoral epiphyses. Dislocated hips. Waddling gait.

ANESTHETIC CONSIDERATIONS

The head must be carefully positioned during laryngoscopy secondary to possible odontoid hypoplasia and atlantoaxial instability. The very short neck may make direct laryngoscopy difficult, particularly in the face of possible atlantoaxial instability. Fiberoptic intubation should be considered as an alternative intubation technique. The patient should be carefully positioned secondary to limited joint mobility and the risk of hip subluxation.

Bibliography:

1. Eguchi M, Kadota Y, Yoshida Y, et al. Anesthetic management of a patient with Dyggve-Melchior-Clausen syndrome [Japanese]. *Masui* 2001;50:1116–1117.
2. Beighton P. Dyggve-Melchior-Clausen syndrome. *J Med Genet* 1990;27:512–515.

Dyschondrosteosis

See Leri-Weill dyschondrosteosis

Dysencephalia Splanchnocystica

See Meckel-Gruber syndrome

Dyskeratosis Congenita

MIM #: 305000, 127550, 224230

This usually X-linked recessive disorder involves dysplasia of the skin, mucous membranes, and bone marrow. Its main features are reticular skin hyperpigmentation, hyperkeratosis, nail dystrophy, generalized leukoplakia, nasolacrimal duct obstruction, and pancytopenia. Except for skin hyperpigmentation (present at birth), the features of this disease do not become apparent until late childhood. However the disease is relentless and most patients die by 30 years of age, primarily from pancytopenia, but also from malignant transformation of the leukoplakia, or opportunistic infections. Although usually inherited in an X-linked recessive fashion, autosomal dominant as well as autosomal recessive inheritance has been documented. The autosomal dominant form tends to result in a milder phenotype. The X-linked type is due to mutations in the gene *DKC1*, which encodes dyskerin, a protein likely involved in the cell cycle and nucleolar function. The autosomal dominant form is due to mutations in the gene *TERC*, which encodes the RNA component of telomerase.

HEENT/AIRWAY: Premalignant leukoplakia on lips, mouth, conjunctivae. Nasolacrimal duct obstruction. May have abnormal hearing. Nasopharyngeal strictures, stenosis. Dental caries, gingival recession, alveolar bone loss, tooth mobility. Esophageal strictures.

NEUROMUSCULAR: Occasional mental deficiency. Intracranial calcifications.

ORTHOPEDIC: Osteoporosis. Avascular necrosis of the femoral head. May have growth deficiency.

GI/GU: Premalignant leukoplakia on the anus, urethra. Occasional hepatic cirrhosis. Ureteral, urethral, vaginal, or anal strictures. Testicular hypoplasia.

OTHER: Skin hyperpigmentation, particularly of the neck, trunk, and upper arms. Palmar and plantar hyperkeratosis. Telangiectasis. Atrophic skin. Nail dystrophy. Thin, sparse hair. Pancytopenia. May have immunologic abnormalities. Leukoplakia often exhibits malignant transformation (squamous cell carcinoma). Other malignancies can develop, including Hodgkin lymphoma, pancreatic adenocarcinoma, cervical carcinoma, and esophageal carcinoma. Patients have shortened telomeres.

MISCELLANEOUS: There may be an increased risk of leukemia in the female carrier of the X-linked gene.

ANESTHETIC CONSIDERATIONS
The teeth should be examined preoperatively for loss or excessive mobility. A complete preoperative blood count should be obtained. The patient should be carefully positioned secondary to osteoporosis and possible bone fragility. Nasotracheal and nasogastric tubes must be placed carefully because of the possibility of nasopharyngeal or esophageal strictures.

Bibliography:
1. Neumann AA, Reddel RR. Telomere maintenance and cancer—look, no telomerase. *Nat Rev Cancer* 2002;2:879–884.
2. Dokal I. Dyskeratosis congenita in all its forms. *Br J Haematol* 2000;110: 768–779.
3. Caux F, Aractingi S, Sawaf MH, et al. Dyskeratosis congenita. *Eur J Dermatol* 1996;6:332–334.

E

Eagle-Barrett Syndrome

See Prune-belly syndrome

Eastman-Bixler Syndrome

See Faciocardiorenal syndrome

Ebstein Anomaly

MIM #: 224700

This anomaly involves abnormal attachment of the septal and posterior leaflets of the tricuspid valve below the valve annulus, somewhere in the right ventricle. A section of the right ventricle above where the leaflets attach becomes "atrialized." This area should have been part of the right ventricle, but because it lies above the level of the tricuspid valve closure, it is physiologically part of the right atrium. The major consequence of the Ebstein anomaly is tricuspid insufficiency. Patients with minimal involvement can remain asymptomatic, and the Ebstein anomaly has been described as an "accidental finding" on autopsies in adults. Almost all cases occur sporadically. Uncommon autosomal recessive cases have been described.

Moderately or severely affected patients are cyanotic at birth. The right-to-left shunt is through a patent foramen ovale or a true atrial septal defect. Severely affected neonates exhibit massive cardiomegaly on chest radiographs. Right atrial pressure is elevated secondary to tricuspid insufficiency and abnormal filling and emptying of the small right ventricle. Right-sided pressures are particularly high in the neonate, where the normally elevated pulmonary vascular resistance is an added burden to right ventricular emptying. Cyanosis often improves with the normal postnatal fall in pulmonary vascular resistance over the first few weeks of life.

Ebstein anomaly is associated with Wolff-Parkinson-White syndrome (see later) approximately 20% of the time. Because of the size of the large right atrium, atrial flutter or fibrillation can also develop. In addition to the auscultatory

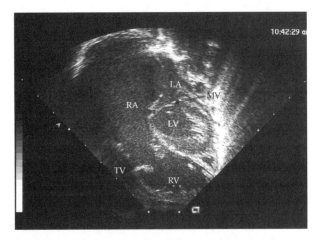

Ebstein anomaly. An echocardiogram of Ebstein anomaly showing redundant tricuspid valve tissue displaced into the right ventricle. There is a massively enlarged right atrium, and the atrial septum can be seen bowing into the left atrium. RA, right atrium; LA, left atrium; MV, mitral valve; TV, tricuspid valve; RV, right ventricle; LV, left ventricle. (From Baum VC. Abnormalities of the atrioventricular valves. In: Lake CL, Booker PD, eds. *Pediatric Cardiac Anesthesia*, Philadelphia: Lippincott Williams & Wilkins. Fourth Edition, 2005.)

and other findings on physical examination of tricuspid insufficiency, these patients may show a "sail sign," a diastolic sound made by redundant tricuspid valve tissue flopping around, similar to a sail flapping freely in the breeze.

CARDIOVASCULAR: During embryonic development, the tricuspid valve leaflets form by a process resembling exfoliation from the ventricular myocardium. This begins distally, and progresses proximally until it reaches the level of the valve annulus, where it halts. If this process is arrested, the valve never completely peels back, or separates from the ventricle, leaving the attachment point of the valve leaflet variably deep in the ventricle. The amount of free septal and posterior tricuspid valve tissue varies widely. The anterior leaflet is normal. Although the typical physiologic consequence is tricuspid insufficiency, occasionally patients will present with tricuspid stenosis because of abnormal chordal attachments. Surgical repair, if needed, is usually by tricuspid valvuloplasty rather than valve replacement. Cyanosis can redevelop during adolescence, presumably from worsening right ventricular failure. Many patients have associated Wolff-Parkinson-White syndrome (see later).

OTHER: Clinical status may deteriorate during pregnancy. Increased intravascular blood volume may worsen the right ventricular function, decreased systemic vascular resistance may increase the right-to-left atrial level shunt, and increased catecholamines may increase a tendency for atrial tachyarrhythmias.

MISCELLANEOUS: First described during the autopsy of a 19-year-old who had had dyspnea, palpitations, and cyanosis for many years. The first diagnosis in a living patient was over 80 years later, in 1949.

Patients with L-transposition of the great arteries (also called congenitally corrected transposition) also have ventricular inversion, or a right-sided anatomic left ventricle pumping to the pulmonary artery, and a left-sided anatomic right ventricle pumping to the aorta. Ebstein anomaly, if it occurs in these patients, occurs in the left-sided tricuspid valve.

ANESTHETIC CONSIDERATIONS

Neonates may need to be maintained on prostaglandin E_1 to maintain ductal patency until pulmonary vascular resistance resolves adequately. Intravenous lines must be kept scrupulously free of air bubbles because of the right-to-left atrial shunt. These hearts tend to be a bit "twitchy" when tickled by an intravascular catheter or wire. Patients with associated Wolff-Parkinson-White syndrome may need their antiarrhythmic medications continued perioperatively. With the very large right atrium and tricuspid insufficiency, swirling of injected induction drugs in the atrium may result in delayed or inadequate induction of anesthesia (3, 6). Rapid decrements in systemic vascular resistance may increase right-to-left shunting, but careful epidural analgesia has been used effectively (2–5). Ergotamine has effects

on the pulmonary vasculature and should be avoided if possible in parturients. Pitocin has been used without problems. Appropriate perioperative antibiotic prophylaxis for endocarditis is indicated.

Bibliography:
1. Lerner M, DiNardo JA, Communale MA. Anesthetic management for repair of Ebstein's anomaly. *J Cardiothorac Vasc Anesth* 2003;17:232–235.
2. Groves ER, Groves JB. Epidural analgesia for labour in a patient with Ebstein's anomaly. *Can J Anaesth* 1995;42:77–79.
3. Halpern S, Gidwaney A, Gates B. Anaesthesia for caesarean section in a pre-eclamptic patient with Ebstein's anomaly. *Can Anaesth Soc J* 1985;32:244–247.
4. Linter SPK, Clarke K. Caesarean section under extradural analgesia in a patient with Ebstein's anomaly. *Br J Anaesth* 1984;56:203–205.
5. Waickman LA, Skorton DJ, Varner MW, et al. Ebstein's anomaly and pregnancy. *Am J Cardiol* 1984;53:357–358.
6. Elsten JL, Kim YD, Hanowell ST, et al. Prolonged induction with exaggerated chamber enlargement in Ebstein's anomaly. *Anesth Analg* 1981;60:909–910.

Ectodermal Dysplasia

See AEC syndrome, EEC syndrome, Ellis-van Creveld syndrome, Marshall syndrome, Rapp-Hodgkin ectodermal dysplasia, pachyonychia congenita, and Rothmund syndrome

Ectrodactyly-Ectodermal Dysplasia-Clefting Syndrome

See EEC syndrome

Edwards Syndrome

See Trisomy 18

EEC Syndrome

SYNONYM: Ectrodactyly-ectodermal dysplasia-clefting syndrome

MIM #: 129900, 602077, 604292

This dysmorphic syndrome is defined by the triad of **E**ctrodactyly ("lobster claw" deformity), **E**ctodermal dysplasia, and **C**left lip and palate. It is likely inherited in an autosomal dominant fashion. There is marked variability in expression; for example, ectrodactyly is not a constant feature. Three forms have been described (EEC 1–3). One form is due to abnormalities in the gene encoding tumor protein p63. Mutations in this gene can also result in the AEC syndrome (see earlier).

HEENT/AIRWAY: Ectodermal dysplasia affects hair, eyes, and teeth. Thin, sparse hair. Maxillary hypoplasia. Lacrimal duct hypoplasia. Dacryocystitis, keratitis, blepharophimosis,

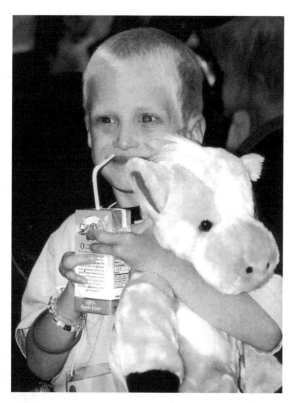

EEC syndrome. This happy young boy has obvious ectrodactyly.

blepharitis and conjunctivitis. Photophobia. May have hearing loss. Small, malformed ears. Occasional choanal atresia. Cleft lip and palate. Hypoplastic teeth, dental caries. Xerostomia. Absence of Stensen duct of the parotid gland.

CHEST: May have recurrent respiratory infections even after repair of cleft lip and palate.

NEUROMUSCULAR: Usually normal intelligence.

ORTHOPEDIC: Ectrodactyly ("lobster-claw" deformity) of the hands and feet. Less severe variants have syndactyly or clinodactyly.

GI/GU: Rare abdominal wall defects, anal atresia. Genitourinary anomalies are frequent, including cryptorchidism, hypospadias, duplicated collecting system, vesicoureteral reflux, hydronephrosis, and renal dysplasia. Bladder diverticulae. Transverse vaginal septum.

OTHER: Ectodermal dysplasia affects skin, sweat glands, nails. Skin is fair and thin, and prone to ulceration. Mild hyperkeratosis. Hypoplasia of the sweat glands. Mild nail dysplasia. Hypoplastic nipples. Patients may be malnourished and anemic secondary to poor oral intake and loss of protein through skin ulcers. Occasional central diabetes insipidus, growth hormone deficiency, or hypogonadotrophic hypogonadism.

ANESTHETIC CONSIDERATIONS

Because of hypoplasia of the sweat glands and abnormal temperature regulation, atropine premedication should be avoided. For the same reason, perioperative hyperthermia may occur. Dental loss and mobility should be documented preoperatively. The eyes need to be protected with ointment because of inadequate tear production. Patients with photophobia may be sensitive to the bright operating room lights. The skin must be well padded because of its fragility. Choanal atresia, if present, precludes the use of a nasal airway or a nasogastric tube. Consider preoperative evaluation of renal function in patients with a history of renal abnormalities, which predispose to renal insufficiency.

Bibliography:

1. Bigata X, Bielsa I, Artigas M, et al. The ectrodactyly-ectodermal dysplasia-clefting syndrome (EEC): report of five cases. *Pediatr Dermatol* 2003;20:113–118.
2. Roelfsema NM, Cobben JM. The EEC syndrome: a literature study. *Clin Dysmorphol* 1996;5:115–127.
3. Buss PW, Hughes HE, Clarke A. Twenty-four cases of the EEC syndrome: clinical presentation and management. *J Med Genet* 1995;32:716–723.
4. Mizushima A, Satoyoshi M. Anaesthetic problems in a child with ectrodactyly, ectodermal dysplasia and cleft lip/palate: the EEC syndrome. *Anaesthesia* 1992;47:137–140.

Ehlers-Danlos Syndrome

MIM #: 130000

There are 10 distinct forms of the Ehlers-Danlos syndrome, varying from mild to severe (type XI, in use for a period of time, is no longer considered a distinct entity). The hallmarks of the syndrome are lax joints, hyperextensibility of the skin, and easy bruising and bleeding. Most types are inherited in an autosomal dominant fashion, with wide variability in expression. At least some cases are caused by mutations in the genes *COL1A1,* or *COL5A1/COL5A2,* the genes encoding types I or V collagen; the gene *PLOD,* which encodes lysyl hydroxylase in collagens and other proteins; and the gene encoding tenascin-X, a noncollagen protein which may regulate collagen synthesis or deposition. Several of the different clinical types are due to different mutations of the same gene, and thus are allelic. Type I is described in detail in the text, and the other types are outlined in Table 1. Type IV disease is associated with premature death, with an estimated median survival of 48 years. Although the above represents the classical description of the Ehlers-Danlos types, a revised nosology divides the syndrome into six types (5).

HEENT/AIRWAY: May have epicanthal folds, blue sclerae, microcornea, keratoconus, glaucoma, dislocated lens, retinal detachment, myopia. Easy upper eyelid eversion (Méténier sign). Hypermobile ears—"lop ears." May have hypoplastic, irregularly spaced teeth. Able to touch tip of nose with tongue (Gorlin sign). May have tracheal dilatation.

TABLE 1. *Types of Ehlers-Danlos syndrome*

Type	Skin hyperextensibility	Joint hypermobility	Skin fragility	Bruising; bleeding	Others	Inheritance	Enzyme defect	MIM #
I. Gravis–severe classic form	Marked	Marked	Marked	Moderate	Prematurity, varicose veins, hernias	Autosomal dominant	Defect in the COL5A1, COL5A2 or COL1A1 genes	130000
II. Mitis–mild classic form	Moderate	Moderate	Moderate	Moderate		Autosomal dominant	Defect in the COL5A1 or COL5A2 genes	130010
III. Benign Hypermobility	Variable	Striking joint hypermobility, frequent joint dislocation, premature osteoarthritis	Soft, but otherwise normal skin	Minimal		Autosomal dominant	Defects in the genes COL3A1 or TNXB	130020
IV. Ecchymotic or vascular type; death before the fifth decade	Minimal	Normal joint mobility, except the small joints of the hands are hypermobile	Thin, translucent skin with easily visible underlying veins/easy bruising	Marked	Characteristic facies with large eyes, a thin, pinched nose and thin lips. Spontaneous carotid- cavernous fistulae, intracranial aneurysms, carotid artery aneurysms. Bowel or arterial rupture leading to death. Uterine rupture during pregnancy	Autosomal dominant and autosomal recessive	Type III collagen gene COL3A1 defect leads to a defect in type III collagen	130050
V. X-linked– clinically similar to type II; female carriers are asymptomatic	Marked	Digits only	Minimal	Minimal		X-linked recessive	Unknown. Lysyl oxidase deficiency has been suggested	305200
VI. Lysyl hydroxylase deficiency	Soft, hyperextensible skin with moderate scarring	Marked	Minimal	Easy bruising	Muscle hypotonia, scoliosis. Corneal and scleral fragility, keratoconus	Autosomal recessive	PLOD gene defect leads to lysyl hydroxylase deficiency, resulting in hydroxylysine-deficient collagen	225400
VII. Procollagen proteinase deficiency	Moderate	Marked joint hypermobility, congenital hip dislocation	Moderate	Moderate	Short stature	Subclassified into three types: EDS VII A, mutation in the COL1A1 gene, autosomal dominant; EDS VII B, mutation in the COL1A2 gene, autosomal dominant; EDS VII C, deficiency in procollagen N-proteinase activity, autosomal recessive		130060 225410
VIII. Ehlers-Danlos syndrome with periodontitis	Minimal	Minimal joint hypermobility except the small joints of the hands show marked hypermobility	Marked	Marked, poor wound healing	Generalized periodontitis	Autosomal dominant	Unknown	130080
IX. Ehlers-Danlos syndrome with occipital horns	Soft, mildly extensible skin				Occipital horn-like exostoses, short humeri, short, broad clavicles. Chronic diarrhea, bladder diverticulae, with a propensity for bladder rupture	X-linked recessive	Defect in alpha peptide of Cu^{2+}-transporting ATPase (same as Menke syndrome)	304150
X. Ehlers-Danlos syndrome with fibronectin defect	Minimal	Joint hypermobility and dislocation	Moderate	Poor wound healing	Platelet aggregation defect that corrects with the addition of fibronectin	Autosomal recessive	Unknown	225310

EDS, Ehlers-Danlos syndrome. (Modified from Arendt-Nielsen L, Kaalund S, Bjerring P. Insufficient effect of local analgesics in Ehlers Danlos type III patients [connective tissue disorder]. *Acta Anaesthesiol Scand* 1990;34:358–361.)

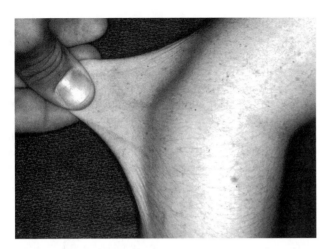

Ehlers-Danlos syndrome. FIG. 1. Marked skin laxity seen in a patient with Ehlers-Danlos syndrome. (Courtesy of Dr. Kenneth E. Greer, Department of Dermatology, University of Virginia Health System.)

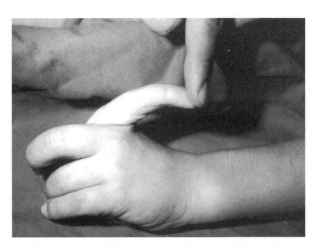

Ehlers-Danlos syndrome. FIG. 2. Ligamentous laxity seen in a patient with Ehlers-Danlos syndrome. (Courtesy of Dr. Kenneth E. Greer, Department of Dermatology, University of Virginia Health System.)

CHEST: Hemoptysis. Downsloping ribs. Lung cysts can be associated with pneumothorax.

CARDIOVASCULAR: Cardiovascular abnormalities include valvular prolapse or insufficiency (usually mitral or tricuspid), a variety of congenital structural defects (most commonly atrial septal defect), and conduction defects. Aortic root dilatation can occur. Aortic dissection secondary to poor vessel integrity has occurred. Intraoperative ischemia from asymptomatic coronary disease in a relatively young adult has been reported (6). Can have postural acrocyanosis. Arterial rupture in type IV disease—teenage boys seem most at risk—can be fatal. The postoperative period is also a high risk period, possibly due to increased collagenase activity.

NEUROMUSCULAR: Rare mental deficiency.

ORTHOPEDIC: Joint laxity with the possibility of dislocation. Joint laxity may also result in spinal or foot deformities. Stiffened joints and arthritis may occur with aging. Slim build, long neck. Mucinoid-containing subcutaneous nodules develop in areas of frequent trauma.

GI/GU: Gastrointestinal bleeding. Inguinal hernias are common. Occasional diaphragmatic hernia, dilatation of the esophagus or intestine, intestinal diverticulae. Umbilical hernia. Spontaneous bowel rupture in type IV disease. Occasional renal tubular acidosis. Uterine rupture in type IV disease.

OTHER: The skin is hyperextensible and fragile. May have acrocyanosis. Wound healing is poor and results in friable "cigarette-paper" scars. Abnormal vessel integrity and platelet dysfunction cause easy bruising or hemarthroses. Premature delivery can be secondary to premature rupture of fragile fetal membranes (affected infant) or lax maternal tissues (affected mother). Other obstetric complications include postpartum hemorrhage, separation of the symphysis pubis, and uterine prolapse.

MISCELLANEOUS: Edvard Ehlers was a Danish dermatologist and Henri Danlos was a French dermatologist at the turn of the last century. This disorder was described by Ehlers several years before Danlos, but in fact there had been several prior descriptions, as early as 1657. The Russian Rschernogobow inferred a systemic defect in connective tissue in 1892. It has been suggested that the famous violinist Paganini may have had Ehlers-Danlos syndrome, thus explaining his unusual dexterity and extensive reach.

ANESTHETIC CONSIDERATIONS

The integrity of the skin and blood vessels is poor. Careful positioning is required to avoid trauma to the skin. Intramuscular medications should be avoided if possible. Untoward hypertension may cause rupture of an unknown vascular aneurysm. Subcutaneous fluids from an infiltrated intravenous catheter may not be discernible because of the extreme distensibility of tissues. Arterial and large central venous catheters should be avoided if possible because of the risk of hematoma formation or arterial aneurysm formation. In addition, the risk of catheter erosion through the vein wall is probably significantly increased. The use of ultrasound for central venous cannulation is suggested to minimize the risk of carotid puncture. Adequate blood should be kept available because blood loss may be out of the ordinary. Prolonged hemorrhage may occur after trauma. Poor tissue integrity can be problematic for the surgeon intraoperatively, and tissue can be torn by routine clamps and sutures. Wound healing is slow and poor. There is an increased risk of wound dehiscence.

Endotracheal intubation carries with it a risk of oral or laryngeal trauma and hematoma formation. If tracheal intubation is required, adequate relaxation is encouraged to minimize the risk of trauma to the airway and to decrease the risk of temporomandibular joint dislocation. Patients may have tracheal dilatation. Airway pressures should be kept as low as possible to minimize the risk of pneumothorax. Spontaneous ventilation, if appropriate, is preferred. Postoperative pleural effusions have been reported in a significant number of patients.

Patients (at least with type III disease) have markedly diminished duration of analgesia with lidocaine infiltration, even with the addition of vasoconstrictors. As a result, they may have inadequate pain relief during dental or cutaneous procedures such as episiotomy repairs. EMLA cream (a eutectic mixture of local anesthetics) also provides inadequate cutaneous analgesia in these patients (9). Although patients are at increased risk for hematoma formation, epidural anesthesia has been used successfully (8, 11).

Patients with structural cardiac defects or mitral valve prolapse with insufficiency require antibiotic prophylaxis as indicated. Intraoperative myocardial ischemia from asymptomatic coronary disease in a relatively young adult has been reported (6).

Bibliography:

1. Solan K, Davies P. Anaesthetic and intensive care management of a patient with Ehlers-Danlos type IV syndrome after laparotomy. *Anaesthesia* 2004;59:1224–1227.
2. Campbell N, Rosaeg OP. Anesthetic management of a parturient with Ehlers Danlos syndrome type IV. *Can J Anaesth* 2002;49:493–496.
3. Pyeritz RE. Ehlers-Danlos syndrome. *N Engl J Med* 2000;342:730–732.
4. Pepin M, Schwarze U, Superti-Furga A, et al. Clinical and genetic features of Ehlers-Danlos syndrome type IV, the vascular type. *N Engl J Med* 2000;342:673–680.
5. Beighton P, De Paepe A, Steinman B, et al. Ehlers-Danlos syndromes: revised nosology, Villefranche, 1997. Ehlers-Danlos national foundation and Ehlers-Danlos support group (UK). *Am J Med Genet* 1998;77:31–37.
6. Price CM, Ford S, St John Jones L, et al. Myocardial ischaemia associated with Ehlers-Danlos syndrome. *Br J Anaesth* 1996;76:464–466.
7. Comunale ME, Moens M, Furlong P, et al. Case 2–1993: cardiopulmonary bypass in a patient with connective tissue disease (Ehlers-Danlos syndrome) and multiple, small arteriovenous fistulae. *J Cardiothorac Vasc Anesth* 1993;7:352–356.
8. Brighouse D, Guard B. Anaesthesia for caesaerean section in a patient with Ehlers Danlos syndrome type IV. *Br J Anaesth* 1992;69:517–519.
9. Arendt-Nielsen L, Kaalund S, Bjerring P. Insufficient effect of local analgesics in Ehlers Danlos type III patients (connective tissue disorder). *Acta Anaesthesiol Scand* 1990;34:358–361.
10. Dolan P, Sisko F, Riley E. Anesthetic considerations for Ehlers Danlos syndrome. *Anesthesiology* 1980;52:266–269.
11. Abouleish E. Obstetric anaesthesia with Ehlers Danlos syndrome. *Br J Anaesth* 1980;52:1283–1285.
12. Leier CV, Call TD, Fulkerson PK, et al. The spectrum of cardiac defects in Ehlers-Danlos syndrome, types I and III. *Ann Intern Med* 1980;92:171–178.

Eisenmenger Syndrome

MIM #: None

Eisenmenger syndrome, also referred to as Eisenmenger physiology, develops when a congenital cardiac defect results in such marked elevations in pulmonary vascular resistance and pulmonary arterial hypertension that a previously purely left-to-right shunt becomes bidirectional or right-to-left. Early on, the changes in the pulmonary vasculature are confined to the arteriolar musculature, and the changes are acutely dynamic and reversible with pharmacologic manipulation, or permanently with surgery. Later the changes become anatomic and fixed. Surgical correction at that point carries a very high mortality rate. Survival until adulthood is likely with Eisenmenger syndrome.

CHEST: Pulmonary hemorrhage can develop.

CARDIOVASCULAR: Fixed elevations in pulmonary vascular resistance result in fixed cardiac output and inability to rapidly increase cardiac output.

NEUROMUSCULAR: Patients are at risk for paradoxical emboli.

MISCELLANEOUS: Eisenmenger described a specific type of nonrestrictive ventricular septal defect, but over the following decades the term became generalized and is used to describe patients with pulmonary vascular disease, regardless of the level of shunt.

ANESTHETIC CONSIDERATIONS
"In conclusion. . . the experience of the anaesthetist is more important than the anaesthetic agent chosen" (5). A protracted preoperative fast should be avoided, both to maintain intravascular volume and to avoid increasing the hematocrit to possibly dangerously high levels. Oxygen saturation routinely increases with the induction of anesthesia, independent of the agent used (5). Intravenous inductions are faster, and inhalational inductions slower than normal, because of the right-to-left shunt. End-tidal carbon dioxide measurements tend to underestimate arterial CO_2 in cyanotic lesions, even in those with increased pulmonary blood flow.

When right ventricular failure secondary to pulmonary hypertension exists, care must be taken to avoid further impairment of right ventricular function, such as can be caused by using anesthetics that are myocardial depressants or by excessively decreasing right ventricular preload (positive pressure ventilation decreases venous return to the right heart). Systemic arterial blood pressure must be maintained to ensure adequate coronary perfusion of the hypertrophied right ventricle and adequate pulmonary blood flow (3). Systemic vasoconstrictors such as phenylephrine should be available for immediate use. Although such alpha agonists will also increase pulmonary vascular resistance (presuming it is not fixed from chronic disease), the increase in systemic vascular resistance will predominate, and pulmonary flow will increase. Intravenous lines must be kept meticulously clear of air bubbles because of the risk of right-to-left shunting. Patients should receive perioperative antibiotic prophylaxis as indicated.

Fixed pulmonary vascular resistance precludes rapid adaptation by the patient to intraoperative hemodynamic changes. Close monitoring of intravascular volume and extremely cautious use of systemic vasodilators, including regional anesthesia, are mandatory. Consideration should be given to the use of an arterial catheter. Decreases in systemic vascular resistance increase right-to-left shunting and decrease systemic oxygen saturation. However, epidural anesthesia, and even incremental spinal anesthesia, **when given slowly**, have been used successfully in some cases (1, 7, 12). Xenon offers a potential advantage for general anesthesia due to its hemodynamic stability (2).

Fixed pulmonary vascular resistance is, by definition, unresponsive to pharmacologic intervention. Nevertheless, it would seem prudent to avoid factors known to increase pulmonary vascular resistance. These include cold, acidosis, hypercarbia, and hypoxia. Since some patients may retain some degree of reactiveness in the pulmonary circulation, they might respond to pulmonary vasodilators such as nitric oxide or inhaled prostacyclin (1).

Although perioperative placement of a pulmonary artery catheter might appear useful, it is of less use than might be expected, and is not without risk, specifically the risk of rupture of the hypertensive pulmonary artery. Both the abnormal intracardiac anatomy and the right-to-left intracardiac shunting may make placement of a flow-directed catheter difficult, if not impossible, without fluoroscopy. The information supplied by the catheter regarding cardiac output will likely be incorrect because of intracardiac shunting. Alternatively, the relative resistances in the pulmonary and systemic circulations are reflected rather directly by changes in systemic arterial saturation, which can be monitored continuously by pulse oximetry. Decreases in systemic vascular resistance or increases in pulmonary vascular resistance increase the right-to-left shunting, decreasing systemic oxygen saturation. Changes in the other direction have the opposite effect.

Bibliography:

1. Heller AR, Litz RJ, Koch T. A fine balance–one-lung ventilation in a patient with Eisenmenger syndrome. *Br J Anaesth* 2004;92:587–590.
2. Hofland J, Gültuna I, Tenbrinck R. Xenon anaesthesia for laparoscopic cholecystectomy in a patient with Eisenmenger's syndrome. *Br J Anaesth* 2001;86:882–886.
3. Sammut MS, Paes ML. Anaesthesia for laparoscopic cholecystectomy in a patient with Eisenmenger's syndrome. *Br J Anaesth* 1997;79:810–812.
4. Raines DE, Liberthson RR, Murray JR. Anesthetic management and outcome following noncardiac surgery in nonparturients with Eisenmenger physiology. *J Clin Anesth* 1996;8:341–347.
5. Lyons B, Motherway C, Casey W, et al. The anaesthetic management of a child with Eisenmenger's syndrome. *Can J Anaesth* 1995;42:904–909.
6. Baum VC, Perloff JK. Anesthetic implications of adults with congenital heart disease. *Anesth Analg* 1993;76:1342–1358.
7. Selsby DS, Sugden JC. Epidural anaesthesia for bilateral inguinal herniorrhaphy in Eisenmenger's syndrome. *Anaesthesia* 1989;44:130–132.
8. Burrows FA, Klinck JR, Rabinovitch M, et al. Pulmonary hypertension in children: perioperative management. *Can Anaesth Soc J* 1986;33:606–628.
9. Kraayenbrink MA, Steven CM. Anaesthesia for carotid body tumor resection in a patient with the Eisenmenger syndrome. *Anaesthesia* 1985;40:1194–1197.
10. Foster JMG, Jones RM. The anaesthetic management of the Eisenmenger syndrome. *Ann R Coll Surg Engl* 1984;66:353–355.
11. Bird TM, Strunin L. Anaesthesia for a patient with Down's syndrome and Eisenmenger's complex. *Anaesthesia* 1984;39:48–50.
12. Spinnato JA, Kraynack BJ, Cooper MW. Eisenmenger's syndrome in pregnancy: epidural anesthesia for elective cesarean section. *N Engl J Med* 1981;304:1215–1217.
13. Lumley J, Whitwam JG, Morgan M. General anesthesia in the presence of Eisenmenger's syndrome. *Anesth Analg* 1977;56:543–547.
14. Weber RK, Buda AJ, Levene DL. General anaesthesia in Eisenmenger's syndrome. *Can Med Assoc J* 1977;117:1413–1414.

Electron Transfer Flavoprotein (ETF) Deficiency

Included in Glutaric aciduria type II

Electron Transfer Flavoprotein:Ubiquinone Oxidoreductase (ETF-QO) Deficiency

Included in Glutaric aciduria type II

Ellis-van Creveld Syndrome

SYNONYM: Chondroectodermal dysplasia

MIM #: 225500

An autosomal recessive dysmorphic syndrome, the Ellis-van Creveld syndrome leads to dwarfism, polydactyly, nail dysplasia, and cardiothoracic malformations. Cardiothoracic malformations are the primary cause of death. The disorder is due to mutations in the gene *EVC*, although it can also be due to a defect in a closely linked gene *EVC2*.

HEENT/AIRWAY: Neonatal teeth, hypoplastic or missing teeth. Alveolar ridge hypoplasia. Multiple maxillary and mandibular frenula attach to the alveolar ridge. Short upper lip ("partial harelip"). May have micrognathia, cleft lip or palate. May have a short trachea.

CHEST: Long, narrow thorax with short ribs. Restrictive lung disease and pulmonary hypoplasia. Bronchial cartilage hypoplasia with lobar emphysema is possible. May have recurrent pneumonia.

CARDIOVASCULAR: Congenital cardiac defects common, especially atrial septal defect (may have single atrium), also ventricular septal defect.

NEUROMUSCULAR: Usually normal intelligence. May have Dandy-Walker malformation.

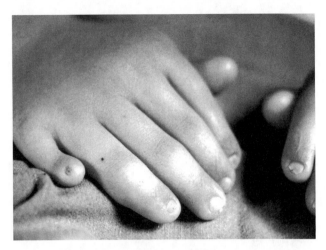

Ellis-van Creveld syndrome. Postaxial polydactyly and dysplastic nails of a child with Ellis-van Creveld syndrome. (Courtesy of Dr. Kenneth E. Greer, Department of Dermatology, University of Virginia Health System.)

ORTHOPEDIC: Short stature, predominantly due to short legs. Progressive shortening of the long bones, predominantly the distal segments. Postaxial polydactyly. Cone-shaped epiphyses of phalanges 2 to 5. Genu valgum. Dysplastic nails. Patients often have limited hand function. Pelvic dysplasia.

GI/GU: May have renal agenesis. May have epispadias, hypospadias, cryptorchidism.

MISCELLANEOUS: The first case of Ellis-van Creveld syndrome was probably reported in 1670, in a description of a "polydactylous monster" found drowned in an Amsterdam canal. The name "six-fingered dwarfism" was proposed at one time to describe this syndrome. This synonym has fallen into disuse in favor of more tactful ones.

This disorder is named after Richard WB Ellis of Guy's Hospital, London, and Simon van Creveld of the University of Amsterdam. The anecdotal story is that Ellis and van Creveld met fortuitously in a railway car on their way to a medical meeting and during the course of their conversation realized they were both considering publication of the same disorder. They decided to publish jointly, with Ellis's name first for reasons of alphabetization and euphony.

In 1941 the Nazis removed Simon van Creveld from his position as Chair of Paediatrics at the University of Amsterdam and condemned him to a concentration camp. He survived his incarceration and at the end of the war was reinstated to his former position.

ANESTHETIC CONSIDERATIONS
Dental abnormalities are common, and should be noted preoperatively in the event of a difficult intubation with possible dental damage. A short trachea may result in inadvertent endobronchial intubation (5). Patients may have significant restrictive lung disease. Patients with congenital

heart disease need perioperative antibiotic prophylaxis as indicated.

Bibliography:
1. Digilio MC, Marino B, Giannotti A, et al. Single atrium, atrioventricular canal/postaxial hexodactyly indicating Ellis-van Creveld syndrome. *Hum Genet* 1995;96:251–253.
2. Wu CL, Litman RS. Anesthetic management for a child with the Ellis-van Creveld syndrome: a case report. *Paediatr Anaesth* 1994;4:335–337.
3. Qureshi F, Jacques SM, Evans MI, et al. Skeletal histopathology in fetuses with chondroectodermal dysplasia (Ellis-van Creveld syndrome). *Am J Med Genet* 1993;45:471–476.
4. Berkowitz I, Raja S, Bender K, et al. Dwarfs: pathophysiology and anesthetic implications. *Anesthesiology* 1990;73:739–759.
5. Wells AL, Wells TR, Landing BH, et al. Short trachea, a hazard in tracheal intubation of neonates and infants: syndromal associations. *Anesthesiology* 1989;71:367–373.

Emery-Dreifuss Muscular Dystrophy

MIM #: 310300

This X-linked muscular dystrophy is differentiated from Duchenne muscular dystrophy by its more benign course and early contractures, and from Becker muscular dystrophy by the presence of contractures and the higher incidence of cardiac problems. It typically presents beginning in the teenage years. Rare cases have been inherited in an autosomal dominant fashion with occurrences in girls (Emery-Dreifuss muscular dystrophy phenotype). There are many distinct mutations of the gene. The gene product of the Emery-Dreifuss muscular dystrophy gene has been termed emerin. It is located on the inner nuclear membrane, but its specific physiologic role is unknown. Autosomal dominant disease can be due to mutations in the gene encoding laminins A and C that, like emerin, are located in the nuclear envelope, on the nucleoplasmic surface of the inner nuclear membrane. Emery-Dreifuss muscular dystrophy may be related to rigid spine syndrome (see later).

HEENT/AIRWAY: Neck flexion can be limited due to contractures of the posterior cervical muscles.

CARDIOVASCULAR: Cardiomyopathy, often presenting as a heart block, typically develops during the third decade of life. Third-degree heart block, which can be fatal, can be preceded by sinus bradycardia or a first-degree heart block. May have atrial standstill. Cardiomyopathy with poor ventricular function is less common than conduction abnormalities. The degree of cardiac involvement does not correlate with the degree of skeletal muscle involvement. Female carriers can have cardiac problems in the absence of any muscle abnormality.

NEUROMUSCULAR: Slowly progressive muscle wasting and weakness with a humeroperoneal distribution in the earliest phases, followed by hip and knee extensors and the proximal upper limb. Progression is slow and patients only rarely lose the ability to walk. Muscle wasting is associated with elevations in creatine kinase, but only three to ten times normal, much lower than in Duchenne muscular dystrophy.

ORTHOPEDIC: Early contractures of the elbows, Achilles tendons (causing toe walking), and posterior cervical muscles. Contractures can appear before muscle weakness. Hypoplasia of the third to fifth cervical vertebral bodies and intervertebral discs with fusion of the apophyseal joints has been described. This is thought to be secondary to the immobilization and disuse caused by stiffness of the posterior cervical muscles.

MISCELLANEOUS: Although reported by Dreifuss and colleagues in the 1960s, it was probably described as early as 1902. Born in Germany, Fritz Dreifuss grew up in New Zealand and was a scarfie (ask your New Zealand colleagues) at the University of Otago in New Zealand. He spent the bulk of his professional career on the neurology faculty at the University of Virginia, where he was uniformly liked and respected. He died in 1997.

ANESTHETIC CONSIDERATIONS

Endotracheal intubation can be difficult because of neck stiffness and decreased cervical mobility. Temporary cardiac pacing must be available at all times perioperatively. Myocardial depressant agents should be avoided in patients with a significant cardiomyopathy. Succinylcholine is contraindicated in this myopathic condition because of the risk of an exaggerated hyperkalemic response. Patients must be carefully positioned perioperatively secondary to multiple joint contractures. Malignant hyperthermia has not been reported in association with this disease. Spinal deformities secondary to myopathy and contractures may make neuraxial techniques difficult.

Bibliography:
1. Aldwinckle RJ, Carr AS. The anesthetic management of a patient with Emery-Dreifuss muscular dystrophy for orthopedic surgery. *Can J Anaesth* 2002;49:467–470.
2. Shende D, Agarwal R. Anaesthetic management of a patient with Emery-Dreifuss muscular dystrophy. *Anaesth Intensive Care* 2002;30:372–375.
3. Jensen V. The anaesthetic management of a patient with Emery-Dreifuss muscular dystrophy. *Can J Anaesth* 1996;43:968–971.
4. Morrison P, Jago RH. Emery-Dreifuss muscular dystrophy. *Anaesthesia* 1991;46:33–35.

Encephalocraniocutaneous Lipomatosis

See also Proteus syndrome

MIM #: 176920 (Proteus syndrome)

This dysmorphic syndrome of unknown etiology has as its main features unilateral craniofacial lipomatosis with ipsilateral cerebral atrophy. There is controversy as to whether this is a distinct syndrome or part of a clinical spectrum that includes Proteus syndrome. It may represent somatic mosaicism of a dominant mutation that is lethal in its nonmosaic state.

HEENT/AIRWAY: Unilateral craniofacial lipomatosis can cause craniofacial asymmetry. Nodules of connective tissue form on the upper inner eyelid and can cause lid retraction. Can have microphthalmia, coloboma, corneal opacity. Epibulbar choristomas. Aniridia has been reported. May have odontomas.

CARDIOVASCULAR: Rare cardiac lipomatosis.

NEUROMUSCULAR: Ipsilateral cerebral atrophy and porencephalic cyst formation. Ipsilateral meningeal lipomatosis. Bony defect may overlie the cerebral abnormality. Extracranial extension of an intracranial lipoma through the foramen ovale has been reported. Variable mental retardation. Marked motor delay. Seizures. May have hydrocephalus. Extradural spinal cord lipomas.

OTHER: Alopecia and skin hypoplasia occur over the craniofacial lipomas.

ANESTHETIC CONSIDERATIONS

Chronic use of anticonvulsant medications may affect the metabolism of some anesthetic drugs. Care needs to be taken in patients with eyelid retraction.

Bibliography:
1. Gawel JS, Schwartz RA, Jozwiak S. Encephalocraniocutaneous lipomatosis. *J Cutan Med Surg* 2003;7:61–65.
2. Romiti R, Rengifo JA, Arnone M, et al. Encephalocraniocutaneous lipomatosis: a new case report and review of the literature. *J Dermatol* 1999;26:808–812.
3. Kodsi SR, Bloom KE, Egbert JE, et al. Ocular and systemic manifestations of encephalocraniocutaneous lipomatosis. *Am J Ophthalmol* 1994;118:77–82.
4. Rizzo R, Pavone L, Micali G, et al. Encephalocraniocutaneous lipomatosis, Proteus syndrome, and somatic mosaicism. *Am J Med Genet* 1993;47:653–655.
5. McCall S, Ramzy MI, Cure JK, et al. Encephalocraniocutaneous lipomatosis and the Proteus syndrome: distinct entities with overlapping manifestations. *Am J Med Genet* 1992;43:662–668.

Engelmann-Camurati Syndrome

See Camurati-Engelmann syndrome

Eosinophilic Granuloma

Included in Langerhans cell histiocytosis

Epidermal Nevus Syndrome

See Nevus sebaceus of Jadassohn

Epidermolysis Bullosa

MIM #: Many

This disease of the epidermis and mucous membranes results in separation of skin layers with formation of bullae after even trivial local trauma. The disease is due to abnormalities in one of several attachment complexes anchoring the epidermis to the underlying dermis. There are over 20 separate subtypes described, both autosomal dominant and recessive, which are divisible into three main groups. In simplex types, the pathologic process occurs above the basement membrane layer of skin, and lesions heal without scarring. In junctional and dystrophic types, the disease occurs at or below the basement membrane, and lesions of the dystrophic types heal with scarring (Table 2). In a recently described type, the hemidesmosomal variant, tissue separation occurs at the basal cell-lamina lucida interface at the hemidesmosomes.

HEENT/AIRWAY: Disease involving the corneal epithelium can lead to bullae that cause corneal ulceration or perforation. In the severe forms, scarring of healed bullae in the oral cavity can limit mouth opening and limit tongue mobility by adhering the tongue to the floor of the mouth. Acute pharyngeal bullae can cause airway obstruction or hemorrhage. Teeth may be dysplastic and prone to caries. Older patients are typically edentulous. Glottic or subglottic bullae or scarring may require tracheostomy. Even though the tracheal epithelium is histologically different, tracheal bullae and scarring can occur.

CARDIOVASCULAR: May be associated with mitral valve prolapse. A case of cardiomyopathy secondary to presumed dietary selenium deficiency has been reported.

NEUROMUSCULAR: One type, caused by abnormalities in the gene *PLEC1*, an adhesion protein found in epidermis and sarcolemma, is associated with late-onset muscular dystrophy.

ORTHOPEDIC: Pseudosyndactyly of the fingers.

GI/GU: Esophageal strictures, diverticulae, and perforation may occur. Gastroesophageal reflux. Esophageal scarring resulting in dysmotility. There may also be anal involvement, often causing chronic constipation. One specific type, caused by mutations in specific integrin genes, is associated with congenital pyloric atresia. Glomerulonephritis may develop from streptococcal skin infections.

OTHER: There may be neoplastic degeneration of skin lesions. Patients may be malnourished and hypoalbuminemic, and develop anemia of chronic disease. The anemia is not responsive to treatment with iron, but has responded to therapy with iron and erythropoietin. Hair and nails may be atrophic.

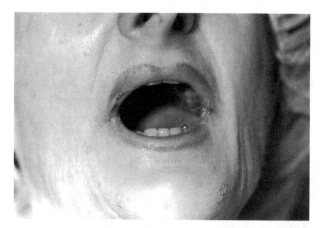

Epidermolysis bullosa. FIG. 1. Photograph of a 62-year-old woman with epidermolysis bullosa showing markedly diminished maximal mouth opening. (Courtesy of Dr. Alison S. Carr, Department of Anaesthesia, Derriford Hospital, Plymouth, England.)

MISCELLANEOUS: A presumed association with porphyria was probably because porphyria cutanea tarda was misdiagnosed as epidermolysis bullosa.

ANESTHETIC CONSIDERATIONS

Tape should not be used to attach monitors or catheters, and adhesive patches from electrocardiograph leads and pulse oximeter probes should be removed (or clip-on oximeter probes should be used). If only stick-on oximeter probes are available, the finger can be covered first with non-adhesive plastic film. Monitors and intravenous catheters can be secured with Webril, Kerlix, or Coban (crinkly, stretchy tape that adheres to itself without adhesive). The blood pressure cuff should be cushioned with flannel gauze. Orthopedic limb tourniquets can be used if well padded (8). Chronic scarring of the

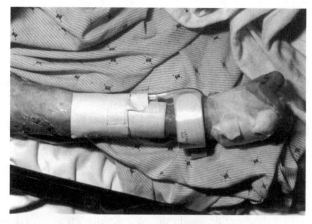

Epidermolysis bullosa. FIG. 2. Photograph of the same patient as in Figure 1 showing markedly atrophic skin on the arms with atrophy and pseudosyndactyly of the fingers. (Courtesy of Dr. Alison S. Carr, Department of Anaesthesia, Derriford Hospital, Plymouth, England.)

hands and feet can result in fusion of the fingers and toes (pseudosyndactyly), so that the pulse oximeter may need to be placed on the ear. Scarring of the hands and arms with parchment-like skin may make venous access difficult. Wiping the skin during preparation for placing vascular or epidural catheters should be avoided. A tourniquet used to aid in intravenous catheter placement may cause bullae. The internal and external jugular veins have been used without any problems. Central venous and arterial cannulae should be sutured rather than taped in place. Patients should position themselves on the operating table to minimize trauma. Pressure points (including heels) must be well padded and lubricated. The operating table must be well padded by a sheepskin or other padding. Skin traction (e.g., for restraining an infant) must be avoided—intramuscular or rectal inductions may be preferred.

Pressure from a face mask or hands holding a face mask can cause facial bullae. Mask cuffs should be covered with Xeroform or Vaseline gauze. Hands holding a face mask should be gloved to decrease skin trauma, and the chin should be padded. Oral scarring may limit mouth opening and laryngoscopy and intubation may be very difficult or impossible. Fiberoptic nasal intubation is often needed in these patients. Nasotracheal tubes may be affixed to a headwrap and foam block, or secured by Coban tape tied to the tube and wrapped around the head. An oral RAE tube might be easier to keep in place when untied or untaped (3). Placement of oral airways, endotracheal intubation, or oropharyngeal suctioning can result in oropharyngeal, lingual, or tracheal bullae. Oropharyngeal suctioning should be done, if at all, under direct vision without touching the mucosa. Laryngoscope blades should be well lubricated with a water-soluble gel and the endotracheal tube should be well lubricated, undersized, and uncuffed. In

several large series, as a result of good care, there were no major tracheal complications from airway management or intubation (3, 6, 23), although there were new oral lesions. Tracheal tube cuffs, if present, should be inflated gently and carefully. The laryngeal mask airway (LMA) has been used successfully (4) and if possible it should be removed in young children prior to awakening to minimize airway trauma.

Good premedication allowing the placement of an intravenous catheter before induction, or a slow inhalation induction allowing spontaneous ventilation, may help bypass the need for positive-pressure ventilation by mask. Ketamine infusion has been used to avoid tracheal intubation if muscle relaxants are not required (12), and total intravenous anesthesia with blow-by oxygen is an attractive alternative if clinically appropriate.

Esophageal disease may increase the risk of aspiration and is an indication for a rapid sequence induction with cricoid pressure (using a lubricated gloved hand and lubrication to the neck). Pressure must be applied with no sideways movement. Nasogastric tubes are relatively contraindicated because of the risk of causing pharyngeal and esophageal bullae.

Contractures about the eyes may prevent complete eye closure during anesthesia. The eyes should be protected with a pad of gel if possible rather than with tape. Upon emergence, patients may rub the eye ointment into their eyes and blur their vision. Despite theoretical risks, caudal (9), brachial plexus (16), and lateral cutaneous nerve of the thigh blocks have been used in children, and regional techniques have been used in adults (10, 14, 17, 18). However, contracted limbs may limit appropriate access, and care needs to be taken to avoid skin trauma during skin preparation. There is a single case report of an epidural catheter in a child that was tunneled and sutured to avoid skin tape. Subcutaneous infiltration

TABLE 2. *Types of epidermolysis bullosa*

Name	Synonym(s)	Features
Nonscarring		
Epidermolysis bullosa simplex- generalized	Koebner type	Onset at birth or in infancy. Generalized bullae without scarring. Normal teeth and nails. Autosomal dominant inheritance.
Epidermolysis bullosa simplex- localized	Weber-Cockayne type	Onset after infancy. Bullae on limbs only without oral lesions. No scarring. Autosomal dominant inheritance.
Junctional epidermolysis bullosa	Herlitz type	Onset at birth or in infancy. Generalized bullae with minimal or no scarring. Minimal involvement of hands and feet. Mucosal, scalp and perioral involvement. Secondary infections with granuloma formation can lead to scarring. Severe anemia and growth failure. Death before 2 years of age common. Autosomal recessive inheritance.
Scarring		
Epidermolysis bullosa dystrophica, dominant	Hyperplastic type, dystrophic type	Onset at birth. Limb but not oral involvement. Bullae heal with scarring, which may be hypertrophic. Autosomal dominant inheritance.
Epidermolysis bullosa dystrophica, recessive	Hallopeau-Siemens type	Onset at birth. Generalized bullae, particularly of the limbs, and may develop acquired syndactyly. Esophageal involvement common. Healed, scarred bullae can be atrophic. Dystrophic nails. Dysplastic teeth. Autosomal recessive inheritance.

(Modified from Holzman RS, Worthen HM, Johnson KL. Anaesthesia for children with junctional epidermolysis bullosa [letalis]. *Can J Anaesth* 1987;34:395–399.)

with local anesthetics should be avoided, but intramuscular injections have not been associated with the formation of bullae. Rectal analgesics must be carefully administered because of the risk of perianal trauma.

Fasciculations from succinylcholine might be capable of causing skin trauma, but one large series reported no significant skin trauma after the use of succinylcholine (8). Hypoalbuminemia and decreased protein binding may necessitate decreased doses of drugs that are protein bound, such as muscle relaxants.

Bleeding oropharyngeal bullae can be treated with the application of epinephrine-soaked sponges (1:200,000).

Bibliography:
1. Doi S, Horimoto Y. Subcutaneous tunneling of an epidural catheter in a child with epidermolysis bullosa [Letter]. *Acta Anaesthesiol Scand* 2006;50:395.
2. Herod J, Denyer J, Goldman A, et al. Epidermolysis bullosa in children: pathophysiology, anaesthesia and pain management. *Paediatr Anaesth* 2002;12:388–397.
3. Iohom G, Lyons B. Anaesthesia for children with epidermolysis bullosa: a review of 20 years' experience. *Eur J Anaesthesiol* 2001;18:745–754.
4. Ames WA, Mayou BJ, Williams K. Anaesthetic management of epidermolysis bullosa. *Br J Anaesth* 1999;82:746–751.
5. Ishimura H, Minami K, Sata T, et al. Airway management for an uncooperative patient with recessive dystrophic epidermolysis bullosa. *Anaesth Intensive Care* 1998;26:110–111.
6. Yonker-Sell AE, Connolly LA. Twelve hour anaesthesia in a patient with epidermolysis bullosa. *Can J Anaesth* 1995;42:735–739.
7. Lin AN, Lateef F, Kelly R, et al. Anesthetic management in epidermolysis bullosa: review of 129 anesthetic episodes in 32 patients. *J Am Acad Dermatol* 1994;30:412–416.
8. Griffin RP, Mayou BJ. The anaesthetic management of patients with dystrophic epidermolysis bullosa. *Anaesthesia* 1993;48:810–815.
9. Yee LL, Gunter JB, Manley CB. Caudal epidural anesthesia in an infant with epidermolysis bullosa. *Anesthesiology* 1989;70:149–151.
10. Boughton R, Crawford MR, Vonwillwe JB. Epidermolysis bullosa: a review of 15 years' experience, including experience with combined general and regional techniques. *Anaesth Intensive Care* 1988;16:260–264.
11. Hagen R, Langenbert C. Anaesthetic management in patients with epidermolysis dystrophica. *Anaesthesia* 1988;43:482–485.
12. Idvall J. Ketamine monoanesthesia for major surgery in epidermolysis bullosa. *Acta Anaesthesiol Scand* 1987;31:658–660.
13. Holzman RS, Worthen HM, Johnson KL. Anaesthesia for children with junctional epidermolysis bullosa (letalis). *Can J Anaesth* 1987;34:395–399.
14. Broster T, Placek R, Eggers GWN. Epidermolysis bullosa: anesthetic management for cesarean section. *Anesth Analg* 1987;66:341–343.
15. Kaplan R, Strauch B. Regional anaesthesia in a child with epidermolysis bullosa. *Anesthesiology* 1987;67:262–264.
16. Kelly RE, Koff HD, Rothaus KO, et al. Brachial plexus anesthesia in eight patients with recessive dystrophic epidermolysis bullosa. *Anesth Analg* 1987;66:1318–1320.
17. Spielman FJ, Mann ES. Subarachnoid and epidural anaesthesia for patients with epidermolysis bullosa. *Can Anaesth Soc J* 1984;31:549–551.
18. Rowlingson JC, Rosenblum SM. Successful regional anesthesia in a patient with epidermolysis bullosa. *Reg Anesth* 1983;8:81–83.
19. Tomlinson AA. Recessive dystrophic epidermolysis bullosa. *Anaesthesia* 1983;38:485–491.
20. James I, Wark H. Airway management during anesthesia in patients with epidermolysis bullosa dystrophica. *Anesthesiology* 1982;56:323–326.
21. Berryhill RE, Benumof JL, Saidman LJ, et al. Anesthetic management of emergency cesarean section in a patient with epidermolysis bullosa dystrophica polydysplastica. *Anesth Analg* 1978;57:281–283.
22. Lee C, Nagel EL. Anesthetic management of a patient with recessive epidermolysis bullosa dystrophica. *Anesthesiology* 1975;43:122–123.
23. Reddy ARR, Wong DHW. Epidermolysis bullosa: a review of anesthetic problems and case reports. *Can Anaesth Soc J* 1972;19:536–548.

Epstein Syndrome

Included in Fechtner syndrome

Escobar Syndrome

See Multiple pterygium syndrome

Essential Fructosuria

SYNONYM: Fructosuria; fructokinase deficiency

MIM #: 229800

This autosomal recessive disorder is due to deficient activity of hepatic fructokinase (ketohexokinase). This enzyme catalyzes the conversion of fructose to fructose-1-phosphate, the first step in the metabolism of fructose. This enzyme is actually better termed a hexokinase because it is not specific for fructose. Accumulation of fructose in this disease is benign. It is the accumulation of fructose-1-phosphate, as occurs in hereditary fructose intolerance (see later), that leads to toxicity.

GI/GU: Reducing substance (fructose) in the urine.

MISCELLANEOUS: These patients are asymptomatic and are usually discovered fortuitously when a reducing substance is found in the urine. This may happen less frequently now that urine test strips that measure reducing sugars have been replaced by test strips that are specific for glucose.

ANESTHETIC CONSIDERATIONS
There are no specific anesthetic considerations.

Bibliography:
1. Hommes FA. Inborn errors of fructose metabolism. *Am J Clin Nutr* 1993;58:788S–795S.

Eulenburg Disease

See Paramyotonia congenita

Exstrophy of the Bladder Sequence

MIM #: 600057

Abnormal development of the anterior abdominal wall mesoderm is the cause of this developmental defect. Failure of the infraumbilical mesenchyme to migrate into the infraumbilical region gives rise to a midline defect of the lower abdominal wall, with exposed bladder, failed fusion of the symphysis pubis, incomplete fusion of the genital tubercles, often with epispadias, and sometimes inguinal hernias. The defects can be surgically repaired, and there are usually no persistent genitourinary abnormalities. Occasional autosomal dominant occurrences have been reported. Pseudoexstrophy of the bladder is a rare occurrence of a healed omphalocele with a defect in the hypogastric area, but an intact bladder.

MISCELLANEOUS: The word exstrophy derives from the Greek ekstriphein, which translates "turn inside out."

ANESTHETIC CONSIDERATIONS
There are no specific anesthetic considerations for this developmental defect.

Bibliography:
1. Messelink EJ, Aronson DC, Knuist M, et al. Four cases of bladder exstrophy in two families. *J Med Genet* 1994;31:490–492.
2. Jeffs RD. Exstrophy, epispadias, and cloacal and urogenital sinus abnormalities. *Pediatr Clin North Am* 1987;34:1233–1257.

Exstrophy of the Cloaca Sequence

SYNONYM: OEIS complex

MIM #: 258040

This developmental disorder is caused by defects in the mesenchyme that will form the lower abdominal wall, the cloacal septum and the lumbosacral vertebrae. As a result, there is a midline defect of the lower abdominal wall, and defects of the lower genitourinary tract and pubis. It has also been referred to as the OEIS complex- for **O**mphalocele, **E**xstrophy of the cloaca, **I**mperforate anus, and **S**pinal defects. The defects can be surgically ameliorated, but there are likely to be persistent genitourinary and sometimes gastrointestinal abnormalities such as urinary incontinence and malnutrition in patients with significantly shortened bowel; and there will also be a need to consider gender reassignment in severely affected patients.

ORTHOPEDIC: Failed fusion of the symphysis pubis. Incomplete development of the lumbosacral vertebrae with hydromyelia. May have anomalies of the lower extremities, including limb hypoplasia, congenital hip dislocation, clubfoot and other deformities.

GI/GU: May occasionally have an omphalocele. Imperforate anus. Short bowel syndrome. Exstrophy of the cloaca (failure of cloacal division with persistence of a single exit point for the ureters and the hindgut), failed fusion of the genital tubercles with severe epispadias. Cryptorchidism. Renal anomalies, including renal agenesis and polycystic kidneys.

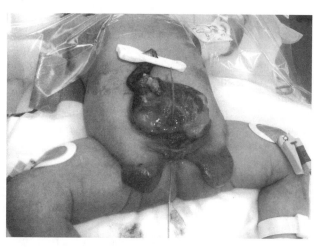

Exstrophy of the cloaca sequence. This neonate with exstrophy of the cloaca still has remnants of the mesenchymal membrane covering the defect. There is a small open bladder connecting to a prolapsed bladder neck (due to the widened symphysis pubis). There is also a common epispadias, bifid scrotum, and an unusual skin bridge across the two pubic tubercles. There is also an imperforate anus, not well seen here. (Courtesy Dr. R. Cartland Burns, Department of Surgery, University of Virginia Health System.)

MISCELLANEOUS: The word exstrophy derives from the Greek ekstriphein, which translates "turn inside out."

ANESTHETIC CONSIDERATIONS
Lower lumbar and caudal anesthesia/analgesia may be technically difficult. In the absence of severe malnutrition or renal disease, there are no other anesthetic considerations for this developmental defect.

Bibliography:
1. Keppler-Noreuil KM. OEIS complex (omphalocoele-exstrophy-imperforate anus-spinal defects): a review of 14 cases. *Am J Med Genet* 2001;99:271–279.
2. Smith NM, Chambers HM, Furness ME, et al. The OEIS complex (omphalocele-exstrophy-imperforate anus-spinal defects): recurrence in sibs. *J Med Genet* 1992;29:730–732.
3. Hurwitz RS, Manzoni GA, Ransley PG, et al. Cloacal exstrophy: a report of 34 cases. *J Urol* 1987;138:1060–1064.

F

Fabry Disease

SYNONYM: Alpha-galactosidase A deficiency; Anderson-Fabry disease

MIM #: 301500

This X-linked disorder, caused by deficient lysosomal alpha-galactosidase A, typically presents in boys during puberty or adolescence. This enzyme splits galactose from the cerebroside ceramide trihexoside, and its deficiency results in the storage of glycolipids with terminal alpha-galactosyl moieties in a variety of tissues, particularly vascular endothelium and smooth muscle. It is closely related to other sphingolipidoses, such as Gaucher disease, in which glucose cannot be split from cerebroside. Because of random X chromosome inactivation, some girls may have some of the manifestations of the disease, such as pain in the extremities (acroparesthesia) and skin lesions (angiokeratoma). On rare occasions, girls can be as severely affected as boys. Death occurs usually in adulthood from renal, cardiac, or cerebrovascular complications. There is also a cardiac variant, where vascular disease is absent. Success has been obtained with recombinant human alpha-galactosidase A replacement therapy; and residual enzyme activity has been enhanced in the cardiac variant, and cardiac function improved with infusions of galactose.

HEENT/AIRWAY: Corneal and lens opacities. Whorl-like corneal epithelial changes visible by slit-lamp examination. These changes are typical of this disease and are alone almost diagnostic. Tortuous retinal and conjunctival vessels with aneurysmal dilatations of venules seen on the conjunctivae. There may be involvement of the temporomandibular joint with limitation of movement.

CHEST: Rare chronic bronchitis or dyspnea. Elderly patients may have abnormal pulmonary function tests with an obstructive pattern and decreased diffusing capacity.

CARDIOVASCULAR: Endothelial accumulation leading to ischemia and infarction. Ischemic cardiovascular disease. Sometimes the electrocardiographic changes consistent with infarction are not because of ischemia, but because of glycolipid deposition in the myocardium. Renovascular hypertension, left ventricular asymmetric hypertrophy with hypertrophic obstructive cardiomyopathy. Valvular abnormalities, including mitral valve prolapse and insufficiency. Conduction abnormalities, including short PR interval and episodic supraventricular tachycardia secondary to progressive glycolipid deposition in the AV node and bundle of His. Cerebrovascular disease. Cardiac disease in the cardiac variant presents as milder disease at an older age, but is progressive and eventually fatal.

NEUROMUSCULAR: Recurrent pain crises of the extremities, characterized by burning pain of the palms and soles. With time, pain may radiate to the proximal extremities and to other parts of the body. These pain crises are provoked by cold, exertion, fever, emotional stress, or rapid changes in temperature or humidity. They tend to diminish in intensity and frequency with aging. In some patients the pain can be excruciating. Acroparesthesias. Abnormal temperature sensation in the extremities. Crises of pain in the extremities are probably due to accumulation of glycolipid in the autonomic nervous system ganglion cells. Chronic

diphenylhydantoin or carbamazepine may be used for pain. Cerebrovascular disease may cause transient ischemic attacks or stroke.

ORTHOPEDIC: Arthralgia. Lymphedema of the legs (without hypoproteinemia), presumably caused by glycolipid deposition in lymphatic vessels. There are multiple ossifications at the insertion of fibrous structures to bone, and articular erosions. A typical defect is the limited extension of the distal interphalangeal joints. There can be avascular necrosis of the head of the femur or the talus, and small infarction-like areas of involvement of the metatarsals, metacarpals, and temporomandibular joint.

GI/GU: Diarrhea, hemorrhoids, and episodic flank pain. The pain is presumably due to deposition in the small intestinal vessels or the autonomic ganglia. Priapism. Renal insufficiency beginning with proteinuria, and hyposthenuria (inability to concentrate urine), progressing to uremia and hypertension.

OTHER: Hypohidrosis (decreased sweating), probably due to accumulation of glycolipid in autonomic nervous system ganglion cells. Angiokeratoma skin lesions are characteristic, although not diagnostic, because they also occur in other lysosomal storage disorders. Angiokeratomas are due to blood vessel ectasia, and are most commonly found between the lower abdomen and the knees, and on the mucous membranes of the mouth and the cornea. They are small dark red to blue-black, slightly raised, superficial, nonblanching lesions. Episodes of pain can be associated with fever and an elevated erythrocyte sedimentation rate.

MISCELLANEOUS: Fabry, a German dermatologist, was probably not the first to describe this disorder. Fabry's description of the skin lesions as "purpura papulosa haemorrhagica Hebrae" implies that it was previously described by Hebra (Hebra was Moriz Kaposi's father-in-law). Anderson described this disorder in the same year. A third case was described in an Egyptian man who had scrotal lesions. Madden, the physician, was unable to make a diagnosis, but consulted Osler, who was then convalescing in Egypt. He also could not make a diagnosis, but suggested that scrotal irradiation might be helpful (ouch!). The typical corneal lesions are identical to those seen with chronic chloroquine or amiodarone therapy.

ANESTHETIC CONSIDERATIONS
Attacks of abdominal pain may be incorrectly ascribed to a surgical abdomen or renal colic. Anticholinergic drugs may exacerbate hypohidrosis, and are best avoided perioperatively. Limited mouth opening can occur secondary to temporomandibular joint disease, and may make direct laryngoscopy more difficult. Cardiac status should be carefully evaluated preoperatively. The possibility of ischemic neurovascular disease should be considered. Renal insufficiency

affects perioperative fluid management and the metabolism of renally excreted drugs. Patients may have polyuria, making urine output a poor indicator of intravascular volume status. Chronic diphenylhydantoin or carbamazepine therapy, used to alleviate pain in the extremities, may affect the metabolism of some anesthetic drugs. Such recurrent pain may be a relative contraindication to regional techniques.

Bibliography:
1. Desnick RJ, Brady RO. Fabry disease in childhood. *J Pediatr* 2004;144: S20–S26.
2. Eng CM, Guffon N, Wilcox WC, et al. Safety and efficacy of recombinant human α-galactose A replacement therapy in Fabry's disease. *N Engl J Med* 2001;345:9–16.
3. Brown LK, Miller A, Bhuptani A, et al. Pulmonary involvement in Fabry disease. *Am J Respir Crit Care Med* 1997;155:1004–1010.
4. Shelley ED, Shelley WB, Kurczynski TW. Painful fingers, heat intolerance, and telangiectases of the ear: easily ignored childhood signs of Fabry disease. *Pediatr Dermatol* 1995;12:215–219.

Facioauriculovertebral Syndrome

See Goldenhar syndrome

Faciocardiorenal Syndrome

SYNONYM: Eastman-Bixler syndrome

MIM #: 227280

This autosomal recessive disorder involves anomalies of the face, the heart, and the kidneys. Because of the small number of patients described, it is not clear if the additional findings are specific to this syndrome. The responsible gene and gene product are not known.

HEENT/AIRWAY: Facial anomalies, including broad nasal bridge, open mouth, large chin.

CARDIOVASCULAR: Cardiac anomalies, including conduction defects, endocardial fibroelastosis, cardiomegaly.

NEUROMUSCULAR: Severe mental retardation. Hyperactive reflexes, ankle clonus. Bilateral Babinski reflex.

ORTHOPEDIC: May have growth retardation.

GI/GU: Renal anomalies, including horseshoe kidney.

OTHER: May have growth hormone deficiency.

ANESTHETIC CONSIDERATIONS

The perioperative electrocardiogram should be monitored closely for evidence of conduction abnormalities. Patients with endocardial fibroelastosis may have diminished myocardial function. Renal disease affects perioperative fluid management and the choice of anesthetic drugs.

Bibliography:
1. Nevin NC, Hill AE, Carson DJ. Facio-cardio-renal (Eastman-Bixler) syndrome. *Am J Med Genet* 1991;40:31–33.

Faciodigitogenital Syndrome

See Aarskog syndrome

Faciogenitopopliteal Syndrome

See Popliteal pterygium syndrome

Facioscapulohumeral Muscular Dystrophy

SYNONYM: Landouzy-Dejerine disease

MIM #: 158900

This autosomal dominant disease is the most clinically benign of the muscular dystrophies. The name indicates the areas of major involvement. The incidence is only 1/50 that of Duchenne muscular dystrophy. The disorder is highly variable. Weakness usually first involves the face and scapulae followed by the foot flexors and the hip girdle.

HEENT/AIRWAY: Weakness of the orbicularis oris and oculi muscles with ptosis. Weakness of the perioral muscles leads to, for example, inability to whistle or blow through a straw. Protruding lips, a result of facial muscle weakness, have been termed "tapir's mouth." Facial muscle weakness leads to a relatively inanimate face, with decreased ability to frown or smile. Retinal vasculopathy with telangiectases, microaneurysms, and capillary leak. Sensorineural hearing loss.

CARDIOVASCULAR: Absence of electrocardiographic and other cardiac findings differentiates this dystrophy from the other forms of muscular dystrophy.

NEUROMUSCULAR: The primary muscles involved are those of the face, neck, shoulder, and upper arms. The lower abdominal muscles, as well as the peroneal and proximal muscles of the leg, can also be involved. The bulbar, extraocular, and respiratory muscles are spared. Intelligence is normal.

ORTHOPEDIC: Kyphoscoliosis. The clavicles slope downward, resulting in drooping shoulders. Winged scapula.

MISCELLANEOUS: Duchenne actually differentiated the infantile form of this disease from the typical Duchenne muscular dystrophy 20 years before its description by Landouzy and Dejerine. Joseph Landouzy was a French physician who became Dean of Medicine at the University of Paris in 1901. Joseph Dejerine was a French neuropathologist. The autopsy results of one of their original patients (from 1886) were reported in 1964. At that time, the pedigree extended through seven generations.

Anesthetic Considerations

Muscular dystrophy places these patients at risk for hyperkalemic arrest with the administration of succinylcholine. Although sensitivity to atracurium was normal in a single patient, reported recovery was faster (1). Baseline weakness of the neck muscles means that the ability to sustain a head lift may not be an appropriate marker of adequate reversal of muscle relaxation. Malignant hyperthermia has not been reported in association with this disease.

Bibliography:

1. Dresner DL, Ali HH. Anaesthetic management of a patient with facioscapulohumeral muscular dystrophy. *Br J Anaesth* 1989;62:331–334.

Factor V Leiden Mutation

MIM #: 227400

Factor V Leiden mutation is the most common cause of hereditary thrombophilia, a familial propensity to develop venous thromboembolism. It is present in approximately 5% to 8% of people of European descent. The factor V Leiden mutation involves a substitution of glutamine for arginine in the 506 position of factor V. This point mutation stops the cleavage of the procoagulant factor Va by activated protein C (APC). The mutated factor V protein exhibits normal procoagulant function *in vitro* but is resistant to inactivation by APC in a PTT assay. It is the most frequent cause of APC resistance. Most affected patients are heterozygous for the factor V Leiden mutation. Homozygotes are at higher thrombotic risk. Also at higher risk are heterozygous patients for the factor V Leiden mutation combined with mutations in the genes for protein C, protein S, or antithrombin III. The genes for factor V and antithrombin III are both located on the long arm of chromosome 1, and are not infrequently inherited together. Approximately 10% of persons carrying the factor V Leiden mutation experience clinically significant thrombosis in their lifetime.

Cardiovascular: Recurrent venous thrombosis, cerebral sinus thrombosis, renal transplant rejection, venous thrombosis during pregnancy/delivery. Risk of thromboembolism is increased in the presence of other risk factors (smoking, pregnancy, contraceptive pill use, surgery, trauma, immobilization, malignancy). There appears to be no increased risk of arterial thrombotic events.

Miscellaneous: In 1987, investigators from Leiden launched the Leiden Thrombophilia Study, a large case–control study designed to define the risk of venous thromboembolism associated with protein C deficiency in the Dutch population. But the study is better remembered (and credited) for identifying this important cause of venous thromboembolism.

Factor V Leiden mutation is so rare as to be essentially nonexistent in persons of Chinese, Japanese, black African, or Native American descent. Because of its genetic distribution, it has been estimated that the mutation must have originated approximately 30,000 years ago, after the evolutionary divergence of European, African, and Asian populations.

Anesthetic Considerations

Venous thrombosis is an important cause of postoperative morbidity and occasionally also mortality. Factor V Leiden mutation is potentially an additive risk factor for this postoperative complication. However, it appears that its contribution is so small as to be clinically insignificant in the face of other perioperative risk factors (especially pregnancy, trauma, surgery, immobility) and in particular in the presence of prophylactic perioperative anticoagulation. It is unnecessary to screen for Factor V Leiden mutation preoperatively, as there is currently no recommended alteration in anesthetic management. Factor V Leiden mutation may decrease the risk of blood loss in patients undergoing cardiopulmonary bypass (7), but at the same time it may be a contributing factor to accelerated graft occlusion after coronary artery bypass grafting. Pregnant patients could be on low molecular weight heparin, making the timing of epidural catheter placement an issue. Transition to unfractionated heparin late in pregnancy has been suggested. Parturients have been reported to be at increased risk for deep vein thrombosis. Increased risk of abruption, preeclampsia, and pregnancy loss have also been reported.

Bibliography:

1. Harnett MJ, Walsh ME, McElrath TF, et al. The use of central neuraxial techniques in parturients with factor V Leiden mutation. *Anesth Analg* 2005;101:1821–1823.
2. Johnson CM, Mureebe L, Silver D. Hypercoagulable states: a review. *Vasc Endovascular Surg* 2005;39:123–133.
3. Donahue BS. Factor V Leiden and perioperative risk. *Anesth Analg* 2004;98:1623–1634.
4. Edmonds MJ, Crichton TJ, Runciman WB, et al. Evidence-based risk factors for postoperative deep vein thrombosis. *ANZ J Surg* 2004;74:1082–1097.
5. Castoldi E, Rosing J. Factor V Leiden: a disorder of factor V anticoagulant function. *Curr Opin Hematol* 2004;11:176–181.
6. Kotaka M, Kohchi A. Perioperative management of a patient with factor V Leiden mutation [Japanese]. *Masui* 2003;52:409–411.
7. Donahue BS, Gailani D, Higgins MS, et al. Factor V Leiden protects against blood loss and transfusion after cardiac surgery. *Circulation* 2003;107:1003–1008.
8. Wahlander K, Larson G, Lindahl TL. et al. Factor V Leiden (G1691A) and prothrombin gene G20210A mutations as potential risk factors for venous thromboembolism after total hip or total knee replacement surgery. *Thromb Haemost* 2002;87:580–585.
9. Ravin AJ, Edwards RPA, Krohn M. et al. The factor V Leiden mutation and the risk of venous thromboembolism in gynecologic oncology patients. *Obstet Gynecol* 2002;100:1285–1289.

10. Caprini JA, Arcelus JI, Reyna JJ. Effective risk stratification of surgical and nonsurgical patients for venous thromboembolic disease. *Semin Hematol* 2001;38:12–19.
11. Blaszyk H, Bjornsson J. Factor V leiden and morbid obesity in fatal postoperative pulmonary embolism. *Arch Surg* 2000;135:1410–1413.
12. Wilder-Smith E, Kothbauer-Margreiter I, Lammle B, et al. Dural puncture and activated protein C resistance: risk factors for cerebral venous sinus thrombosis. *J Neurol Neurosurg Psychiatry* 1997;63:351–356.

Fahr Disease

MIM #: 213600

This disease is characterized by nonatherosclerotic calcification of multiple (probably demyelinated) areas of the brain, with degeneration of function and eventual decerebration. Some cases of Fahr disease are clearly inherited, but it has been suggested that this may also be a disease of defective iron transport or the sequela of a fetal viral infection. Hypoparathyroidism may be a causative factor in some cases.

The mineralizations contain not only calcium, but aluminum, zinc, and iron. The differences in mineral content between pericapillary and nonvascular, and between the globus pallidus and dentate nucleus of the cerebellum suggest that mineralization is a secondary process. Single-photon emission computed tomography scans show decreased blood flow to the affected areas.

HEENT/AIRWAY: Small, round head. Prolongation of visual evoked potentials. Optic atrophy. Retinitis pigmentosa.

NEUROMUSCULAR: Calcification (actually mineralization) of widely scattered areas of the brain, including the cortex, basal ganglia, and cerebellum. Mineralization is both perivascular and within the brain substance. Progressive deterioration of mental and motor function. Basal ganglia changes lead to athetosis. Cerebellar dysarthria. Symmetric spastic paralysis. Seizures, dementia, and psychiatric disturbances. Memory problems. Astrocytoma may develop.

OTHER: Hypoparathyroidism.

MISCELLANEOUS: Fahr's original patient probably did not have his eponymous disorder.

ANESTHETIC CONSIDERATIONS

Patients with dysarthria may be at increased risk for aspiration. Hypocalcemia from hypoparathyroidism should be excluded before surgery (but is specifically excluded in a narrow delineation of the disease). Chronic use of anticonvulsant medications may alter the metabolism of some anesthetic drugs. Succinylcholine is contraindicated in patients with advanced spastic paralysis.

Bibliography:

1. Manyam BV, Bhatt MH, Moore WD, et al. Bilateral striopallidodentate calcinosis: cerebrospinal fluid, imaging, and electrophysiological studies. *Ann Neurol* 1992;31:379–384.
2. Beall SS, Patten BM, Mallette L, et al. Abnormal systemic metabolism of iron, porphyrin, and calcium in Fahr's syndrome. *Ann Neurol* 1989;26:569–575.

Fairbank Type Multiple Epiphyseal Dysplasia

Included in Multiple epiphyseal dysplasia

Familial Adenomatous Polyposis

See Gardner syndrome

Familial Dysautonomia

See also Congenital insensitivity to pain and anhydrosis (familial dysautonomia, type II)

SYNONYM: Riley-Day syndrome; Hereditary sensory and autonomic neuropathy (HSAN III)

MIM #: 223900

This autosomal recessive disorder affects both sensory and autonomic neurons, causing abnormalities in multiple organ systems. The pathogenesis is not clear, although there is demyelination in the brainstem and posterior columns of the spinal cord, and degeneration of the autonomic ganglia. Almost all cases are mutations in the gene *IKBKAP*. This disorder is characterized by lack of tearing, absent corneal reflexes, excessive sweating, cold hands and feet, peripheral sensory neuropathy, absent deep tendon reflexes, hypotonia, cardiovascular lability, and emotional lability. It is seen almost entirely in people of Ashkenazic Jewish descent. The causes of death are typically respiratory failure, renal failure, or unexplained sudden death.

HEENT/AIRWAY: Lack of tears, absent corneal reflexes. Corneal ulcerations can develop. The tongue is smooth secondary to the absence of fungiform papillae. Impaired gag reflex. Drooling.

CHEST: Respiratory drive in response to hypercapnia and hypoxia is blunted. Recurrent aspiration leads to chronic lung disease. May also have restrictive lung disease from hypotonia and kyphoscoliosis.

CARDIOVASCULAR: Sympathetic and parasympathetic instability with profound fluctuations in vasomotor response and blood pressure. Paroxysmal hypertension is common. Hypersensitivity to endogenous and exogenous catecholamines. Vasovagal reflex may be exaggerated. Postural hypotension.

NEUROMUSCULAR: Normal intelligence. Speech delay. Decreased pain and temperature perception, followed later by decreased vibratory sensation. Emotional lability and immature behavior. Decreased sensitivity to taste. Peripheral sensory neuropathy, absent deep tendon reflexes. Poor coordination. May have seizures. Decreased myelinated and unmyelinated small nerve fibers, large myelinated fibers, sympathetic ganglia neurons, and neurons in dorsal horns.

ORTHOPEDIC: Kyphoscoliosis. Peripheral sensory neuropathy eventually leads to Charcot type neuropathic joints.

GI/GU: Difficulties in swallowing, with abnormal esophageal and gastrointestinal motility. High incidence of gastroesophageal reflux, aspiration, protracted episodes of vomiting, abdominal pain. Constipation. Poor control of bladder function.

OTHER: Excessive sweating, blotching of the skin, cold hands and feet, acrocyanosis. Impairment of temperature regulation, episodic fever. Diabetes mellitus can develop.

ANESTHETIC CONSIDERATIONS

Emotional lability and immature behavior may be especially apparent preoperatively. Judicious use of premedication (avoiding narcotic-induced hypoventilation—see later) attenuates the stress response to preoperative anxiety. Lack of tears and the absence of corneal reflexes means that these patients are at increased risk of corneal injuries. Meticulous perioperative eye care is necessary. Impairment of the gag reflex, difficulties in swallowing, and abnormal esophageal motility place these patients at very high risk for perioperative aspiration. Pretreatment with an H_2-receptor antagonist may be considered. Patients should have a rapid sequence induction, and the airway should be protected with an endotracheal tube. Careful assessment of the patient's preoperative hydration status is necessary because patients may be dehydrated secondary to difficulties in swallowing or excessive sweating. Patients may be incapable of responding appropriately to intraoperative hypovolemia.

Sympathetic and parasympathetic instability may lead to profound fluctuations in blood pressure, and paroxysmal hypertension is common. Patients are hypersensitive to endogenous and exogenous catecholamines. Inotropes should be avoided unless absolutely necessary. An arterial catheter may be helpful. Premedication with a phenothiazine or a beta blocker has been recommended to minimize the blood pressure response to circulating catecholamines perioperatively. The vasovagal reflex may be exaggerated. Cardiovascular autonomic instability may make accurate assessment of the anesthetic depth difficult. Epidural anesthesia has been used as an adjunct to general anesthesia and was thought to provide additional cardiovascular stability (3).

Respiratory drive in response to hypercapnia and hypoxia is blunted. Patients may be unable to compensate for narcotic-induced hypoventilation. Intraoperative assisted or controlled ventilation is recommended (5). Patients may have chronic lung disease secondary to recurrent aspiration

or restrictive lung disease secondary to kyphoscoliosis. Extubation in the operating room has resulted in an increased incidence of postoperative atelectasis (5).

Patients may require lower than expected concentrations of volatile anesthetics, probably secondary to decreased muscle tone and decreased peripheral pain sensation. There is no specific contraindication to the use of succinylcholine or nondepolarizing muscle relaxants. Temperature regulation is impaired. Patients may become hypothermic or hyperthermic intraoperatively, hence body temperature must be monitored and controlled as well as possible.

Postoperative complications include persistent vomiting, aspiration, orthostatic hypotension and syncope, paroxysmal hypertension, hypoxemia, hypoventilation, and hyperthermia. There is decreased need for postoperative analgesics secondary to decreased peripheral pain sensation. Chlorpromazine has been used in the past to control postoperative nausea, hyperthermia, and hypertension (5). Diazepam is the drug of choice for the treatment of dysautonomic crises.

Bibliography:
1. Axelrod FB. Familial dysautonomia. *Muscle Nerve* 2004;29: 352–363.
2. Benardi L, Hilz M, Stemper B, et al. Respiratory and cerebrovascular responses to hypoxia and hypercapnia in familial dysautonomia. *Am J Respir Crit Care Med* 2003;167:141–149.
3. Challands JF, Facer EK. Epidural anaesthesia and familial dysautonomia (the Riley-Day-syndrome): three case reports. *Paediatr Anaesth* 1998;8:83–88.
4. Dell'oste C, Vincenti E, Torre G. Multiple and various anaesthetics, ketamine included, in a young patient with familial dysautonomia, case report. *Minerva Pediatr* 1996;48:113–116.
5. Axelrod FB, Donenfelf RF, Danziger F, et al. Anesthesia in familial dysautonomia. *Anesthesiology* 1988;68:631–635.
6. Fishbein D, Grossman RF. Pulmonary manifestations of familial dysautonomia in an adult. *Am J Med* 1986;80:709–712.
7. Beilin B, Maayan CH, Vatashsky E, et al. Fentanyl anesthesia in familial dysautonomia. *Anesth Analg* 1985;64:72–76.
8. Stenquist O, Sigurdsson J. The anaesthetic management of a patient with familial dysautonomia. *Anaesthesia* 1982;37:929–932.

Familial Hyperkalemic Periodic Paralysis

See Familial periodic paralysis

Familial Hypokalemic Periodic Paralysis

See Familial periodic paralysis

Familial Hyperlysinemia

SYNONYM: Hyperlysinemia

MIM #: 238700

This autosomal recessive disease is due to a defect in the enzyme alpha-aminoadipic semialdehyde synthase (AASS).

This enzyme catalyzes the deamination of lysine as a first step in the metabolism of excess lysine through the Krebs cycle to produce energy. This enzyme is present in many tissues. It actually catalyzes two separate steps in the metabolic pathway (and was previously thought to be two separate enzymes). Deficiency of this enzyme also results in saccharopinemia, an increase in saccharopine, which is another intermediary metabolite. Familial hyperlysinemia may, in fact, not have any clinical significance, because early cases were identified from among patients referred for medical care for developmental or neurologic problems, and later patients identified prospectively have not had problems.

HEENT/AIRWAY: Ectopia lentis.

NEUROMUSCULAR: Mental retardation, seizures, hypotonia.

ORTHOPEDIC: Lax ligaments.

GI/GU: Significant lysinuria.

OTHER: Mild anemia.

MISCELLANEOUS: Hyperlysinemia itself is not toxic, as evidenced by the lack of effects on the fetus of a mother with the disease (lysine freely traverses the placenta).

ANESTHETIC CONSIDERATIONS

Chronic use of anticonvulsant medications may alter the metabolism of some anesthetic drugs. Patients must be carefully positioned perioperatively secondary to ligamentous laxity.

Bibliography:

1. Dancis J, Hutzler J, Ampola MG, et al. The prognosis of hyperlysinemia: an interim report. *Am J Hum Genet* 1983;35:438–442.

Familial Mediterranean Fever

MIM #: 249100

This autosomal recessive disease, found predominantly in patients of Eastern Mediterranean ancestry, is characterized by recurrent bouts of fever and serositis. Acute attacks last from 1 to 4 days and can occur from several times per week to yearly. The frequency and intensity of attacks tend to lessen with aging. The disease can be accompanied by amyloidosis, even in the absence of these crises. The disease often becomes apparent in early childhood. It is treated with colchicine, which not only controls the symptoms but can arrest the development of amyloidosis. Colchicine will not abort an ongoing crisis. The disorder is due to abnormalities in the gene *MEVF*, which encodes pyrin. Pyrin is found only in mature granulocytes. Pyrin is thought to regulate the inflammatory response at the level of the leukocyte cytoskeleton.

HEENT/AIRWAY: Transient conjunctivitis. Temporomandibular arthritis has been reported.

CHEST: Recurrent pleuritis, transient pleural effusion.

CARDIOVASCULAR: Self-limiting pericarditis.

NEUROMUSCULAR: Uncommon, benign, recurrent, aseptic meningitis. Myalgia during an attack. Migraine headaches during attacks have been described.

ORTHOPEDIC: Mild arthralgia or recurrent arthritis, monoarticular or polyarticular.

GI/GU: Recurrent abdominal pain. Recurrent peritonitis. Children often have associated diarrhea. Splenic amyloidosis. Recurrent orchitis. Progressive renal amyloidosis with proteinuria, eventually leading to renal failure, which can occur without overt crises.

OTHER: Attacks are accompanied by fever as high as 39° to 40°C. Many patients have an erysipelas-like skin rash, typically of the lower leg or foot. Pregnancy is associated with remission of symptoms, which resume postpartum. Leukocytosis. Elevated erythrocyte sedimentation rate. The thyroid can be involved.

MISCELLANEOUS: Pyrin has also been called marenostrin, from the Latin for Mediterranean Sea (*mare nostrum*).

ANESTHETIC CONSIDERATIONS

Recurrent abdominal pain can be incorrectly diagnosed as an acute abdomen. In one series of children, one-third were subjected to needless surgery, most often laparotomies (4). Some physicians suggest prophylactic laparoscopic appendectomy early in the course of the disease to prevent misdiagnosis of true appendicitis later. Peritoneal irritation during surgery rarely provokes an attack. Recurrent peritonitis does not result in peritoneal adhesions.

Tetrahydrocannabinol was used successfully in a patient with recurrent abdominal pain to decrease the requirement of analgesics (3). Temporomandibular arthritis, a rare manifestation, may impair opening of the mouth and make direct laryngoscopy more difficult. Renal failure can affect perioperative fluid management and the metabolism of some anesthetic drugs.

Bibliography:

1. Samuels J, Aksentijevich I, Torosyan T. Familial mediterranean fever at the millennium. Clinical spectrum, ancient mutations, and a survey of 100 American referrals to the national institutes of health. *Medicine (Baltimore)* 1998;77:268–297.
2. Ben-Chetrit E, Levy M. Familial mediterranean fever. *Lancet* 1998;351:659–664.
3. Holdcroft A, Smith M, Jacklin A, et al. Pain relief with oral cannabinoids in familial Mediterranean fever. *Anaesthesia* 1997;52:483–486.
4. Majeed HA, Barakat M. Familial Mediterranean fever (recurrent hereditary polyserositis) in children: analysis of 88 cases. *Eur J Pediatr* 1989;148:636–641.

Familial Periodic Paralysis

SYNONYM: Periodic paralysis. (Includes Hyperkalemic periodic paralysis and Hypokalemic periodic paralysis)
  See also Paramyotonia congenita

MIM #: 170400, 170500, 311700

This spectrum of disorders includes hypokalemic, normokalemic, and hyperkalemic periodic paralysis, although it is unclear whether normokalemic paralysis is a distinct entity. **Hyperkalemic periodic paralysis** is due to mutations in the *SCN4A* (alpha subunit, skeletal muscle sodium channel) gene. Hypopolarization of the membrane does not allow activation of the sodium channel. **Hypokalemic periodic paralysis** is due to mutations in *CACNL1A3* (the dihydropyridine-sensitive calcium channel) gene, the *SCN4A* gene, or the *KCNE3* gene [a subunit of the slow potassium channel I (Ks)]. Both diseases are autosomal dominant. In general, hypokalemic attacks are nocturnal or occur in the early morning and are prolonged, whereas hyperkalemic attacks occur during the daytime and are of a shorter duration. Between episodes, the serum potassium is normal in both variants.

CARDIOVASCULAR: Can be associated with arrhythmias. Concurrent use of digoxin increases the risk of arrhythmias associated with hypokalemia.

NEUROMUSCULAR: Profound weakness can be precipitated by exercise, exposure to cold, or with rest after exercise. The diaphragm is spared. Menses and pregnancy have been reported to exacerbate the condition. Respiratory and cranial muscles tend to be spared except during the worst attacks. Muscle tone is normal in the absence of an episode of weakness. Myotonia has been associated with hyperkalemic paralysis, although the myotonia may be detectable only electromyographically.

OTHER: Excessive intake of dietary sodium or carbohydrate can provoke an attack of weakness in hypokalemic patients.

MISCELLANEOUS: The names "hyperkalemic" and "hypokalemic" periodic paralysis are to an extent misnomers, because although the serum potassium rises or falls during an episode of weakness, it may remain within normal limits. The diagnosis of hyperkalemic periodic paralysis is made on the basis of provocation through an oral potassium load. Hypokalemia in patients with hypokalemic periodic paralysis is produced by administration of insulin and glucose.

ANESTHETIC CONSIDERATIONS
Hyperkalemic paralysis: Prolonged preoperative fasting and administration of potassium containing intravenous fluids should be avoided. Intraoperative fluids should provide some dextrose and no potassium. Old banked blood can present a significant potassium load. Utilizing washed red cells may be considered, if appropriate. Hyperkalemic paralysis may present during general anesthesia or in the postanesthesia care unit. Perioperative decreases in body temperature can provoke an attack. Episodic measures of plasma potassium should be performed perioperatively, and the patient's electrocardiogram should be monitored continuously for evidence of hyperkalemic changes. Once a hyperkalemic attack is in progress, treatment options include glucose and insulin, beta agonists, glucagon, and calcium chloride, as well as kaliuretics such as furosemide. Succinylcholine is contraindicated in patients with a hyperkalemic variant. During an episode of paralysis, a nerve stimulator will unreliably reflect the state of neuromuscular blockade. There is no contraindication to using nondepolarizing muscle relaxants, although neostigmine has been reported to increase myotonia. Spinal and epidural anesthesia have been used successfully.

Hypokalemic paralysis: Hypokalemic paralysis can also be precipitated by perioperative stress or hypothermia. It has been suggested that anxiety can precipitate an attack of weakness, hence appropriate premedication may be warranted. Infusions of glucose and large carbohydrate meals should be avoided in hypokalemic patients. Hyperventilation (as during delivery) could decrease serum potassium levels. Beta-adrenergic agents can decrease blood potassium levels. Perioperative potassium concentrations must be monitored closely, and intravenous potassium supplementation used. Routine oral potassium supplementation should be resumed when practical. The patient's electrocardiogram should be monitored continuously for evidence of hypokalemic changes. Hypokalemic weakness responds to an infusion of potassium. Spinal anesthesia and epidurals have been used as the sole anesthetic without complication, despite the small decrease in serum potassium accompanying conduction block (3, 5). Postoperative muscle weakness has been reported after depolarizing neuromuscular blockade, but nondepolarizing agents have not been problematic.

Malignant hyperthermia with equivocal *in vitro* contracture tests has been reported (6, 11), and there has been a report of a single patient with positive halothane and caffeine contracture tests, but with inconclusive genetic analysis of *CACNL1A3* and *SCN4A* (1). However, most information indicates that familial periodic paralysis is not associated with malignant hyperthermia. Myotonia has been associated with hyperkalemic paralysis. A single patient has been described with hypokalemic/normokalemic paralysis and myotonia, which made intubation impossible (7).

Bibliography:
1. Rajabally YA, El Lahawi M. Hypokalemic pereiodic paralysis associated with malignant hyperthermia. *Muscle Nerve* 2002;25:453–455.
2. Weller JF, Elliott RA, Pronovost PJ. Spinal anesthesia for a patient with familial hyperkalemic periodic paralysis. *Anesthesiology* 2002;97:259–260.
3. Viscomi CM, Ptacek L, Dudley D. Anesthetic management of familial hypokalemic periodic paralysis during parturition. *Anesth Analg* 1999;88:1081–1082.

4. Bunting HE, Allen RW. Prolonged muscle weakness following emergency tonsillectomy in a patient with familial periodic paralysis and infectious mononucleosis. *Paediatr Anaesth* 1997;7:171–175.
5. Hecht ML, Valtysson B, Hogan K. Spinal anesthesia for a patient with a calcium channel mutation causing hypokalemic periodic paralysis. *Anesth Analg* 1997;84:961–964.
6. Lambert C, Blanloeil Y, Horber RK. Malignant hyperthermia in a patient with hypokalemic periodic paralysis. *Anesth Analg* 1994;79: 1012–1014.
7. Neuman GG, Kopman AE. Dyskalemic periodic paralysis and myotonia. *Anesth Analg* 1993;76:426–428.
8. Ashwood EM, Russell WJ, Burrow DD. Hyperkalemic periodic paralysis and anaesthesia. *Anaesthesia* 1992;47:579–584.
9. Lema G, Urzua J, Moran S, et al. Successful anesthetic management of a patient with hypokalemic familial periodic paralysis undergoing cardiac surgery. *Anesthesiology* 1991;74:373–375.
10. Laurito CE, Becker GL, Miller PE. Atracurium use in a patient with familial periodic paralysis. *J Clin Anesth* 1991;3:225–228.
11. Lehmann-Horn F, Iazzo PA. Are myotonias and periodic paralysis associated with susceptibility to malignant hyperthermia? *Br J Anaesth* 1990;65:692–697.
12. Aarons JJ, Moon RE, Camporesi EM. General anesthesia and hyperkalemic periodic paralysis. *Anesthesiology* 1989;71:303–304.
13. Rooney RT, Shanahan EC, Sun T, et al. Atracurium and hyperkalemic familial periodic paralysis. *Anesth Analg* 1988;67:782–783.
14. Rollman JE, Dickson CM. Anesthetic management of a patient with hypokalemic familial periodic paralysis for coronary artery bypass surgery. *Anesthesiology* 1985;63:526–527.
15. Horton B. Anesthetic experiences in a family with hypokalemic familial periodic paralysis. *Anesthesiology* 1977;47:308–310.

Fanconi Anemia

MIM #: 227650, 300514

This mostly autosomal recessive entity (one of the types is X-linked) is due to a defect in a DNA repair mechanism, and the hallmarks are bone marrow failure, susceptibility to cancer, and skeletal defects. It is distinct from Fanconi syndrome (see later). The marrow is primarily affected, along with the heart, kidney, and limbs. The disorder is related to abnormalities in one of several Fanconi anemia complementation group genes, *FANCA* through *FANCM*. Bone marrow transplantation has been curative, but patients are overly sensitive to the conditioning regimen. Patients may or may not have associated dysmorphic features. Male heterozygotes have a three- to fourfold elevated risk of malignancy. DNA repair mechanisms are abnormal in four other inherited diseases: ataxia—telangiectasia, xeroderma pigmentosum, Bloom syndrome, and Cockayne syndrome.

HEENT/AIRWAY: Microcephaly. Ptosis, strabismus, nystagmus, microphthalmia. Atresia of the external auditory canal.

NEUROMUSCULAR: Hydrocephalus or ventriculomegaly, absent septum pellucidum and neural tube defects have been reported.

ORTHOPEDIC: Short stature. Hallmark findings are small or aplastic thumbs and radial aplasia. Clinodactyly, syndactyly, occasional radial abnormalities. Rib and vertebral defects. Congenital hip dislocation.

GI/GU: Small penis, small testes, cryptorchidism. Hydronephrosis, absent or ectopic kidneys.

OTHER: Hypoplastic and eventually aplastic bone marrow. Pancytopenia, typically thrombocytopenia followed by anemia and neutropenia. Hexokinase deficiency (see later) has been reported as part of Fanconi anemia. Increased risk of malignancies—particularly acute myelogenous leukemia (AML) as a child, and solid tumors if a person survives up to adulthood. Uneven hyperpigmentation of the skin. Patients can have a variety of endocrinopathies, including growth hormone deficiency, hypothyroidism, glucose intolerance, and clinical diabetes.

MISCELLANEOUS: Fanconi was a Swiss pediatrician of international renown. His name has been attached to more than 15 diseases or genetic syndromes. Bone marrow transplantation is curative only for marrow failure and prevention of AML. There is still the risk of solid tumors of a variety of types, including squamous cell carcinomas.

ANESTHETIC CONSIDERATIONS
The hematocrit and platelet count must be evaluated before surgery. Neutropenia suggests that special attention should be paid to good aseptic technique. Radial abnormalities may exclude radial artery catheter placement. Patients may have renal dysfunction, which has implications for perioperative fluid management and the choice of anesthetic drugs.

Bibliography:
1. Collins N, Kupfer GM. Molecular pathogenesis of Fanconi anemia. *Int J Hematol* 2005;82:176–183.
2. Alter BP. Fanconi's anaemia and its variability. *Br J Haematol* 1993;85:9–14.
3. Alter BP. Fanconi's anemia: current concepts. *Am J Pediatr Hematol Oncol* 1992;14:170–176.

Fanconi Syndrome

SYNONYM: de Toni-Debre-Fanconi syndrome

MIM #: 134600

This is a distinct entity from Fanconi anemia (see earlier). Fanconi syndrome is a disorder of proximal renal tubular dysfunction with impaired reabsorption of amino acids, glucose, phosphate, urate, potassium, and bicarbonate, as well as a vitamin D-resistant metabolic bone disease. It is a consequence of a variety of genetic diseases and toxins, and as such can be inherited (autosomal dominant) or acquired. It can be seen with cystinosis, Wilson disease, galactosemia, tyrosinemia, cytochrome *c* oxidase deficiency, von Gierke disease, hereditary fructose intolerance, Lowe syndrome, and amyloidosis. It can also be caused by a variety of toxins, including outdated tetracycline, cadmium, valproate, Lysol, multiple myeloma protein (Bence-Jones protein) and quite a few others. The specific gene and gene product of the autosomal dominant type are not known, and it is possible that a primary, idiopathic, autosomal dominant form does not really exist.

NEUROMUSCULAR: Severe potassium depletion from urinary losses can cause muscle weakness.

ORTHOPEDIC: Short stature. Renal phosphate loss presents as vitamin D-resistant rickets in children and osteomalacia in adults. Adults may have pathologic fractures.

GI/GU: Proximal renal tubular dysfunction, with generalized aminoaciduria, normoglycemic glycosuria, hyperphosphaturia with hypophosphatemia, and excessive urinary loss of potassium, bicarbonate, and water, resulting in polyuria and polydipsia. Chronic renal failure can eventually develop.

OTHER: Chronic hyperchloremic metabolic acidosis from renal bicarbonate loss (renal tubular acidosis), hypokalemia.

MISCELLANEOUS: Fanconi was a Swiss pediatrician of international renown. His name has been attached to more than 15 diseases or genetic syndromes. Fanconi syndrome was of course first described by Abderhalden. Fanconi synthesized the similarities between his case and those of de Toni and Debre in the next few years. A similar disease occurs in Basenji dogs. Fanconi syndrome from cadmium toxicity in postwar Japan was known as "Itai-Itai" or "ouch-ouch" disease.

ANESTHETIC CONSIDERATIONS
Patients have proximal renal tubular dysfunction, with aminoaciduria, glycosuria, hyperphosphaturia, and excessive urinary loss of potassium bicarbonate, and water. Careful attention must be paid to the volume of the patient's urinary output, electrolyte, and acid–base status. Urine volume may be an inadequate indicator of intravascular volume. Chronic renal failure develops in some patients, which affects the metabolism of renally excreted drugs. Patients with metabolic bone disease may be at increased risk for pathologic fractures, so careful perioperative positioning is imperative.

Bibliography:
1. Foreman JW, Roth KS. Human renal Fanconi syndrome: then and now. *Nephron* 1989;51:301–306.
2. Joel M, Rosales JK. Fanconi syndrome and anesthesia. *Anesthesiology* 1981;55:455–456.

Farber Disease

SYNONYM: Disseminated lipogranulomatosis

MIM #: 228000

This autosomal recessive storage disease is due to deficiency of the lysosomal enzyme ceramidase, which results in the accumulation of ceramide in the lysosomes of a wide variety of tissues. Symptoms begin in infancy. Patients with type I disease usually die by 2 years of age of airway and ventilation problems. There are four additional types. Patients with types II and III disease have a more benign course, and most of them have normal intelligence. Patients with type IV disease present malignant-like histiocytosis and have severe hepatosplenomegaly. Patients with type V disease have predominantly nervous system involvement, with visceral sparing. Hematopoietic stem cell transplantation has been used successfully in type II/III disease.

HEENT/AIRWAY: Cherry-red spot on the macula. Granulomas of the conjunctivae. Granulomas occur in the oral cavity, epiglottis, and larynx causing upper airway obstruction and difficulty in swallowing. The tongue may be enlarged. Involvement of the larynx may cause a hoarse voice, progressing to aphonia.

CHEST: Pulmonary involvement may cause obstructive disease. Recurrent pulmonary consolidation with fever, possibly secondary to aspiration.

CARDIOVASCULAR: Granulomatous lesions of the cardiac valves.

NEUROMUSCULAR: Profound psychomotor retardation, secondary to accumulation of ceramide in neurons and glial cells. Peripheral neuropathy with diminished deep tendon reflexes, hypotonia, and muscle wasting. Muscle denervation.

ORTHOPEDIC: Multiple, progressive, painful arthropathies with eventual contractures. Swelling over bony protuberances.

GI/GU: Episodic vomiting, poor appetite. Hepatomegaly. Rare splenomegaly. May have nephropathy.

OTHER: Subcutaneous nodules, lymphadenopathy. Very rare cases associated with *in utero* hydrops.

MISCELLANEOUS: Sidney Farber, of the Boston Children's Hospital, was one of the founders of pediatric pathology. The Sidney Farber Cancer Institute and the Dana-Farber Cancer Institute, both located in Boston, are named in his honor.

ANESTHETIC CONSIDERATIONS
Direct laryngoscopy and tracheal intubation may be difficult secondary to the presence of airway granulomas or an enlarged tongue. Even mild post-extubation laryngeal edema can compromise an already narrowed airway. Patients are at risk for hyperkalemia with the administration of succinylcholine because of the presence of denervation myopathy. Patients must be carefully positioned and padded because they have poor tissue mass and prominent subcutaneous nodules. Temperature maintenance during surgery is difficult in these patients, as they typically have a thin body habitus. Patients with cardiac valve involvement need perioperative antibiotic prophylaxis as indicated.

Bibliography:
1. Asada A. The anesthetic implications of a patient with Farber's granulomatosis. *Anesthesiology* 80;1994:206–209.
2. Pilz H, Heipertz R, Seidel D. Basic findings and current developments in sphingolipidoses. *Hum Genet* 1979;47:113–134.

Fazio-Londe Disease

MIM #: 211500

This progressive bulbar palsy is usually inherited in an autosomal recessive fashion, although it has been suggested that one of its three subtypes is autosomal dominant. Progressive deterioration of the anterior horn cells of the cranial nerves occurs, with little or no spinal cord involvement. The affected gene(s) and gene product(s) are not known.

HEENT/AIRWAY: Weakness of the periorbital muscles with ptosis. Involvement of the extraocular muscles is very rare. Facial weakness. Absent gag reflex. Stridor. Vocal cords may be almost immobile.

CHEST: Decreased diaphragmatic movement.

NEUROMUSCULAR: Bulbar palsy. The seventh cranial nerve is almost always affected. Hyperreflexia. Pyramidal tracts are uninvolved. Trunk and limb muscles also become involved as the disease progresses.

GI/GU: Swallowing difficulties.

ANESTHETIC CONSIDERATIONS
Patients are at increased risk for aspiration secondary to an absent gag reflex and swallowing difficulties. Patients often have stridor at baseline, and need to be observed closely perioperatively, and more so postoperatively for airway obstruction. Succinylcholine is relatively contraindicated in this neuropathy with associated muscle weakness because of the risk of an exaggerated hyperkalemic response.

Bibliography:
1. McShane MA, Boyd S, Harding B. Progressive bulbar paralysis of childhood: a reappraisal of Fazio-Londe disease. *Brain* 1992;115:1889–1900.

Fechtner Syndrome

(Includes May-Hegglin anomaly, Sebastian syndrome, and Epstein syndrome)

MIM #: 153640

This autosomal dominant disease is due to mutations in the gene encoding nonmuscle myosin heavy chain-9. It is marked by thrombocytopenia with giant platelets, sensorineural hearing loss and renal insufficiency. Thus, it is similar to Alport syndrome with additional hematologic findings. It is thought that Fechtner syndrome and the similar **May-Hegglin anomaly, Sebastian syndrome,** and **Epstein syndrome** are allelic expressions of the same entity.

HEENT/AIRWAY: Congenital cataracts. High tone sensorineural hearing loss.

GI/GU: Nephritis, ranging from microscopic hematuria to end stage renal failure requiring dialysis.

OTHER: Giant platelets, symptomatic thrombocytopenia, small pale blue inclusions in neutrophils and eosinophils. Variable bleeding diathesis due to abnormal platelet–vessel wall and platelet–platelet interactions. One patient has been described who had coexisting von Willebrand disease (2).

MISCELLANEOUS: Fechtner was the name of the first reported family.

ANESTHETIC CONSIDERATIONS
May have excessive surgical bleeding and/or need a transfusion of platelets perioperatively. Patients may have developed alloimmunization from multiple prior transfusions.

Bibliography:
1. Seri M, Pecci A, Di Bari F, et al. MYH9-related disease: May-Hegglin anomaly, Sebastian syndrome, Fechtner syndrome, and Epstein syndromes are not distinct entities but represent a variable expression of a single illness. *Medicine (Baltimore)* 2003;82:203–215.
2. Mertzlufft F, Koster A, Steinhart H, et al. Fechtner's syndrome: considerations and anesthetic management. *Anesth Analg* 2000;90:1372–1375.

Femoral Hypoplasia–Unusual Facies Syndrome

MIM #: 134780

This usually sporadic, possibly autosomal dominant, syndrome is characterized by severe femoral hypoplasia, up-slanting palpebral fissures, a short nose and cleft palate. Although the significance is unknown, many of these patients are infants of diabetic mothers.

HEENT/AIRWAY: May have craniosynostosis. Up-slanting palpebral fissures. Short nose with a broad tip, hypoplastic alae nasi. Long philtrum, thin upper lip. Cleft palate. Low-set or malformed ears. Micrognathia.

CHEST: May have Sprengel deformity, or fused or missing ribs.

CARDIOVASCULAR: May have cardiac defect, including ventricular septal defect, pulmonary stenosis, or truncus arteriosus.

NEUROMUSCULAR: Normal intelligence.

ORTHOPEDIC: Short stature and short thighs secondary to femoral hypoplasia. Femoral hypoplasia is severe and often asymmetric. A case with femoral aplasia has been reported. Variable and often asymmetric hypoplasia of the tibia and fibula. May have abnormal pelvis with hypoplastic acetabulae, large obturator foramina and vertical ischial axis. May have humeral hypoplasia with decreased mobility at the shoulder or elbow. May have radioulnar and radiohumeral synostosis. Preaxial polydactyly. Syndactyly of the toes. Scoliosis. Vertebral dysplasia. Caudal dysplasia, similar to the caudal regression syndrome (see earlier). Clubfoot deformity.

GI/GU: Inguinal hernias. Cryptorchidism. Small penis, testes, or labia majora. Polycystic kidneys, absent kidneys, abnormal collecting system.

ANESTHETIC CONSIDERATIONS

Micrognathia may make direct laryngoscopy and tracheal intubation more difficult. Fiberoptic intubation through a laryngeal mask airway (LMA) has been successful in an infant. Patients must be carefully positioned perioperatively due to restricted joint mobility. Significant renal disease has implications for perioperative fluid management and the choice of anesthetic drugs.

Bibliography:

1. Iohom G, Lyons B, Casey W. Airway management in a baby with femoral hypoplasia-unusual facies syndrome. *Paediatr Anaesth* 2002;12:461–464.
2. Baraitser M, Reardon W, Oley C. et al. Femoral hypoplasia unusual facies syndrome with preaxial polydactyly. *Clin Dysmorphol* 1994;3:40–45.
3. Johnson JP, Carey JC, Gooch WM, et al. Femoral hypoplasia-unusual facies syndrome in infants of diabetic mothers. *J Pediatr* 1983;102:866–872.

Femur-Fibula-Ulna Syndrome

MIM #: 228200

This sporadically occurring disorder involves femoral defects in association with several rare defects of the upper extremities including unilateral or bilateral amelia (absence of the limb), peromelia (severe malformation of the limb), humeroradial synostosis, and ulnar defects. Defects are more likely to be unilateral than bilateral, and are more likely to be right-sided. The upper limbs are usually more severely affected than the lower limbs. The particular upper limb abnormalities associated with this syndrome are rarely seen in association with other multiple malformation syndromes, lending credence to the belief that this is a unique malformation syndrome. The cause is unknown.

ORTHOPEDIC: Femoral defects, including peromelia at the level of the femur. Fibular defects. Unilateral or bilateral amelia or peromelia of the upper extremities. Humeroradial synostosis. Ulnar defects.

ANESTHETIC CONSIDERATIONS

Limb abnormalities may make vascular access more challenging. Ultrasound has been used in a child with femur-fibula-ulna syndrome to perform a local anesthetic block of the brachial plexus at the level of the interscalenes.

Bibliography:

1. van Geffen GJ, Tielens L, Gielen M. Ultrasound-guided intrascalene brachial plexus block in a child with femur fibula ulna syndrome. *Paediatr Anaesth* 2006;16:330–332.
2. Lenz W, Zygulska M, Horst J. FFU complex: an analysis of 491 cases. *Hum Genet* 1993;91:347–356.

Fetal Akinesia/Hypokinesia Sequence

SYNONYM: Pena-Shokeir syndrome, type I

MIM #: 208150

This usually sporadic or autosomal recessive disorder is marked by arthrogryposis and pulmonary hypoplasia. Most patients are stillborn or die in the neonatal period as a consequence of pulmonary hypoplasia. Although this disorder can be inherited in an autosomal recessive fashion, it is clear that the clinical features of the syndrome can also occur when there has been decreased fetal movement for any reason. Thus this syndrome is etiologically heterogeneous and could be considered a fetal akinesia deformation sequence. The pathophysiology of this disorder may be related to abnormalities of the cortical motor neurons, anomalies of the spinal cord, neurogenic muscle atrophy, intrinsic muscle dysfunction, or restrictive dermopathy. Decreased fetal movement impairs normal development of the joints. Dysfunction of the diaphragm and intercostal muscles leads to pulmonary hypoplasia.

HEENT/AIRWAY: Rigid, expressionless face. Hypertelorism, prominent eyes, epicanthal folds. Ptosis. Simple, posteriorly rotated ears. Flattened nasal tip. Small mouth, high-arched palate. May have cleft palate. Micrognathia. Apparent short neck.

CHEST: Pulmonary hypoplasia. Small thorax. Thin ribs.

CARDIOVASCULAR: May have congenital cardiac defect.

NEUROMUSCULAR: May have hydrocephalus, microgyri, cerebellar hypoplasia, absent septum pellucidum.

ORTHOPEDIC: Arthrogryposis of multiple joints, including elbows, hips, knees, and ankles. May have osseous hypoplasia. Ulnar deviation of the hands. Clenched hand positioning, similar to that seen with trisomy 18. Camptodactyly. Rockerbottom feet, clubfeet. Can have perinatal fractures of thin, gracile long bones.

GI/GU: Short bowel syndrome with malabsorption. Cryptorchidism.

OTHER: Polyhydramnios secondary to impaired swallowing of amniotic fluid. Intrauterine growth retardation. A case with thymic and lymphoid hyperplasia has been reported.

ANESTHETIC CONSIDERATIONS

Micrognathia and short neck may make direct laryngoscopy and tracheal intubation more difficult. Patients are likely to have significant pulmonary hypoplasia. Careful perioperative positioning is necessary secondary to multiple contractures.

Bibliography:

1. Chen H, Blackburn WR, Wertelecki W. Fetal akinesia and multiple perinatal fractures. *Am J Med Genet* 1995;55:472–477.
2. Katzenstein M, Goodman RM. Pre- and postnatal findings in Pena Shokeir I syndrome: case report and a review of the literature. *J Craniofac Genet Dev Biol* 1988;8:111–126.

Fetal Alcohol Syndrome

MIM #: None

Alcohol is the most common teratogen in our society. It leads to a variety of craniofacial, growth, and central nervous system defects. The characteristic facies of fetal alcohol syndrome involve maxillary hypoplasia, short palpebral fissures, a short, upturned nose, a thin upper lip, and a long, smooth philtrum. In general, the frequency and severity of the various anomalies are dose dependent. However, it is possible to have central nervous system effects without obvious involvement of other organs (2).

HEENT/AIRWAY: Mild to moderate microcephaly, maxillary hypoplasia. Short palpebral fissures, ptosis, microphthalmia. Posteriorly rotated, prominent ears. May have hearing loss. Eustachian tube dysfunction. Short, upturned nose. Thin upper lip with long, smooth philtrum. Malocclusion, cleft lip or palate. Micrognathia. Short neck.

CHEST: Rib anomalies.

CARDIOVASCULAR: Ventricular septal defects common. Atrial septal defects, tetralogy of Fallot, and coarctation of the aorta have also been reported.

NEUROMUSCULAR: Mild to moderate mental retardation. Poor fine motor coordination, hypotonia. Irritability in infancy and hyperactivity in childhood. May have tremor. May have absent corpus callosum, cerebellar anomalies, meningomyelocele.

ORTHOPEDIC: Growth deficiency, of prenatal onset. Cervical vertebral anomalies. Abnormal palmar creases, short fourth and fifth metacarpals, small distal phalanges, small fifth fingernails, clinodactyly. Abnormal joint position or function.

GI/GU: Hypoplastic labia majora.

OTHER: Strawberry hemangiomas. Failure to thrive.

MISCELLANEOUS: It has been estimated that 10% to 20% of people with IQs in the range of 50 to 80 have fetal alcohol syndrome.

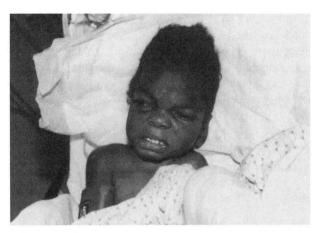

Fetal alcohol syndrome. This 5-year-old boy with fetal alcohol syndrome has typical facies. He also has hypoplasia of tooth enamel, and a fibrous trachea, sternocleidomastoid and hyoid. He has markedly diminished neck extension. A laryngeal mask airway could not be placed successfully. The nares were small and only one side would accept a 2.7 mm fiberoptic bronchoscope, but a nasotracheal tube could not be advanced. The anaesthesia was administered by mask ventilation.

ANESTHETIC CONSIDERATIONS

Preoperative management may be challenging secondary to mental retardation and hyperactivity. Direct laryngoscopy and tracheal intubation may be difficult secondary to micrognathia and a short neck. Patients with congenital heart disease need antibiotic prophylaxis as indicated.

Bibliography:

1. Wattendorf DJ, Muenke M. Fetal alcohol spectrum disorders. *Am Fam Physician* 2005;72:279–282.
2. Mattson SN, Riley EP, Gramling L, et al. Heavy alcohol exposure with or without physical features of fetal alcohol syndrome leads to IQ deficits. *J Pediatr* 1997;131:718–721.
3. Streissguth AP, Aase JM, Clarren SK, et al. Fetal alcohol syndrome in adolescents and adults. *JAMA* 1991;265:1961–1967.

Fetal Cocaine Effect

MIM #: None

The prevalence of cocaine use in the obstetric population has been reported to be as high as 10%. Although a variety of isolated congenital anomalies have been reported in infants who were exposed to cocaine *in utero,* fetal cocaine exposure has not been associated with any specific pattern of teratogenesis. The underlying pathogenesis of the various anomalies is probably related to the vascular effects of cocaine, which causes uterine, placental, or fetal vasoconstriction. Disruption of the blood supply leads to altered morphogenesis of the developing structures.

HEENT/AIRWAY: May have microcephaly. May have cleft lip.

CARDIOVASCULAR: Increased heart rate and systemic blood pressure, and decreased cardiac output have been documented in cocaine-exposed newborns. May have atrial and ventricular arrhythmias. May have cardiac anomalies, including pulmonary stenosis, transposition of the great vessels, hemopericardium. May have vascular anomalies.

NEUROMUSCULAR: May have delayed fine and gross motor skills, hypotonia, irritability, abnormal reflexes, electroencephalographic abnormalities, and seizures. May have cavitary central nervous system lesions. Most neurophysiologic findings are limited to infancy and early childhood.

ORTHOPEDIC: May have limb reduction defects or other skeletal defects.

GI/GU: May have intestinal atresia or infarction. May have genitourinary anomalies. May have renal dysfunction.

OTHER: Increased incidence of intrauterine growth retardation and prematurity—probably secondary to uteroplacental insufficiency from cocaine-induced vasoconstriction. If the mother's cocaine use is recent, the infant might undergo a neonatal abstinence syndrome—hyperflexion, prolonged periods of scanning eye movements, excessive irritability, and tachypnea. Fetal cocaine syndrome may be associated with an increased risk of sudden infant death syndrome.

ANESTHETIC CONSIDERATIONS

Cocaine-exposed newborns have increased heart rate and systemic blood pressure and decreased cardiac output compared to other newborns, consistent with either transplacental passage of maternal catecholamines, or transplacental passage of cocaine, which then results in increased levels of circulating catecholamines in the newborn. These cardiovascular changes are resolved by the second day of life (4). Therefore, if an infant of a cocaine-using mother is born with a congenital anomaly that requires surgery, that surgery, unless it is urgently required, should be postponed to at least the second postnatal day, in order to allow the effects of cocaine to abate. It has been suggested that fetal exposure might lead to diminished ability of the neonatal heart to respond to inotropic drugs.

Bibliography:

1. Vidaeff AC, Mastrobattista JM. *In utero* cocaine exposure: a thorny mix of science and mythology. *Am J Perinatol* 2003;20:165–172.
2. Little BB, Wilson GN, Jackson G. Is there a cocaine syndrome? Dysmorphic and anthropometric assessment of infants exposed to cocaine. *Teratology* 1996;54:145–149.
3. Kain ZN, Rimar S, Barash PG. Cocaine abuse in the parturient and effects on the fetus and neonate. *Anesth Analg* 1993;77:835–845.
4. van de Bor M, Walther FJ, Ebrahimi M. Decreased cardiac output in infants of mothers who abused cocaine. *Pediatrics* 1990;85:30–32.
5. Hoyme HE, Jones KL, Dixon SD, et al. Prenatal cocaine exposure and fetal vascular disruption. *Pediatrics* 1990;85:743–747.
6. Madden JD, Payne TF, Miller S. Maternal cocaine abuse and effect on the newborn. *Pediatrics* 1986;77:209–211.

Fetal Coumarin Syndrome

See Fetal warfarin syndrome

Fetal Dilantin Syndrome

See Fetal hydantoin syndrome

Fetal Face Syndrome

See Robinow syndrome

Fetal Hydantoin Syndrome

SYNONYM: Fetal Dilantin syndrome

MIM #: None

This syndrome is usually caused by *in utero* exposure to phenytoin (Dilantin), although a variety of anticonvulsants (including carbamazepine, mysoline, and phenobarbital) have been implicated in the etiology of this syndrome. Severity may be altered by inherited differences in fetal detoxification pathways. Exposure to multiple agents increases fetal risk. Approximately 10% of infants exposed *in utero* have the full-blown syndrome, and an additional one-third have some features. There is no known safe upper limit for maternal dosing (see also the fetal valproate syndrome, later).

HEENT/AIRWAY: Microcephaly, wide anterior fontanelle, ridging of the metopic suture. Hypertelorism, strabismus, coloboma, glaucoma. Midface hypoplasia. Broad flat nasal bridge, short nose. Cleft lip and palate. Short neck, webbed neck, low-set hairline.

CHEST: Rib anomalies, widely spaced nipples.

CARDIOVASCULAR: A variety of cardiac defects have been described.

NEUROMUSCULAR: Occasional mild mental retardation, which may improve in childhood. Pilonidal sinus.

ORTHOPEDIC: Mild to moderate growth retardation, usually with prenatal onset. Hypoplastic distal phalanges with small nails, digitalized thumb, syndactyly, polydactyly. Hypoplastic toenails. Congenital hip dislocation.

GI/GU: Inguinal and umbilical hernias, single umbilical artery. Pyloric stenosis, duodenal atresia, anal atresia. Hypospadias, micropenis, or ambiguous genitalia. Renal malformations.

OTHER: Hirsutism with coarse scalp hair. Children may be at increased risk for development of cancer. Neonatal hypocalcemia has been reported.

ANESTHETIC CONSIDERATIONS
Patients with congenital heart disease need appropriate perioperative antibiotic prophylaxis as indicated. A short neck may make direct laryngoscopy and tracheal intubation more difficult.

Bibliography:
1. Patel J, Neff SPW. Airway management in a patient with occipitocervical fusion [Letter]. *Anaesth Intensive Care* 1999;27:222–223.
2. Buehler BA, Rao V, Finnell RH. Biochemical and molecular teratology of fetal hydantoin syndrome. *Neurol Clin* 1994;12:741–748.
3. Hanson JW. Teratogen update: fetal hydantoin effects. *Teratology* 1986; 33:349–353.

Fetal Hyperphenylalaninemia Syndrome

See Maternal PKU syndrome

Fetal Rubella Syndrome

SYNONYM: Congenital rubella syndrome

MIM #: None

Maternal rubella infection during the first trimester is associated with up to a 50% risk of the fetal rubella syndrome, which is characterized by microcephaly, mental retardation, cataracts, glaucoma, hearing loss, and cardiac defects. Maternal rubella infection during the second trimester still carries some risk, particularly for mental retardation and hearing loss.

HEENT/AIRWAY: Microcephaly. Cataracts, corneal opacity, glaucoma, chorioretinitis, microphthalmia, strabismus. Sensorineural hearing loss.

CHEST: Interstitial pneumonia as a neonate.

CARDIOVASCULAR: A variety of congenital heart defects, particularly patent ductus arteriosus, peripheral pulmonic stenosis, ventricular septal defect, and atrial septal defect.

NEUROMUSCULAR: Mental and psychomotor retardation. May have meningomyelocele.

ORTHOPEDIC: Growth deficiency.

GI/GU: Neonatal hepatosplenomegaly, hepatitis. Cryptorchidism, hypospadias.

OTHER: Neonatal anemia. Neonatal thrombocytopenia, resulting in the so-called "blueberry muffin" appearance of some neonates. Hypopituitarism. Diabetes mellitus develops in up to 40% of survivors.

ANESTHETIC CONSIDERATIONS
Neonates may be quite ill secondary to interstitial pneumonia, anemia, or thrombocytopenia. Patients with congenital heart disease need perioperative antibiotic prophylaxis as indicated. The presence of diabetes mellitus requires appropriate perioperative management of glucose and insulin. Infants require contact isolation for at least 1 year, unless nasopharyngeal and urine cultures are negative after 3 months of age.

Bibliography:
1. Banatvala JE, Brown DW. Rubella. *Lancet* 2004;363:1127–1137.
2. Zgorniak-Nowosielska I, Zawilinska B, Szostek S. Rubella infection during pregnancy in the 1985–86 epidemic: follow-up after seven years. *Eur J Epidemiol* 1996;12:303–308.
3. McIntosh ED, Menser MA. A fifty-year follow-up of congenital rubella. *Lancet* 1992;340:414–415.

Fetal Valproate Syndrome

MIM #: None

This dysmorphic syndrome is due to maternal use of the anticonvulsant valproic acid during pregnancy. *In utero* exposure to multiple anticonvulsant agents increases the risk to the fetus (see also the fetal hydantoin syndrome, earlier). Only a small number of prenatally exposed infants are affected, and the occurrence of the syndrome in several sets of twins suggests a hereditary susceptibility.

HEENT/AIRWAY: Narrow head, high forehead. Metopic suture synostosis, trigonocephaly. Epicanthal folds. Myopia. Low nasal bridge, short nose with anteverted nostrils. Long upper lip with shallow philtrum. Small mouth, cleft lip. May have cleft palate. May have micrognathia.

CHEST: Broad chest, bifid ribs. Supernumerary nipples.

CARDIOVASCULAR: A variety of congenital cardiac defects, including left-sided obstructive lesions, ventricular septal defect, atrial septal defect, and pulmonary atresia.

NEUROMUSCULAR: Meningomyelocele, spina bifida.

ORTHOPEDIC: Long, thin fingers and toes, polydactyly, triphalangeal thumbs, radial anomalies. Growth retardation.

GI/GU: Inguinal and umbilical hernias. Hypospadias.

ANESTHETIC CONSIDERATIONS
Radial anomalies may make placement of a radial arterial catheter more difficult. Patients with congenital heart disease need perioperative antibiotic prophylaxis as indicated.

Bibliography:
1. Kozma C. Valproic acid embryopathy: report of two siblings with further expansion of the phenotypic abnormalities and a review of the literature. *Am J Med Genet* 2001;98:168–175.

2. Clayton-Smith J, Donnai D. Fetal valproate syndrome. *J Med Genet* 1995;32:724–727.
3. DiLiberti JH, Farndon PA, Dennis NR, et al. The fetal valproate syndrome. *Am J Med Genet* 1984;19:473–481.

Fetal Warfarin Syndrome

SYNONYM: Fetal coumarin syndrome

MIM #: None

This dysmorphic syndrome is due to the teratogenic effects of maternal warfarin use during pregnancy. Approximately one-third of fetuses exposed during the first trimester to coumarin derivatives are affected. The effects of exposure during the second and third trimesters are unclear. Warfarin appears to inhibit the activity of aryl sulfatase E, the deficiency of which causes chondrodysplasia punctata, X-linked recessive type (*MIM #* 302950). Not surprisingly, the fetal warfarin syndrome is phenotypically similar to chondrodysplasia punctata.

HEENT/AIRWAY: Microcephaly. Depressed nasal bridge with nasal hypoplasia. May have upper airway obstruction.

CARDIOVASCULAR: Congenital heart defects.

NEUROMUSCULAR: Severe mental retardation. Seizures. Hydrocephalus, Dandy-Walker malformation, agenesis of the corpus callosum.

ORTHOPEDIC: Rhizomelia. Calcified stippling of uncalcified epiphyses, which disappears after the first year. Mild nail hypoplasia and shortened fingers.

OTHER: Low birth weight with catch-up growth postnatally.

ANESTHETIC CONSIDERATIONS
Infants may present with upper airway obstruction, which can be relieved by an oral airway. Patients with congenital heart disease need antibiotic prophylaxis as indicated. Chronic use of anticonvulsant medications may alter the metabolism of some anesthetic drugs.

Bibliography:
1. Greaves M. Anticoagulants in pregnancy. *Pharmacol Ther* 1993;59:311–327.
2. Iturbe-Alessio I, Fonseca MC, Mutchinik O, et al. Risks of anticoagulant therapy in pregnant women with artificial heart valves. *N Engl J Med* 1986;315:1390–1393.
3. Hall JG, Pauli RM, Wilson KM. Maternal and fetal sequelae of anticoagulation during pregnancy. *Am J Med* 1980;68:122–140.

FG Syndrome

SYNONYM: Opitz-Kaveggia syndrome

MIM #: 305450

This X-linked recessive disorder is characterized by mental retardation, macrocephaly with a prominent forehead, imperforate anus, and congenital hypotonia. It is a genetically heterogeneous disorder.

HEENT/AIRWAY: Macrocephaly. Prominent forehead, large anterior fontanelle. Plagiocephaly. Hypertelorism, epicanthal folds, down-slanting palpebral fissures, strabismus. Small, simple ears. May have sensorineural hearing loss. Prominent facial wrinkles, long philtrum, prominent lower lip. Narrow palate. May have choanal atresia, cleft lip/palate, short neck. High-pitched voice.

CARDIOVASCULAR: Occasional cardiac defect.

NEUROMUSCULAR: Congenital hypotonia. Usually severe mental deficiency and motor delay. Seizures. May have hydrocephalus. Agenesis of the corpus callosum. Tethered spinal cord. Pleasant personality, with attention deficit and hyperactivity.

ORTHOPEDIC: Short stature. Broad thumbs and great toes. Clinodactyly, camptodactyly, syndactyly. Simian crease. Persistent fetal finger pads. Lax joints in infancy. Multiple joint contractures.

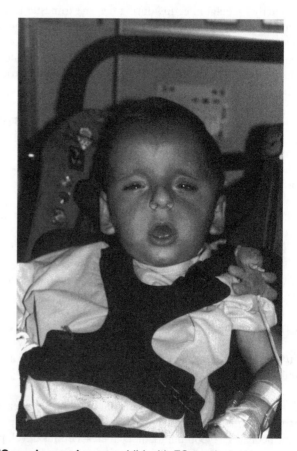

FG syndrome. A young child with FG syndrome.

GI/GU: Imperforate anus, anal stenosis, or anteriorly placed anus. May have umbilical hernia. Severe constipation. May have pyloric stenosis or malrotation. Cryptorchidism, hypospadias.

OTHER: Fine, thin hair. Frontal cowlick. Sociable personality.

MISCELLANEOUS: The term "FG" comes from Opitz's use of a patient's initials to refer to this syndrome.

ANESTHETIC CONSIDERATIONS

Although patients are usually severely mentally retarded, they may nonetheless cooperate with induction because of a generally easy-going personality. Choanal atresia, if present, precludes the use of a nasal airway or a nasogastric tube. Patients must be carefully positioned secondary to multiple joint contractures. Patients with cardiac defects need antibiotic prophylaxis as indicated.

Bibliography:

1. Zwamborn-Hanssen AMN, Schrander-Stumpel CTRM, Smeets E, et al. FG syndrome: the triad mental retardation, hypotonia and constipation reviewed. *Genet Couns* 1995;6:313–319.
2. Romano C, Baraitser M, Thompson E. A clinical follow-up of British patients with FG syndrome. *Clin Dysmorphol* 1994;3:104–114.

Fibrodysplasia Ossificans Progressiva Syndrome

SYNONYM: Myositis ossificans progressiva

MIM #: 135100

This syndrome is characterized by abnormal fibrous tissue in which there is progressive ectopic ossification. Inheritance is autosomal dominant, with most cases representing fresh mutations. The fibrodysplasia becomes apparent in most affected individuals by the age of 5 years. The initial ectopic ossification center is usually located in the neck, spine, or shoulder. Ectopic ossification usually progresses from proximal to distal and from cranial to caudal. By their mid-teens, most patients have severely limited mobility in the upper extremities secondary to ectopic ossification. Most patients experience alternating periods of exacerbations and remissions. Ectopic ossification of soft tissues can occur after trauma or surgery. Patients are often misdiagnosed, with an average time from onset of symptoms to correct diagnosis being greater than 4 years. Attempts to surgically remove the ossifications have resulted in massive new bone formation.

HEENT/AIRWAY: Ectopic ossifications develop in the neck, spine, and shoulders, which may result in severely limited mobility. These begin as tumor-like swellings. May have secondary torticollis. Involvement of the masticatory muscles leads to limited ability to open the mouth. Abnormal temporomandibular joints with dislocation have been reported.

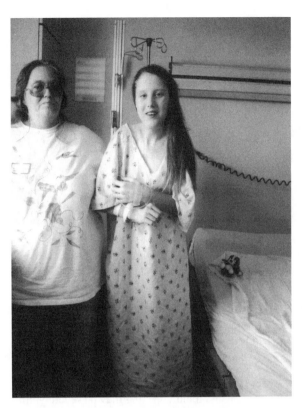

Fibrodysplasia ossificans progressiva. FIG. 1. This 19-year-old with fibrodysplasia ossificans progressiva has such muscle stiffness that she cannot bend enough to sit and cannot brush her teeth. She walks on the tips of her toes. She has essentially no flexion or extension of her neck and required a nasal fiberoptic intubation.

CHEST: Restrictive lung disease may develop secondary to ankylosis of the costovertebral joints, which limits respiratory excursion. The diaphragm is usually unaffected. The most common cause of death is pneumonia.

CARDIOVASCULAR: Approximately 30% have an abnormal electrocardiogram, with right bundle branch block, inferior lead T-wave inversion, left axis deviation, or supraventricular tachycardia.

NEUROMUSCULAR: Although the spine may be severely affected, nerve compression has not occurred.

ORTHOPEDIC: Short big toes with hallux valgus are an invariable feature of this syndrome. Initially there is pain and swelling, followed by ossification, which occurs in fascia, tendons, ligaments, joint capsules, and muscles. Joint mobility often becomes limited. There may be severe spinal involvement with cervical fusion and marked limitation of motion. Scoliosis. There may be secondary osteoporosis. Pathologic fractures may occur.

GI/GU: May have inguinal hernias.

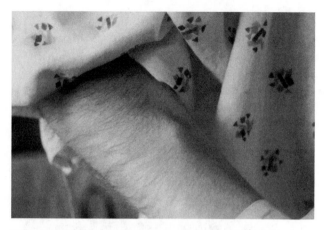

Fibrodysplasia ossificans progressiva. FIG. 2. A bony forearm nodule in the young woman in Figure 1.

MISCELLANEOUS: First described in 1692 by Patin, who noted a woman *"qui est devenue dure comme du bois"* ("who had become hard like wood").

ANESTHETIC CONSIDERATIONS

Head extension and mouth opening may be severely limited because of involvement of the neck, spine, and the muscles of the jaw. Direct laryngoscopy may be very difficult. Tracheostomy may also be difficult because of neck flexion, and should be avoided because the stoma can calcify. Patients can have severe restrictive lung disease. Poor cough requires good postoperative chest physiotherapy; however, excessive tissue injury can result in traumatic ossification.

A significant percentage of these patients have cardiac conduction abnormalities, usually right bundle branch block or supraventricular tachycardia. Patients are often on steroids to ameliorate the pain and swelling, and perioperative stress doses of steroids should be considered. Biopsies, minor trauma, intramuscular injections, other injections (e.g., dental analgesia) and intravenous catheters can all serve as a nidus for calcification. For that reason, and because spinal abnormalities may be present, regional anesthesia is relatively contraindicated.

Bibliography:

1. Kitterman JA, Kantanie S, Rocke DM, et al. Iatrogenic harm caused by diagnostic errors in fibrodysplasia ossificans progressiva. *Pediatrics* 2005;116:e654–e661.
2. Singh A, Ayyalapu A, Keochekian A. Anesthetic management in fibrodysplasia ossificans progressiva (FOP): a case report. *J Clin Anesth* 2003;15:211–213.
3. Smith R, Athanasou NA, Vipond SE. Fibrodysplasia (myositis) ossificans progressiva: clinicopathological features and natural history. *Q J Med* 1996;89:445–456.
4. Cohen RB, Hahn GV, Tabas JA, et al. The natural history of heterotopic ossification in patients who have fibrodysplasia ossificans progressiva. *J Bone Joint Surg Am* 1993;75:215–219.
5. Newton MC, Allen PW, Ryan DC. Fibrodysplasia ossificans progressiva. *Br J Anaesth* 1990;64:246–250.
6. Stark WH, Krechel SW, Eggers GW. Anesthesia in "stone man" myositis ossificans progressiva. *J Clin Anesth* 1990;2:332–335.
7. Lininger TE, Brown EM, Brown M. General anesthesia and fibrodysplasia ossificans progressiva. *Anesth Analg* 1989;68:175–176.

Floating-Harbor Syndrome

MIM #: 136140

This syndrome of unknown etiology is characterized by short stature, distinctive facies with a bulbous nose, and abnormalities in the acquisition of expressive language. The distinctive facial appearance is best appreciated in mid-childhood. Most cases are sporadic.

HEENT/AIRWAY: Triangular facies. May have trigonocephaly. Bulbous nose, large nares. Eyes appear deep-set secondary to a very prominent nasal bridge. Posteriorly rotated ears. Short philtrum. Wide mouth with thin lips. May have supernumerary upper incisor. Low posterior hairline. Short neck.

CARDIOVASCULAR: Rare pulmonary valvular stenosis.

NEUROMUSCULAR: Abnormalities in the acquisition of expressive language result in delayed speech development. Mild mental retardation. No motor delay.

ORTHOPEDIC: Short stature with prenatal onset. Delayed bone age, joint laxity. Clinodactyly, brachydactyly, broad thumbs. May have finger clubbing.

GI/GU: May have celiac disease.

OTHER: Hirsutism.

MISCELLANEOUS: The name Floating-Harbor syndrome comes from a combination of the names of the two hospitals where the first two patients were observed (Boston Floating Hospital in Boston, Massachusetts and Harbor General Hospital in Torrance, California).

ANESTHETIC CONSIDERATIONS

Other than communication problems associated with expressive language delay, there are no specific anesthetic considerations with this syndrome.

Bibliography:

1. Midro AT, Olchowik B, Rogowska M, et al. Floating Harbor syndrome: case report and further syndrome delineation. *Ann Genet* 1997;40:133–138.
2. Lacombe D, Patton MA, Elleau C, et al. Floating-Harbor syndrome: description of a further patient, review of the literature, and suggestion of autosomal dominant inheritance. *Eur J Pediatr* 1995;154:658–661.
3. Houlston RS, Collins ALDennis NR, et al. Further observations on the Floating-Harbor syndrome. *Clin Dysmorphol* 1994;3:143–149.

Focal Dermal Hypoplasia

See Goltz syndrome

Forbes Disease

See Debrancher deficiency

Forney Syndrome

MIM #: 157800

This autosomal dominant disorder is characterized by mitral insufficiency, deafness and bony fusion. The responsible gene and gene product are not known.

HEENT/AIRWAY: Freckling of the iris. Congenital deafness from fixation of the stapes.

CARDIOVASCULAR: Congenital mitral insufficiency.

ORTHOPEDIC: Short stature. Fusion of cervical vertebrae, carpal bones and tarsal bones.

OTHER: Facial freckling.

ANESTHETIC CONSIDERATIONS

Recall that patients are likely to be deaf. Cervical vertebral fusion may make direct laryngoscopy and tracheal intubation difficult. Patients with mitral insufficiency require perioperative antibiotic prophylaxis as indicated.

Bibliography:

1. There are no recent references.

Fragile X Syndrome

SYNONYM: Martin-Bell syndrome. (Includes fragile XE syndrome and X-associated tremor/ataxia syndrome)

MIM #: 309550

This X-linked syndrome is characterized by moderate to severe mental retardation, large ears, and macroorchidism. The syndrome gets its name from the fragility of the X chromosome when cells are cultured in certain media. The fragile site on the X chromosome is marked by repeats of the trinucleotide CGG. The gene at this locus is termed *FMR1*. When the repeats are long (normal allele—30 repeats, affected individuals—mean of 230 repeats), the gene becomes hypermethylated and is not transcribed. Carriers of intermediate alleles have smaller but still excessive numbers of repeats. The product of this gene, termed FMRP, is an RNA-binding protein and may be associated with neuronal plasticity. Although most of the identified patients are male, girls can be affected. This syndrome is relatively common. Up to 6% of mentally retarded boys (and 0.3% of mentally retarded girls) have this disorder. Presumably, fewer girls with full complements of CGG repeats manifest the full syndrome because of X-chromosome inactivation (lyonization). Fragility of the X chromosome (at Xq27.3) in these patients is caused by folate deficiency or folate antagonists. An additional gene, the **fragile XE syndrome** gene (*FMR2*), is located downstream from the fragile X syndrome gene. The much less common fragile XE syndrome is a less severe disease, with mild mental retardation and speech delay, but without physical or behavioral problems. These syndromes are also known as FMR1 (fragile X) and FMR2 (fragile XE), for fragile X mental retardation.

HEENT/AIRWAY: Macrocephaly in early childhood, dolichocephaly, coarse acromegalic facies. Epicanthal folds, pale blue iris, nystagmus, strabismus, myopia. Large ears with soft cartilage. Thickened nasal bridge. Thick lips. Crowding of teeth. Submucous cleft palate. Prognathism (actually a prominent mandibular symphysis, or square chin). High-pitched voice. Torticollis.

CHEST: Pectus excavatum.

CARDIOVASCULAR: Mitral valve prolapse, aortic dilatation.

NEUROMUSCULAR: Moderate to severe mental retardation, which declines with aging due to decreased ability to acquire adaptive behaviors. Cluttered speech, or complete lack of speech in those severely affected. Decreased short term abstract visual memory. Attention deficit disorder with hyperactivity. Behavioral problems with hand flapping or biting. Poor social interaction with peers. Poor eye contact. Autism. Seizures. Hypotonia. Small cerebellar vermis and enlarged fourth ventricle. A subset of males with smaller numbers of excessive repeats can present at age ranging from 50 to 70 years with progressive intention tremor or ataxia and Parkinsonian symptoms. This is called **X-associated tremor/ataxia syndrome**. Depression in women with greater than 100 repeats.

ORTHOPEDIC: Accelerated growth rate in early years. Kyphoscoliosis. Hyperextensible fingers, flat feet.

GI/GU: Macroorchidism, particularly noticeable after puberty. Women with smaller numbers of excessive repeats can have premature ovarian failure.

MISCELLANEOUS: Martin and Bell described X-linked mental retardation, but it was not until 26 years later that karyotype analysis allowed a description of the fragile X chromosomes. Julia Bell remained active until her death at the age of 100, even publishing an original paper at 80. She retired at 86. When James Martin and Marjorie Blandy (another physician) married in 1922 in England, they initially kept their marriage a secret, because in that era women in England were forced to give up their careers after marriage.

Nucleic acid base triplet repeats are also the etiology of other diseases, including Friedreich ataxia, spinocerebellar ataxia type I, and Joseph disease.

ANESTHETIC CONSIDERATIONS

Attention deficit, hyperactivity and behavioral problems may make preoperative management and induction challenging. Chronic use of anticonvulsant medications may alter the metabolism of some anesthetic drugs. Patients in whom mitral insufficiency accompanies mitral valve prolapse need perioperative antibiotic prophylaxis as indicated.

Bibliography:
1. Visootsak J, Warren ST, Anido A, et al. Fragile X syndrome: an update and review for the primary pediatrician. *Clin Pediatr* 2005;44:371–381.
2. Rosenberg RN. DNA triplet repeats and neurologic disease. *N Engl J Med* 1996;335:1222–1224.

Fragile XE Syndrome

Included in Fragile X syndrome

Franceschetti-Klein Syndrome

See Treacher Collins syndrome

Fraser Syndrome

SYNONYM: Cryptophthalmos syndrome; Cryptophthalmos-syndactyly syndrome

MIM #: 219000

This autosomal recessive syndrome involves cryptophthalmos, auricular and nasal malformations, syndactyly, and genital anomalies. It can be caused by mutations in the genes *FRAS1* or *FREM2*. *FRAS1* and *FREM2* are both likely to encode an extracellular matrix protein. Cryptophthalmos is a condition in which the palpebral fissures are absent, and skin covers the eyeballs. Often there are associated eyebrow and ocular defects. Because cryptophthalmos is a variable feature, this syndrome is most appropriately called Fraser syndrome. Isolated cryptophthalmos, without the other features of Fraser syndrome, has also been reported. Nearly half of the patients with Fraser syndrome are stillborn or die in the first year of life, chiefly from renal or laryngeal anomalies. It is interesting to note that some of the anomalies in this syndrome occur when areas that are temporarily fused *in utero* fail to separate (eyelids, digits, vagina).

HEENT/AIRWAY: Hair from the temples grows onto the lateral forehead. Cryptophthalmos. Often have associated ocular anomalies with abnormal vision. May have eyebrow anomalies. Hypertelorism. Lacrimal duct defects. Ear anomalies include microtia, stenosis or atresia of the external auditory canal, low-set ears, cup-shaped ears, absent pinna, conductive hearing loss. Nasal anomalies include narrow, notched nares, coloboma of the *alae nasi*, beaked nose. High-arched palate. May have cleft lip or palate. Choanal stenosis or atresia. Micrognathia. Laryngeal or tracheal stenosis, webbing, hypoplasia, or atresia. Fusion of the vocal cords.

CHEST: Occasional pulmonary hyperplasia, probably secondary to retention of amniotic fluid in the fetal lung because of laryngeal or tracheal stenosis. Widely spaced nipples.

CARDIOVASCULAR: Associated with a variety of congenital cardiac defects.

NEUROMUSCULAR: Mental retardation not uncommon. May have meningomyelocele, encephalocele.

ORTHOPEDIC: Cutaneous syndactyly. Widely spaced symphysis pubis. Clubfeet.

GI/GU: May have umbilical anomaly, anal stenosis or atresia, malrotation of the gut. Genital anomalies include hypospadias, cryptorchidism, bicornuate uterus, vaginal atresia, enlarged clitoris. Renal agenesis or hypoplasia. May have hypoplastic bladder, urethral valves.

MISCELLANEOUS: The syndrome was first described as cryptophthalmos ("hidden eye") in 1872; Fraser's contribution in 1962 was the recognition that the syndrome was also associated with a variety of other malformations. Chiari in the 19th century was the first to note the association of laryngeal atresia and cryptophthalmos.

ANESTHETIC CONSIDERATIONS

Because of stenosis, atresia, or webbing of the larynx or trachea, laryngoscopy and tracheal intubation may be very difficult or impossible. Infants may be asymptomatic but have significant subglottic stenosis (1,4,6). Choanal stenosis or atresia precludes placement of a nasal airway, nasal intubation, or placement of a nasogastric tube. Patients with cardiac defects need perioperative antibiotic prophylaxis as indicated. Patients with renal disease need careful titration of perioperative fluids, and avoidance of or reduced dosages of renally excreted drugs.

Bibliography:
1. Crowe S, Westbrook A, Bourke M, et al. Impossible laryngeal intubation in an infant with Fraser syndrome. *Paediatr Anaesth* 2004;14:276–278.
2. Franks L. Miracle Kid. *New Yorker* 1999;17:68–77.
3. Jagtap SR, Malde AD, Pantvaidya SH. Anaesthetic considerations in a patient with Fraser syndrome. *Anaesthesia* 1995;50:39–41.
4. Saito M, Higuchi A, Kamitani K, et al. Anesthetic management of a patient with a cryptophthalmos syndactyly syndrome and subglottic stenosis [Japanese]. *Masui* 1994;43:415–417.
5. Stevens CA, McClanahan C, Steck A, et al. Pulmonary hyperplasia in the Fraser cryptophthalmos syndrome. *Am J Med Genet* 1994;52:427–431.
6. Rose JB, Kettrick RG. Subglottic stenosis complicating the anaesthetic management of newborn with Fraser syndrome. *Paediatr Anaesth* 1993;3:383–385.

Frasier Syndrome

MIM #: 136680

This autosomal dominant disease is closely related to the Drash syndrome (see earlier), which is associated with Wilms tumor. Frasier syndrome is thought to be due to a somatic mutation in the *WT1* (Wilms tumor) gene. Rather than an abnormal protein, with this mutation there is an abnormal ratio of the two splice isoforms. Despite the defect in the Wilms tumor gene, Wilms tumor is not associated with Frasier syndrome.

GI/GU: Streak gonads, male pseudohermaphroditism. Renal failure. Nephrotic syndrome. Gonadoblastoma.

ANESTHETIC CONSIDERATIONS

Renal function should be evaluated preoperatively. Patients with renal dysfunction need careful titration of perioperative fluids, and avoidance of or reduced dosages of renally excreted drugs. A certain degree of sensitivity is required when speaking with patients (or families of patients) with intersex disorders.

Bibliography:

1. Auber F, Lortat-Jacob S, Sarnacki S, et al. Surgical management and genotype/phenotype correlations in WT1 gene-related diseases (Drash, Frasier syndromes). *J Pediatr Surg* 2003;38:124–129.
2. Barbaux S, Niaudet P, Gubler M, et al. Donor splice-site mutations in WT1 are responsible for Frasier syndrome. *Nat Genet* 1997;17:467–470.

Freeman-Sheldon Syndrome

See Whistling face syndrome

Friedreich Ataxia

MIM #: 229300

This autosomal recessive syndrome is characterized by neurologic degeneration with ataxia and cardiomegaly. The mean age at onset of symptoms is 15 years, but can be as early as 2 years and as late as 50 years, with clumsiness or gait instability. The degree of cardiac involvement does not necessarily mirror the degree of neurologic involvement. This syndrome is due to a mutation in the gene *FRDA*, encoding frataxin, a protein whose function is unknown. The disorder is due to a variable number of repeats of the triplet GAA in the gene. The age at onset, the severity of the disease and the risk of nonneurologic involvement are inversely related to the number of GAA triplets. An additional locus has been mapped to 9p. There is loss of the large sensory neurons of the dorsal root ganglia, and loss of peripheral branches with loss of large myelinated fibers. There is degeneration of the posterior columns.

HEENT/AIRWAY: Retinal pigmentation. Optic atrophy later in life. Fixation instability. May have nystagmus. Can develop sensorineural hearing loss later in life.

CHEST: Severe kyphoscoliosis may result in decreased pulmonary function.

CARDIOVASCULAR: Cardiomyopathy is eventually present in almost all patients, although it may remain asymptomatic in a few. There is symmetric, concentric hypertrophy. A small proportion of patients may have cardiac findings similar to hypertrophic cardiomyopathy, with asymmetric hypertrophy. The severity of the left ventricular hypertrophy is related to the number of repeats of the sequence GAA in the frataxin gene. Patients are at risk of sudden death and may have had placement of an implanted cardioverter-defibrillator.

NEUROMUSCULAR: There is degeneration of the corticospinal and spinocerebellar tracts most prominently, but also of the dorsal columns, pyramidal tracts, and, to a lesser extent, the cerebellum and medulla, so that sensory loss and lack of position and vibration sense are cardinal features. Ataxia, particularly of the legs. Dysarthria. Intention tremor. Skeletal muscle weakness. Diminished or absent deep tendon reflexes. Babinski sign.

ORTHOPEDIC: Kyphoscoliosis. Pes cavus.

OTHER: Diabetes mellitus has been reported in some patients, and some other patients have been reported to be carbohydrate intolerant.

MISCELLANEOUS: Nikolaus Friedreich succeeded Virchow to the Chair of Pathologic Anatomy at Wurzburg. Nucleic acid base triplet repeats are also apparently the etiology of other diseases, including fragile X syndrome, spinocerebellar ataxia type I, and Joseph disease. Frataxin bears homology with gram negative, but not gram positive bacteria, and may be a mitochondrial gene originally derived from protomitochondrial bacteria, which then shifted to the nucleus.

ANESTHETIC CONSIDERATIONS

Hyperkalemia has been reported after the use of succinylcholine. Atracurium, *d*-tubocurarine and rocuronium have been used successfully (1, 3, 8) with normal responses in terms of onset time and duration, although with typical interpatient variability. Most patients have some degree of cardiomyopathy. Severe kyphoscoliosis may result in decreased pulmonary function. Spinal and regional anesthesia have been used successfully, although they may be more difficult with scoliosis (6).

Bibliography:

1. Schmitt HJ, Wick S, Münster. Rocuronium for muscle relaxation in two children with Friedreich's ataxia. *Br J Anaesth* 2004;92:592–596.
2. Delatycki MB, Williamson R, Forrest SM. Friedreich ataxia: an overview. *J Med Genet* 2000;37:1–8.
3. Mouloudi H, Katsanoulas C, Frantzeskos G. Requirements for muscle relaxation in Friedreichs ataxia. *Anaesthesia* 1998;53:177–180.

4. Durr A, Cossee M, Agid Y, et al. Clinical and genetic abnormalities in patients with Friedreich's ataxia. *N Engl J Med* 1996;335:1169–1175.
5. Rosenberg RN. DNA-triplet-repeats and neurologic disease. *N Engl J Med* 1996;335:1222–1224.
6. Kubal K, Pasricha SK, Bhargava M. Spinal anesthesia in a patient with Friedreich's ataxia. *Anesth Analg* 1991;72:257–258.
7. Campbell AM, Finley GA. Anaesthesia for a patient with Friedreich's ataxia and cardiomyopathy. *Can J Anaesth* 1989;36:89–93.
8. Bell CF, Kelly JM, Jones RE. Anesthesia for Friedreich's ataxia. *Anaesthesia* 1986;41:296–301.

Frontometaphyseal Dysplasia

SYNONYM: Gorlin-Cohen syndrome

MIM #: 305620

This X-linked recessive disorder results in abnormalities in multiple organ systems. It is due to mutations in the gene *FLNA*, which encodes filamin A. Filamin A crosslinks actin filaments and aids in anchoring membrane proteins. The most common features are prominent supraorbital ridges, metaphyseal dysplasia, progressive joint contractures, and restricted joint mobility. Boys are more severely affected than girls.

HEENT/AIRWAY: Frontal hyperostosis leading to prominent supraorbital ridges. Wide nasal bridge. Incomplete sinus development. Hypertelorism. Down-slanting palpebral fissures. Conductive and sensorineural hearing loss. Long, thick philtrum. High-arched palate. Missing permanent teeth, retained deciduous teeth. Hypoplasia of the mandibular ramus. Small, pointed chin. May have subglottic stenosis, tracheal web. May have tracheoesophageal fistula.

CHEST: Thoracic scoliosis and rib cage deformities may lead to restrictive lung disease. Malformation of the bronchial tree can result in respiratory compromise.

CARDIOVASCULAR: May have primary pulmonary hypertension. May have right bundle branch block. May have mitral valve prolapse.

NEUROMUSCULAR: Cervical vertebral anomalies or fusion. Wide foramen magnum. Anteriorly placed odontoid. May have mental retardation. Wasting of muscles in arms and legs, especially hypothenar and interosseous muscles of the hands.

ORTHOPEDIC: Metaphyseal dysplasia. Progressive joint contractures (fingers, wrists, elbows, knees, and ankles), and restricted joint mobility. Arachnodactyly. Winged scapula. Flared pelvis. Thoracic scoliosis.

GI/GU: Obstructive uropathy. Cryptorchidism.

OTHER: Hirsutism of buttocks and thighs.

ANESTHETIC CONSIDERATIONS

Facial anomalies may make direct laryngoscopy and tracheal intubation difficult. A smaller endotracheal tube may be necessary if the patient has subglottic stenosis. Patients may have a history of recurrent respiratory tract infections or chronic lung disease, and are at risk for postoperative pulmonary complications. Dental abnormalities (especially missing teeth) should be documented preoperatively. Patients must be carefully positioned secondary to the presence of contractures.

Bibliography:
1. Franceschini P, Guala A, Licata D, et al. Esophageal atresia with distal tracheoesophageal fistula in a patient with fronto-metaphyseal dysplasia. *Am J Med Genet* 1997;73:10–14.
2. Mehta Y, Schou H. The anaesthetic management of an infant with frontometaphyseal dysplasia (Gorlin-Cohen syndrome). *Acta Anaesthesiol Scand* 1988;32:505–507.
3. Fitzsimmons JS, Fitzsimmons EM, Barrow M, et al. Frontometaphyseal dysplasia: further delineation of the clinical syndrome. *Clin Genet* 1982; 22:195–205.

Frontonasal Dysplasia Sequence

See Median cleft face syndrome

Fructokinase Deficiency

See Essential fructosuria

Fructose-1,6-Diphosphatase Deficiency (Fructose-1,6-Biphosphatase Deficiency)

MIM #: 229700

This autosomal recessive disorder is due to mutations in the gene encoding fructose-1,6-diphosphatase. This enzyme is one of four rate-limiting enzymes of hepatic gluconeogenesis. In this autosomal recessive disorder, the liver is unable to convert fructose, lactate, glycerol, or amino acids into glucose. Onset of symptoms with episodic metabolic acidosis and hypoglycemia is often in the first year of life. Half of affected children have their first episode within the first 4 days of life. Later, episodes are often triggered by fasting or febrile illnesses. Episodes have caused apnea and cardiac arrest.

CHEST: Hyperventilation will often be the first sign of metabolic acidosis in infants.

NEUROMUSCULAR: Normal intelligence. Hypotonia. Episodes can be signaled by trembling, lethargy, and coma. May have hypoglycemic seizures.

GI/GU: Hepatomegaly with fatty changes in the liver.

OTHER: Failure to thrive. Recurrent episodes of hypoglycemia and metabolic ketoacidosis precipitated by stress, infection, the ingestion of fructose or sucrose, or prolonged fasting. Severe lactic acidosis can develop during an acute episode. A glucose-insulin infusion may be needed during severe episodes. Episodes of hypoglycemia and metabolic ketoacidosis occur more rarely as the patient ages. Ketonuria. Tolerance of fasting also improves with age. Prolonged thrombin time with decreased factor VII has been reported, which normalized with infusion of glucose.

MISCELLANEOUS: Unlike patients with hereditary fructose intolerance (see later), these patients do not have an aversion to fructose-containing foods. Glycerol can also cause a response similar to a load of fructose.

ANESTHETIC CONSIDERATIONS

Fructose should already have been eliminated from the diet. It is important to avoid any oral premedicant syrup that contains fructose. Patients also have a reduced tolerance to sorbitol, which can also be found in oral medications. Postoperatively, sucrose should be avoided (sucrose is a disaccharide of glucose and fructose). Preoperative fasting should be minimized because of the risk of hypoglycemia and metabolic ketoacidosis. Intravenous glucose should be provided perioperatively, and the amount of glucose needed may exceed normal maintenance requirements. Blood glucose levels should be monitored perioperatively. Persistent lactic acidemia indicates that glucose needs are not being met.

Glycerol is sometimes used to treat cerebral edema. In some countries glycerol preparations are prepared with 5% fructose and their use in these patients has been associated with worsening cerebral edema.

FIGURE: See **Appendix E**

Bibliography:
1. van den Berghe G. Disorders of gluconeogenesis. *J Inherit Metab Dis* 1996;19:470–477.
2. Hashimoto Y, Watanabe H, Satou M. Anesthetic management of a patient with hereditary fructose-1,6-diphosphatase deficiency. *Anesth Analg* 1978;57:503–506.

Fructose-1-Phosphate Aldolase B Deficiency

See Hereditary fructose intolerance

Fructosuria

See Essential fructosuria

Fryns Syndrome

MIM #: 229850

This autosomal recessive syndrome has as its main features diaphragmatic defects, lung hypoplasia, cleft lip or palate, distal limb abnormalities, and genital anomalies. Most patients are stillborn or die in early infancy. The responsible gene and gene product are not known.

HEENT/AIRWAY: Coarse facies. Optic anomalies. Malformed ears. Olfactory anomalies. Broad, flat nasal bridge, anteverted nares. Large mouth. Cleft lip or palate. Retrognathia. Micrognathia.

CHEST: Congenital diaphragmatic defects (usually hernia). Lung hypoplasia. Can have broad clavicles.

CARDIOVASCULAR: Ventricular septal defects, aortic arch anomalies.

NEUROMUSCULAR: Severe mental retardation. Myoclonus. May have Dandy-Walker malformation, hydrocephalus, agenesis of the corpus callosum, arhinencephaly.

ORTHOPEDIC: Distal limb abnormalities including digital hypoplasia and nail dysplasia. Camptodactyly.

GI/GU: Delayed gastric emptying. May have omphalocele, malrotation of the gut, pyloric stenosis, duodenal atresia, anteriorly placed or imperforate anus. Genital anomalies include cryptorchidism, hypospadias, bifid scrotum, uterine and cervical atresia, bicornuate uterus, duplicated vagina. Renal dysplasia. Ureteral dilation.

ANESTHETIC CONSIDERATIONS

Most patients exhibit severe respiratory distress at birth secondary to diaphragmatic hernia or lung hypoplasia. Microretrognathia may make direct laryngoscopy and intubation difficult. Patients have delayed gastric emptying and are at risk for perioperative aspiration. Significant renal disease has implications for perioperative fluid management and the choice of anesthetic drugs. Patients with hydrocephalus may warrant precautions for increased intracranial pressure, although this may not necessarily be so for young infants with open sutures. Patients with cardiac defects need perioperative antibiotic prophylaxis as indicated.

Bibliography:
1. Slavotinek AM. Fryns syndrome: a review of the phenotype and diagnostic guidelines. *Am J Med Genet A* 2004;124:427–433.
2. Van Hove JL, Spiridigliozzi GA, Heinz R, et al. Fryns syndrome survivors and neurologic outcome. *Am J Med Genet* 1995;59:334–340.
3. Cunniff C, Jones KL, Saal HM, et al. Fryns syndrome: an autosomal recessive disorder associated with craniofacial anomalies, diaphragmatic hernia and distal digital hypoplasia. *Pediatrics* 1990;85:499–504.

G

G Syndrome

See Hypertelorism-hypospadias syndrome

G6PD Deficiency

See Glucose-6-phosphate dehydrogenase deficiency

Galactocerebrosidase Deficiency

See Krabbe disease

Galactokinase Deficiency

MIM #: 230200

This autosomal recessive disorder is due to an abnormality in the enzyme galactokinase. Galactokinase converts galactose to galactose-1-phosphate in the pathway that ultimately converts galactose to glucose. This enzyme deficiency is occasionally included in the term "galactosemia" (see later). Galactose is in the diet as lactose, a disaccharide of glucose and galactose. Nuclear cataracts are the only consistent clinical finding. The cataracts are thought to be due to a reduction of galactose to galactitol.

HEENT/AIRWAY: Nuclear cataracts. Neonatal diagnosis and removal of dietary galactose can result in clearing of cataracts.

NEUROMUSCULAR: Pseudotumor cerebri has been reported.

GI/GU: Neonatal jaundice.

OTHER: Elevated blood galactose. Galactosuria.

MISCELLANEOUS: Gitzelmann in 1965 was the first to identify a patient with galactokinase deficiency. The patient was 44 years of age, and had a history of galactosuria after the ingestion of milk. Galactosuria had been identified in the patient 33 years earlier when he required treatment for cataracts. At that time, Fanconi had called his condition "galactose diabetes." At age 44 the patient was drinking 3 quarts of milk a day, and was healthy other than for his blindness.

The ability to make a diagnosis of this disorder easily in the early period after birth has been diminished in our modern times because of the substitution of urine glucose test strips that test specifically for glucose (by glucose oxidase) rather than for reducing substances in general (which include galactose). Urine and blood tests will be positive in the newborn only after feedings are well established, and early discharge of the newborn from the nursery means that the samples for the purpose are not readily available.

ANESTHETIC CONSIDERATIONS

There are no specific anesthetic concerns other than consideration of possible vision loss.

Bibliography:

1. Bosch AM, Bakker HD, van Gennip AH, et al. Clinical features of galactokinase deficiency: a review of the literature. *J Inherit Metab Dis* 2002;25:629–634.

Galactose-1-Phosphate Uridyltransferase Deficiency

See Galactosemia

Galactosemia

SYNONYM: Galactose-1-phosphate uridyltransferase deficiency

MIM #: 230400

This autosomal recessive disorder is caused by a deficiency in galactose-1-phosphate uridyltransferase, one of the three enzymes that catalyze the conversion of dietary galactose to glucose. Galactose-1-phosphate uridyltransferase catalyzes the conversion of galactose-1-phosphate (formed by galactokinase) and uridine diphosphate glucose (UDP-glucose) into UDP-galactose and glucose-1-phosphate. Excess galactose-1-phosphate is presumably a substance that is toxic to a wide variety of tissues. Severe disease can present in the first weeks of life with poor feeding, weight loss, vomiting, diarrhea, lethargy, and hypotonia. Partial activity of the galactose-1-phosphate uridyltransferase enzyme leads to milder clinical manifestations of the syndrome. Two other enzyme deficiencies result in elevated blood galactose, but they have distinct clinical presentations (see galactokinase deficiency, earlier; and uridine diphosphate galactose epimerase deficiency, later). These two other enzyme deficiencies are occasionally generically referred to as "galactosemia."

HEENT/AIRWAY: Neonatal cataracts. Retinal and vitreous hemorrhage has been reported, presumably on the basis of coagulopathy from hepatic failure.

NEUROMUSCULAR: Mental retardation, even with appropriate dietary restriction and resolution of acute symptoms.

GI/GU: Vomiting or diarrhea. Hepatomegaly or acute hepatic failure in the neonatal period, progressing to periportal fibrosis, cirrhosis and decreased hepatic function. Ascites as a preterminal finding. Renal tubular acidosis, albuminuria and aminoaciduria. Ovarian failure.

OTHER: Failure to thrive. Bleeding diathesis, some patients may have hemolysis. Susceptibility to *Escherichia coli* sepsis as a neonate if untreated. Hypergonadotropic hypogonadism with gonadal failure in females.

MISCELLANEOUS: In most states, neonates are routinely screened for galactosemia. Abnormal urine levels of galactose are not identified by current urine test strips because they use glucose oxidase, which is specific for glucose. Older tablet techniques identified all reducing sugars, including galactose. Interestingly, the diagnosis of galactosemia, particularly of variants with partial activity and false-positive diagnoses, increases during the summer months. This is presumably due to the degradation of enzyme activity in the blood samples in hot mailrooms and delivery trucks.

ANESTHETIC CONSIDERATIONS

Recall that patients may have impaired vision. Neonates may have a significant bleeding diathesis. Hepatic dysfunction may affect the binding or the metabolism of some anesthetic drugs. Significant albuminuria may make urine output a poor indicator of intravascular volume.

Bibliography:
1. Segal S. Galactosemia unsolved. *Eur J Pediatr* 1995;154:S97–S102.
2. Holton JB, de la Cruz F, Levy HL. Galactosemia: the uridine diphosphate galactose deficiency- uridine treatment controversy. *J Pediatr* 1993;123:1009–1014.
3. Holton JB. Galactose disorders: an overview. *J lnherit Metab Dis* 1990;13:476–486.

Galactosialidosis

MIM #: 256540

This autosomal recessive lysosomal storage disease is due to mutations in the gene encoding cathepsin A. This protein is a serine protease which protects beta-galactosidase (the cause of GM_1 gangliosidosis, see later) and alpha-neuraminidase from intralysosomal proteolysis. This results in the accumulation of lysosomal polysaccharide. Three types of disease have been described—early infantile, the most severe form, which is associated with early death (average age of death is 7 months), late juvenile, and juvenile/adult, which are slowly progressive. Children with the late juvenile type tend to have milder neurologic but more severe cardiac disease, have growth retardation, and do not die young. Most juvenile/adult patients are Japanese.

HEENT/AIRWAY: Coarse, "gargoyle" facies. Conjunctival telangiectasis. Corneal clouding, macular cherry-red spot. Conductive hearing loss. Macroglossia. Small mouth opening, malocclusion.

CHEST: Barrel chest.

CARDIOVASCULAR: Thickened mitral and aortic valves with stenosis and/or insufficiency. Cardiomyopathy.

NEUROMUSCULAR: Cervical spine instability, atlantoaxial instability. Mental retardation, seizures.

ORTHOPEDIC: Skeletal dysplasias and dysostosis. Short stature.

GI/GU: May have hepatosplenomegaly.

OTHER: Widespread angiokeratomas, particularly in juvenile/adult type. In the extreme it can cause hydrops fetalis. Can develop hemophagocytosis.

ANESTHETIC CONSIDERATIONS

Macroglossia, combined with cervical spine instability can make laryngoscopy and tracheal intubation difficult. The difficulty is likely to worsen with aging, as with other lysosomal storage disorders, in which laryngoscopy and intubation can be exceedingly difficult. The laryngeal mask airway (LMA) has been used successfully in patients with other lysosomal storage diseases. Nasal fiberoptic intubation has been used successfully, but with difficulty (1). Cardiac status should be evaluated preoperatively, and patients with valve disease will require perioperative antibiotic prophylaxis as indicated.

Bibliography:
1. Friedhoff RJ, Rose SH, Brown MJ, et al. Galactosialidosis: a unique disease with significant clinical implications during perioperative anesthesia management. *Anesth Analg* 2003;97:53–55.
2. Bursi F, Osranek M, Seward JB, et al. Mitral and aortic valve thickening associated with galactosialidosis: echocardiographic features of a lysosomal storage disease. *Echocardiography* 2003;20:605–606.
3. Kleijer WJ, Geilen GC, Janse HC, et al. Cathepsin a deficiency in galactosialidosis: studies of patients and carriers in 16 families. *Pediatr Res* 1996;39:1067–1071.

Gardner Syndrome

SYNONYM: Familial adenomatous polyposis

MIM #: 175100

This autosomal dominant disorder involves extensive adenomatous polyposis of the colon and upper gastrointestinal tract. The responsible gene, called the *APC* gene, has been mapped to the long arm of chromosome 5. The gene product has not yet been identified. This disorder is accompanied by a high incidence of colorectal cancer, but a variety of other malignancies can also occur. Individually, polyps are indistinguishable from those that appear in the general population, and are no more likely to become cancerous. However, their massive number almost guarantees that some will. In the past, Gardner syndrome specifically referred to patients with extracolonic manifestations, but "Gardner syndrome" and "familial adenomatous polyposis" are now considered synonyms.

HEENT/AIRWAY: Skull osteomas, with overlying fibromas of the skin. Pigmented retinal lesions (congenital hypertrophy of retinal pigment) which can rarely become malignant. Jaw cysts, mandibular osteomas, dental abnormalities.

NEUROMUSCULAR: Central nervous system cancers.

ORTHOPEDIC: Osteosarcoma.

GI/GU: Extensive adenomatous polyposis, primarily of the colon, but also of the upper gastrointestinal tract, including gastric and duodenal polyposis. The incidence of gastric carcinoma is higher in Japan. Malignant transformation of the polyps leads to colorectal carcinoma, periampullary carcinoma, bile duct carcinoma, and hepatoblastoma. There is a high incidence of colorectal cancer in early adult life. Mesenteric fibromatosis (desmoid tumors) can occur after surgery. Adrenal carcinoma.

OTHER: Thyroid carcinoma. Sebaceous and epidermoid cysts of skin, particularly on the back.

MISCELLANEOUS: Eldon Gardner made major contributions in *Drosophila* genetics.

ANESTHETIC CONSIDERATIONS
Prophylactic colectomy may be indicated. Because of the incidence of mandibular and dental anomalies, dentition should be carefully assessed preoperatively. Nonsteroidal anti-inflammatory drugs have been shown to suppress the development of adenomatous polyps and can cause regression of existing polyps, so patients may be put on one of these drugs, including aspirin.

Bibliography:

1. Foulkes WD. A tale of four syndromes: familial adenomatous polyposis, Gardner syndrome, attenuated APC and Turcot syndrome. *Q J Med* 1995;88:853–863.
2. Harned RK, Buck JL, Olmsted WW, et al. Extracolonic manifestations of the familial adenomatous polyposis syndromes. *AJR Am J Roentgenol* 1991;156:481–485.

Gaucher Disease

SYNONYM: Glucosyl cerebroside lipidosis; Glucocerebrosidase deficiency

MIM #: 230800

This most common of the lysosomal storage diseases is an autosomal recessive defect of the lysosomal enzyme beta-glucosidase with consequent glycolipid (glucosylceramide) storage. The major features are hematologic abnormalities, hypersplenism, and bone lesions. Three subgroups have been described in the past (infantile, juvenile, and adult types), but symptoms can begin in infancy in all three. There is great interpatient variability. Death is usually by 1 year of age in the infantile type. Life expectancy is normal in those with the adult form who are mildly affected. The juvenile group is more varied. The current nosology is to categorize the disease as types 1, 2, and 3. The most common type is the nonneuropathic type 1, formerly classified as the adult type. Type 2, similar to the infantile form, has infantile onset and severe neurologic findings. Type 3, similar to the juvenile form, is also nonneuropathic, but signs usually begin later in the first decade and progress more slowly than in type 1.

The characteristic Gaucher cells are found in the marrow and in reticuloendothelial cells. These are large, lipid-laden histiocytes whose appearance has been likened to wrinkled

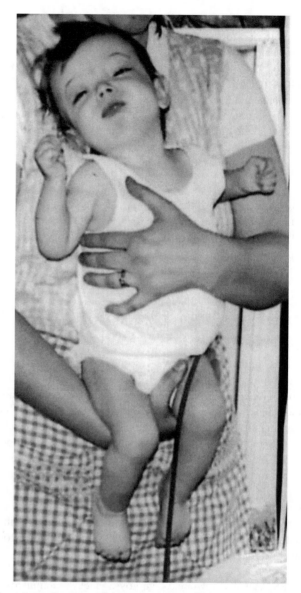

Gaucher disease. This young boy with Gaucher disease died shortly after this photo was taken. Note retroflexion and hypertonia.

tissue paper. Treatment with alglucerase (Ceredase), a mannose-substituted enzyme replacement, is available.

HEENT/AIRWAY: Strabismus and trismus in type 2. Pingueculae can occur with greater frequency, but are not collections of Gaucher cells. Can have accumulation of brown Gaucher cells at corneoscleral limbus.

CHEST: Pulmonary infiltration can lead to pulmonary hypertension and cor pulmonale. May develop right to left intrapulmonary shunting as a consequence of hepatic disease. Treatment with alglucerase can be associated with pulmonary arterial hypertension in a small percentage of patients. Bronchoscopy with bronchial washing may show typical Gaucher cells in the aspirate. A small number of patients may have pulmonary disease with hypoxia. Kyphoscoliosis may cause restrictive lung disease.

CARDIOVASCULAR: Cardiac involvement is rare, and occurs particularly in a subtype of type 3, which has a specific mutation. Calcification of the aortic and mitral valves and the ascending aorta has been reported.

NEUROMUSCULAR: Absent in type 1 disease. Cranial nerve involvement, myoclonic jerks, seizures, and apnea in the infantile type. Patients with types 2 and 3 may have trismus and opisthotonos.

ORTHOPEDIC: Decreased bone density of long bones and vertebrae, with risk of pathologic fractures. Vertebral collapse causing kyphoscoliosis. Avascular necrosis of the femoral head. Erlenmeyer flask deformity of distal femur. Episodic painful bony crises in some, which can be associated with fever. Osteolytic lesions can follow within months of splenectomy, suggesting that only partial splenectomies should be done.

GI/GU: Cranial nerve involvement can cause swallowing difficulties. Hepatomegaly can be profound, with normal hepatic function (until late). Portal hypertension with secondary hepatic failure is rare. Splenic infarcts accompanied by pain. Splenomegaly, hypersplenism, which may require splenectomy. Renal involvement is rare.

OTHER: Anemia and thrombocytopenia from hypersplenism. In addition to thrombocytopenia, platelet dysfunction may occur. Anemia can also occur from marrow infiltration by storage material. Enlargement of lymphoid tissue, including lymph nodes, thymus, Peyer patches, and tonsils. There can be a yellow-brown pigmentation over the face or lower legs. A variety of lymphoid and bone tumors have been described.

MISCELLANEOUS: Gaucher, a French dermatologist and venereologist, entered medicine when he failed the university entrance examinations to study natural sciences. He described this particular type of hypersplenism in his doctoral thesis in 1882. One of his more interesting papers (on Salvarsan, an arsenic compound previously used to treat syphilis) was titled "606 or the German Poison."

It has been suggested that heterozygosity for the glucocerebrosidase gene may predispose to the development of Parkinson disease.

ANESTHETIC CONSIDERATIONS

Both lymphoid hyperplasia and trismus have been reported anecdotally to complicate airway management. Trismus and opisthotonos resolve with muscle relaxants. Patients with a history of difficult intubation may become more difficult to intubate with age. Many patients require an endotracheal tube that is smaller than that predicted by age. Patients with

swallowing difficulties are at risk for aspiration, and a rapid sequence induction is recommended. Patients should be evaluated preoperatively for anemia and thrombocytopenia, and may need to be transfused before surgery. Patients with otherwise mild disease may have a bleeding dyscrasia and unexpected perioperative bleeding. Spinal anesthesia has been used successfully (3), but bleeding dyscrasias need to be excluded.

Bibliography:
1. Ioscovich A, Briskin A, Abrahamov A, et al. Uncomplicated outcome after anesthesia for pediatric patients with Gaucher disease. *Can J Anaesth* 2005;52:845–847.
2. Grabowski GA. Gaucher disease: lessons from a decade of therapy. *J Pediatr* 2004;144(5 Suppl):S15–S19.
3. García Collada JC, Pereda Marín RM, Garrote Martínez AI, et al. Subarachnoid anesthesia in a patient with type I Gaucher disease. *Acta Anaesthesiol Scand* 2003;47:106–109.
4. Tobias JD, Atwood RA, Lowe S, et al. Anesthetic considerations in the child with Gaucher disease. *J Clin Anesth* 1993;5:150–153.
5. Mahoney A, Soni N, Vellodi A. Anaesthesia and the lipidoses: a review of patients treated by bone marrow transplantation. *Paediatr Anaesth* 1992;2:205–209.
6. Beutler E. Gaucher's disease. *N Engl J Med* 1991;325:1354–1360.
7. Wark H, Gold P, Overton J. The airway of patients with a lipid storage disease. *Anaesth Intensive Care* 1984;12:343–344.

Geleophysic Dysplasia

MIM #: 231050

This autosomal recessive syndrome is distinguished by characteristic facies, short stature, small hands and feet, and progressive cardiac valvular disease. It has been suggested that geleophysic dysplasia is a lysosomal storage disease, based on the finding of lysosomal storage vacuoles in cells from the skin, tracheal mucosa, cartilage, liver, and heart valves. The responsible gene and gene product, however, are not known.

HEENT/AIRWAY: Characteristic "happy-natured" facies: round face, up-slanting palpebral fissures, thickened ears, short nose with anteverted nares, long smooth philtrum, thin inverted vermilion, wide mouth. Gradual coarsening of facial features. High-pitched voice. Tracheal stenosis can develop.

CHEST: Can have stenosis of the mainstem bronchi. Can have pectus excavatum.

CARDIOVASCULAR: Progressive valvular disease (especially aortic and mitral) with valvular thickening and eventual stenosis or incompetence. Cardiomegaly.

NEUROMUSCULAR: Can have developmental delay, seizures.

ORTHOPEDIC: Short stature. Small hands and feet. Progressive contractures of multiple joints, particularly fingers and wrists. Decreased bone density. Coxa valga. Shortened tubular bones.

GI/GU: Hepatomegaly.

OTHER: Thick skin. Small nails.

MISCELLANEOUS: *Geleos,* meaning "happy," and *physis,* meaning "nature" are combined to describe this syndrome that includes characteristic "happy-natured" facies.

ANESTHETIC CONSIDERATIONS

Tracheal stenosis can be progressive and lead to critical airway narrowing. A smaller-than-expected endotracheal tube invariably is needed. Cardiac valvular disease is progressive, and often causes death secondary to heart failure in early childhood. Patients need appropriate perioperative antibiotic prophylaxis. Joint contractures may make proper positioning difficult.

Bibliography:

1. Santolaya JM, Groninga LC, Delgado A, et al. Patients with geleophysic dysplasia are not always geleophysic. *Am J Med Genet* 1997;72:85–90.
2. Pontz BF, Stoss H, Henschke F, et al. Clinical and ultrastructural findings in three patients with geleophysic dysplasia. *Am J Med Genet* 1996;63:50–54.

Gilbert Disease

MIM #: 143500

This autosomal dominant condition leads to chronic mild unconjugated hyperbilirubinemia. Bilirubin levels can rise during periods of intercurrent illness and with fasting, and can be normal at other times. It is due to deficient activity of the microsomal enzyme uridine diphosphate glucuronyltransferase (UDP-glucuronyltransferase), which catalyzes the conversion of unconjugated bilirubin to conjugated bilirubin. The most common abnormalities are mutations in the promoter region of the gene. Patients are usually asymptomatic, but can have mild, nonspecific complaints such as abdominal pain, diarrhea, fatigue, and malaise. Gilbert disease is the most benign of the diseases of hepatic bilirubin metabolism, which also include Crigler-Najjar, Dubin-Johnson, and Rotor syndromes. Crigler-Najjar syndrome (see earlier) is also due to a defect in UDP-glucuronyltransferase, and these two syndromes are likely allelic. Phenobarbital therapy lowers the serum bilirubin. The response to phenobarbital also suggests that the genetic defect is in a control gene rather than a structural gene.

HEENT/AIRWAY: Scleral icterus.

GI/GU: Chronic but often intermittent, low-grade, unconjugated hyperbilirubinemia. Bilirubin levels are usually less than 3 mg/dL. Urobilinogen is absent, and liver function tests and histologic appearance are normal. Patients may complain of vague abdominal discomfort. Neonates may rapidly acquire normal postnatal levels of hyperbilirubinemia.

OTHER: Factors that can increase serum bilirubin levels include stress, intercurrent illness, infection, exercise, fatigue, alcohol ingestion, fasting, and menstruation.

MISCELLANEOUS: Nicolas Gilbert was a French clinical pathologist—hence the soft "G" in "Gilbert." The Bolivian squirrel monkey (but not the Brazilian squirrel monkey) also gets Gilbert disease.

ANESTHETIC CONSIDERATIONS

Stress, such as with surgery, perioperative fasting, intercurrent illness, infection, exercise, or fatigue can increase the serum bilirubin concentration. Elevated fasting bilirubin concentration is rapidly normalized with the administration of oral or intravenous carbohydrate, but not fat. Postoperative unconjugated hyperbilirubinemia can occur, even in a previously asymptomatic patient. Some drugs, the most common being rifampin, cause enzyme inhibition with increased serum bilirubin levels and jaundice. Although sulfonamides, some cephalosporins, and intravenous contrast agents can increase free bilirubin levels by displacing bilirubin from albumin, no currently used anesthetic agents are known to displace bilirubin to a degree that would contraindicate their use. Morphine is metabolized by a different glucuronyltransferase system, and can be used in these patients.

Bibliography:

1. Kaplan MK, Hammerman C, Maisels MJ. Bilirubin genetics for the nongeneticist: hereditary defects of neonatal bilirubin conjugation. *Pediatrics* 2003;111:886–893.
2. Monaghan G, Ryan M, Seddon R, et al. Genetic variation in bilirubin UPD-glucuronosyltransferase gene promoter and Gilbert's syndrome. *Lancet* 1996;347:578–581.
3. Miyakawa H, Matsumoto K, Matsumoto S, et al. Anesthetic and postoperative management of a patient with Gilbert's syndrome and another with Dubin-Johnson syndrome [Japanese]. *Masui* 1991;40:119–123.
4. Taylor S. Gilbert's syndrome as a cause of postoperative jaundice. *Anaesthesia* 1984;39:1222–1224.

Gilles de la Tourette Syndrome

See Tourette syndrome

Gitelman Syndrome

Included in Bartter syndrome

Globoid-Cell Leukodystrophy

See Krabbe disease

Glucocerebrosidase Deficiency

See Gaucher disease

Glucose Phosphate Isomerase Deficiency

SYNONYM: Phosphohexose isomerase deficiency; phosphoglucoisomerase deficiency

MIM #: 172400

This autosomal recessive disease is caused by a deficiency in the enzyme glucose phosphate isomerase. This enzyme catalyzes the interconversion of glucose-6-phosphate and fructose-6-phosphate, the second step of the Embden-Meyerhof glycolytic pathway. Glucose phosphate isomerase deficiency presents as hemolytic anemia.

NEUROMUSCULAR: Mixed cerebellar and sensory ataxia. Muscle weakness.

GI/GU: Gallstones, cholecystitis, splenomegaly.

OTHER: Hemolytic anemia with spontaneous hemolytic crises. Splenectomy may significantly improve hematocrit and transfusion requirements. Impaired granulocytic function.

ANESTHETIC CONSIDERATIONS

The patient's hematocrit should be evaluated preoperatively. Perioperative hypoglycemia is not a concern.

Bibliography:

1. Arnold H. Inherited glucosephosphate isomerase deficiency: a review of known variants and some aspects of the pathomechanism of the deficiency. *Blut* 1979;39:405–417.
2. Paglia DE, Valentine WN. Hereditary glucosephosphate isomerase deficiency: a review. *Am J Clin Pathol* 1974;62:740–751.

Glucose-6-Phosphatase Deficiency

See von Gierke disease

Glucose-6-Phosphate Dehydrogenase Deficiency

SYNONYM: G6PD deficiency

MIM #: 305900

This X-linked enzyme defect can result in hemolysis in response to a variety of drugs or metabolic insults. Glucose-6-phosphate dehydrogenase (G6PD) deficiency is the most common enzymopathy in humans. G6PD is the first step in the hexose monophosphate shunt, and the only source of NADPH (the reduced form of nicotinamide-adenine dinucleotide phosphate [NADP]) in mature red blood cells, which lack the citric acid cycle. There are about 400 known genetic variants of this disease, and there are several different clinical presentations. In an African form (G6PD A-), young red blood cells have normal levels of the enzyme, hence the increased erythrocyte production in response to hemolysis produces more young cells and therefore limits hemolysis. An enzyme assay done at this time may be normal. In the Mediterranean and Asian forms, there is decreased enzyme activity in both young and old red blood cells, and hemolysis continues as long as the triggering agent or condition is present. Occasional rare types present with chronic, rather than episodic, hemolytic anemia. Because of early X chromosome inactivation, female heterozygotes have two populations of red blood cells, either with or without the enzyme. Total enzyme activity in female heterozygotes ranges from normal to that seen in male hemizygotes, and female heterozygotes can have hemolytic attacks.

Hemolysis after exposure to a triggering agent becomes apparent 2 to 3 days after the exposure. Anemia worsens through the seventh day. The hematocrit begins to recover on the eighth day. There is some discrepancy between the small number of drugs clearly shown to be triggers for hemolysis, and the large number of drugs that have been implicated.

Oxidant drugs are problematic because superoxide ions are normally converted by superoxide dismutase to H_2O_2, and subsequently converted by reduced glutathione to water. NADPH is required to convert glutathione back to the reduced state.

GI/GU: Abdominal pain can occur during hemolytic episodes and the spleen may be palpable. Cholelithiasis and cholecystitis. Hemolysis can cause renal failure, which is more common in adults than it is in children. Most episodes of renal failure are transient, if supported by dialysis.

OTHER: Hemolytic episodes can be caused by infection, presumably secondary to the release of peroxides from activated phagocytes and microbial metabolic products. Neonatal hyperbilirubinemia can be severe. Some patients will have a chronic hemolytic anemia which can worsen during periods of oxidative stress.

MISCELLANEOUS: "Favism" refers to hemolysis after ingestion of fava beans. Its effects were noted long ago. Pythagoras is said to have warned against eating fava beans. G6PD-deficient red blood cells appear to provide some protection against malaria in female heterozygotes.

ANESTHETIC CONSIDERATIONS

Drugs known to trigger hemolysis must be avoided (Table 3). Although there have been no reports of complications with the use of a eutectic mixture of local anesthetic (EMLA) cream, prilocaine, which is found in EMLA cream, is a potential trigger of hemolysis.

TABLE 3. *Drugs and other agents that can cause hemolysis in glucose-6-phosphate dehydrogenase deficiency*

Analgesics
Aspirin (only in very high doses; much of the problem with aspirin is probably due to the underlying infection for which the aspirin is taken)
Phenacetin
Prilocaine (possibly—and in high doses only, due to increased methemoglobin production)
Antibiotics
Nitrofurantoin
Nalidixic acid
Sulfonamides
Antimalarials
Chloroquine
Primaquin
Other
Alpha-methyldopa (Aldomet)
Ascorbic acid (in massive doses)
Dimercaprol (BAL) (maybe)
Fava beans
Glyburide (possibly)
Hydralazine
Methylene blue
Mothballs (naphthalene)(maybe)
Nitrates
Nitroprusside (possibly because of increased methemoglobin production)
Probenecid (maybe)
Vitamin K (water-soluble analogs)
In mediterranean form only
Chloramphenicol
Quinine
Quinidine

BAL, British anti-Lewisite

Bibliography:
1. Maddali MM, Fahr J. Postoperative methemoglobinemia with associated G-6-P-D deficiency in infant cardiac surgery-enigmas in diagnosis and management. *Paediatr Anaesth* 2005;15:334–337.
2. Mehta AB. Glucose-6-phosphate dehydrogenase deficiency. *Postgrad Med J* 1994;70:871–877.
3. Beutler E. Glucose-6-phosphate dehydrogenase deficiency. *N Engl J Med* 1991;324:169–174.
4. Smith CL, Snowdon SL. Anaesthesia and glucose-6-phosphate dehydrogenase deficiency. *Anaesthesia* 1987;42:281–288.

Glucosyl Cerebroside Lipidosis

See Gaucher disease

Glutaric Acidemia Type I (Glutaric Aciduria Type I)

SYNONYM: Glutaryl-CoA dehydrogenase deficiency

MIM #: 231670

This enzyme deficiency results primarily in chronic neurologic deterioration, although there may be metabolic abnormalities during episodes of acute clinical deterioration. It is marked by neuronal loss in the basal ganglia. The enzyme for this autosomal recessive disease catalyzes the conversion of glutaryl-CoA to glutaconyl CoA, and glutaconyl-CoA to crotonyl-CoA, which are intermediates in the eventual metabolism of lysine to acetyl-CoA. The defect affects the degradation of lysine, hydroxylysine, and tryptophan, and the accumulated glutaryl-CoA is esterified with carnitine, which can lead to a severe secondary carnitine deficiency. This enzyme resides in the mitochondria, and it is distinct from glutaric aciduria type II (see later). Treatment is with a protein limited diet, carnitine and riboflavin, a cofactor of the enzyme.

HEENT/AIRWAY: Megalencephaly, often at birth. Opisthotonos.

NEUROMUSCULAR: Rare patients are normal. Extrapyramidal signs (dystonia, choreoathetosis). Eventual spastic quadriparesis. Progressive atrophic signs on brain imaging, particularly of the caudate and putamen. Can have hydrocephalus or arachnoid cysts. Patients may have an acute encephalopathic crisis with intercurrent infection. With recovery, there is a loss of developmental milestones. The etiology of acute crises is unknown. Intellectual function is preserved until late in the course of the disease. Can be associated with acute and chronic subdural hematoma.

GI/GU: Vomiting and hepatomegaly with acute crises. Microvesicular fatty infiltration of the liver and kidney.

OTHER: Metabolic findings are minimal, and are often related to the secondary carnitine deficiency. Can have acute metabolic crises during intercurrent illness, with severe hypoglycemia, ketosis and metabolic acidosis, which can progress to an encephalopathic Reye-like syndrome. Patients respond to glucose, carnitine, and bicarbonate. Association with subdural hematomas makes false allegations of child abuse possible.

ANESTHETIC CONSIDERATIONS

Despite significant neurologic dysfunction that suggests otherwise, children maintain normal intellectual function until late in the disease. Patients can have difficulty swallowing, and are at increased risk for perioperative aspiration. Adequate levels of serum glucose must be ensured perioperatively. Phenothiazines, butyrophenones, and other dopaminergic blockers can exacerbate movement disorders. Metoclopramide can cause extrapyramidal effects, and is best avoided. Ondansetron should be safe as an antiemetic because it does not have antidopaminergic effects. Involuntary movements may be aggravated by valproic acid. Baclofen reduces involuntary movements.

The cysts, subdural fluid collections and hydrocephalus may reflect atrophic brain changes, and a decompressive neurosurgical procedure might worsen the condition. Thus, neurosurgical intervention is undertaken only when there is evidence of raised intracranial pressure.

Bibliography:

1. Hernández-Palazó J, Sánchez-Ródenas L, Martínez-Lage JF. Anesthetic management in two siblings with glutaric aciduria type 1. *Paediatr Anaesth* 2006;16:188–191.
2. Hartley LM, Khwaja OS, Verity CM. Glutaric acidemia type 1 and nonaccidental head injury. *Pediatrics* 2001;107:174–176.
3. Haworth JC, Booth FA, Chudley AE, et al. Phenotypic variability in glutaric aciduria type I: report of fourteen cases in five Canadian Indian kindreds. *J Pediatr* 1991;118:52–58.

Glutaric Aciduria Type II

SYNONYM: Multiple acyl-CoA dehydrogenase deficiency (MADD); Acyl-CoA dehydrogenase deficiency. (Includes Electron transfer flavoprotein (ETF) deficiency; Electron transfer flavoprotein: ubiquinone oxidoreductase (ETF–QO) deficiency)

MIM #: 231680

This disorder differs from glutaric acidemia type I (glutaric aciduria type I) in that in type II, multiple acyl-CoA dehydrogenase deficiencies result in the excretion of a variety of organic acids in addition to glutaric acid. There are several autosomal recessive abnormalities that involve diminished activity of one or more of the acyl-CoA dehydrogenases involved in the transfer of electrons from acyl-CoA dehydrogenase to coenzyme Q in the mitochondrial electron transport chain. These abnormalities result in inhibition of mitochondrial oxidation of fatty acids and some amino acids. Acyl-CoA dehydrogenases are integral to fatty acid oxidation. After mobilization from adipose tissue, fatty acids are taken up by the liver and other tissues, and converted to acyl-CoA esters in the cytoplasm. These enter mitochondria as carnitine esters, and then become reesterified as acyl-CoA esters. Beta oxidation results in the liberation of electrons that are transferred to electron transfer flavoprotein (ETF). As beta oxidation proceeds, the acyl chain is gradually shortened, and this first step in the oxidation process is catalyzed by acyl-CoA dehydrogenases with differing, but overlapping, chain length specificities. There are very-long-chain, long-chain, medium-chain, and short-chain acyl-CoA dehydrogenases. The clinical presentation is variable. Some infants die as neonates, whereas others eventually succumb to cardiac disease. In some, episodes of a Reye-like syndrome develop.

Three clinical phenotypes have been described, which are consistent within families. They are neonatal onset without congenital anomalies, neonatal onset with congenital anomalies, and mild and/or later onset. Infants with congenital anomalies often die on the first day of life.

This disorder can also be caused by abnormalities of the alpha or beta subunit of **electron transfer flavoprotein (ETF)** or by **electron transfer flavoprotein: ubiquinone oxidoreductase (ETF-QO) deficiency.** These proteins carry the electrons generated by a variety of dehydrogenases into the mitochondria and the main electron transport chain.

Treatment with riboflavin has been used in some patients with some success.

HEENT/AIRWAY: Macrocephaly, high forehead, large anterior fontanelle, hypoplastic midface. Hypertelorism, congenital cataracts. Low-set and malformed ears. Flat nasal bridge.

CHEST: Neonatal respiratory distress. Pulmonary hypoplasia with ETF deficiency.

CARDIOVASCULAR: Fatty degeneration of the myocardium. Severe hypertrophic cardiomyopathy can be fatal.

NEUROMUSCULAR: Hypotonia, muscle weakness. Pachygyria, cerebral gliosis.

ORTHOPEDIC: Rocker-bottom feet.

GI/GU: Nausea and vomiting. Abdominal wall defects. Fatty infiltration of the liver with hepatomegaly. Fatty degeneration of the renal tubular epithelium with proximal tubule damage resulting in glycosuria and generalized aminoaciduria. Polycystic kidneys, renal dysplasia. Kidneys can be palpable in affected neonates. External genital anomalies.

OTHER: Nonketotic hypoglycemia, hyperammonemia, hyperuricemia. Neonatal presentation is associated with profound hypoglycemia and metabolic acidosis, and delivery is often premature. Metabolic acidosis associated with an odor of sweaty feet and stale breath.

MISCELLANEOUS: A similar range of organic acids is excreted in the urine in Jamaican vomiting sickness, which is caused by the ingestion of unripe akee. The toxin hypoglycin in unripe akee inhibits several acyl-CoA dehydrogenases.

ANESTHETIC CONSIDERATIONS

Perioperative fasting should be minimized because patients are prone to hypoglycemia and nonketotic metabolic acidosis during periods of fasting. Blood glucose should be followed perioperatively, and patients should receive perioperative intravenous glucose supplementation. Patients with a history of nausea and vomiting may be at increased risk for aspiration. Renal defects may make urine output a poor indicator of intravascular volume. Consideration should be given to avoiding the use of nitroprusside because cyanide inhibits electron transport, although nitroprusside has been used in a patient without apparent injury (1). Patients may have cardiomyopathy.

Bibliography:

1. Farag E, Argalious M, Narouze S, et al. The anesthetic management of ventricular septal defect (VSD) repair in a child with mitochondrial cytopathy. *Can J Anaesth* 2002;49:958–962.

2. Wilson GN, de Chadarevian JP, Kaplan P, et al. Glutaric aciduria type II: review of the phenotype and report of an unusual glomerulopathy. *Am J Med Genet* 1989;32:395–401.
3. Dusheiko G, Kew MC, Joffe BI, et al. Recurrent hypoglycemia associated with glutaric aciduria type II in an adult. *N Engl J Med* 1979;301:1405–1409.

Glutaryl-CoA Dehydrogenase Deficiency

See Glutaric acidemia type I (glutaric aciduria type I)

Glycerol Kinase Deficiency

See Hyperglycerolemia

Glycine Encephalopathy

See Nonketotic hyperglycinemia

Glycogen Storage Disease Type 0

SYNONYM: Glycogen synthase deficiency

MIM #: 240600

This autosomal recessive glycogen storage disease is due to one of several mutations in the gene encoding hepatic glycogen synthase. It is marked by fasting ketotic hypoglycemia and postprandial hyperglycemia and hyperlactatemia. There is a varied presentation and it is likely that many if not most patients with the disease will not have the severe manifestations delineated below. Strictly speaking, this is not a glycogen storage disease, as the disorder results in decreased glycogen stores. Treatment is with frequent protein-rich meals, and nighttime addition of uncooked cornstarch.

NEUROMUSCULAR: Seizures, developmental delay. Morning drowsiness (prior to breakfast).

GI/GU: Hepatic steatosis.

OTHER: Growth failure, small for gestational age. Neonatal hypoglycemia. Fasting ketotic hypoglycemia. Postprandial hyperglycemia, hyperlactatemia, and glycosuria. Episodic hyperglycemia, glycosuria, and ketonuria make a superficial misdiagnosis of diabetes tempting. Hypoglycemic episodes can resolve with aging, except during pregnancy.

ANESTHETIC CONSIDERATIONS

Protracted preoperative fasting should be avoided. Perioperative fluids should contain glucose, and serum glucose should be monitored perioperatively.

Bibliography:
1. Bachrach BE, Weinstein DA, Orho-Melander M, et al. Glycogen synthase deficiency (glycogen storage disease type 0) presenting with hyperglycemia and glucosuria: report of three new mutations. *J Pediatr* 2002;140:781–783.
2. Rutledge SL, Atchison J, Bosshard NU, et al. Liver glycogen synthase deficiency: a cause of ketotic hypoglycemia. *Pediatrics* 2001;108:495–497.

Glycogen Storage Disease Type I (IA and IB)

See von Gierke disease

Glycogen Storage Disease Type II

See Pompe disease

Glycogen Storage Disease Type III

See Debrancher deficiency

Glycogen Storage Disease Type IV

See Brancher deficiency

Glycogen Storage Disease Type V

See McArdle syndrome

Glycogen Storage Disease Type VI

See Hers disease

Glycogen Storage Disease Type VII

SYNONYM: Phosphofructokinase deficiency; Muscle phosphofructokinase deficiency. (Includes Tarui disease)

MIM #: 232800

This autosomal recessive glycogen storage disease is similar to, but more severe than, glycogen storage disease type V (see McArdle syndrome, later). There is involvement of muscle and red blood cell energy metabolism.

Phosphofructokinase catalyzes the conversion of fructose 6-phosphate to fructose 1,6-diphosphate, a rate-limiting step in glycolysis. The enzyme in mammals is a complex isozyme with three subunits each encoded by its own structural gene: L, the major form found in liver and kidney; M, found in liver and the only form found in muscle; and P, the platelet form. Red blood cells contain both L and M subunits, and in general have half the enzyme activity. Because red blood cells have no energy source other than glycolysis, this decrease in enzyme activity is significant and decreases red blood cell half-life. Glucose cannot be utilized, but also lowers free fatty acid levels, the primary energy source of muscles. There is a severe infantile variant of this disease that also includes central nervous system and cardiac muscle abnormalities. In the infantile form, a severe myopathy is present at birth and is often accompanied by arthrogryposis. There is also a late onset myopathic variant. The rare **Tarui disease** consists of myopathy and hemolysis secondary to deficiency of the M type.

CHEST: Death secondary to respiratory complications is common in the severe infantile form.

CARDIOVASCULAR: Cardiomyopathy in the severe infantile form.

NEUROMUSCULAR: Muscle cramps with exertion, muscle weakness. Easy onset of fatigue, especially after high carbohydrate meals. Infants with the neonatal form can have seizures, mental retardation, or other central nervous system manifestations.

ORTHOPEDIC: Arthrogryposis in the neonatal form.

GI/GU: Gallstones. Mild hemolytic anemia. Myoglobinuria with extreme exertion. A case of acute renal failure from rhabdomyolysis after exercise has been reported.

OTHER: There is mild erythrocytosis, thought to be secondary to decreased production of 2,3-diphosphoglycerate. Hemolytic tendency with elevated reticulocyte counts and serum bilirubin. There is no associated hypoglycemia. Hyperuricemia.

MISCELLANEOUS: Relatively common in English springer spaniels.

ANESTHETIC CONSIDERATIONS
Patients with the severe infantile form may have a cardiomyopathy. Muscles are unable to use glucose and do not benefit from glucose or glucagon. Muscle fatigue is worse after a high carbohydrate meal, and exercise tolerance is worse after a glucose infusion (5). The effects of perioperative glucose infusions remain speculative. Succinylcholine may be relatively contraindicated in patients with a myopathy because of the risk of an exaggerated hyperkalemic response. Propofol may increase urinary excretion of uric acid (3), making this a potential consideration when propofol is used for prolonged anesthesia or sedation.

FIGURE: See **Appendix E**

Bibliography:
1. Ronquist G. Glycogenosis type VII (Tarui's disease): diagnostic considerations and late sequelae. *South Med J* 2002;95:1361–1362.
2. Nakajima H, Raben N, Hamaguchi T, et al. Phosphofructokinase deficiency; past, present and future. *Curr Mol Med* 2002;2:197–212.
3. Masuda A, Asahi T, Sakamaki M, et al. Uric acid excretion increases during propofol anesthesia. *Anesth Analg* 1997;85:144–148.
4. Talente GM, Coleman RA, Alter C, et al. Glycogen storage disease in adults. *Ann Intern Med* 1994;120:218–226.
5. Haller RG, Lewis SE. Glucose-induced exertional fatigue in muscle phosphofructokinase deficiency. *N Engl J Med* 1991;324:364–369.

Glycogen Storage Disease Type VIII

SYNONYM: Phosphorylase kinase deficiency; Glycogen storage disease type IX; Hepatic phosphorylase b kinase deficiency

MIM #: 306000

The enzyme deficient in this X-linked recessive disease is involved in phosphorylating glycogen to glucose-1-phosphate. The major finding is hypoglycemia and fasting ketosis in infancy. There is reduction in the severity of the disease with age, such that most adults are asymptomatic. The confusion of the nomenclature (glycogen storage disease VIII vs. IX) is due to the fact that the enzyme complex is encoded on both the X chromosome and on autosomes. About 75% of cases are X-linked. Most adult patients become asymptomatic, despite continued lack of enzyme activity.

Several subtypes have been delineated, depending on which enzyme is missing (hepatic and/or muscle).

CARDIOVASCULAR: A rare cardiac-specific enzyme deficit has been reported with death during infancy with massive cardiac glycogen deposition.

NEUROMUSCULAR: Muscles are not involved. Some patients with an autosomal lack of hepatic and muscle phosphorylase kinase deficiency will have hypotonia. Mild motor delay.

ORTHOPEDIC: Growth retardation, but normal adult height.

GI/GU: Hepatomegaly, elevated liver transaminases. Renal tubular acidosis has been reported.

OTHER: Hypercholesterolemia, hypertriglyceridemia, fasting ketosis, hypoglycemia in infancy.

ANESTHETIC CONSIDERATIONS
Adequate levels of serum glucose must be ensured perioperatively in infants and young children. Patients respond normally to glucagons. There are no specific anesthetic concerns in adults.

FIGURE: See **Appendix E**

Bibliography:
1. Talente GM, Coleman RA, Alter C, et al. Glycogen storage disease in adults. *Ann Intern Med* 1994;120:218–226.
2. Willems PJ, Gerver WJM, Berger R, et al. The natural history of liver glycogenosis due to phosphorylase kinase deficiency: a longitudinal study of 41 patients. *Eur J Pediatr* 1990;149:268–271.

Glycogen Storage Disease Type IX

See Glycogen storage disease type VIII

Glycogen Synthase Deficiency

See Glycogen storage disease type 0

GM₁ Gangliosidosis

MIM #: 230500, 230600, 230650

This autosomal recessive disease is due to a defect in the gene for beta-galactosidase, resulting in the accumulation of GM_1 ganglioside. Infantile, juvenile, and adult forms have been described, due to different mutations of the same gene. The main manifestations are neurologic. Death in the infantile form occurs by the age of 2 to 3 years.

Gangliosides have both a hydrophobic ceramide moiety and a hydrophilic oligosaccharide chain. They are components of the outer cell membrane, with the hydrophobic moiety anchoring it in the membrane and the hydrophilic chain extending into the extracellular space. Although their function is unknown, they have been implicated as binding sites for a variety of viruses, bacterial toxins, growth factors, and interferons.

HEENT/AIRWAY

Infantile form: Coarse facies, frontal bossing. Macular cherry-red spot. Optic atrophy. Corneal clouding. Large, low-set ears. Depressed nasal bridge. Gingival hypertrophy, mild macroglossia. Short neck.

Juvenile form: Late blindness with normal cornea, retina, and macula.

Adult form: Normal vision.

CHEST

Infantile and juvenile forms: Spatulate ribs. Recurrent aspiration pneumonia.

CARDIOVASCULAR

Infantile form: May have cardiomyopathy. May have paroxysmal supraventricular tachycardia.

NEUROMUSCULAR

Infantile form: Severely retarded mental and motor development, hypotonia, hyperreflexia. Seizures. Eventual decerebrate rigidity within a year of life.

Juvenile form: Mental and motor deterioration. Ataxia, choreoathetosis, progressive spasticity, lethargy. Generalized muscle weakness. Seizures. Eventual decerebrate rigidity.

Adult form: Intelligence usually normal or mildly affected. Facial dystonia (grimacing) and dysarthria with normal eye movements are common. Cerebellar dysfunction, ataxia, dystonia which is eventually incapacitating. Seizures are uncommon.

ORTHOPEDIC

Infantile form: Dwarfism, thoracolumbar kyphosis, scoliosis, stiff joints, flexion contractures of knees and elbows. Periosteal new bone formation in a newborn. Hypoplastic vertebral bodies with anterior beaking, osteoporosis of cortex of most bones, iliac flaring, wedge-shaped metacarpals. The bony changes are similar to those seen with the mucopolysaccharidoses.

Juvenile form: Mild changes with inferior beaking of lumbar vertebral bodies, proximal pointing of metacarpals (particularly the fifth), mild remodeling of the pelvis.

Adult form: Minimal radiologic changes.

GI/GU

Infantile form: Hepatosplenomegaly, inguinal hernia.

Juvenile and adult forms: No hepatosplenomegaly.

OTHER

Infantile form: Failure to thrive, edema. Thick, rough, hirsute skin. Angiokeratomas. May have increased incidence of Mongolian spots.

Adult form: Angiokeratomas.

MISCELLANEOUS: This disease also occurs in sheep.

ANESTHETIC CONSIDERATIONS

Although there are no reports in the anesthesia literature, given the phenotypic similarity with the mucopolysaccharidoses, laryngoscopy and tracheal intubation might be difficult. Children should be considered to be at increased risk for perioperative aspiration. Succinylcholine is relatively contraindicated in this disease because of the risk of an exaggerated hyperkalemic response. Chronic use of anticonvulsant medications may affect the metabolism of some anesthetic drugs. Abnormal skin in the infantile form may make vascular access more challenging. Contractures may make proper positioning more difficult. Supraventricular tachycardia in the infantile form has been fatal.

Bibliography:

1. Muthane U, Chickabasaviah Y, Kaneski C, et al. Clinical features of adult GM1 gangliosidosis: report of three Indian patients and review of 40 cases. *Mov Disord* 2004;19:1334–1341.
2. Suzuki Y, Sakuraba H, Oshima A, et al. Clinical and molecular heterogeneity in hereditary beta-galactosidase deficiency. *Dev Neurosci* 1991;13:299–303.

GM₂ Gangliosidosis

See Sandhoff disease and Tay-Sachs disease

Goldenhar Syndrome

SYNONYM: Facioauriculovertebral syndrome; Hemifacial microsomia; Oculoauriculovertebral syndrome

MIM #: 164210

The main features of this sporadically occurring phenotypically variable syndrome are developmental anomalies of the first and second branchial arches, ocular anomalies and vertebral anomalies. The anomalies are usually unilateral, or at least asymmetric, hence the term "hemifacial microsomia." Epibulbar dermoids are common. This syndrome may represent the sequelae of a fetal vascular accident affecting the first and second branchial arches. Most cases are sporadic, but there are instances where inheritance is consistent with either autosomal dominant or autosomal recessive inheritance.

HEENT/AIRWAY: Unilateral or asymmetric hypoplasia of the facial bones and muscles. Epibulbar dermoids. May have upper lid coloboma, subconjunctival lipoma, strabismus, microphthalmia. Microtia and conductive hearing loss. Preauricular skin tags or pits. May have limited mouth opening, deviation of the mandible to the affected side, micrognathia. May have cleft palate or high-arched palate. Abnormal tongue and palatal function. Parotid gland dysfunction. May have branchial cleft remnants in the neck. Occasional laryngeal anomaly, including tracheoesophageal fistula. May develop obstructive sleep apnea.

CHEST: May have rib anomalies. Rare pulmonary hypoplasia or aplasia.

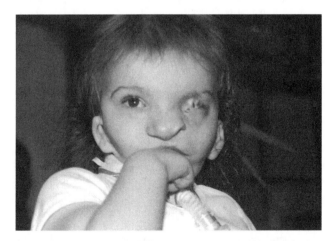

Goldenhar syndrome. FIG. 1. A young girl with Goldenhar syndrome. She has required a tracheostomy, and the eye findings are apparent.

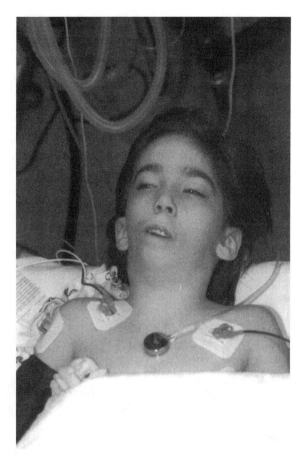

Goldenhar syndrome. FIG. 2. The facial asymmetry in this young girl was more apparent after the induction of anesthesia. She has significant micrognathia with markedly diminished mouth opening. Tracheal intubation was very difficult.

CARDIOVASCULAR: May have congenital cardiac defect, including ventricular septal defect, patent ductus arteriosus, tetralogy of Fallot, or coarctation.

NEUROMUSCULAR: Intelligence is usually normal. May have Arnold-Chiari malformation or hydrocephalus.

ORTHOPEDIC: Vertebral anomalies, especially of the cervical vertebrae, including hemivertebrae or hypoplasia. May have radial anomalies.

GI/GU: Renal anomalies include agenesis, ectopia, or dysplasia. May have ureteral duplication, vesicoureteral reflux.

ANESTHETIC CONSIDERATIONS
Craniofacial and vertebral anomalies can make laryngoscopy and tracheal intubation exceedingly difficult (1,2,4,7,10,13). The difficult airway often gets progressively worse with age. Correct mask fit may be difficult because of facial asymmetry. Introducing the laryngoscope into the unaffected side of the mouth, where there is more room to displace the tongue, may help. Intubation through a laryngeal mask

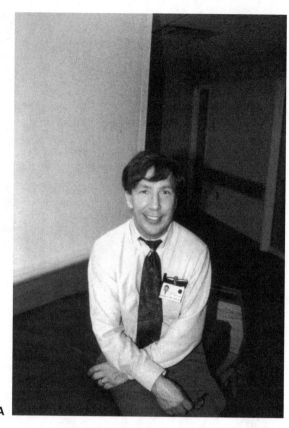 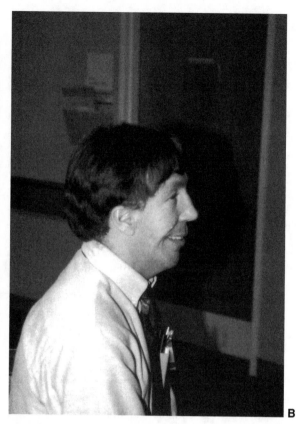

A B

Goldenhar syndrome. FIG. 3. A, B. This physician has had surgery in the past where tracheal intubation could not be done by direct visualization and he required fiberoptic intubation. Other manifestations of the syndrome include an eye coloboma, an ear tag, and slight micrognathia, none of which is immediately apparent.

airway has been reported, and the laryngeal mask airway has resolved airway obstruction when inserted into an awake infant after nebulization of lidocaine (6).

It has been suggested that preoperative radiographs of the mandible are predictive of the degree of difficulty for laryngsocopy (2). Mandibles that were merely small were least likely to be associated with a difficult intubation. Absent ramus, condyle, and temporomandibular joint had a high association with difficult intubation. Radiologic grading was not as useful with bilateral involvement. Prior mandibular lengthening was still associated with difficult intubating conditions, and prior surgery should not be considered reassuring.

Airway abnormalities can predispose to obstructive sleep apnea. One review of patients with Goldenhar syndrome found the incidence of obstructive sleep apnea to be nearly 24% (3). Care should be taken, particularly in the postanesthesia care unit, to avoid perioperative airway obstruction.

Patients can have hydrocephalus (10) and if they do so, they will require appropriate management of intracranial pressure. Radial anomalies may make placement of a radial arterial catheter more difficult. Patients with renal disease have altered metabolism of renally excreted drugs. Patients

with congenital heart disease need perioperative antibiotic prophylaxis as indicated.

Bibliography:

1. Chen PP, Cheng CK, Abdullah V, et al. Tracheal intubation using suspension laryngoscopy in an infant with Goldenhar's syndrome. *Anaesth Intensive Care* 2001;29:548–551.
2. Nargozian C, Ririe DG, Bennun RD, et al. Hemifacial microsomia: anatomical prediction of difficult intubation. *Paediatr Anaesth* 1999;9:393–398.
3. Cohen SR, Levitt CA, Simms C, et al. Airway disorders in hemifacial microsomia. *Plast Reconstr Surg* 1999;103:27–33.
4. Perkins JA, Sie KC, Milczuk H, et al. Airway management in children with craniofacial anomalies. *Cleft Palate Craniofac J* 1997;34: 135–140.
5. Fan SZ, Lee TS, Chen LK, et al. Long-term propofol infusion and airway management in a patient with Goldenhar's syndrome. *Acta Anaesthesiol Sin* 1995;33:233–236.
6. Sutphen R, Galan-Gomez E, Cortada X, et al. Tracheoesophageal anomalies in oculoauriculovertebral (Goldenhar) spectrum. *Clin Genet* 1995;48:66–71.
7. Johnson CM, Sims C. Awake fibreoptic intubation via a laryngeal mask in an infant with Goldenhar's syndrome. *Anaesth Intensive Care* 1994;22:194–197.
8. Ritchey ML, Norbeck J, Huang C, et al. Urologic manifestations of Goldenhar syndrome. *Urology* 1994;43:88–91.
9. Morrison PJ, Mulholland HC, Craig BG, et al. Cardiovascular abnormalities in the oculo-auriculo-vertebral spectrum (Goldenhar syndrome). *Am J Med Genet* 1992;44:425–428.
10. Madan R, Trikha A, Venkataraman RK, et al. Goldenhar's syndrome: an analysis of anaesthetic management. *Anaesthesia* 1990;45:49–52.

11. Aoe T, Kohchi T, Mizuguchi T. Respiratory inductance plethysmography and pulse oximetry in the assessment of upper airway patency in a child with Goldenhar's syndrome. *Can J Anaesth* 1990;37:369–371.
12. Scholtes JL, Veyckemans F, Van Obbergh L, et al. Neonatal anaesthetic management of a patients with Goldenhar's syndrome with hydrocephalus. *Anaesth Intensive Care* 1987;15:338–340.
13. Cooper CMS, Murray-Wilson A. Retrograde intubation. *Anaesthesia* 1987;42:1197–1200.
14. Rollnick BR, Kaye CI, Nagatoshi K, et al. Oculoauriculovertebral dysplasia and variants: phenotypic characteristics of 294 patients. *Am J Med Genet* 1987;26:361–375.

Goltz Syndrome

SYNONYM: Focal dermal hypoplasia; Goltz-Gorlin syndrome

MIM #: 305600

This X-linked dominant disorder is a disease of mesoectodermal development, with primary manifestations in skin, nails, hair, bones, and teeth. Specifically, patients exhibit pigmentary and atrophic skin changes, nail dystrophy, thin hair, syndactyly, bone hypoplasia, and small teeth with dental hypoplasia. Over 80% of affected individuals are female, suggesting that the disorder is lethal in male hemizygotes. The Goltz and Aicardi syndromes (see earlier) may be contiguous gene syndromes on the short arm of the X chromosome.

Note that Goltz syndrome is also known as Goltz-Gorlin syndrome. Gorlin syndrome, also known as Gorlin-Goltz syndrome, is a different syndrome that involves nevoid basal cell carcinomas (see Basal cell nevus syndrome, earlier).

HEENT/AIRWAY: May have facial asymmetry, microcephaly. Strabismus, colobomas of the iris or choroid, microphthalmia, aniridia. Low-set ears with thin ear helix. May have hearing loss. Broad nasal tip with notched alae nasi. Small teeth with enamel hypoplasia. Delayed tooth eruption, hypodontia, oligodontia. High-arched palate. Pointed chin. Papillomas of the lip, buccal mucosa, and gingivae. Esophageal or laryngeal papillomas, which can be obstructive. May have cleft lip or palate.

CHEST: Midclavicular hypoplasia or aplasia, rib hypoplasia. Supernumerary nipples. Asymmetric breasts. May have diaphragmatic hernia.

CARDIOVASCULAR: May have a congenital cardiac defect.

NEUROMUSCULAR: Occasional mental retardation. May have spina bifida occulta.

ORTHOPEDIC: Nail dystrophy. Sparse, brittle hair. Patchy alopecia. Syndactyly, clinodactyly, brachydactyly, polydactyly, adactyly. Aplasia or hypoplasia of the clavicles. Failure of fusion of the pelvic bones. Striated long bones. Scoliosis. Hypermobile joints. Skeletal asymmetry. May have short stature. Congenital dislocation of the hip.

GI/GU: Gastroesophageal reflux. Umbilical and inguinal hernias. Anal and vulvar papillomas. May have renal dysplasia, horseshoe kidney, bifid ureter. May have labial or clitoral hypoplasia. May have cryptorchidism.

OTHER: Pigmentary and atrophic skin changes. Herniation of fat through areas of severe dermal atrophy. Hyperhidrosis. Telangiectasis. Palmar hyperkeratosis. Multiple skin and mucous membrane papillomas. Thin, brittle hair. Alopecia.

MISCELLANEOUS: Robert Goltz is a preeminent dermatopathologist and a past president of the American Academy of Dermatology.

ANESTHETIC CONSIDERATIONS
Laryngeal papillomas can obstruct the glottic opening. Airway obstruction is so severe in some patients as to require a tracheostomy. Teeth should be examined preoperatively for number and stability. Gastroesophageal reflux is common, so precautions should be taken to minimize the risk of aspiration. Clavicular anomalies may make placement of a subclavian venous catheter difficult. Patients should be carefully positioned and padded secondary to dermal hypoplasia and joint hypermobility.

Bibliography:
1. Bellosta M, Trespiolli D, Ghiselli E, et al. Focal dermal hypoplasia: report of a family with 7 affected women in 3 generations. *Eur J Dermatol* 1996;6:499–500.
2. Goltz RW. Focal dermal hypoplasia syndrome: an update (Editorial). *Arch Dermatol* 1992;128:1108–1111.
3. Holzman RS. Airway involvement and anesthetic management in Goltz's syndrome. *J Clin Anesth* 1991;3:422–425.

Goltz-Gorlin Syndrome

See Goltz syndrome

Goodman Syndrome

SYNONYM: Acrocephalosyndactyly type IV

MIM #: None

Many believe that this autosomal recessive syndrome is a variant of Carpenter syndrome (see earlier). The primary findings are acrocephaly and syndactyly. A few have argued that it is a distinct entity based on the presence of clinodactyly, camptodactyly, and ulnar deviation. See Carpenter syndrome for a more detailed clinical description.

HEENT/AIRWAY: Acrocephaly. Craniosynostosis.

CARDIOVASCULAR: May have congenital heart disease. Eisenmenger syndrome has been described.

NEUROMUSCULAR: May have elevated intracranial pressure if craniosynostosis is severe.

ORTHOPEDIC: Syndactyly, clinodactyly, camptodactyly, polydactyly. Ulnar deviation.

ANESTHETIC CONSIDERATIONS

Patients may have elevated intracranial pressure, in which case precautions should be taken to avoid further elevations in pressure. Antibiotic prophylaxis may be indicated if there is associated congenital heart disease.

Bibliography:
1. Gershoni-Baruch R. Carpenter syndrome: marked variability of expression to include the Summitt and Goodman syndromes. *Am J Med Genet* 1990;35:236–240.
2. Cohen DM, Green JG, Miller J, et al. Acrocephalopolysyndactyly type II-Carpenter syndrome: clinical spectrum and an attempt at unification with Goodman and Summitt syndromes. *Am J Med Genet* 1987;28:311–324.

Gorham Syndrome

SYNONYM: Gorham-Stout disease

MIM #: 123880

This is an autosomal dominant disease of massive osteolysis with replacement of bone with fibrovascular tissue resulting in pathologic fractures and secondary complications. The etiology is not currently understood. Onset in most cases is in the second or third decade of life, but may be as early as 1 to 2 years of age. Impairment of the spine or lungs can prove fatal. Bone grafts have not proven successful, but resection and replacement with artificial bone materal has been effective, as has radiation therapy.

HEENT/AIRWAY: Can have destruction of maxillary or mandibular bones, as well as orbital and cranial bones.

CHEST: Relapsing pleural effusions. Respiratory failure from restrictive disease or pleural effusions. Chylothorax, which carries an approximately 50% mortality rate.

CARDIOVASCULAR: May have chylopericardium.

NEUROMUSCULAR: May have neurologic complications from spine involvement.

ORTHOPEDIC: Massive osteolysis. In most patients several adjacent bones are involved. The spine may be severely affected.

OTHER: May have hypoproteinemia secondary to chylothorax. Bone changes can be preceded by vascular skin changes.

ANESTHETIC CONSIDERATIONS

Pulmonary function and cervical spine integrity should be evaluated preoperatively. Succinylcholine should be avoided in patients with severely osteolytic bones because of a risk of bone fracture secondary to succinylcholine-induced fasciculations. Patients may have cervical spine involvement requiring intubation with midline stabilization or fiberoptic techniques. Maxillary or mandibular involvement may make mask ventilation difficult.

Bibliography:
1. Czabo C, Habre W. Gorham syndrome: anaesthetic management. *Anaesthesia* 2000;55:157–159.
2. Mangar D, Murtha PA, Aquilina TC, et al. Anesthesia for a patient with Gorham's syndrome. *Anesthesiology* 1994;80:466–468.

Gorham-Stout disease

See Gorham Syndrome

Gorlin Syndrome

See Basal cell nevus syndrome

Gorlin-Cohen Syndrome

See Frontometaphyseal dysplasia

Gorlin-Gold Syndrome

See Basal cell nevus syndrome

Grebe Syndrome

MIM #: 200700

This autosomal recessive syndrome is characterized by marked distal limb reduction and polydactyly, and is thus a type of acromesomelic dysplasia. This chondrodysplasia results from a mutation in the gene *CDMP1*, which encodes cartilage-derived morphogenetic protein 1, a member of the transforming growth factor-beta superfamily of growth factor/signaling proteins. *CDMP1* is primarily expressed at sites of skeletal development. Heterozygotes have a milder phenotype. Two other acromesomelic dysplasias, those of Hunter-Thompson and Maroteaux (see acromesomelic dysplasia, earlier), are allelic disorders.

HEENT/AIRWAY: Normal facies.

NEUROMUSCULAR: Normal intelligence.

ORTHOPEDIC: Small stature due to limb reduction. Distal limb reduction (bones are shortened)—lower extremities affected more than upper extremities, distal bones more severely affected than proximal bones. The very short fingers resemble toes. Polydactyly. Short feet are in valgus position.

OTHER: May be stillborn.

MISCELLANEOUS: Grebe is pronounced "GRAY-beh." Hans Grebe was a university colleague of Mengele, a pupil of the racial hygienist Otmar Freiherr von Verschuer, and himself an advocate of the Nazi racial doctrines.

ANESTHETIC CONSIDERATIONS
Peripheral vascular access is difficult secondary to marked limb reduction defects. Otherwise there are no specific anesthetic implications.

Bibliography:
1. Costa T, Ramsby G, Cassia F, et al. Grebe syndrome: clinical and radiographic findings in affected individuals and heterozygous carriers. *Am J Med Genet* 1998;75:523–529.
2. Thomas JT, Kilpatrick MW, Lin K, et al. Disruption of human limb morphogenesis by a dominant negative mutation in CDMP1. *Nat Genet* 1997;17:58–64.
3. Kumar D, Curtis D, Blank CE. Grebe chondrodysplasia and brachydactyly in a family. *Clin Genet* 1984;25:68–72.

Greig Cephalopolysyndactyly Syndrome

MIM #: 175700

This autosomal dominant syndrome is distinguished by a characteristic skull shape (high forehead with frontal bossing), polydactyly, and syndactyly. This disorder is caused by mutations in the gene *GLI3,* which maps to chromosome 7. *GLI3* is homologous to the *Drosophila* cubitus interruptus gene, and this syndrome is homologous to the mouse mutant "extra toes." Frameshift mutations in this same gene result in the Pallister-Hall syndrome (see later), making these two disorders allelic.

HEENT/AIRWAY: High forehead with frontal bossing, macrocephaly. Apparent hypertelorism, may have down-slanting palpebral fissures. Broad nasal root.

NEUROMUSCULAR: Normal intelligence. May have craniosynostosis. May have mild hydrocephalus. May have agenesis of the corpus callosum.

ORTHOPEDIC: Postaxial polydactyly in the hands, preaxial polydactyly in the feet. Syndactyly. Broad thumbs and halluces. Camptodactyly. May have hip dislocation.

MISCELLANEOUS: Greig was a Scottish surgeon who described this entity during his tenure as the curator of the Museum of the Royal College of Surgeons of Edinburgh. He collected over 300 skulls during his lifetime, which he donated to the College Museum. Greig is pronounced "Gregg."

ANESTHETIC CONSIDERATIONS
There are no specific anesthetic considerations with this syndrome.

Bibliography:
1. Debeer P, Peeters H, Driess S, et al. Variable phenotype in Greig cephalopolysyndactyly syndrome: clinical and radiological findings in 4 independent families and 3 sporadic cases with identified GLI3 mutations. *Am J Med Genet A* 2003;120:49–58.
2. Ausems MG, Ippel PF, Renardel de Lavalette PA. Greig cephalopolysyndactyly syndrome in a large family: a comparison of the clinical signs with those described in the literature. *Clin Dysmorphol* 1994;3:21–30.

H

Hajdu-Cheney Syndrome

SYNONYM: Arthrodentoosteo dysplasia; Acroosteolysis syndrome

MIM #: 102500

This autosomal dominant disorder is characterized by acroosteolysis (dissolution of bone in the distal phalanges of the fingers and toes), lax joints, and early dental loss. There is a connective tissue abnormality, primarily affecting the development of skeletal tissue. Although the disorder begins in childhood, the diagnosis is often delayed. Patients frequently present with pain in the affected fingers, weakness, or pathologic fractures. The responsible gene and gene product are not currently known.

HEENT/AIRWAY: Bathrocephaly. Cranial sutures may fail to ossify. Thickened cranium with wormian bones. Thick, straight scalp hair, prominent eyebrows and eyelashes. Synophrys. Absent frontal sinus. Down-slanting palpebral fissures. Low-set, prominent ears. Hearing loss. Broad nose, anteverted nares, long philtrum. High, narrow palate. May have low-pitched voice. Hypoplasia of the mandibular ramus. Early dental loss. Short neck.

NEUROMUSCULAR: Progressive basilar impaction against the foramen magnum may result in brainstem dysfunction. Hydrocephalus.

ORTHOPEDIC: Short stature that may be aggravated by vertebral osseous compression. Rare cervical instability secondary to cervical osteolysis. Biconcave vertebrae, vertebral osteopenia that may lead to collapse, narrow intervertebral disc spaces. Kyphoscoliosis. Lax joints. Dislocation of the radial head ("nursemaid's elbow"). Patellar dislocation. Acroosteolysis (shrinking fingers and toes), short distal phalanges, short nails. Genu valgus, fibular bowing. May have osteoporosis and pathologic fractures.

GI/GU: Inguinal hernias. May have cystic renal disease.

OTHER: Hirsutism.

ANESTHETIC CONSIDERATIONS

Short neck and hypoplasia of the mandibular ramus may make direct visualization of the larynx difficult. Cervical instability may be present. Dental loss should be documented preoperatively. There is a report of vocal cord paralysis in a patient with Hajdu-Cheney syndrome (2). Patients must be carefully positioned to avoid hyperextension of lax joints or causing/aggravating pathologic fractures. Renal function should be assessed preoperatively in patients suspected of having cystic renal disease.

Bibliography:

1. Brennan AM, Pauli RM. Hajdu-Cheney syndrome: evolution of phenotype and clinical problems. *Am J Med Genet* 2001;100:292–310.
2. Fryns JP, Stinckens C, Feenstra L. Vocal cord paralysis and cystic kidney disease in Hajdu-Cheney syndrome. *Clin Genet* 1997;51:271–274.
3. O'Reilly MAR, Shaw DG. Hajdu-Cheney syndrome. *Ann Rheum Dis* 1994;53:276–279.

Hallermann-Streiff Syndrome

SYNONYM: Oculomandibulofacial dyscephaly

MIM #: 234100

This sporadic disorder is characterized by birdlike facies, ocular defects, mandibular hypoplasia, tracheomalacia, and hypotrichosis.

HEENT/AIRWAY: Small, birdlike facies with a large cranial vault and frontal bossing. Ocular defects include microphthalmia, cataracts, coloboma, nystagmus, strabismus, glaucoma, and retinal degeneration. Sparse eyebrows and eyelashes. Hypoplastic, pointed (beaked) nose with septal deviation. Malar hypoplasia. Absence of mandibular condyles. Mandibular hypoplasia and anterior displacement of the temporomandibular joints, making the mouth appear open. High-arched palate. Narrow upper airway. Neonatal, missing, supernumerary, or hypoplastic teeth. Tracheomalacia.

CHEST: Rib hypoplasia. A narrow upper airway combined with tracheomalacia frequently results in respiratory complications, including respiratory distress, obstructive sleep apnea, and recurrent infection.

CARDIOVASCULAR: Chronic upper airway obstruction and respiratory insufficiency can lead to cor pulmonale. May have congenital heart disease.

NEUROMUSCULAR: Intelligence is usually normal but may have mental retardation. May have spina bifida, hyperactivity, choreoathetosis, seizures.

ORTHOPEDIC: Proportionate short stature. Thin, slender long bones. Clavicular hypoplasia. Hyperextensible joints. May have scoliosis, osteoporosis.

OTHER: Low birth weight. Hypotrichosis. Focal areas of skin atrophy over the nose and scalp.

ANESTHETIC CONSIDERATIONS

Major craniofacial abnormalities make endotracheal intubation difficult. The hypoplastic nose with deviated septum may make nasotracheal intubation difficult. The temporomandibular joints may be weak, allowing dislocation during laryngoscopy. Neonatal teeth (teeth present at birth) as well as deciduous and permanent teeth are brittle and can be broken easily during laryngoscopy.

Patients with significant upper airway obstruction may need a tracheostomy. Patients with recurrent respiratory infections may have chronic lung disease. These patients in particular are at risk for postoperative pulmonary complications. Patients with congenital heart disease need perioperative antibiotic prophylaxis as indicated. Clavicular anomalies may make placement of a subclavian venous catheter more difficult. Care needs to be taken in positioning patients with hyperextensible joints.

Bibliography:

1. Cheong KF, Tham SL. Anaesthetic management of a child with Hallermann-Streiff Francois syndrome. *Paediatr Anaesth* 2003;13: 274–275.
2. Malde AD, Jagtap SR, Pantvaidya SH. Hallermann-Streiff syndrome: airway problems during anaesthesia. *J Postgrad Med* 1994;40:216–218.
3. Cohen MM. Hallermann-Streiff syndrome: a review. *Am J Med Genet* 1991;41:488–499.
4. Robinow M. Respiratory obstruction and cor pulmonale in the Hallermann-Streiff syndrome. *Am J Med Genet* 1991;41:515–516.
5. Salbert BA, Stevens CA, Spence JE. Tracheomalacia in Hallermann-Streiff syndrome. *Am J Med Genet* 1991;41:521–523.
6. Ravindran R, Stoops CM. Anesthetic management of a patient with Hallermann-Streiff syndrome. *Anesth Analg* 1979;58:254–255.

Hallervorden-Spatz Disease

MIM #: 234200

Hallervorden-Spatz disease is an autosomal recessive neurologic disease. Its pathologic hallmark is iron deposition, particularly in the globus pallidus, caudate and substantia nigra. It typically presents in childhood with movement disorders and may rarely present in adults as Parkinsonism and dementia. It is due to mutations in the gene *PANC2*, which encodes pantothenate kinase. This enzyme is important in the synthesis of coenzyme A. Patients with the classic form have onset of signs in the first decade of life. There are also subtypes with early onset and slow progression, and late onset with rapid progression. Patients with early onset tend to have pigmentary retinopathy while those with late onset tend to have speech and psychiatric disorders. Abnormalities in this gene are also responsible for the allelic HARP syndrome, not discussed in this text.

HEENT/AIRWAY: Optic atrophy, retinitis pigmentosa. Oromandibular rigidity from dystonia. Dysarthria and difficulty in swallowing.

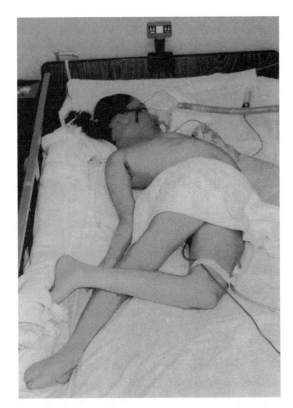

Hallervorden-Spatz disease. A 21-year-old woman with Hallervorden-Spatz disease. Scoliosis and dystonia are apparent. She had torticollis and trismus that prevented any mouth opening. Hypertonicity, including oromandibular hypertonicity and torticollis, resolved with halothane. (Courtesy of Dr. Raymond C. Roy, Department of Anesthesiology, Wake Forest University School of Medicine.)

CHEST: Risk of recurrent aspiration pneumonia.

NEUROMUSCULAR: Choreoathetosis. Dystonia with torticollis is common. Parkinsonian features including tremor and rigidity. Rigidity is progressive and begins in the lower extremities before progressing to the upper. Behavioral problems. Psychiatric problems. Progressive dementia. Spasticity. T_2-weighted MRI demonstrates a specific pattern of hyperintensity within the generally hypointense globus pallidus ("eye of the tiger sign").

ORTHOPEDIC: Scoliosis is common from dystonia. Equinovarus foot deformity.

MISCELLANEOUS: Both Hallervorden and Spatz were Nazi war criminals. A majority of the brains they investigated during the Nazi period were victims of euthanasia, and there is good evidence that Hallervorden in particular was present at the killing of many of these people. Because of concerns regarding the origins of Hallervorden's personal pathological collection, the collection has been removed from the Edinger Institute. It has also been suggested that this eponymous disease be renamed (1).

ANESTHETIC CONSIDERATIONS
With the induction of anesthesia (even with volatile agents alone) muscle tone diminishes, and leads to relaxation of oromandibular rigidity and resolution of torticollis. Nondepolarizing muscle relaxants can be used. Succinylcholine is contraindicated in these patients who may be bedridden and who may have unpredictable lesions involving upper motor neurons.

A patient has been reported in whom apparent neuroleptic malignant syndrome developed perioperatively, presumably secondary to decreased dopaminergic activity in the substantia nigra and the nigrostriatal projections (3).

Bibliography:
1. Shevell M. Hallervorden and history. *N Engl J Med* 2003;348:3–4.
2. Hayflick SJ, Westaway SK, Levinson B, et al. Genetic, clinical, and radiographic delineation of Hallervorden-Spatz syndrome. *N Engl J Med* 2003;348:33–40.
3. Hayashi K, Chihara E, Sawa T, et al. Clinical features of neuroleptic malignant syndrome: spontaneous presentation in a patient with Hallervorden-Spatz disease in the absence of neuroleptic drugs. *Anaesthesia* 1993;48:499–502.
4. Roy RC, McLain S, Wise A, et al. Anesthetic management of a patient with Hallervorden-Spatz disease. *Anesthesiology* 1983;58:382–384.

Hand-Schüller-Christian Disease

Included in Langerhans cell histiocytosis

Hanhart Syndrome

See Oromandibular-limb hypogenesis

Happy Puppet Syndrome

See Angelman syndrome

HARD(E) Syndrome

See Walker-Warburg syndrome

Hartnup Disorder

MIM #: 234500

This autosomal recessive disorder involves impairment of neutral amino acid transport in the kidneys and the small bowel. Some patients can have renal involvement only, others have bowel involvement only. Because tryptophan is required for niacin synthesis, reduced tryptophan absorption and increased renal losses lead to secondary niacin deficiency. The skin and neurologic findings are similar to those of pellagra (the four Ds of niacin deficiency: Diarrhea, Dermatitis, Dementia, and Death). There is significant phenotypic variability. Many patients diagnosed by neonatal screening remain asymptomatic, as do most siblings of identified patients. The disorder is due to mutations in the gene *SLC6A19*.

HEENT/AIRWAY: Nystagmus, diplopia.

NEUROMUSCULAR: Intermittent cerebellar ataxia, tremors, episodic emotional instability, seizures, psychosis. Mild mental retardation. Most patients, however, are normal.

GI/GU: Diarrhea. Aminoaciduria. The pattern of aminoaciduria differs from the generalized hyperaminoaciduria of, for example, the Fanconi syndrome or cystinuria. Tests of renal function are otherwise normal.

OTHER: Pellagra-like, light-sensitive skin rash on exposed areas of the body. The rash initially blisters, and eventually is scaly and depigmented. Maternal Hartnup disorder does not affect the fetus. A patient has been reported in whom a pellagra-like rash developed coincident with lactation and breast-feeding.

MISCELLANEOUS: This disorder was named not after Dr. Hartnup, but rather the Hartnup family, in whom it was first described. It is thought that the full-blown syndrome is not often seen in the United States because of the generally superadequate diet. Treatment with niacin or nicotinamide can often clear the rash and improve the neurologic findings, if treatment is thought necessary.

ANESTHETIC CONSIDERATIONS
Adequate hydration must be ensured in these patients who have frequent diarrhea. A protracted perioperative fast without adequate protein intake could worsen the symptoms of this disorder.

Bibliography:
1. Seow HF, Broer S, Broer A, et al. Hartnup disorder is caused by mutations in the gene encoding the neutral amino acid transporter SLC6A19. *Nat Genet* 2004;36:1003–1007.
2. Wilcken B, Yu JS, Brown DA. Natural history of Hartnup disease. *Arch Dis Child* 1977;52:38–40.

Hay-Wells Ectodermal Dysplasia

See AEC syndrome

Heart-Hand Syndrome

See Holt-Oram syndrome

Hecht Beals Syndrome

See Dutch-Kentucky syndrome

Hecht Syndrome

See Dutch-Kentucky syndrome

Hemifacial Microsomia

See Goldenhar syndrome

Hemoglobin H Disease

Included in Thalassemia

Hemoglobin S-Thalassemia

Included in Thalassemia

Hemophilia

See Hemophilia A or Hemophilia B

Hemophilia A

MIM #: 306700

This X-linked disorder is due to mutations or deletions of the gene that encodes clotting factor VIII. Over 370 distinct mutations in the gene have been described. This disorder cannot be clinically differentiated from hemophilia B (Christmas disease, see later), which is due to deficient activity of factor IX. Acquired hemophilia A is a rare condition caused by the acquisition of autoantibodies against factor VIII.

Patients with less than 1% factor VIII activity are said to have severe disease, those with 1% to 5% activity have moderate disease, and those with 5% to 25% activity have mild disease. Patients with severe disease can have spontaneous bleeding, whereas patients with mild disease usually have bleeding only after surgery or major trauma. However, life-threatening bleeding can occur in all groups. Of the approximately 17,000 people with hemophilia A in the United States, approximately 30% have the mild form, and may not be aware that they have hemophilia. Female carriers usually have normal coagulation, but in some instances can have severe bleeding as well.

HEENT/AIRWAY: Subgaleal hematoma or cephalohematoma can be seen in the newborn. Bleeding after dental procedures or trauma to the lip or tongue can be severe (saliva has significant fibrinolytic activity). Antifibrinolytics such as epsilon aminocaproic acid (Amicar) or tranexamic acid are useful for control of bleeding in the mouth.

NEUROMUSCULAR: Central nervous system bleeding, usually after trauma, but can also be spontaneous. Severity of the bleeding may not become apparent until several days after the trauma.

ORTHOPEDIC: Hemarthrosis is the most common type of bleeding, especially in the knees, elbows, and ankles, but also in the shoulders, hips, and wrists. Cold packs, brief immobilization and early physiotherapy are indicated for hemarthrosis. Joints only rarely need to be aspirated. Recurrent bleeding can damage synovia, cartilage, and bone, destroying joint function. Epiphyseal damage can cause abnormal bone growth. Bone cysts are a late complication.

GI/GU: Gastrointestinal abnormalities can be associated with excessive gastrointestinal bleeding. Retroperitoneal bleeding. Painless hematuria. Antifibrinolytics such as epsilon aminocaproic acid should be avoided in patients with hematuria to avoid causing clot formation in the ureters.

OTHER: Platelet function and bleeding time are normal. Previously, there was a high incidence of hepatitis B infection and human immunodeficiency virus (HIV) infection because of inadequate testing of blood and factor products and the frequency with which these patients required blood products. This occurs rarely now due to the use of recombinant factor replacement.

MISCELLANEOUS: Hemophilia was a scourge to the male offspring of Queen Victoria. It has been suggested that this was a paternal age effect because there had been no previous hemophilia in the family and her father was 52 years old when she was born.

ANESTHETIC CONSIDERATIONS

Orotracheal intubation is preferred because of the increased risk of bleeding with nasotracheal intubation. Hemostasis after venipuncture or catheter placement in large veins may be a problem. Intramuscular injections should be avoided or given only after treatment with factor VIII. Regional anesthesia is relatively contraindicated, and certainly so without prior treatment with factor VIII and documentation of normal factor level and activated partial thromboplastin time (1). Although newly diagnosed hemophiliacs are now given the hepatitis B vaccine, there was a high incidence of hepatitis B in hemophiliacs in the past. A large number of hemophiliacs were also tragically infected with HIV before adequate testing of blood supplies began. Now that a recombinant preparation is available, viral infections will be less problematic.

Specific therapy may vary slightly, and the following are offered as guidelines only:

For *minor surgery,* patients should receive a loading dose of human factor VIII concentrate of 50 units/kg followed by an infusion of 4 units/kg/hour for 24 hours postoperatively to maintain a factor VIII level of 100%. After 24 hours,

the dosage is changed to every 8 hours for 7 days. For *major surgery,* patients should receive a loading dose of 50 units/kg of human factor VIII concentrate followed by an infusion of 4 units/kg/hour for 7 days. Because of the variable rate of decay of the recombinant factor, levels must be monitored and factor dosing adjusted based on these levels.

For minor nonsurgical soft tissue bleeding, factor VIII activity should be replaced to 20% of normal; for hemarthroses or severe soft tissue bleeds, factor VIII activity should be replaced to at least 40% of normal; for extensive dental work, factor VIII activity should be replaced to at least 70% of normal; for central nervous system bleeds, factor VIII activity should be replaced to 80% to 100% of normal. For central nervous system or retroperitoneal bleeds, treatment may be needed for 7 to 14 days.

One unit of factor VIII per kilogram weight increases the circulating factor VIII activity by 2%. The half-life of factor VIII is 8 hours for the first dose and 12 hours thereafter. There is individual variation, so specific dosing may need to be determined by measuring blood levels.

Factor VIII is available in several preparations:

1. Fresh frozen plasma: 1 unit/mL. This requires the use of excessive volumes.
2. Cryoprecipitate: 80 to 120 units/bag.
3. Human recombinant factor VIII: the concentration of factor VIII varies (usually approximately 40 units/mL).

Desmopressin (DDAVP) has been used in a dose of 0.3 µg/kg for mild (and only mild) cases. DDAVP stimulates the release of von Willebrand factor, which is needed for the proper functioning of factor VIII. The dose of epsilon aminocaproic acid (Amicar) is a loading dose of 100 to 200 mg/kg followed by 75 to 100 mg/kg every 4 to 6 hours orally to a daily maximum of 30 g. The intravenous dose is 100 mg/kg followed by an infusion of 10 to 20 mg/kg/hour. The dose of tranexamic acid is 25 mg/kg every 4 to 6 hours orally. The intravenous dose is 100 mg/kg followed by an infusion of 10 mg/kg/hour. In patients in whom high titers of inhibitors have developed, the use of activated factor VII can be considered.

Bibliography:
1. Shar P, Abramovitz S, DiMichele D, et al. Management of pregnancy in a patient with severe haemophilia A. *Br J Anaesth* 2003;91:432–435.
2. Bolton-Maggs PH, Pasi KJ. Haemophilias A and B. *Lancet* 2003;361:1801–1809.
3. Baujard C, Gouyet L, Murat I. Diagnosis and anaesthesia management of haemophilia during the neonatal period. *Paediatr Anaesth* 1998;8:245–247.
4. Kobayashi M, Matsushita M, Nishikimi N, et al. Treatment for abdominal aortic aneurysm in a patient with hemophilia A: a case report and review of the literature. *J Vasc Surg* 1997;25:945–948.
5. DiMichele D. Hemophilia 1996: new approach to an old disease. *Pediatr Clin North Am* 1996;43:709–736.
6. Zieg PM, Cohn SM, Beardsley DS. Nonoperative management of a splenic tear in a Jehovah's Witness with hemophilia. *J Trauma* 1996;40:299–301.

Hemophilia B

SYNONYM: Christmas disease

MIM #: 306900

This type of hemophilia is due to a defect in the gene that encodes factor IX. It is inherited as an X-linked recessive trait. Female carriers are almost never clinically affected. The clinical manifestations are identical to those of hemophilia A (factor VIII deficiency). See Hemophilia A (earlier) for a discussion of the clinical findings. The activated partial thromboplastin time may be normal in patients with factor IX levels in the 20% to 30% range.

MISCELLANEOUS: The second report of this disease appeared in the December 27 (Christmas) issue of *The British Medical Journal,* and reported a 5-year-old boy with the family name of Christmas (as well as other patients).

ANESTHETIC CONSIDERATIONS
See Hemophilia A (earlier) for a discussion of the general perioperative treatment of hemophilia. Specific treatment for hemophilia B requires the administration of factor IX. This is available in a variety of preparations. A recombinant factor IX preparation (BeneFIX) as well as several plasma-derived preparations are now available. One unit of factor IX per kilogram weight should increase the circulating factor IX activity by 1%. However, preliminary experience with the recombinant preparation suggests that more than this is required. One unit/kg raises the plasma level by 0.4% to 1.4%, and allergic reactions can occur. Treatment will need to be continued postoperatively. The half-life is 18 to 24 hours. Factor IX levels can be measured with a relatively short turnaround time. Hypercoagulability has not been a problem with recombinant factor IX replacement, even when combined with antifibrinolytics. In patients in whom high titers of inhibitors have developed, use of activated factor VII can be considered. The use of fibrin sealants has helped surgical hemostasis and the requirement for protracted postoperative treatment.

For muscle, soft tissue, mucous membrane, or urinary tract bleeding, factor IX activity should be replaced to 40% of normal; for joint bleeding, factor IX activity should be replaced to 60% of normal; for surgery or head or neck trauma, factor IX activity should be replaced to 100% of normal. In general, a loading dose is given to reach the targeted level, followed by an infusion of 8 units/kg/hr.

Bibliography:

1. Bolton-Maggs PH, Pasi KJ. Haemophilias A and B. *Lancet* 2003;361: 1801–1809.
2. Donahue BS, Emerson CW, Slaughter TF. Case 1–1999. Elective and emergency cardiac surgery on a patient with hemophilia B. *J Cardiothorac Vasc Anesth* 1999;13:92–97.
3. Cahill MR, Colvin BT. Haemophilia. *Postgrad Med J* 1997;73:201–206.

Henoch-Schönlein Purpura

SYNONYM: Schönlein-Henoch purpura

MIM #: None

This small-vessel vasculitis is often postinfectious. It causes deposition of immune complexes, primarily IgA and C3, in many organs. The primary findings are a nonthrombocytopenic purpuric rash of the lower abdomen and legs, arthritis, abdominal pain and nephritis. Most cases are self-limited and last approximately 4 weeks. Younger children usually have a shorter course and fewer recurrences. Recurrences can uncommonly occur as late as 2 years after the onset, although renal relapses are not seen after the urine becomes clear.

HEENT/AIRWAY: Patients may have dependent edema. In infants, this tends to be scalp edema.

CHEST: Pulmonary hemorrhage is rare but can be fatal.

NEUROMUSCULAR: Seizures and intracranial hemorrhage are uncommon.

ORTHOPEDIC: Arthritis or arthralgia, particularly of the feet and ankles, and also the knees. This is a periarticular process rather than a true synovitis. Dependent edema.

GI/GU: Colicky abdominal pain. Uncommon complications are intussusception, bowel infarction or perforation, and gastrointestinal tract bleeding. Steroids decrease abdominal pain and probably decrease the incidence of intussusception. Hematuria, proteinuria. Nephritis and progressive renal failure is less common. May have orchitis.

OTHER: Fever, malaise. Nonthrombocytopenic purpuric rash over the lower extremities, less commonly on the arms or face. Onset of the rash can follow the arthritis or abdominal pain. Nonpitting edema of the hands, feet, and face. Anemia. Normal coagulation.

MISCELLANEOUS: Henoch initially had a poor opinion of modern bacteriology, calling it Bakterienschwindel (the swindle of bacteria) in the first edition of his primary work *Vorlesungen über Kinderkrankheiten.* Subsequent editions did not include this opinion. Schönlein published only two papers, and they were only one and three pages long respectively. Nonetheless, it was Schönlein who coined the term "haemophilia."

Osler incorrectly thought this disorder was a consequence of anaphylaxis, and for many years it was referred to as anaphylactoid purpura.

ANESTHETIC CONSIDERATIONS
Peripheral venous access can be difficult secondary to edema. Patients may be whole-body fluid overloaded secondary to

edema, but may be intravascularly hypovolemic. Renal function should be evaluated preoperatively. Renal dysfunction can affect the metabolism of some anesthetic drugs and has implications for the perioperative titration of fluids. Patients may be quite uncomfortable, and may much appreciate care in positioning. Patients taking steroids need to receive perioperative stress doses of steroids.

Bibliography:
1. Saulsbury FT. Henoch-Schönlein purpura in children. Report of 100 patients and review of the literature. *Medicine (Baltimore)* 1999;78:395–409.
2. Tizard EJ. Henoch-Schönlein purpura. *Arch Dis Child* 1999;80:380–383.
3. Piette WW. What is Schönlein-Henoch purpura, and why should we care? *Arch Dermatol* 1997;133:515–518.
4. Szer IS. Henoch-Schönlein purpura: when and how to treat. *J Rheumatol* 1996;23:1661–1665.

Hepatic Phosphorylase b Kinase Deficiency

See Glycogen storage disease type VIII

Hepatolenticular Degeneration

See Wilson disease

Hereditary Angioedema

SYNONYM: C1 esterase inhibitor deficiency; Hereditary angioneurotic edema

MIM #: 106100

This autosomal dominant disorder is due to a deficiency of the serum inhibitor of the first component of complement (C1 esterase inhibitor, C1EI), allowing uncontrolled activation of the classic complement cascade. Type I disease has decreased levels of normal C1EI, whereas the less common type 2 disease has normal or increased levels of a functionally abnormal C1EI. Appropriate biologic activity is confirmed by normal C4 levels in the blood. Abnormal subepithelial edema can form in the skin, abdominal organs, and the upper airway and larynx. Attacks progress over 1 to 2 days and regress over the next 2 or 3 days. Trauma to an extremity, tonsillectomy, and tooth extraction are common initiating events, although often there will be no identifiable initiating event.

Less commonly, the deficiency can be acquired. The acquired form is more common in females than in males, and can be associated with autoimmune or low-grade lymphoproliferative disorders where it is due to increased catabolism of the protein.

Long-term prophylaxis is with the modified androgens danazol (50 to 300 mg/day in adults) or stanazol (also spelled stanozol) (1 to 4 mg/day in adults). Stanazol has fewer side effects. These increase hepatic synthesis of C1EI.

C1EI (obtained from pooled plasma) can be used for acute prophylaxis.

HEENT/AIRWAY: Episodes of airway edema can be precipitated by trauma or emotional upset. Edema can involve the tongue, oral cavity, soft palate, pharynx, and larynx, but not the bronchi, presumably because of local breakdown of kinins by angiotensin-converting enzyme in the lungs. Prophylactic androgens and C1 esterase inhibitors for exacerbations have essentially eliminated airway deaths and airway-related intensive care unit admissions.

GI/GU: Recurrent abdominal pain is a common complaint, sometimes accompanied by nausea and vomiting, or severe diarrhea. Decreased motility can be severe enough to cause a functional bowel obstruction. One-third of patients undergo unnecessary appendectomies or laparotomies. Hypovolemic shock can develop secondary to fluid loss into the peritoneum or bowel wall. There is an increased incidence of polycystic ovaries.

OTHER: Erythema marginatum during an attack. Attacks can occur with menses. The incidence appears to decrease after the first trimester of pregnancy and after menopause. The disease can be exacerbated during adolescence. Dental surgery is more likely to trigger an attack than abdominal surgery. Hypercoagulability (based on the thromboelastogram) was documented in one patient who had coronary artery surgery (3).

MISCELLANEOUS: First described by Quincke, the hereditary nature of the disease was first recognized by Sir William Osler. Before the development of modern therapeutic approaches, there was a significant incidence of fatal laryngeal edema after dental extractions, and one-third of the patients eventually died secondary to airway obstruction. Stanazol figured prominently in the recent steroid abuse scandal in American major league baseball.

ANESTHETIC CONSIDERATIONS

Dental, ear/nose/throat, and endoscopic manipulations are known to have precipitated episodes of edema. Endotracheal intubation should be avoided if possible. Edema can develop hours to days after surgery. Mask general anesthesia and regional anesthesia have not been reported to cause problems, and should be considered preferable if clinically appropriate. There are no apparent contraindications to any routinely used anesthetic drugs. The effect of the laryngeal mask airway (LMA) is not known, but in the absence of further information it should be considered as a source of potential airway trauma, and in any event would not circumvent obstruction from laryngeal edema.

Antihistamines, epinephrine, and steroids are not effective in the treatment of episodes of edema or for emergency preoperative prophylaxis. Perioperative prophylaxis includes increasing the dose of androgen from 6 days before surgery until 3 days after surgery (danazol 600 mg/day in adults or stanazol 6 mg/day in adults). If immediate prophylaxis or treatment of an exacerbation is required, or if androgens are contraindicated, as in pregnancy, C1EI (obtained from pooled plasma) can be used. The dose is 25 units/kg in adults, and the effect lasts 4 to 5 days, but it is currently not available in the United States. Fresh frozen plasma (two units in adults) has been used in lieu of C1EI, but the use of fresh frozen plasma in an emergency is controversial. It does supply C1EI, but it also supplies C2 and C4, which provide additional substrate, and levels of C1EI can be at the same time inadequate. Treatment of an acute episode is limited in the absence of commercially available C1EI. Fresh frozen plasma could be considered in this clinical setting.

If an emergency intubation is required, assistance from an otolaryngologist should be obtained, as an emergency tracheostomy is possible.

Both cardiopulmonary bypass and heparin-protamine complexes activate complement, which can be disastrous, and hemodilution will dilute low but adequate levels of C1EI. Mortality related to complement activation during bypass has been reported (8). However, successful cardiopulmonary bypass has been undertaken after preoperative treatment as outlined previously (7), and off-pump coronary artery surgery is a viable alternative (2).

C1 esterase inhibitor has been used successfully to treat nonhereditary angioedema, such as from angiotensin-converting enzyme (ACE) inhibitors (1).

Bibliography:

1. Nielsen EW, Gramstad S. Angioedema from angiotensin-converting enzyme (ACE) inhibitor treated with complement 1 (C1) inhibitor concentrate. *Acta Anaesthesiol Scand* 2006;50:120–122.
2. Bainbridge DT, Mackensen GB, Newman MF, et al. Off-pump coronary artery bypass surgery in a patient with C1 esterase inhibitor deficiency. *Anesthesiology* 2001;95:795–796.
3. Chaney JD, Adair TM, Lell WA, et al. Hemostatic analysis of a patient with hereditary angioedema undergoing coronary artery bypass grafting. *Anesth Analg* 2001;93:1480–1482.
4. Nzeako UC, Frigas E, Tremaine WJ. Hereditary angioedema: a broad review for clinicians. *Arch Intern Med* 2001;161:2417–2429.
5. Jensen NF, Weiler JM. C1 esterase inhibitor deficiency, airway compromise, and anesthesia. *Anesth Analg* 1998;87:480–488.
6. Cax M, Holdcroft A. Hereditary angioneurotic oedema: current management in pregnancy. *Anaesthesia* 1995;50:547–549.
7. Haering JM, Comunale ME. Cardiopulmonary bypass in hereditary angioedema. *Anesthesiology* 1993;79:1429–1433.
8. Bonser RS, Dave J, Morgan J, et al. Complement activation during bypass in acquired C1 esterase deficiency. *Ann Thorac Surg* 1991;52:541–543.
9. Wall RT, Frank M, Hahn M. A review of 25 patients with hereditary angioedema requiring surgery. *Anesthesiology* 1989;71:309–311.
10. Poppers PJ. Anaesthetic implications of hereditary angioneurotic oedema. *Can J Anaesth* 1987;34:76–78.
11. Smith GB, Shribman AJ. Anaesthesia and severe skin disease. *Anaesthesia* 1984;39:443–455.
12. Hopkinson RB, Sutcliffe J. Hereditary angioneurotic oedema. *Anaesthesia* 1979;34:183–186.
13. Abada RP, Owens WD. Hereditary angioneurotic edema, an anesthetic dilemma. *Anesthesiology* 1977;46:428–430.
14. Gibbs PS, LoSasso AM, Moorthy SS, et al. The anesthetic and perioperative management of a patient with documented hereditary angioneurotic edema. *Anesth Analg* 1977;56:571–573.
15. Hamilton AG, Bosley ARJ, Bowen DJ. Laryngeal oedema due to hereditary angioedema. *Anaesthesia* 1977;32:265–267.

Hereditary Angioneurotic Edema

See Hereditary angioedema

Hereditary Sensory and Autonomic Neuropathy (HSAN)

See Congenital insensitivity to pain and anhydrosis (HSAN IV) and Familial dysautonomia (HSAN III)

Hereditary Fructose Intolerance

SYNONYM: Fructose-1-phosphate aldolase B deficiency

MIM #: 229600

This autosomal recessive disease is caused by the inability to split fructose-1-phosphate into dihydroxyacetone phosphate and glyceraldehyde. This has several sequelae: fructose cannot be converted into glucose in the organs containing this pathway (liver, renal cortex, small bowel mucosa), and there is increased activity of the proximal enzyme in the pathway, fructokinase, so that any fructose causes accumulation of fructose-1-phosphate, which inhibits gluconeogenesis as well as glycogenolysis, causing hypoglycemia and depletion of adenosine triphosphate and guanosine triphosphate stores. Ingestion of fructose is followed shortly by severe hypoglycemia and emesis.

Patients are asymptomatic as long as there is no fructose in the diet, so infants do well while breast-fed, but experience problems when cow's milk formula sweetened with sucrose is added, or when they are fed fruits or vegetables. Patients (or their parents) typically are aware of which foods to avoid, and maintain themselves asymptomatic. The younger the child and the larger the fructose load, the more severe the symptoms. Infants receiving only bottle feedings sweetened with fructose or sucrose can have a fatal reaction. The disease can be encountered occasionally in children with a Reye syndrome-like presentation. Extensive disease in older children or adults is rare.

NEUROMUSCULAR: Lethargy, dizziness, apathy, myoclonic jerks, eventually seizures.

GI/GU: Gastrointestinal discomfort, abdominal distention, diarrhea. Gastrointestinal bleeding. Hepatomegaly, jaundice, ascites. Proximal renal tubule dysfunction with renal tubular acidosis (aminoaciduria, glycosuria, phosphaturia, bicarbonaturia).

OTHER: Hypoglycemia (uncommon and short-lived after fructose ingestion), lactic acidosis. Hyperuricemia when fructose is not restricted. Failure to thrive, nausea, pallor. Bleeding dyscrasia. Growth retardation with chronic ingestion. Can have transient hypermagnesemia from break-down of Mg^{2+} ATP with fructose ingestion.

MISCELLANEOUS: Approximately one half of adult patients are completely without dental caries, presumably from decreased dietary sucrose. Strange food phobias may on occasion be considered to be a psychiatric problem. The first case reported was that of a 24-year-old "spinster." Times change.

ANESTHETIC CONSIDERATIONS
Oral medications that are suspended or dissolved in syrup sweetened with sucrose, fructose, or sorbitol must be avoided. Inadvertent postoperative infusions of fructose, sorbitol, or invert sugar in the past have been fatal, and have been reported primarily in the German literature. Hypoglycemia is unresponsive to glucagon. Fresh frozen plasma or exchange transfusion may be needed for a severe bleeding dyscrasia.

Bibliography:
1. Cox TM. The genetic consequences of our sweet tooth. *Nat Rev Genet* 2002;3:481–487.
2. Cox TM. Aldolase B and fructose intolerance. *FASEB J* 1994;8:62–71.
3. Willems PJ, Gerver WJM, Berger R, et al. The natural history of liver glycogenosis due to phosphorylase kinase deficiency: a longitudinal study of 41 patients. *Eur J Pediatr* 1990;149:268–271.
4. Cox TM. Hereditary fructose intolerance. *Q J Med* 1988;68:585–594.

Hereditary Hemorrhagic Telangiectasia

See Osler-Weber-Rendu syndrome

Hereditary Onychoosteodysplasia

See Nail-patella syndrome

Hereditary Spherocytosis

SYNONYM: Congenital spherocytosis; Spherocytosis

MIM #: 182900

Hereditary spherocytosis is a genetically heterogeneous autosomal dominant form of hemolytic anemia. There is incomplete penetrance with variability in the severity of disease, and 25% of cases are sporadic. The disorder is characterized by mild to moderately severe anemia, spherocytosis on the peripheral blood smear, and marked improvement after splenectomy. Most cases of hereditary spherocytosis are caused by mutations in the genes encoding for ankyrin and/or spectrin, proteins critical to the integrity of the red cell membrane. Ankyrin is the principal binding site for spectrin on the membrane. Deficiencies in ankyrin and/or spectrin lead to abnormal red cell membrane permeability to sodium, a

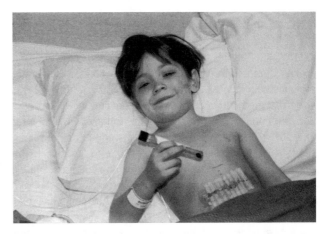

Hereditary spherocytosis. A young boy with congenital spherocytosis posing with his gallstones following a chole-cystectomy and partial splenectomy. His hematocrit was 22 and his total bilirubin 10.4 mg/dL (direct fraction 0.8 mg/dL).

loss of red cell membrane lipids, a decrease in red cell membrane surface area and the formation of the characteristic spherocytes. These cells are rigid and osmotically fragile. The abnormal red blood cells are in turn removed from circulation by the spleen, leading to a clinical picture of anemia and splenomegaly.

GI/GU: Splenomegaly.

OTHER: Mild to moderately severe anemia. Characteristic spherocytes in peripheral blood smear. Neonatal jaundice. May have clinically significant iron overload and formation of bilirubinate gallstones. May have leg ulcers. Clinical symptoms improve significantly after splenectomy.

MISCELLANEOUS: Hereditary spherocytosis was first described by Vanlair and Masius in 1871, and then rediscovered 20 years later by Wilson and Minkowski.

ANESTHETIC CONSIDERATIONS
The patient's hematocrit should be evaluated preoperatively and consideration should be given to the potential need for perioperative transfusion.

Bibliography:
1. Bolton-Maggs PHB, Stevens RF, Dodd NJ, et al. Guidelines for the diagnosis and management of hereditary spherocytosis. *Br J Haematol* 2004;126:455–474.
2. Roth U, Conzen P. Anesthesia and hyperbilirubinemia. *Anaesthesist* 1999;48:654–656.
3. Gallagher PG, Forget BG. Hematologically important mutations: spectrin and ankyrin variants in hereditary spherocytosis. *Blood Cells Mol Dis* 1998;24:539–543.

Hereditary Xanthinuria

See Xanthinuria

Hermansky-Pudlak Syndrome

MIM #: 203300

The hallmarks of this autosomal recessive disorder are oculocutaneous albinism, a bleeding diathesis, and abnormal pigmented reticuloendothelial cells with lysosomal accumulation of ceroid lipofuscin primarily in the lungs and gut. There can be granulomatous colitis or pulmonary fibrosis. The disorder appears to be due to an abnormality of the membranes of lysosomes, melanosomes, and platelet dense bodies. Platelet dense bodies trigger the secondary aggregation of platelets. The responsible gene has been recently identified, and named *HPS*. The gene product has not yet been identified, but it is likely to be a transmembrane protein that is a component of multiple organelles.

HEENT/AIRWAY: Congenital nystagmus, ocular albinism, visual loss (approximately 20/200). Epistaxis. Excessive bleeding after dental extractions.

CHEST: Can have pulmonary fibrosis, which is progressive, beginning with restrictive disease and often becoming fatal in the fourth or fifth decade of life.

CARDIOVASCULAR: May have cardiomyopathy.

GI/GU: Inflammatory bowel disease, especially granulomatous colitis. Abnormal pigmented hepatic reticuloendothelial cells, renal failure.

OTHER: Albinism with variable cutaneous hypopigmentation. Bleeding diathesis, easy bruisability, platelets lack dense bodies and have abnormal aggregation studies. Pigmented reticular cells in bone marrow and lymph glands, lysosomal accumulation of ceroid lipofuscin.

MISCELLANEOUS: The disorder is particularly common in northwest Puerto Rico, and in a small isolated Swiss Alpine village.

ANESTHETIC CONSIDERATIONS

Although pulmonary and cardiac abnormalities are uncommon, a careful evaluation of these organ systems is required preoperatively. Restrictive lung disease can occur. Nasal intubation or the placement of a nasogastric tube should be undertaken with caution because of the increased risk of bleeding. Medications containing aspirin must be avoided. Desmopressin (DDAVP) may be useful in controlling bleeding by improving platelet function. Patients may require perioperative platelet transfusions. Patients who are on chronic steroid therapy require perioperative stress doses of steroids.

Bibliography:
1. Poddar RK, Coley S, Pavord S. Hermansky-Pudlak syndrome in a pregnant patient. *Br J Anaesth* 2004;93:740–742.

2. Huizing M, Anikster Y, Gahl WA. Hermansky-Pudlak syndrome and Chediak-Higashi syndrome: disorders of vesicle formation and trafficking. *Thromb Haemost* 2001;86:233–245.
3. Gahl WA, Brantly M, Kaiser-Kupfer MI, et al. Genetic defects and clinical characteristics of patients with a form of oculocutaneous albinism (Hermansky-Pudlak syndrome). *N Engl J Med* 1998;338:1258–1264.
4. Mahadeo R, Markowitz J, Fisher S, et al. Hermansky-Pudlak syndrome with granulomatous colitis in children. *J Pediatr* 1991;118:904–906.

Hers Disease

SYNONYM: Glycogen storage disease type VI; Liver phosphorylase deficiency; Phosphorylase b kinase deficiency

MIM #: 232700

The taxonomy of the glycogen storage diseases is particularly confusing here. This disorder is caused by an autosomal recessive defect in liver phosphorylase (which can be partially or completely absent). This enzyme is involved in the degradation of glycogen. In the past, Hers disease has also included the X-linked type VIII glycogen storage disease, which has also been called type VIa glycogen storage disease. Previously, hepatic phosphorylase deficiency was called type VIII glycogen storage disease. This is a relatively benign disorder, and most patients with Hers disease do not require specific treatment.

CARDIOVASCULAR: The heart is unaffected.

NEUROMUSCULAR: Normal development and intelligence. Muscles are unaffected with liver phosphorylase deficiency.

ORTHOPEDIC: Growth retardation.

GI/GU: Prominent hepatomegaly with the potential for the development of hepatic adenomas or malignancies. Hepatomegaly usually resolves with age and disappears around the time of puberty. Cirrhosis can develop.

OTHER: Patients may have mild to moderate hypoglycemia and mild ketosis. There is no hyperuricemia.

ANESTHETIC CONSIDERATIONS

A prolonged preoperative fast should be avoided. Serum glucose levels should be monitored perioperatively and adequate perioperative glucose should be ensured. Patients respond normally to glucagon.

FIGURE: See **Appendix E**

Bibliography:
1. Talente GM, Coleman RA, Alter C, et al. Glycogen storage disease in adults. *Ann Intern Med* 1994;120:218–226.

Heterotaxy Syndrome

See Asplenia or Polysplenia

Hexokinase Deficiency

MIM #: 235700

Like phosphofructokinase and pyruvate kinase, hexokinase catalyzes a rate-limiting step in glycolysis. Hexokinase catalyzes the conversion of glucose and adenosine triphosphate to glucose-6-phosphate. Glycolysis is the only energy source available to red blood cells, and deficiency of hexokinase results in a chronic hemolytic anemia. The enzyme has four isozymes, each encoded by its own gene. A variety of alleles for this autosomal recessive disorder have been reported.

GI/GU: Cholelithiasis, cholecystitis. Splenomegaly.

OTHER: Chronic hemolytic anemia with jaundice. A transfusion requirement may be partly ameliorated by splenectomy.

MISCELLANEOUS: Hexokinase deficiency has also been reported as part of Fanconi anemia, but that defect also involves deficient platelet and white blood cell hexokinase, which are normal in this hexokinase deficiency. A model in the mouse is called "downeast anemia."

ANESTHETIC CONSIDERATIONS
The patient's hematocrit should be evaluated preoperatively, and consideration should be given to the potential need for perioperative transfusions.

Bibliography:
1. Gelsanz F, Meyer E, Paglia DE, et al. Congenital hemolytic anemia due to hexokinase deficiency. *Am J Dis Child* 1978;132:636–637.
2. Beutler E, Dyment PG, Matsumoto E. Hereditary nonspherocytic hemolytic anemia and hexokinase deficiency. *Blood* 1978;51:935–940.

HHH Syndrome

SYNONYM: Hyperornithinemia-hyperammonemia-homocitrullinuria syndrome

MIM #: 238970

This autosomal recessive disorder is due to mutations in the gene *SLC25A15*. This gene encodes a transporter (ORNT1) which moves ornithine across the inner mitochondrial membrane from cytosol to mitochondrial matrix. Infants do well until breast-feeding is discontinued and a protein-rich diet begun. Patients often self-select a low-protein diet and avoid milk and meat. Symptoms are related to hyperammonemia, and are similar to the urea cycle defects. It is likely that early intervention with arginine, ornithine, or citrulline may effect a favorable neurologic prognosis (3). Onset can be from childhood to adulthood. A second mitochondrial transporter, ORNT2, when overexpressed, can minimize the effects of the disorder.

HEENT/AIRWAY: Retinal depigmentation.

NEUROMUSCULAR: Periodic neurologic symptoms develop with high protein intake and include episodic confusion, lethargy, ataxia, and choreoathetosis. Delayed milestones. Progressive spastic paraplegia-hypotonia early, with spasticity late. Seizures. Intelligence is low normal to severely retarded.

GI/GU: Episodic vomiting.

OTHER: Failure to thrive, growth failure. Hyperornithinemia, postprandial hyperammonemia, homocitrullinuria. A bleeding diathesis has been described in a few patients.

ANESTHETIC CONSIDERATIONS
Patients should be maintained on a low-protein diet perioperatively. Succinylcholine may be contraindicated in patients with muscle disuse because of the risk of an exaggerated hyperkalemic response. An orogastric tube or throat packs should be placed if the surgery has the potential to cause oral or intestinal bleeding because blood in the gastrointestinal tract provides a protein load that may lead to the development of hyperammonemia. Chronic use of anticonvulsant medications may alter the metabolism of some anesthetic drugs.

FIGURE: See **Appendix C**

Bibliography:
1. Muhling J, Dehne MG, Fuchs M, et al. Conscientious metabolic monitoring on a patient with hyperornithinemia-hyperammonemia-homocitrullinemia (HHH) syndrome undergoing anaesthesia. *Amino Acids* 2001;21:303–318.
2. Urea Cycle Disorders Conference group. Consensus statement from a conference for the management of patients with urea cycle disorders. *J Pediatr* 2001;138(S1–5).
3. Zammarchi E, Ciani F, Pasquini E, et al. Neonatal onset of hyperornithinemia-hyperammonemia-homocitrullinuria syndrome with favorable outcome. *J Pediatr* 1997;131:440–443.
4. Lemay JF, Lambert MA, Mitchell GA, et al. Hyperammonemia-hyperornithinemia-homocitrullinuria syndrome: neurologic, ophthalmologic, and neuropsychologic examination of 6 patients. *J Pediatr* 1992;121:725–730.

Hirschsprung Disease

MIM #: 142623

Hirschsprung disease is colonic aganglionosis, which results in a functional rectal or colonic obstruction. The normal *in utero* craniocaudal progression of neural crest cells is arrested in this disorder, with subsequent absence of distal myenteric and submucosal ganglia. The diagnosis can be made on rectal biopsy. In infants, a colostomy is done for decompression, followed approximately a year later by a definitive "pull-through" procedure. The affected segment, of variable length, is chronically contracted.

Although long thought to be inherited as an autosomal recessive trait, defects in one or more genes, both autosomal dominant and autosomal recessive, can be responsible for this disease. These include the *RET* gene, the gene for endothelin receptor type B, the gene for endothelin-3, and the gene for glial cell line-derived neurotrophic factor. There is a male predominance.

There is an association of Hirschsprung disease with Ondine's curse, or central hypoventilation syndrome (see later). Although only a small number of patients with Hirschsprung disease have Ondine's curse, approximately 50% of children with Ondine's curse can have Hirschsprung disease. There is also an increased incidence of Hirschsprung disease in a variety of neurocristopathy and nonneurocristopathy syndromes, such as Down syndrome, Bardet-Biedl syndrome, Smith-Lemli-Opitz syndrome, and Waardenburg syndrome (1), among others.

HEENT/AIRWAY: Bicolored iris has been described.

NEUROMUSCULAR: Central hypoventilation ("Ondine's curse") has been reported.

GI/GU: Colonic or rectal aganglionosis. Failure to pass neonatal meconium. Vomiting on the first day or two of life. Patients may present with enterocolitis resembling sepsis or necrotizing enterocolitis. The affected segment is of variable length, and may be very short, which makes the clinical diagnosis more challenging. A barium enema in neonates may not show the typical transition of normal to abnormal bowel seen in older patients. Therapy is an initial colostomy followed approximately a year later by a definitive pull-through operation, although earlier definitive repair has been proposed.

May have Meckel diverticulum. Increased incidence of megaureter, megacystis, cryptorchidism, cystic renal disease, bladder diverticulae, hypoplastic uterus.

MISCELLANEOUS: The high incidence of Hirschsprung disease in association with the central hypoventilation syndrome ("Ondine's curse") has led to the suggestion that Ondine-Hirschsprung disease is a synonym for this disease, and a mutation in the receptor tyrosine kinase (RET) protooncogene has been documented in a child with Ondine-Hirschsprung syndrome.

Harald Hirschsprung was the first Danish pediatrician. He was appointed as director of the Queen Louisa Hospital for Children. Queen Louisa requested that Biblical texts be placed over each bed. When Hirschsprung insisted on placing pictures of animals there, the Queen refused to enter the hospital. Hirschsprung frequently offered his medical lectures only on Sunday mornings, to be certain that only those students who were truly interested would attend.

ANESTHETIC CONSIDERATIONS

Neonates frequently present with vomiting, and are at risk for dehydration and perioperative aspiration. Adequate preoperative intravenous rehydration should occur and a rapid sequence induction of anesthesia should be undertaken.

Bibliography:
1. Swenson O. Hirschsprung's disease: a review. *Pediatrics* 2002;109:914–918.
2. Coran AG, Teitelbaum DH. Recent advances in the management of Hirschsprung's disease. *Am J Surg* 2000;180:382–387.
3. Croaker GD, Shi E, Simpson E, et al. Congenital central hypoventilation syndrome and Hirschsprung's disease. *Arch Dis Child* 1998;78:316–322.
4. Passarge E. Wither polygenic inheritance: mapping Hirschsprung disease. *Nat Genet* 1993;4:325–326.

Histidinemia

MIM #: 235800

This autosomal recessive disease is due to deficient activity of the enzyme histidine ammonia-lyase (histidase). This enzyme catalyzes the first step in the deamination of histidine, the conversion of histidine to *trans*-urocanic acid. Urocanic acid has been proposed to have an ultraviolet protective effect, and urocanase is not present in the epidermis.

Contrary to earlier suggestions, it is now thought that this is a benign disease. Histidinemia might potentiate the central nervous system effects of other processes, such as perinatal hypoxia, explaining the abnormal findings in some patients. Alternatively, ascertainment bias is possible, because earlier cases were identified in patients who came to medical attention for other problems, such as developmental disorders. Later cases have been ascertained by neonatal screening and there has been no increased incidence of clinical abnormalities. A histidine restricted diet has been shown to have no effect.

MISCELLANEOUS: This disorder is particularly common among French-Canadians and the Japanese.

ANESTHETIC CONSIDERATIONS
There are no specific anesthetic considerations.

Bibliography:
1. Lam WK, Cleary MA, Wraith JE, et al. Histidinaemia: a benign metabolic disorder. *Arch Dis Child* 1996;74:343–346.

Histiocytosis X

See Langerhans cell histiocytosis

Holocarboxylase Synthetase Deficiency

SYNONYM: Multiple carboxylase deficiency

MIM #: 253270

This autosomal recessive disease is closely related to biotinidase deficiency (the other multiple carboxylase deficiency, see earlier). Biotin, a B vitamin, is a cofactor for four carboxylases: pyruvate carboxylase, propionyl CoA carboxylase, beta-methylcrotonyl CoA carboxylase, and acetyl CoA carboxylase. Holocarboxylase synthetase attaches biotin to the inactive apoenzyme. Abnormalities in this enzyme result in defective activity of all of these carboxylases, and holocarboxylase synthetase deficiency is thus a cause of multiple carboxylase deficiency. Biotinidase liberates biotin from a proteolytic enzyme degradation product. While there is some overlap, holocarboxylase synthetase deficiency presents in the neonatal period, and is usually fatal if untreated, while biotinidase deficiency typically presents after several months of life. Acute episodes are triggered by intercurrent infection or increased protein intake, and involve ketoacidosis and hyperammonemia. Treatment with biotin should correct all symptoms (unless fixed, such as optic atrophy), although some poorly biotin-responsive forms have been reported. Isolated abnormalities in the carboxylase enzymes have been reported and are biotin unresponsive.

HEENT/AIRWAY: Conjunctivitis, optic atrophy, myopia, abnormal retinal pigment. Auditory nerve atrophy with hearing loss. Laryngeal stridor has been reported in the closely related biotinidase deficiency.

CHEST: Tachypnea and Kussmaul breathing from ketoacidosis.

NEUROMUSCULAR: Lethargy, hypotonia, ataxia, seizures, coma during acute episodes. May have psychomotor developmental delay. May have subependymal cysts.

GI/GU: Feeding difficulty, vomiting. Odd smelling urine.

OTHER: Potentially fatal episodes of ketoacidosis, lactic acidosis and hyperammonemia. Organic aciduria. Hypothermia. Bright red, scaly rash over the body, particularly in the diaper and intertriginous areas. Alopecia totalis. Abnormal T-cell and B-cell function.

ANESTHETIC CONSIDERATIONS
Treatment with biotin should be continued perioperatively. It is not known whether perioperative stress and catabolism can provoke an acute episode in this disorder. Patients are at risk for perioperative aspiration because of the increased risk of feeding difficulties and vomiting. Good aseptic technique is indicated in these patients who are likely to have T- and B-cell dysfunction. Chronic use of anticonvulsant medications may alter the metabolism of some anesthetic drugs. Intravenous hyperalimentation must include biotin.

Bibliography:
1. Morrone A, Malvagia S, Donati MA, et al. Clinical findings and biochemical and molecular analysis of four patients with holocarboxylase synthetase deficiency. *Am J Med Genet* 2002;111:10–18.
2. Sweetman L, Nyhan WL. Inheritable biotin-treatable disorders and associated phenomena. *Annu Rev Nutr* 1986;6:317–343.

Holoprosencephaly Sequence

MIM #: 236100

Most cases of holoprosencephaly are sporadic and the exact cause remains unknown. Association with at least 12 genetic loci has been proposed. Anomalous development of the prechordal mesoderm leads to failure of cleavage of the prosencephalon, which results in midline facial defects and defects in the development of the forebrain into two hemispheres. A spectrum of anomalies can result, which can vary from severe (cyclopia with a severely malformed forebrain) to mild (hypotelorism, varying degrees of forebrain malformation). Cleft lip and palate are a frequent manifestation of the midline facial defect. Although most cases of holoprosencephaly are sporadic, this developmental disorder can be secondary to teratogenic effects, such as is seen among infants of diabetic mothers, who are at increased risk for holoprosencephaly. In addition, some cases of holoprosencephaly are genetic, due to abnormalities in one of several genes, one of which is the gene *sonic hedgehog*. There is an autosomal dominant form of holoprosencephaly. Also, holoprosencephaly has been seen in association with trisomy 13, trisomy 18, some of the deletion syndromes, CHARGE syndrome, Meckel-Gruber syndrome, Pallister-Hall syndrome, Smith-Lemli-Opitz syndrome, and velocardiofacial syndrome.

HEENT/AIRWAY: Cebocephaly ("monkey-like" head—hypotelorism, nasal defects). Microcephaly. Variable defects of midline facial development, including hypotelorism, nasal defects, absence of the philtrum, absence of the superior labial frenulum, cleft lip and palate, bifid uvula, and a single central maxillary incisor. In its most severe manifestation, cyclopia with a proboscis above the single eye.

CARDIOVASCULAR: Cardiac defects include dextrocardia and ventricular septal defects.

NEUROMUSCULAR: Arhinencephaly (absence of the rhinencephalon). Intellectual development may be extremely limited. Apnea. Seizures. Can have pituitary deficiency or absence.

GI/GU: Can have malrotation of the gut, bile duct stenosis.

ANESTHETIC CONSIDERATIONS
The oral and median facial defects may make both mask ventilation and endotracheal intubation very difficult. Perioperative temperature instability, seizures and periodic apnea may all affect anesthetic management. Hypernatremia from acute worsening of underlying subclinical diabetes insipidus following surgical stress has been reported (1). Chronic use of anticonvulsant medications may alter the metabolism of some anesthetic drugs.

Bibliography:

1. Tung A, Anderson J, Daves S, et al. Hypernatremia after cleft lip repair in a patient with holoprosencephaly [Letter]. *Anesth Analg* 2006;103:965–966.
2. Goodman FR. Congenital abnormalities of body patterning: embryology revisited. *Lancet* 2003;362:651–662.
3. Corsello G, Buttitta P, Cammarata M, et al. Holoprosencephaly: examples of clinical variability and etiologic heterogeneity. *Am J Med Genet* 1990;37:244–249.
4. Katende RS, Herlich A. Anesthetic considerations in holoprosencephaly. *Anesth Analg* 1987;66:908–910.

Holt-Oram Syndrome

SYNONYM: Cardiac-limb syndrome; Heart–hand syndrome

MIM #: 142900

This autosomal dominant disorder is characterized by cardiac anomalies, primarily atrial septal defect, and upper limb defects. There is marked variability of expression, with some affected people having only radiographic evidence of the syndrome. The severity of the limb defects does not correlate with the severity of the cardiac defect. Patients with only limb defects can have children with the full syndrome. This syndrome is due to a mutation in the gene T-box 5 (*TBX5*). Members of the T-box gene family act as transcription factors, whose expression is tissue specific. The product of *TBX5* promotes cardiomyocyte differentiation. Different mutations can apparently result in the full syndrome, or solely cardiac or limb manifestations.

HEENT/AIRWAY: May have hypertelorism.

CHEST: May have pectus excavatum, thoracic scoliosis.

CARDIOVASCULAR: Various cardiac anomalies, primarily atrial septal defect (ostium secundum type), but also ventricular septal defect, patent ductus arteriosus, mitral valve prolapse, aortic stenosis, pulmonic stenosis, and others. May have conduction abnormalities.

ORTHOPEDIC: Variable, often asymmetric, upper limb defects, including absent, hypoplastic, or triphalangeal thumbs, hypoplastic digits, syndactyly, polydactyly, absent carpal ossification centers, hypoplastic radius, decreased mobility at the elbows, and phocomelia. Shoulders are narrow and sloping. May have vertebral anomalies. May have absent pectoralis major muscle.

MISCELLANEOUS: Mary Holt was Samuel Oram's assistant. Oram said that her name preceded his as she was a lady, and it seemed only proper.

ANESTHETIC CONSIDERATIONS

Even patients with only minimal upper limb defects should receive a cardiac examination and possibly an echocardiogram because the severity of the limb defects does not correlate with the severity of the cardiac defect. Peripheral vascular access may be difficult in patients with significant limb anomalies. Upper limb defects may make fixation of an appropriate-sized blood pressure cuff difficult, and falsely high pressures may be displayed by noninvasive monitors. An appropriate blood pressure cuff should cover two-thirds of the upper arm. Patients with congenital heart disease need perioperative antibiotic prophylaxis as indicated, bearing in mind that isolated secundum atrial septal defect does not require prophylaxis.

Bibliography:

1. Li QY, Newbury-Ecob RA, Terrett JA, et al. Holt-Oram syndrome is caused by mutations in TBX5, a member of the Brachyury (T) gene family. *Nat Genet* 1997;15:21–29.
2. Newbury-Ecob RA, Leanage R, Raeburn JA, et al. Holt-Oram syndrome: a clinical genetic study. *J Med Genet* 1996;33:300–307.
3. Sletten LJ, Pierpont ME. Variation in severity of cardiac disease in Holt-Oram syndrome. *Am J Med Genet* 1996;65:128–132.
4. Hasson CT, Cowley GS, Solomon SD, et al. The clinical and genetic spectrum of the Holt-Oram syndrome (heart-hand syndrome). *N Engl J Med* 1994;330:885–891.

Homocystinuria

MIM #: 236200

Homocystinuria is the second most common disease of amino acid metabolism. There are three types of homocystinuria. The most common or classic type (type I) is an autosomal recessive disease due to a defect in cystathionine synthetase, which catalyzes the synthesis of cystathionine from homocysteine and serine. This results in a defect in transsulfuration of the precursors of cysteine, which in turn results in the weakened cross-linking of collagen. There are two variants of type I (classic) homocystinuria, one which is vitamin B_6 (pyridoxine) responsive, and the other which is unresponsive. Homocystinuria can also be caused by defects in the enzymes tetrahydrofolate methyltransferase (type II) or tetrahydrofolate reductase (type III), which are also involved in the metabolism of methionine to cystathionine.

Low methionine diets, although likely beneficial, are relatively unpalatable and poorly tolerated. There has been interest shown in treatment with betaine, a methyl donor, increasing homocysteine methylation.

HEENT/AIRWAY: Lens dislocation is common, and uniform after 10 years of age. Myopia. Less commonly, can have glaucoma, optic atrophy, retinal degeneration, cataracts. High-arched palate.

CHEST: Pectus excavatum. Spontaneous pneumothorax, though rare, has been reported in pyridixine-unresponsive patients.

CARDIOVASCULAR: Increased risk of premature coronary vascular disease with myocardial infarction. Thrombi in major arteries and veins. Thromboembolic events can occur

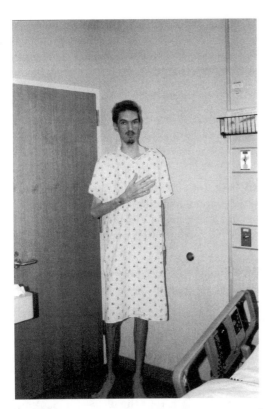

Homocystinuria. This 19-year-old with homocystinuria and scoliosis has an obvious Marfanoid habitus. He is 6″ 7″ (201 cm) tall; his father is only 6′ (183 cm).

during childhood and adolescence. Hypertrophy of the carotid wall.

NEUROMUSCULAR: May have mental retardation; intelligence normal in approximately one-third. Seizures. Risk of cerebrovascular accidents. Cerebral angiography has been associated with fatal thrombosis.

ORTHOPEDIC: Marfanoid habitus. Osteoporosis beginning in childhood or adolescence, scoliosis.

GI/GU: Pancreatitis with pseudocyst formation has been reported. The urine can have a foul odor.

OTHER: Spontaneous thromboemboli, presumably from either fraying of collagen in vessel media with loss of overlying endothelium, or from activation of Hageman factor by homocysteine. These can be arterial or venous. This is a cause of early death. Hypercoagulability has been shown on thromboelastography. Hypopigmentation, reversible in pyridoxine-responsive disease.

There is hyperinsulinemia from pancreatic exposure to elevated levels of sulfur-containing amino acids such as methionine. There can be secondary hypoglycemia.

The disease is diagnosed by the presence of homocysteine and elevated levels of methionine in the urine. Also, when tested with nitroprusside, the urine turns magenta in color.

MISCELLANEOUS: Phenotypically somewhat similar to Marfan syndrome. One differentiating feature is that mental retardation can be associated with homocystinuria. Another differentiating feature is that the optic lens dislocates down in homocystinuria, and up in Marfan syndrome.

The incidence of premature vascular disease in homocystinuria prompted a prospective study that associated elevated homocysteine levels with increased risk of mortality in (nonhomocystinuric) adult patients with coronary artery disease (3).

ANESTHETIC CONSIDERATIONS
The cardiovascular status and risk of coronary artery disease should be evaluated preoperatively. Because of the risk of hypoglycemia in type I disease, prolonged preoperative fasting should be avoided and patients should receive glucose-containing intravenous fluid perioperatively.

Because of the risk of thromboembolism, factors encouraging tissue perfusion (good cardiac output, adequate hydration, avoidance of stasis, pneumatic stockings, early ambulation) should be encouraged. Perioperative dextran infusions have been used in an effort to decrease perioperative thrombosis. Heparin appears to be ineffective. Dipyridamole may help normalize platelet dysfunction, but results have been mixed.

Nitrous oxide inhibits the activity of the enzyme methionine synthase, which converts homocysteine to methionine, and thereby raises homocysteine levels. It has been suggested that, at least for anesthetics of longer duration, nitrous oxide not be used (4), and a fatal outcome in a patient with type III has been reported.

Bibliography:
1. Yamada T, Hamada H, Mochizuki S, et al. General anesthesia for patient [sic] with type III homocystinuria (tetrahydrofolate reductase deficiency. *J Clin Anesth* 2005;17:565–567.
2. Selzer RR, Rosenblatt DS, Laxova R, et al. Adverse effect of nitrous oxide in a child with 5,10-methylenetetrahydrofolate reductase deficiency. *N Engl J Med* 2003;349:49–50.
3. Nygard O, Nordrehaug JE, Refsum H, et al. Plasma homocysteine levels and mortality in patients with coronary artery disease. *N Engl J Med* 1997;337:230–236.
4. Koblin DD. Homocystinuria and administration of nitrous oxide [Letter]. *J Clin Anesth* 1995;7:176.
5. Lowe S, Johnson DA, Tobias JD. Anesthetic implications of the child with homocystinuria. *J Clin Anesth* 1994;6:142–144.
6. Paris MCV, Quimby CW. Anesthetic considerations for the patient with homocystinuria. *Anesth Analg* 1982;61:708–710.

Hunter Syndrome

SYNONYM: Mucopolysaccharidosis II

MIM #: 309900

This X-linked recessive disorder is caused by the absence of the lysosomal enzyme iduronate sulfatase, with subsequent storage of dermatan sulfate and heparan sulfate in a wide variety of tissues. Characteristics of the disease usually become

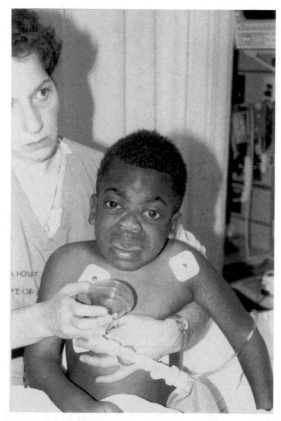

Hunter syndrome. This 7-year-old boy required anesthesia for a magnetic resonance imaging scan. He has a history of obstructive sleep apnea and very difficult intubations. His macroglossia is easily appreciated. He also has pebbled skin, a thickened, prolapsed mitral valve, and recurrent otitis media. The anesthetic was performed easily using a laryngeal mask airway.

apparent by 2 to 4 years of age. Severe Hunter syndrome can be differentiated from the phenotypically similar Hurler syndrome (mucopolysaccharidosis IH, see later) by having generally less mental retardation, joint disease, and organ involvement, as well as clear corneas, no gibbus deformity of the spine, and a more gradual onset of the physical characteristics. A milder disease, similar to Hurler/Scheie or Scheie syndromes (see later), it can be differentiated by normal intelligence and slower progression of disease.

HEENT/AIRWAY: Macrocephaly, scaphocephaly, coarse facial features. Atypical retinitis pigmentosa. Hearing loss and recurrent ear infections. Patients often have macroglossia and are mouth breathers. The soft tissues of the mouth and lips are often stiff and can be manipulated only with difficulty. There can be hypertrophy of the adenoids and tonsils and copious oral secretions. The temporomandibular joints are stiff. Infiltration of soft tissues can limit neck mobility. There is mucopolysaccharide deposited in the tissues of the upper airway. The larynx appears to be shifted anteriorly and cephalad with the continued mucopolysaccharide deposition that occurs with aging.

CHEST: Pectus excavatum or carinatum, spatulated ribs. Recurrent upper respiratory tract infections. Patients with a mucopolysaccharidosis are susceptible to pulmonary hemorrhage after bone marrow transplantation. May have sleep apnea.

CARDIOVASCULAR: Can have coronary artery narrowing and ischemic cardiac disease. Can have thickening of cardiac valves.

NEUROMUSCULAR: Progressive mild mental retardation, or can have normal intelligence. Communicating hydrocephalus due to meningeal thickening. Can have cervical spinal canal narrowing with cord compression.

ORTHOPEDIC: Stiff joints, carpal tunnel syndrome, kyphosis, beaking of the lumbar vertebrae.

GI/GU: Hepatosplenomegaly, prominent abdomen. Inguinal and umbilical hernias. Chronic diarrhea.

OTHER: Hypertrichosis, "pebbled" skin.

MISCELLANEOUS: Charles Hunter was a Scotsman who practiced medicine in Winnipeg, Manitoba. He was for a period of time Professor of Medicine at the University of Manitoba, but objected to the bureaucratic administrative side of the position and resigned, but continued to teach and maintain a private practice.

ANESTHETIC CONSIDERATIONS

Laryngoscopy and tracheal intubation can be extraordinarily difficult secondary to a variety of airway problems, including copious oral secretions, macroglossia, hypertrophy of the adenoids and tonsils, stiff temporomandibular joints, limited neck mobility, and mucopolysaccharide deposits in the tissues of the upper airway and larynx. An oropharyngeal airway can worsen airway obstruction by pushing down a long, high epiglottis over the larynx. A nasopharyngeal airway may help, but on occasions advancement is difficult because of mucopolysaccharide deposits. The laryngeal mask airway (LMA) has been used successfully in patients with mucopolysaccharidoses (4); however, a case of airway obstruction from a LMA pushing down a large laryngeal polyp has also been reported (2). Consideration should be given to administering anticholinergic premedication to dry up oral secretions. Patients should be observed closely in the postanesthesia care unit for evidence of airway compromise. Postobstructive pulmonary edema has been reported.

A case of delayed awakening after a single, small dose of fentanyl has been reported (6). Patients must be carefully positioned intraoperatively secondary to stiff joints. Patients with cardiac valve involvement require perioperative antibiotic prophylaxis as indicated.

Bibliography:

1. Walker RWM, Colovic V, Robinson DN, et al. Postobstructive pulmonary oedema during anaesthesia in children with mucopolysaccharidoses. *Paediatr Anaesth* 2003;13:441–447.
2. Busoni P, Fognani G. Failure of the laryngeal mask to secure the airway in a patient with Hunter's syndrome (mucopolysaccharidosis type II). *Paediatr Anaesth* 1999;9:153–155.
3. Yoskovitch A, Tewfik TL, Brouillette RT, et al. Acute airway obstruction in Hunter syndrome. *Int J Pediatr Otorhinolaryngol* 1998;44:273–278.
4. Walker RWM, Allen DL, Rothera MR. A fibreoptic intubation technique for children with mucopolysaccharidoses using the laryngeal mask airway. *Paediatr Anaesth* 1997;7:421–426.
5. Moores C, Rogers JG, McKenzie IM, et al. Anaesthesia for children with mucopolysaccharidoses. *Anaesth Intensive Care* 1996;24:459–463.
6. Kreidstein A, Boorin MR, Crespi P, et al. Delayed awakening from general anaesthesia in a patient with Hunter syndrome. *Can J Anaesth* 1994;41:423–426.
7. Walker RWM, Darowski M, Morris P. Anaesthesia and mucopolysaccharidoses: a review of airway problems in children. *Anaesthesia* 1994;49:1078–1084.
8. Diaz JH, Belani K. Perioperative management of children with mucopolysaccharidoses. *Anesth Analg* 1993;77:1261–1270.
9. Mahoney A, Soni N, Vellodi A. Anaesthesia and the mucopolysaccharidoses: a review of patients treated by bone marrow transplantation. *Paediatr Anaesth* 1992;2:317–324.
10. Berkowitz I, Raja S, Bender K, et al. Dwarfs: pathophysiology and anesthetic implications. *Anesthesiology* 1990;73:739–759.
11. Herrick IA, Rhine EJ. The mucopolysaccharidoses and anaesthesia: a report of clinical experience. *Can J Anaesth* 1988;35:67–73.
12. Sjogren P, Pedersen T, Steinmetz H. Mucopolysaccharidoses and anaesthetic risks. *Acta Anaesthesiol Scand* 1987;31:214–218.
13. King DH, Jones RM, Barrett MB. Anaesthetic considerations in the mucopolysaccharidoses. *Anaesthesia* 1984;39:126–131.
14. Baines D, Kenneally J. Anaesthetic management of the mucopolysaccharidoses: a fifteen-year experience in a children's hospital. *Anaesth Intensive Care* 1983;11:198–202.
15. Kempthorne PM, Brown TCK. Anaesthesia and the mucopolysaccharidoses: a survey of techniques and problems. *Anaesth Intensive Care* 1983;11:203–207.

Hurler Syndrome

SYNONYM: Mucopolysaccharidosis IH

MIM #: 607014

This autosomal recessive disorder is due to an abnormality in alpha-L-iduronidase, which is involved in the degradation of glycosaminoglycans (mucopolysaccharides). Deficiency of alpha-L-iduronidase can result in three related clinical syndromes with significant phenotypic variability: (a) Hurler, (b) Scheie and (c) the intermediate Hurler-Scheie syndromes (see later for both), and these more correctly represent a spectrum of mucopolysaccharidosis I, with Hurler syndrome at the severe end of the spectrum, Scheie at the mild end, and Hurler-Scheie intermediate. Hurler syndrome can be differentiated from the phenotypically similar Hunter syndrome (mucopolysaccharidosis II, see earlier) by showing a greater degree of mental retardation, joint disease, and organ involvement, as well as corneal opacities, a gibbus deformity of the spine, and a more rapid onset of the physical characteristics.

Death is usually at several years of age from obstructive airway disease, respiratory infection, or cardiac

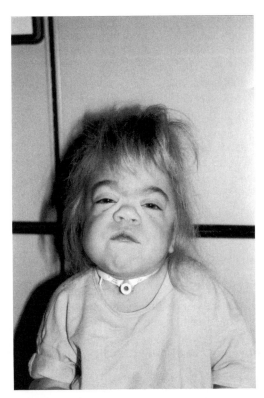

Hurler syndrome. This 4-year-old girl with Hurler syndrome had a recent tracheostomy.

complications. Treatment with recombinant human alpha-L-iduronidase can significantly improve some clinical manifestations of the disease, and bone marrow transplantation has provided very good long-term results. It is expected that a larger number of older patients will be seen with this disease due to these treatments (1). Cord blood transplantation has also been used successfully, with improved results when patients are under 2 years of age. Bone marrow transplantation appears to have minimal effect on the progression of skeletal disease.

HEENT/AIRWAY: Macrocephaly, scaphocephaly, coarse facies. Corneal opacities. Can develop glaucoma. Hearing loss (combination of both sensorineural and conductive). Recurrent middle ear infections. The tongue, tonsils, adenoids, and lips are large. The sphenoid can approximate the hard palate, and the nasopharynx can be further occluded by adenoidal tissue. Patients are often mouth breathers and have copious nasal discharge. The teeth are widely spaced and peg-like, and there are dental cysts. The trachea can be narrowed and flattened. Granulomatous tissue can be present in the trachea and lower respiratory tract. Obstructive sleep apnea. The epiglottis may be situated higher than normal because of small cervical vertebrae, and the epiglottis and aryepiglottic folds may be infiltrated. Short neck.

CHEST: Oar-like ribs (broad at the sternal ends). Spine deformities and hepatosplenomegaly can inhibit pulmonary function. Recurrent upper respiratory tract infections. Glycosaminoglycan deposition in the lower airway and pulmonary interstitium can cause obstructive disease and a diffusion defect. Distal tracheal obstruction may develop and be extremely problematic. Patients with a mucopolysaccharidosis are susceptible to pulmonary hemorrhage after bone marrow transplantation.

CARDIOVASCULAR: Can have coronary artery narrowing and ischemic cardiac disease. Since coronary artery involvement is diffuse, the extent of the disease may be underestimated by coronary angiography. Valvular defects, particularly mitral valve thickening. Infants with fatal cardiomyopathy have been reported.

NEUROMUSCULAR: Mental retardation. Enlarged, "J"-shaped sella turcica. Communicating hydrocephalus, usually associated with increased intracranial pressure. Can have thickened meninges resulting in hydrocephalus or myelopathy from cord compression.

ORTHOPEDIC: Small stature. Can have a hypoplastic odontoid with atlantoaxial subluxation. Joint contractures. Early kyphoscoliosis, lumbar lordosis. Thoracolumbar gibbus deformity. Deformed lower thoracic and upper lumbar vertebrae, pelvic dysplasia, shortened tubular bones, expanded diaphyses with dysplastic epiphyses. Brachydactyly. Coxa valga with poorly formed pelvis and small femoral heads. Flexion deformity of the hip.

GI/GU: Hepatosplenomegaly. Inguinal and umbilical hernias. Alternating constipation and diarrhea.

OTHER: Thick skin, hypertrichosis.

MISCELLANEOUS: Gertrud Hurler pronounced her name "Hooler." This mispronunciation has apparently even extended to German physicians, which has been bemoaned (11). The first case was actually presented to the Munich Pediatric Society by her chief, Pfaundler, but was written by Hurler (described by Wiedemann as "ambitious"). A defect in lysosomal alpha-L-iduronidase also occurs in Plott hound dogs.

ANESTHETIC CONSIDERATIONS
Hurler syndrome is "the worst airway problem in pediatric anesthesia" (19). Because of the abnormal facies, a regular pediatric mask may not fit adequately, and it has been suggested that in these cases the mask be applied upside-down, with the narrower nasal bridge over the mouth (9). Thickening of the soft tissues, an enlarged tongue, a short, immobile neck, and limited mobility of the cervical spine and temporomandibular joints make laryngoscopy extremely difficult. Laryngoscopy may become more difficult with age, particularly after approximately 2 years of age. There is a high incidence of difficult or failed intubation. An oral airway has been reported to displace the epiglottis downward,

impairing flow though the larynx. Nasal airways have proven to be more effective without this complication (17), but on occasion advancement is difficult because of mucopolysaccharide deposits in the nose. Fiberoptic intubation of older patients has been reported (1, 13), and the laryngeal mask airway (LMA) has been used successfully (6, 8), although a case of inability to ventilate or intubate through an LMA due to abnormal laryngeal anatomy has been reported (4). Neck manipulation to improve the airway is risky in the presence of cervical spine instability. Bone marrow transplantation may decrease the difficulty of intubation when transplantation is done in the first 2 years of life (2). A case of failed epidural block despite good placement of the catheter has been reported and ascribed to possible deposition of mucopolysaccharide in the epidural space or on the nerve sheaths (5). Postoperative respiratory complications are common, and patients should be observed closely in the postanesthesia care unit for evidence of airway compromise. Postobstructive pulmonary edema has been reported.

Patients must be carefully positioned intraoperatively secondary to joint contractures. Patients with valvar cardiac disease need perioperative antibiotic prophylaxis as indicated.

Bibliography:

1. Ard JL, Bekker A, Frempong-Boadu K. Jr. Anesthesia for an adult with mucopolysaccharidosis I. *J Clin Anesth* 2005;17:624–626.
2. Ramchandani LM, Grewal SS, Beebe DS, et al. Anesthesia risks before and after hematopoietic stem cell transplant (HSCT) in Hurler syndrome [Abstract]. *Anesthesiology* 2004;101:A1442.
3. Walker RWM, Colovic V, Robinson DN, et al. Postobstructive pulmonary oedema during anaesthesia in children with mucopolysaccharidoses. *Paediatr Anaesth* 2003;13:441–447.
4. Khan FA, Khan FH. Use of the Laryngeal Mask Airway™ in mucopolysaccharidoses. *Paediatr Anaesth* 2002;12:468.
5. Vas L, Naregal F. Failed epidural anaesthesia in a patient with Hurler's disease. *Paediatr Anaesth* 2000;10:95–98.
6. Walker RWM, Allen DL, Rothera MR. A fibreoptic intubation technique for children with mucopolysaccharidoses using the laryngeal mask airway. *Paediatr Anaesth* 1997;7:421–426.
7. Moores C, Rogers JG, McKenzie IM, et al. Anaesthesia for children with mucopolysaccharidoses. *Anaesth Intensive Care* 1996;24:459–463.
8. Walker RWM, Darowski M, Morris P. Anaesthesia and mucopolysaccharidoses: a review of airway problems in children. *Anaesthesia* 1994;49:1078–1084.
9. Diaz JH, Belani K. Perioperative management of children with mucopolysaccharidoses. *Anesth Analg* 1993;77:1261–1270.
10. Mahoney A, Soni N, Vellodi A. Anaesthesia and the mucopolysaccharidoses: a review of patients treated by bone marrow transplantation. *Paediatr Anaesth* 1992;2:317–324.
11. Wiedemann HR. Otto Ullrich and his syndromes. *Am J Med Genet* 1991;41:128–133.
12. Berkowitz I, Raja S, Bender K, et al. Dwarfs: pathophysiology and anesthetic implications. *Anesthesiology* 1990;73:739–759.
13. Wilder RT, Belani KG. Fiberoptic intubation complicated by pulmonary edema in a 12-year-old child with Hurler syndrome. *Anesthesiology* 1990;72:205–207.
14. Herrick IA, Rhine EJ. The mucopolysaccharidoses and anaesthesia: a report of clinical experience. *Can J Anaesth* 1988;35:67–73.
15. Sjogren P, Pedersen T, Steinmetz H. Mucopolysaccharidoses and anaesthetic risks. *Acta Anaesthesiol Scand* 1987;31:214–218.
16. King DH, Jones RM, Barrett MB. Anaesthetic considerations in the mucopolysaccharidoses. *Anaesthesia* 1984;39:126–131.
17. Kempthorne PM, Brown TCK. Anaesthesia and the mucopolysaccharidoses: a survey of techniques and problems. *Anaesth Intensive Care* 1983;11:203–207.

18. Baines D, Kenneally J. Anaesthetic management of the mucopolysaccharidoses: a fifteen-year experience in a children's hospital. *Anaesth Intensive Care* 1983;11:198–202.
19. Smith RM. *Anesthesia for Infants and Children*, 4th ed. St. Louis: CV Mosby, 1980:533–536.

Hurler-Scheie Syndrome

SYNONYM: Mucopolysaccharidosis I H/S

MIM #: 252800

This is an autosomal recessive disorder of alpha-L-iduronidase, which is involved in the degradation of glycosaminoglycans (mucopolysaccharides). This disorder represents a phenotype intermediate between Hurler (see earlier) and Scheie syndromes (see later), both of which are also due to a deficiency of alpha-L-iduronidase. There is significant variability between these syndromes, which more correctly represents a spectrum of mucopolysaccharidosis I. Treatment with recombinant human alpha-L-iduronidase can significantly improve some clinical manifestations of the disease, and bone marrow transplantation has provided very good long-term results. Cord blood transplantation has also been used successfully, with improved results when patients are under 2 years of age. Bone marrow transplantation appears to have minimal effects on the progression of skeletal disease.

HEENT/AIRWAY: Corneal clouding, deafness (both sensorineural and conduction loss). Some patients have had micrognathia. Accumulation of mucopolysaccharides in the oropharynx, tongue, epiglottis, aryepiglottic folds, and tracheal wall. Short neck.

CHEST: Pectus carinatum, clubbed ribs. May have sleep apnea. Patients with a mucopolysaccharidosis are susceptible to pulmonary hemorrhage after bone marrow transplantation.

CARDIOVASCULAR: Valvular stenosis or insufficiency. The mitral valve is most commonly affected, followed by the aortic and tricuspid valves.

NEUROMUSCULAR: Varying degrees of mild mental retardation, but many have normal intelligence. May have cervical cord compression from dural mucopolysaccharide accumulation ("pachymeningitis cervicalis"). Communicating hydrocephalus is rare in patients with normal intelligence. Compression of lower spinal cord from spondylolisthesis.

ORTHOPEDIC: Dwarfism, thoracic kyphoscoliosis, lumbar gibbus, stiff joints.

GI/GU: Hepatosplenomegaly.

MISCELLANEOUS: A defect in lysosomal alpha-L-iduronidase also occurs in Plott hound dogs. Treatment with recombinant human alpha-L-iduronidase can significantly improve some clinical manifestations of this disease.

ANESTHETIC CONSIDERATIONS

Accumulation of mucopolysaccharides in the oropharynx, tongue, epiglottis, aryepiglottic folds, and tracheal wall, in conjunction with a short neck and possible micrognathia conspire to make the airway difficult or impossible to intubate antegrade, even in the best of hands using multiple techniques. In addition, distortion of the anatomy may not allow identification of the cricothyroid membrane for retrograde techniques (7). The laryngeal mask airway (LMA) has been used with success in patients with mucopolysaccharidoses (2). Airway involvement is progressive with increasing age. Postoperative respiratory complications are common, and patients should be observed closely in the postanesthesia care unit for evidence of airway compromise. Postobstructive pulmonary edema has been reported.

Spinal anesthesia has been used successfully, and is an option if otherwise appropriate. Patients must be carefully positioned intraoperatively secondary to stiff joints. Patients with cardiac valve involvement require perioperative antibiotic prophylaxis as indicated.

Bibliography:
1. Walker RWM, Colovic V, Robinson DN, et al. Postobstructive pulmonary oedema during anaesthesia in children with mucopolysaccharidoses. *Paediatr Anaesth* 2003;13:441–447.
2. Walker RWM, Allen DL, Rothera MR. A fibreoptic intubation technique for children with mucopolysaccharidoses using the laryngeal mask airway. *Paediatr Anaesth* 1997;7:421–426.
3. Moores C, Rogers JG, McKenzie IM et al. Anaesthesia for children with mucopolysaccharidoses. *Anaesth Intensive Care* 1996;24:459–463.
4. Walker RWM, Darowski M, Morris P. Anaesthesia and mucopolysaccharidoses: a review of airway problems in children. *Anaesthesia* 1994;49:1078–1084.
5. Diaz JH, Belani K. Perioperative management of children with mucopolysaccharidoses. *Anesth Analg* 1993;77:1261–1270.
6. Mahoney A, Soni N, Vellodi A. Anaesthesia and the mucopolysaccharidoses: a review of patients treated by bone marrow transplantation. *Paediatr Anaesth* 1992;2:317–324.
7. Nicolson SC, Black AE, Kraras CM. Management of a difficult airway in a patient with Hurler-Scheie during cardiac surgery. *Anesth Analg* 1992;75:830–832.
8. Berkowitz I, Raja S, Bender K, et al. Dwarfs: pathophysiology and anesthetic implications. *Anesthesiology* 1990;73:739–759.
9. Sjogren P, Pedersen T, Steinmetz H. Mucopolysaccharidoses and anaesthetic risks. *Acta Anaesthesiol Scand* 1987;31:214–218.
10. Sjogren P, Pedersen T. Anaesthetic problems in Hurler-Scheie syndrome. *Acta Anaesthesiol Scand* 1986;30:484–486.
11. King DH, Jones RM, Barrett MB. Anaesthetic considerations in the mucopolysaccharidoses. *Anaesthesia* 1984;39:126–131.
12. Baines D, Kenneally J. Anaesthetic management of the mucopolysaccharidoses: a fifteen-year experience in a children's hospital. *Anaesth Intensive Care* 1983;11:198–202.
13. Kempthorne PM, Brown TCK. Anaesthesia and the mucopolysaccharidoses: a survey of techniques and problems. *Anaesth Intensive Care* 1983;11:203–207.

Hutchinson-Gilford Syndrome

See Progeria

Hydantoin

See Fetal hydantoin syndrome

Hydroxyacyl-CoA Dehydrogenase Deficiency

See Long-chain acyl-CoA dehydrogenase deficiency

Hydroxydicarboxilic Acidemia

See Long-chain acyl-CoA dehydrogenase deficiency

Hydroxymethylglutaric Aciduria

SYNONYM: Hydroxymethyl glutaryl-CoA lyase deficiency; 3-hydroxy-3-methylglutaryl-CoA lyase deficiency

MIM #: None

This autosomal recessive disorder results in the accumulation of 3-hydroxy-3-methylglutaric acid in the urine. Deficiency of hydroxymethyl glutaryl-CoA lyase leads to the hydrolysis of 3-hydroxy-3-methylglutaryl-CoA to form 3-hydroxy-3-methylglutaric acid, which is excreted in the urine. 3-hydroxy-3-methylglutaryl-CoA is derived from the catabolism of leucine and from the synthetic pathway of ketone bodies from fatty acid oxidation. Patients present with signs similar to those of Reye syndrome. Patients have been known to self-select a low-protein diet, although the limitation of dietary fat has been shown to be more effective in lowering the excretion of metabolites. There are some patients who have hydroxymethylglutaric aciduria with normal enzyme activity, and the pathogenesis of this disorder is unknown.

HEENT/AIRWAY: Microcephaly.

NEUROMUSCULAR: Hypotonia and lethargy that may progress to coma or seizures during an acute episode. Cerebral atrophy. Most are developmentally normal.

GI/GU: Vomiting. Hepatomegaly, elevated transaminases.

OTHER: Metabolic acidosis, which can be profound. There is never any ketosis because this enzyme is required for ketone production. However, lactic acidosis can develop in patients during severe episodes. Hyperammonemia, sometimes severe. Hypoglycemia, which can be fatal. There can be secondary carnitine deficiency. Two children who became very ill after immunizations have been reported.

ANESTHETIC CONSIDERATIONS
Extended perioperative fasts must be avoided because fasting causes hypoglycemia and increases fatty acid oxidation. Patients must receive adequate perioperative glucose. Acute exacerbations should be treated with glucose and bicarbonate.

FIGURE: See **Appendix D**

Bibliography:
1. Wysocki SJ, Hahnel R. 3-Hydroxy-3-methylglutaryl-CoA lyase deficiency: a review. *J Inherit Metab Dis* 1986;9:225–233.

Hydroxymethyl Glutaryl-CoA Lyase Deficiency

See Hydroxymethylglutaric aciduria

Hydroxyprolinemia

SYNONYM: Hyperhydroxyprolinemia

MIM #: 237000

This disorder is distinct from hyperprolinemia (see later). Hydroxyproline is derived from the breakdown of collagen. Hydroxyprolinemia is an autosomal recessive disorder due to deficient activity of hydroxyproline oxidase. Hydroxyproline oxidase is involved in the catabolism of hydroxyproline, catalyzing the conversion of 4-hydroxy-L-proline to delta-1-pyrroline-3-hydroxy-5-carboxylic acid. Proline oxidation is unaffected.

Although clinical manifestations were ascribed to the disorder in early reports, this likely reflects an ascertainment bias because these patients first came to medical attention for a clinical problem, probably unrelated. It is unclear whether this disorder has any clinical manifestations.

NEUROMUSCULAR: Possibly mental retardation or psychiatric problems.

GI/GU: Possibly microscopic hematuria.

ANESTHETIC CONSIDERATIONS
There are no specific anesthetic implications.

Bibliography:
1. Kim SZ, Varvogli L, Waisbren S, et al. Hydroxyprolinemia: comparison of a patient and her unaffected twin sister. *J Pediatr* 1997;130:437–441.

Hyperekplexia (Hyperexplexia)

See Stiff baby syndrome

Hyperglycerolemia

SYNONYM: Glycerol kinase deficiency

MIM #: 307030

This X-linked disease is due to a deficiency of glycerol kinase, and is marked by hyperglycerolemia and glyceroluria. Glycerol kinase catalyzes the first step in glycerol catabolism, the phosphorylation of glycerol to glycerol-3-phosphate. There are three clinical phenotypes: (a) an infantile form due to a microdeletion, (b) a juvenile form that is associated with vomiting, acidosis, and stupor in the toddler age group, and (c) an adult or benign form. There is considerable clinical heterogeneity. Glycerol-limited diets appear to be of benefit in symptomatic patients. The adult form is typically detected by "pseudohypertriglyceridemia." Laboratories may measure triglyceride levels by quantitation of glycerol after lipolysis, and these patients have elevated levels of blood glycerol unrelated to triglyceride levels.

This gene is closely linked to the genes for Duchenne muscular dystrophy and congenital adrenal hypoplasia (note: hypoplasia, not hyperplasia), and patients with all three have been described as part of the microdeletion manifestations associated with the infantile form.

HEENT/AIRWAY: Esotropia.

NEUROMUSCULAR: Mental retardation. Episodes of somnolence or stupor progressing to coma. May be associated with Duchenne muscular dystrophy, but the myopathy may be relatively mild.

ORTHOPEDIC: Osteoporosis, pathologic fractures.

GI/GU: Vomiting, poor growth.

OTHER: Acidemia. Adults with the benign form can have mild diabetes mellitus.

MISCELLANEOUS: Glycerol (the same as glycerin) derives its name from the Greek *glykeros* ("sweet"), by way of the French glycerine.

ANESTHETIC CONSIDERATIONS

Perioperative medications should be checked to ensure that they do not include glycerol (glycerin) as a component of the vehicle.

Adrenal function should be assessed in patients with the infantile form. Patients with associated adrenal hypoplasia should be on steroid replacement therapy with a glucocorticoid and a mineralocorticoid, and require perioperative stress doses of steroids. Adequate perioperative sources of glucose should be assured. Patients must be carefully positioned secondary to osteoporosis and the risk of pathologic fractures.

Given the association between the infantile form and Duchenne muscular dystrophy, it would seem safest to proceed as if these patients had Duchenne muscular dystrophy, particularly younger boys who may not yet show clinical manifestations of the muscular dystrophy (see Duchenne muscular dystrophy, earlier).

Bibliography:
1. Matsumoto T, Kondoh T, Yoshimoto M, et al. Complex glycerol kinase deficiency: molecular-genetic, cytogenetic, and clinical studies of five Japanese patients. *Am J Med Genet* 1988;31:603–616.
2. McCabe ER, Seltzer WK. Glycerol kinase deficiency: compartmental considerations regarding pathogenesis and clinical heterogeneity. *Adv Exp Med Biol* 1986;194:481–493.

Hyperglycinemia (Nonketotic)

See Nonketotic hyperglycinemia

Hyperhydroxyprolinemia

See Hydroxyprolinemia

Hyperimmunoglobulin E Syndrome

See Job syndrome

Hyperkalemic Periodic Paralysis

See Familial periodic paralysis

Hyperlysinemia

See Familial hyperlysinemia

Hyperornithinemia with Gyrate Atrophy of the Choroid and Retina

See Ornithine delta-aminotransferase deficiency

Hyperornithinemia-Hyperammonemia-Homocitrullinuria Syndrome

See HHH syndrome

Hyperoxaluria

See Oxalosis

Hyperprolinemia Type I

SYNONYM: Proline oxidase (dehydrogenase) deficiency

MIM #: 239500

This autosomal recessive disorder of proline metabolism is due to deficient activity of proline oxidase. This enzyme catalyzes the first step in proline catabolism, the conversion of proline to pyrroline-5-carboxylate. The enzyme is tightly bound to the inner mitochondrial membrane. The proline oxidase gene is located on chromosome 22, immediately adjacent to, or very close to the region involved in DiGeorge syndrome (see earlier). A case of hyperprolinemia type I has been described in a patient with CATCH 22 (DiGeorge) syndrome.

Initially, patients with this syndrome were reported to have various associated clinical findings. However, this was likely due to ascertainment bias because these patients came to medical attention because they had other medical problems. Patients who have been identified prospectively (through neonatal screening programs) do not appear to exhibit any clinical findings that are specific to this disorder.

GI/GU: Maternal disease has had no apparent effect on offspring.

MISCELLANEOUS: This gene is a homologue of the "*sluggish-A*" gene in *Drosophila*. It has been suggested that at least some mutations in this gene might be a risk factor for the development of schizophrenia.

ANESTHETIC CONSIDERATIONS
There are no specific anesthetic considerations associated with this disorder.

Bibliography:

1. Humbertclaude V, Rivier F, Roubertie A, et al. Is hyperprolinemia type I actually a benign trait? Report of a case with severe neurologic involvement and vigabatrin intolerance. *J Child Neurol* 2001;16:622–623.
2. Jaeken J, Goemans N, Fryns JP, et al. Association of hyperprolinemia type I and heparin cofactor II deficiency with CATCH 22 syndrome: evidence for a contiguous gene syndrome locating the proline oxidase gene. *J Inherit Metab Dis* 1996;19:275–277.
3. Potter JL, Waickman FJ. Hyperprolinemia: I. Study of a large family. *J Pediatr* 1973;83:635–638.

Hyperprolinemia Type II

MIM #: 239510

This autosomal recessive disorder is due to deficient activity of delta-1-pyrroline-5-carboxylic acid dehydrogenase. This enzyme catalyzes a terminal step in proline catabolism, the conversion of glutamate-gamma-semialdehyde to glutamate, with the production of nicotinamide adenine dinucleotide (NADH).

Although early reports listed clinical manifestations of this disease, these were likely due to ascertainment bias because patients were identified only after coming to medical attention for other problems. Prospectively identified patients (through neonatal screening programs) have exhibited only one consistent finding: there appears to be an increased risk for the development of neonatal seizures. It has been hypothesized that excess proline can contribute to the multifactorial pathogenesis of these seizures because proline is known to have neuromodulatory properties.

NEUROMUSCULAR: Neonatal seizures. Possible mental retardation.

GI/GU: Maternal disease has had no apparent effect on offspring.

MISCELLANEOUS: Hyperprolinemic mice have learning deficits.

ANESTHETIC CONSIDERATIONS
There are no specific anesthetic considerations associated with this disorder, although chronic use of anticonvulsant medications can alter metabolism of some anesthetic drugs.

Bibliography:

1. Farrant RD, Walker V, Mills GA, et al. Pyridoxal phosphate deactivation by pyrroline-5-carboxylic acid. Increased risk of vitamin B6 deficiency and seizures in hyperprolinemia type II. *J Biol Chem* 2001;276:15107–15116.
2. Geraghty MT, Vaughn D, Nicholson AJ, et al. Mutations in the Delta1-pyrroline 5-carboxylate dehydrogenase gene cause type II hyperprolinemia. *Hum Mol Genet* 1998;7:1411–1415.

Hyperprostaglandin E Syndrome

See Bartter syndrome

Hypertelorism-Hypospadias Syndrome

SYNONYM: Opitz syndrome; Opitz-Frias syndrome; Telecanthus-hypospadias syndrome; G syndrome

MIM #: 145410, 300000

This syndrome is distinguished by hypertelorism and hypospadias. There is a predominance of affected male patients, which suggests X-linked inheritance or autosomal dominant inheritance with partial sex limitation. In fact, genetic heterogeneity has been established, with an X-linked form that maps to the short arm of the X chromosome and an autosomal dominant form that maps to the long arm of chromosome 22. There are no significant phenotypic differences between the two forms. The X chromosome gene has been identified as *MID 1* (midline 1). Its product has been termed midin, and associates itself with microtubules.

Boys are usually more severely affected than girls. This is a disorder of midline development.

HEENT/AIRWAY: Hypertelorism, telecanthus. Prominent occiput, posterior scalp defects. Slight slanting of palpebral fissures, epicanthal folds (in X-linked form only), strabismus. Protruding and posteriorly rotated ears. Broad nasal bridge, anteverted nares. Short lingual frenulum. High-arched palate. Cleft lip or palate (in X-linked form only). Bifid uvula. Micrognathia. Can have hypoplastic epiglottis, laryngotracheal cleft or hypoplasia/malformation of the larynx. Can have high carina in the most severely affected patients. Can have tracheoesophageal fistula, which is more common and more severe in boys.

CHEST: Stridor with a weak cry. Rare pulmonary alveolar and vascular hypoplasia. Esophageal abnormalities can result in recurrent aspiration.

CARDIOVASCULAR: Can have congenital cardiac defect, especially coarctation of the aorta and atrial septal defects.

NEUROMUSCULAR: Can have mild mental retardation. Hypotonia. Can have agenesis of the corpus callosum, hypoplasia of the cerebellar vermis, enlarged cisterna magna, cortical atrophy.

GI/GU: Dysphagia and swallowing difficulties, achalasia, hiatal hernia. Imperforate anus. Hypospadias, cryptorchidism, bifid scrotum, splayed labia majora. Can have renal anomalies.

OTHER: Increased incidence of monozygotic twinning.

MISCELLANEOUS: Opitz called this "G syndrome," using the initials of the family in which he first described this syndrome. In the mouse, several exons of the homologous gene are located on the X chromosome, while some are located on both the X and Y chromosomes.

ANESTHETIC CONSIDERATIONS

Micrognathia and laryngeal anomalies may make direct laryngoscopy and tracheal intubation difficult. Laryngeal hypoplasia can limit the size of endotracheal tube that may be passed. Inadvertent endobronchial intubation is more likely in patients with a high carina. Because of dysphagia and swallowing difficulties, these patients are at risk for perioperative aspiration. Patients may have limited pulmonary reserve secondary to recurrent aspiration or pulmonary hypoplasia.

Bibliography:

1. So J, Suckow V, Kijas Z, et al. Mild phenotypes in a series of patients with Opitz GBBB syndrome with MID1 mutations. *Am J Med Genet A* 2005;132:1–7.
2. de Falco F, Cainarca S, Andolfi G, et al. X-linked Opitz syndrome: novel mutations and redefinition of the clinical spectrum. *Am J Med Genet A* 2003;120:222–228.
3. Robin NH, Opitz JM, Muenke M. Opitz G/BBB syndrome: clinical comparisons of families linked to Xp22 and 22q, and a review of the literature. *Am J Med Genet* 1996;62:305–317.
4. Brooks JK, Leonard CO, Coccaro PJ. Opitz (BBB/G) syndrome: oral manifestations. *Am J Med Genet* 1992;43:595–601.
5. Bolsin SN, Gillbe C. Opitz-Frias syndrome. *Anaesthesia* 1985;40:1189–1193.

Hypochondroplasia

MIM #: 146000

This autosomal dominant disorder is often confused with achondroplasia. Like achondroplasia, this syndrome involves short stature and caudal narrowing of the spinal canal. Unlike achondroplasia, there are no significant craniofacial abnormalities, very infrequent cervical spinal cord abnormalities, and only mild abnormalities of the hands. Most cases of hypochondroplasia are caused by mutations in the gene for fibroblast growth factor receptor-3 (*FGFR3*). Mutations of this same gene cause achondroplasia. Thus, in many instances the two disorders are allelic. However, some cases of hypochondroplasia have been shown to be caused by defects in the insulin-like growth factor I gene (*IGF1*), and are not allelic with achondroplasia.

HEENT/AIRWAY: Macrocephaly, brachycephaly. Mild frontal bossing. Ptosis, esotropia, cataracts.

NEUROMUSCULAR: Caudal narrowing of the spinal canal. May have learning disabilities.

ORTHOPEDIC: Short stature. Lumbar lordosis. Narrow vertebral interpedicular distance. Proportionately short limbs. Short hands and feet, without trident hand. May have brachydactyly, polydactyly. Marked bowing of the legs. Fibulae relatively longer than the tibiae may cause inversion of the feet. Small ilia.

ANESTHETIC CONSIDERATIONS

As in achondroplasia, cesarean section is often preferable in hypochondroplastic women because of lumbar lordosis and relatively small ilia. Regional anesthesia may be technically difficult secondary to spinal abnormalities. There are no specific concerns about the airway or the stability of the cervical spine, as there are with achondroplasia.

Bibliography:

1. Prinster C, Carrera P, Del Maschio M, et al. Comparison of clinical-radiological and molecular findings in hypochondroplasia. *Am J Med Genet* 1998;75:109–112.
2. Rousseau F, Bonaventure J, Legeai-Mallet L, et al. Clinical and genetic heterogeneity of hypochondroplasia. *J Med Genet* 1996;33:749–752.

Hypoglossia-Hypodactyly Syndrome

See Oromandibular-limb hypogenesis

Hypohidrotic Ectodermal Dysplasia, Autosomal Dominant Type

See Rapp-Hodgkin ectodermal dysplasia

Hypokalemic Periodic Paralysis

See Familial periodic paralysis

Hypomelanosis of Ito

SYNONYM: Incontinentia pigmenti achromians

MIM #: 300337

Hypomelanosis of Ito has been used to describe areas of skin hypopigmentation that form a characteristic whorl or streak pattern on the trunk or limbs. The characteristic skin lesions have multiple etiologies, but may be a nonspecific marker for chromosomal mosaicism, and may be associated with craniofacial, limb, or neurologic anomalies. The skin lesions are somewhat like a negative of the hyperpigmented lesions in classic incontinentia pigmenti (see later), and do not undergo evolutionary changes as in incontinentia pigmenti.

HEENT/AIRWAY: Macrocephaly. Hypertelorism. Epicanthal folds, strabismus, abnormal retinal pigmentation. Abnormal ears. Cleft lip/palate. Dental dysplasia and irregularities.

NEUROMUSCULAR: Can have mental retardation, seizures, hypotonia, cerebral atrophy.

ORTHOPEDIC: Short stature. Kyphoscoliosis/lordosis. Syndactyly, polydactyly, clinodactyly, ectrodactyly, triphalangeal thumb. Genu valgum.

OTHER: Areas of skin hypopigmentation form a characteristic whorl or streak pattern on the trunk or limbs. Alopecia. Hypertrichosis.

ANESTHETIC CONSIDERATIONS

Careful preoperative examination of the teeth is necessary. Chronic use of anticonvulsant medications can affect the metabolism of some anesthetic drugs.

Bibliography:

1. Ruggieri M, Pavone L. Hypomelanosis of Ito: clinical syndrome or just phenotype? *J Child Neurol* 2000;15:635–644.
2. Kuster W, Konig A. Hypomelanosis of Ito: no entity, but a cutaneous sign of mosaicism. *Am J Med Genet* 1999;85:346–350.
3. Fujino O, Hashimoto K, Fujita T, et al. Clinico-neuropathological study of incontinentia pigmenti achromians: an autopsy case. *Brain Dev* 1995;17:425–427.

Hypophosphatasia

MIM #: 241500, 241510

This usually autosomal recessive disorder is characterized by a severe deficiency of skeletal mineralization. The syndrome is called "hypophosphatasia" because there is deficient alkaline phosphatase activity in serum, tissues, and organs. There is wide variability in the clinical expression of this syndrome, with severe infantile and milder childhood onset diseases. Some patients are asymptomatic, whereas others suffer from recurrent fractures, and severely affected patients die *in utero*. Clinically, this syndrome often resembles rickets. However, traditional therapy for rickets (vitamin D) must be avoided in these patients because they have normal levels of vitamin D. Excessive vitamin D exacerbates the hypercalcemia and hypercalciuria seen with this syndrome. Some patients can present solely with dental abnormalities. The disorder is due to a defect in the *ALPL* gene (alkaline phosphatase, liver/bone/kidney type), and many specific mutations have been described, mostly missense mutations.

HEENT/AIRWAY: Underossified cranial bones give the appearance of widely separated sutures in severely affected neonates. Can have brachycephaly. Can have mild hypertelorism, proptosis, blue sclerae. Aplasia or hypoplasia of dental cementum with premature loss of deciduous teeth. Early loss of adult teeth in milder, adult form.

CHEST: Respiratory insufficiency from rachitic disease of the chest. Recurrent pneumonia. Harrison's groove (a classic finding in rickets)—a horizontal depression at the attachment point of the anterior diaphragm to the chest wall.

NEUROMUSCULAR: Hypotonia. Children with infantile onset have functional craniosynostosis due to defective ossification, which can cause elevated intracranial pressure, papilledema. Seizures, periodic apnea in severe cases. Can have muscle weakness, particularly of the thighs.

ORTHOPEDIC: Short stature. In the most severe form, there is almost complete lack of skeletal mineralization at birth with short, deformed limbs and abnormal long bone spurs. Rachitic changes of wrist, knees, and costochondral junctions ("rachitic rosary"). Scoliosis. Bowed legs, waddling gait. Poorly healing fractures. Osteomalacia, stress fractures and pseudofractures in adults. Adults can have arthritis from deposition of calcium phosphate crystals.

GI/GU: Extramedullary hepatic hematopoiesis. Nephrocalcinosis, renal stones.

OTHER: Anemia, possibly secondary to marrow cavity encroachment by osteoid. Can have symptomatic hypercalciuria, with or without hypercalcemia. Can have increased incidence of primary hyperparathyroidism.

ANESTHETIC CONSIDERATIONS

There is premature loss of deciduous teeth in children and permanent teeth in adults, so dental abnormalities should be documented preoperatively. Patients must be adequately hydrated perioperatively to avoid encouragement of hypercalciuric stone formation. Patients should be positioned carefully, although the bones are not as fragile as they are in osteogenesis imperfecta. Precautions to avoid further increases in intracranial pressure must be taken in patients with increased intracranial pressure. Severely affected infants need close observation of their postoperative respiratory status.

Bibliography:

1. Fallon MD, Teitelbaum SL, Weinstein RS, et al. Hypophosphatasia: clinicopathologic comparison of the infantile, childhood, and adult forms. *Medicine (Baltimore)* 1984;63:12–24.

I

I-Cell Disease

SYNONYM: Mucolipidosis II

MIM #: 252500

This autosomal recessive disease is related to the mucopolysaccharidoses. Before the biochemistry of the mucolipidoses was understood, it was recognized that these patients had features of both the mucopolysaccharidoses and the sphingolipidoses, hence the name "mucolipidosis." The term "I-cell" was coined to refer to "inclusion-cell." This syndrome is characterized by abnormal lysosomal enzyme transport in cells of mesenchymal origin, resulting in enzymes being released into the extracellular stroma rather than being stored in lysozymes. The deficient enzyme is N-acetylglucosaminyl-1-phosphotransferase (also deficient in pseudo-Hurler syndrome, or mucolipidosis III; see later). This enzyme catalyzes the formation of mannose 6-phosphate that is required for targeting lysosomal hydrolases to the lysosome. The phenotype resembles Hurler syndrome (see earlier), but with an earlier onset. The presence of gingival hypertrophy in I-cell disease also differentiates the two. Death is often by 5 to 8 years of age, but some can survive into adolescence.

HEENT/AIRWAY: Coarse facies. Corneal opacities. Puffy eyelids. Hearing loss. Anteverted nostrils. The base of the tongue, epiglottis, and larynx can be thickened. Hyperplastic gums. The adenoids and tonsils can be involved and enlarged. The jaw and neck can be stiff. Short neck.

CHEST: The tracheal wall can be thickened. Thoracic deformities. Respiratory infections.

CARDIOVASCULAR: The myocardium is normal, but the valves can be thickened because of numerous vacuolated fibroblasts. Aortic insufficiency.

NEUROMUSCULAR: Severely retarded psychomotor development. Hypotonia.

ORTHOPEDIC: Kyphoscoliosis, lumbar gibbus deformity, anterior beaking of vertebral bodies, Congenital hip dislocation. Carpal tunnel syndrome, claw hand. Stiff joints. Intrauterine fractures. Congenital dislocation of the hip. Growth failure.

GI/GU: Abdominal distension with hepatomegaly. Inguinal hernias, diastasis recti, umbilical hernia. Constipation alternating with diarrhea.

OTHER: Hydrops fetalis in the most severely affected.

ANESTHETIC CONSIDERATIONS

The anesthetic implications are similar to those of the mucopolysaccharidoses, such as Hunter syndrome (see earlier). When meeting the patient before surgery, confirm whether they have hearing loss. Direct laryngoscopy and tracheal intubation may be very difficult, and may become more difficult as the patient ages. It may be difficult to maintain a patent airway with a mask, even with an oral airway. In one case, a laryngeal mask airway helped, and in another it did not (2). If the patient's tracheal wall is thickened, an endotracheal tube that is smaller than predicted may be required. Patients with chronic airway obstruction should be observed closely postoperatively. Patients must be carefully positioned secondary to stiff joints. Patients with valvular heart disease require perioperative antibiotic prophylaxis as indicated.

Bibliography:

1. Beck M, Barone R, Hoffmann R, et al. Inter- and intrafamilial variability in mucolipidosis II (I-cell disease). *Clin Genet* 1995;47:191–199.
2. Baines DB, Street N, Overton JH. Anaesthetic implications of mucolipidosis. *Paediatr Anaesth* 1993;3:303–306.
3. King DH, Jones RM, Barrett MB. Anaesthetic considerations in the mucopolysaccharidoses. *Anaesthesia* 1984;39:126–131.
4. Baines D, Kenneally J. Anaesthetic management of the mucopolysaccharidoses: a fifteen-year experience in a children's hospital. *Anaesth Intensive Care* 1983;11:198–202.
5. Kempthorne PM, Brown TC. Anaesthesia and the mucopolysaccharidoses: a survey of techniques and problems. *Anaesth Intensive Care* 1983;11:203–207.

Ichthyosis

(Includes Collodion membranes)

MIM #: Many

"Ichthyosis" is a general term used to describe any skin disorder that results in dry, scaly (fish-like) skin. Skin involvement may vary from mild to severe. Most cases

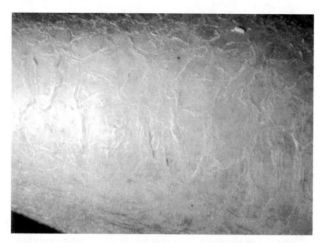

Ichthyosis. Typical lamellar scales. (Courtesy of Dr. Kenneth E. Greer, Department of Dermatology, University of Virginia Health System.)

of ichthyosis are congenital, but ichthyosis can also occur secondary to chronic diseases such as hypothyroidism, renal insufficiency, malabsorption, or lymphoma. The pathogenesis of ichthyosis involves overproduction of keratin, excessive retention of keratin in the stratum corneum layer, or the production of abnormal keratin. Congenital ichthyoses can be divided into four major forms, and a fifth form that is exceedingly rare:

1. **Ichthyosis vulgaris** (also called **ichthyosis simplex**) is the mildest and most common form of ichthyosis. It is inherited in an autosomal dominant fashion, and is noted for the sparing of the flexural surfaces. It is usually not present at birth, and is first noted in childhood. It involves large, lamellar scales, and sometimes smaller white scales. This form tends to subside with age.

2. **Sex-linked ichthyosis** is inherited in an X-linked recessive fashion and is therefore seen primarily in male patients. It is first noted in infancy (usually by 3 months of age). Some infants have a collodion-like (parchment-like) membrane at birth. The palms and soles, central face, and flexural areas are spared. It involves large, brownish scales, which is why it is also known as **ichthyosis nigricans.** Corneal opacities develop in some patients. This form remains stable or worsens with age.

3. **Lamellar ichthyosis** is much rarer, and is inherited in an autosomal recessive fashion. It presents at birth or in early infancy. At birth, most patients have a **collodion membrane** (a parchment-like membrane with cracking), the so-called "collodion baby." The collodion membrane fissures and desquamates over several weeks. Sheet-like layers are shed, leaving residual redness and hyperkeratosis. This form of ichthyosis involves large, quadrangular, gray-brown scales. The scales are adherent centrally and the edges are raised, such that they resemble armor plates. The scales are more common in the flexural areas, palms, and soles. The cheeks are often spared. The nails may be involved. Ectropion develops in some patients. This form remains stable or worsens with age.

4. **Epidermal hyperkeratosis** is inherited in an autosomal dominant fashion. It involves thick, gray-brown, verruciform scales, particularly in the flexural and intertriginous areas. Palms and soles are involved. Bullae appear shortly after birth and are replaced by hyperkeratosis by 3 months of age. This form remains stable or worsens with age.

5. The most dramatic form of congenital ichthyosis is the exceedingly rare **harlequin fetus,** in which the child is covered by thick plates of stratum corneum separated by deep fissures at birth. The skin is hard and thick, with the feel of bark. The skin restricts respiratory movements. The joints are contractured. All infants die in the neonatal period, usually in the first week. Death is a consequence of hypoventilation and pneumonia, or sepsis stemming from cutaneous infection. The name is derived from the deep purple fissures that divide the thickened gray or yellow skin into geometric plaques, giving the appearance of a harlequin's costume.

ANESTHETIC CONSIDERATIONS

Treatment of ichthyosis is aimed at reducing or softening the scale by the application of lubricants or keratinolytic agents. The oily base in these agents prevents adhesives from sticking to the skin. Perioperatively, tubes and catheters may need to be sewn or tied into place. Peripheral intravenous access may be difficult. In severe ichthyosis, temperature regulation is impaired. The collodion baby has severe restrictive lung disease, may be difficult to intubate secondary to limited mouth opening and facial distortion, may have protein and electrolyte losses and dehydration, and is at risk for the development of sepsis.

Bibliography:
1. Francis JS. Genetic skin diseases. *Curr Opin Pediatr* 1994;6:447–453.
2. Buyse L, Graves C, Marks R, et al. Collodion baby dehydration: the danger of high transepidermal water loss. *Br J Dermatol* 1993;129:86–88.
3. Ran RE, Baden HP. The ichthyoses: a review. *J Am Acad Dermatol* 1983;8:285–305.

Immotile Cilia Syndrome

See Kartagener syndrome

Incontinentia Pigmenti

SYNONYM: Bloch-Sulzberger syndrome

MIM #: 308300

This X-linked dominant disease is lethal in hemizygous males. The major findings are eye anomalies and characteristic skin changes. The disorder is due to mutations in the gene *IKK-gamma*, also known as *NEMO*, the nuclear

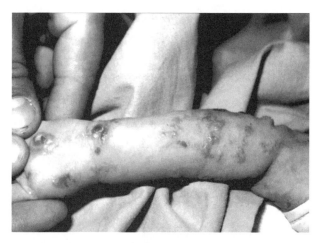

Incontinentia pigmenti. FIG. 1. Relatively early skin lesions of incontinentia pigmenti. (Courtesy of Dr. Kenneth E. Greer, Department of Dermatology, University of Virginia Health System.)

factor (NF)-kappa-B essential modulator gene. In females, cells expressing the mutated gene are selectively eliminated around the time of birth, so that X-inactivation is not random.

HEENT/AIRWAY: Microcephaly. Strabismus, cataracts, optic atrophy, uveitis, keratitis, retinal vascular and pigmentary abnormalities, retinal detachment. Delayed dentition with pointed or absent teeth.

CHEST: Occasional unilateral breast aplasia or hypoplasia.

NEUROMUSCULAR: Mental retardation. Spasticity, hemiparesis, seizures. Dilated ventricles.

ORTHOPEDIC: Mild dystrophy of the nails.

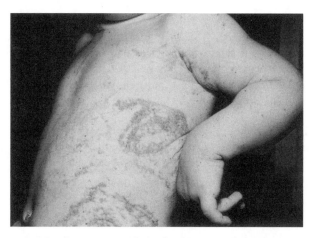

Incontinentia pigmenti. FIG. 2. Relatively later skin lesions of incontinentia pigmenti. (Courtesy of Dr. Kenneth E. Greer, Department of Dermatology, University of Virginia Health System.)

OTHER: The hallmark finding is so-called autochthonous tattooing of the skin in a swirl pattern (resembling the pattern in a marble cake). The skin is initially erythematous with vesicles and pustules, followed by papules, verrucous lesions with hyperkeratosis, hyperpigmentation, and, finally, pallor, atrophy, and scarring. The hyperpigmentation typically fades by adulthood. The pigmented swirl lesions can also occur in areas not obviously affected by the inflammatory changes. Spotty alopecia. Can have abnormal nails.

MISCELLANEOUS: The name is derived from the early belief that the basal layer of epidermis was "incontinent" of melanin. The progression of the skin lesions has been interpreted as representing the gradual replacement of cells containing an abnormal gene on the X chromosome with cells containing a normal gene on the X chromosome (the Lyon hypothesis). X-linked dominance with lethality in male hemizygotes is supported by the presence of this disease in a male patient with Klinefelter syndrome (XXY).

ANESTHETIC CONSIDERATIONS
Dental abnormalities should be documented preoperatively. Confirm whether patients have visual impairment. Chronic use of anticonvulsant medications can alter the metabolism of some anesthetic drugs. Succinylcholine may be contraindicated in patients with hemiparesis or spasticity because of the risk of hyperkalemia.

Bibliography:
1. Berlin AL, Paller AS, Chan LS. Incontinentia pigmenti: a review and update on the molecular basis of pathophysiology. *J Am Acad Dermatol* 2002;47:169–187.
2. Francis JS, Sybert VP. Incontinentia pigmenti. *Sem Cutan Med Surg* 1997;16:54–60.
3. Landy SJ, Donnai D. Incontinentia pigmenti (Bloch-Sulzberger syndrome). *J Med Genet* 1993;30:53–59.

Incontinentia Pigmenti Achromians

See Hypomelanosis of Ito

Infantile Autism

See Autism

Infantile Cortical Hyperostosis

See Caffey disease

Infantile Refsum Disease

Included in Refsum disease

Isovaleric Acidemia

SYNONYM: Isovaleryl-CoA dehydrogenase deficiency

MIM #: 243500

This autosomal recessive disease is due to a defect in the enzyme isovaleryl-CoA dehydrogenase. Isovaleryl-CoA dehydrogenase catalyzes a step in the catabolism of leucine. Patients present either in the neonatal period with an often fatal episode of severe metabolic acidosis, or later in infancy with a chronic intermittent metabolic acidosis. Both forms have the same biochemical defect, and this difference may be nothing more than an indication of the period of imposed metabolic stress, because neonates who survive an episode at birth can go on to have the chronic intermittent form. Episodes of the chronic intermittent form are associated with intercurrent infection or increased dietary protein. Patients often self-select a protein-restricted diet. Chronic therapy with glycine and carnitine may be helpful. These chemicals work by enhancing the excretion of the major abnormal metabolite, isovaleryl-CoA, as nontoxic isovalerylglycine and isovaleryl carnitine. Isovaleryl carnitine is excreted in the urine at a rate greater than the body's ability to synthesize carnitine, so these patients may have low carnitine levels.

NEUROMUSCULAR: Psychomotor development is usually normal, but some have mild or occasionally severe mental retardation. Episodes of lethargy may progress to coma, hypothermia, seizures.

GI/GU: Episodic severe vomiting, episodic pancreatitis, diarrhea, hepatomegaly.

OTHER: Episodes of metabolic acidosis, with hyperammonemia and mild ketosis. Hypocalcemia. Occasional hyperglycemia. There is an odor of sweaty feet from elevated isovaleric acid levels, particularly during acute episodes. Hypoplastic bone marrow. Thrombocytopenia, neutropenia with acute episodes. May have associated carnitine deficiency.

MISCELLANEOUS: Isovaleric acidemia was the first inborn error of metabolism to be diagnosed by gas chromatography-mass spectrometry of metabolites. In its chronic state it is treated with a protein-restricted diet, carnitine, and glycine. In the acute state it is treated with the provision of glucose and protein restriction.

ANESTHETIC CONSIDERATIONS

Patients must receive adequate perioperative glucose to minimize protein catabolism. Protein-restricted diets should be continued perioperatively. An orogastric tube or throat packs should be placed if the surgery has the potential to cause oral or intestinal bleeding because blood aspirated into the gastrointestinal tract after oral or nasal surgery might present an excessive protein load, and trigger an acute decompensation.

A case of intraoperative arrhythmia thought to be associated with bupivacaine toxicity has been reported (1). It was speculated to have been related to a lowered arrhythmia threshold because of the associated carnitine deficiency.

FIGURE: See **Appendix D**

Bibliography:
1. Weinberg GL, Laurito CE, Geldner P, et al. Malignant ventricular dysrhythmias in a patient with isovaleric acidemia receiving general and local anaesthesia for suction lipectomy. *J Clin Anesth* 1997;9:668–670.
2. Shih VE, Aubert RH, Degrade G, et al. Maternal isovaleric acidemia. *J Pediatr* 1984;105:77–78.

Isovaleryl-CoA Dehydrogenase Deficiency

See Isovaleric acidemia

Ivemark Syndrome

See Asplenia or Polysplenia

J

Jacobsen Syndrome

See 11q-syndrome

Jansen Type Metaphyseal Dysplasia

See Metaphyseal chondrodysplasia, Jansen type

Jarcho-Levin Syndrome

SYNONYM: Spondylothoracic dysplasia

MIM #: 277300

This autosomal recessive form of dwarfism is distinguished by a short trunk with a short, malformed thoracic cage. It can be due to abnormalities in the genes *DLL3* or *MESP2*. The disorder is apparently one of inappropriate segmentation.

HEENT/AIRWAY: Wide forehead, prominent occiput, low posterior hairline. Upslanting palpebral fissures. Wide nasal bridge, anteverted nares. Can have cleft palate. Short neck, with limited mobility.

CHEST: Short thoracic cage with an increased anteroposterior diameter and ribs that fan out, giving the thorax a crab-like appearance on radiography. Rib anomalies, including absent ribs, hemivertebrae, posterior rib fusion. Pectus carinatum. Pulmonary hypoplasia in the most severely affected.

CARDIOVASCULAR: Can have congenital heart disease.

NEUROMUSCULAR: Can have meningomyelocele.

ORTHOPEDIC: Short trunk dwarfism—extremities are normal in length. Multiple thoracic vertebral defects, including hemivertebrae, vertebral fusions. Kyphoscoliosis, lordosis.

GI/GU: Protuberant abdomen. Can have cryptorchidism, hypospadias, ureteral or urethral obstruction.

MISCELLANEOUS: Abnormalities in *DLL3* in mice result in the "pudgy" phenotype. Jarcho and Levin misidentified the first cases as Klippel-Feil syndrome.

ANESTHETIC CONSIDERATIONS

Patients have severe restrictive lung disease secondary to limited thoracic volume, limited chest excursion, and recurrent infection. Many patients die in infancy secondary to respiratory insufficiency. Direct laryngoscopy and tracheal intubation can be difficult because of a short neck with limited extension. Patients with congenital heart disease need perioperative antibiotic prophylaxis as indicated.

Bibliography:

1. Cornier AS, Ramirez N, Arroyo S, et al. Phenotype characterization and natural history of spondylothoracic dysplasia syndrome: a series of 27 new cases. *Am J Med Genet A* 2004;128:120–126.
2. McCall CP, Hudgins L, Cloutier M, et al. Jarcho-Levin syndrome: unusual survival in a classical case. *Am J Med Genet* 1994;49:328–332.

Jansky-Bielschowsky Disease

SYNONYM: Late infantile ceroid lipofuscinosis

MIM #: 204500

This autosomal recessive disorder is one of several, perhaps eight, lipofuscinoses, which are lysosomal disorders with profound central nervous system degeneration. Others include juvenile onset Spielmeyer-Vogt disease, Batten disease, Spielmeyer-Vogt disease (see later under Spielmeyer-Vogt disease), and Santavuori-Haltia and Kuf diseases (not discussed in this text). These neurodegenerative disorders are marked by the accumulation of an autofluorescent pigment in the brain and other tissues. Jansky-Bielschowsky disease is late infantile lipifuscinosis, and is due to mutations in the gene *CLN2,* which probable encodes a lysosomal peptidase. This form of lipofuscinosis presents at 2 to 4 years of age and death occurs at 10 to 15 years of age. Major problems include seizures, myoclonus, mental retardation, and ataxia.

HEENT/AIRWAY: Progressive visual loss leading to blindness, retinal degeneration, absent electroretinogram.

NEUROMUSCULAR: Drug-resistant grand mal and myoclonic seizures, ataxia, mental retardation, cerebral atrophy, autofluorescent lipigment in neurons and extraneuronal cells.

OTHER: Autonomic dysregulation, including abnormal thermal regulation.

ANESTHETIC CONSIDERATIONS

Patients may be bedridden with muscle atrophy, so succinylcholine should be avoided and volatile anesthetics alone may provide adequately relaxed muscles. Intraoperative hypothermia can result from abnormal thermal regulation (2). Seizures can be difficult to control and can occur perioperatively. Chronic use of anticonvulsant medications can alter the metabolism of some anesthetic drugs.

Bibliography:

1. Rust RS, Karluk D. Case records of the Massachusetts general hospital. Weekly clinicopathological exercises. Case 27–2002. A $5\frac{1}{2}$-year-old boy with seizures and progressive deterioration of cognitive and motor function. *N Engl J Med* 2002;347:672–680.
2. Yamada Y, Doi K, Sakura S, et al. Anesthetic management for a patient with Jansky-Bielschowsky disease. *Can J Anaesth* 2002;49:81–83.
3. Defalque RJ. Anesthesia for a patient with Kuf's disease. *Anesthesiology* 1990;73:1041–1042.

Jervell-Lange-Nielson Syndrome

Included in Long QT syndrome

Jeune Syndrome

SYNONYM: Asphyxiating thoracic dystrophy; Thoracic-pelvic-phalangeal dystrophy

MIM #: 208500

This autosomal recessive disorder is characterized by severe thoracic hypoplasia and deformity, short limbs, and hypoplastic iliac wings. Death in infancy is common. In long-term survivors, chronic renal failure is common.

HEENT/AIRWAY: Can have progressive retinal degeneration. Occasional cleft lip or palate.

CHEST: Severe deformity of the thoracic cage prevents adequate respiratory excursion in the neonate. In the most severe cases, there is also pulmonary hypoplasia. Persistent pulmonary hypertension has been reported in some neonates. Early infant death is common, secondary to asphyxia or pneumonia. Chest radiographs show a typical, very narrow thorax with short horizontal ribs. Survivors usually exhibit progressive growth of the thoracic cage. Attempts at surgical expansion of the thoracic cage have met with variable success.

CARDIOVASCULAR: Cor pulmonale secondary to restrictive lung disease or chronic hypoxemia. Myocardial failure has been reported in older patients.

NEUROMUSCULAR: Rare mental retardation. Rare mild congenital hydrocephalus.

ORTHOPEDIC: Short stature. Short limbs, especially marked in the hands. Occasional polydactyly. Hypoplastic iliac wings.

GI/GU: Occasional direct hyperbilirubinemia. Hepatic cirrhosis has been observed in some children, and portal hypertension that required transplantation has been described. Occasional pancreatic fibrosis or cysts. Intestinal malabsorption has been reported. Cystic renal disease or renal fibrosis can lead to chronic renal failure by late infancy or early childhood in patients who have survived the neonatal period.

MISCELLANEOUS: Expandable titanium rib prostheses have been proposed for these children, and there is evidence of rib growth and ossification which is not ultimately dependent on the prosthetic ribs.

ANESTHETIC CONSIDERATIONS

Most patients have severe respiratory insufficiency. If not already hypoxic at rest, patients will likely desaturate with agitation secondary to asynchronous rib and abdominal motion superimposed on small lung volumes. Intraoperatively, peak airway pressures must be maintained as low as possible to avoid barotrauma and the effects of high airway pressures on pulmonary arterial blood flow. After thoracoplasty, most infants require long-term mechanical ventilation. Renal disease has implications for perioperative fluid management and the choice of anesthetic drugs. Hepatic insufficiency may affect the binding or metabolism of some anesthetic agents. It is thought that modern neonatal care will improve mortality.

Bibliography:

1. Kajantie E, Andersson S, Kaitila I. Familial asphyxiating thoracic dysplasia: clinical variability and impact of improved neonatal intensive care. *J Pediatr* 2001;139:130–133.
2. Hudgins L, Rosengren S, Treem W, et al. Early cirrhosis in survivors with Jeune thoracic dystrophy. *J Pediatr* 1992;120:754–756.
3. Borland LM. Anesthesia for children with Jeune's syndrome (asphyxiating thoracic dystrophy). *Anesthesiology* 1987;66:86–88.
4. Okerlaid F, Danks DM, Mayne V, et al. Asphyxiating thoracic dystrophy. *Arch Dis Child* 1977;52:758–765.

Job Syndrome

SYNONYM: Hyperimmunoglobulin E syndrome

MIM #: 243700

This autosomal dominant and autosomal recessive syndrome of unknown etiology results in the overproduction of immunoglobulin E (IgE) and deficient neutrophil and monocyte chemotaxis. The responsible gene and gene product are not known. The gene responsible for the recessive form is thought to reside on chromosome 4.

HEENT: May have craniosynostosis. Facial asymmetry, prominent forehead, deep-set eyes, broad nasal bridge with wide fleshy tip, and thickened ears. Full lower lip. Rough facial skin with prominent pores. Mild prognathism. Failure or delayed shedding of primary teeth due to deficient root resorption. May have mucocutaneous candidiasis.

CHEST: Recurrent bacterial infections of the sinopulmonary tract, usually due to *Staphylococcus aureus*. Patients present frequently for abscess drainage. There is a very high incidence of empyema. Large pneumatoceles can form.

NEUROMUSCULAR: Strokes and lymphocytic encephalitis. A variety of central nervous system problems in the recessive type.

ORTHOPEDIC: May have scoliosis. Hyperextensible joints, bone fractures with minimal trauma in the dominant type.

OTHER: Eczema is common. Patients often have red hair. Serum IgE levels are at least 10 times normal. Eosinophilia. Neutrophil and monocyte chemotaxis is deficient. Recurrent bacterial infections of the skin. Abscesses may form, which are often quite large. Bacteremia or deep infections of viscera or the central nervous system are uncommon. The recessive type has been associated with small vessel vasculitis.

MISCELLANEOUS: "So went Satan forth from the presence of the Lord, and smote Job with sore boils from the sole of his foot unto his crown" (Job II,7).

ANESTHETIC CONSIDERATIONS

Placing an epidural or spinal needle through chronically infected skin may increase the infection risk of epidural or spinal anesthesia. Because abscesses in this syndrome do not elicit a local inflammatory response, an epidural abscess, should it form, would not become apparent until it has caused neurologic compromise. Patients must be carefully positioned because of joint hyperextensibility. A single case of prolonged succinylcholine effect in a patient with normal plasma cholinesterase activity has been reported (3).

Bibliography:

1. Renner ED, Puck JM, Holland SM, et al. Autosomal recessive hyperimmunoglobulin E syndrome: a distinct disease entity. *J Pediatr* 2004;144:93–99.
2. Grimbacher B, Holland SM, Gallin JI, et al. Hyper-IgE syndrome with recurrent infections—an autosomal dominant multisystem disorder. *N Engl J Med* 1999;340:692–702.
3. Guzzi LM, Stamatos JM. Job's syndrome: an unusual response to a common drug. *Anesth Analg* 1992;75:139–140.
4. Miller FL, Mann DL. Anesthetic management of a pregnant patient with the hyperimmunoglobulin E (Job's) syndrome. *Anesth Analg* 1990;70:454–456.
5. Tapper JB, Giesecke AH. Spinal anaesthesia in a child with Job's syndrome, pneumatocoeles and empyema. *Anaesthesia* 1990;45:378–380.

Johanson-Blizzard Syndrome

MIM #: 243800

This autosomal recessive disease affects a variety of organ systems. The disorder is due to abnormalities in the gene

UBR1, involved in the degradation of damaged proteins or those with a short half-life.

HEENT/AIRWAY: Microcephaly. High forehead. Lateral hairline can extend onto the forehead. Midline scalp defects. Can have strabismus. Missing eyelashes and eyebrows. Nasolacrimal duct–cutaneous fistulae or aplasia. Low set ears. Congenital deafness. Hypoplasia or aplasia of the alae nasi with beaked nose. Hypoplastic deciduous and absent permanent teeth. Can have micrognathia.

CARDIOVASCULAR: May have congenital heart disease.

NEUROMUSCULAR: Intelligence can be normal, but can have mild retardation. Can have hypopituitarism.

ORTHOPEDIC: Postnatal growth retardation. Clinodactyly. Simian crease.

GI/GU: Malabsorption. Anorectal anomalies, including imperforate anus. Can have malrotation. Can have exocrine pancreatic insufficiency. Urogenital abnormalities, including double vagina, double uterus, and rectovaginal fistula. Cryptorchidism. Abnormalities of renal pelvis with hydronephrosis.

OTHER: Hypothyroidism, hypopituitarism, pancreatic exocrine insufficiency. Deficiency of fat soluble vitamins due to pancreatic insufficiency. Can have diabetes. A patient with insulin resistance has been reported. Alopecia. Sparse blond hair. Can have failure to thrive. Can have situs inversus.

MISCELLANEOUS: Robert Blizzard was the Chairman of the Department of Pediatrics at the University of Virginia.

ANESTHETIC CONSIDERATIONS
Dental abnormalities should be documented preoperatively. Airway management can be challenging due to micrognathia and abnormal facies. Obtaining a proper mask fit may be difficult. Patients are at risk for postoperative airway obstruction (1). Nasolacrimal duct abnormalities may lead to accelerated drying of the cornea under general anesthesia. Consider preoperative evaluation of renal function in patients with a history of renal abnormalities which predispose to renal insufficiency. Hypothyroidism, when present, could result in delayed gastric emptying, alterations in drug metabolism, and impaired temperature regulation. When meeting the patients before surgery, confirm whether they have hearing loss. Children with congenital heart disease require perioperative antibiotic prophylaxis as clinically indicated.

Bibliography:
1. Fichter CR, Johnson GA, Braddock SR, et al. Perioperative care of the child with the Johanson-Blizzard syndrome. *Paediatr Anaesth* 2003;13: 72–75.
2. Gershoni-Baruch R, Lerner A, Braun J, et al. Johanson-Blizzard syndrome: clinical spectrum and further delineation of the syndrome. *Am J Med Genet* 1990;35:546–551.

Joseph Disease

SYNONYM: Machado-Joseph disease; Spinocerebellar ataxia type 3

MIM #: 109150

This autosomal dominant neurologic disease often does not become apparent until adulthood. It is characterized by loss of neurons and gliosis in a variety of locations, including the substantia nigra, the nuclei of the vestibular and cranial nerves and the anterior horns. The responsible gene, *MJD1* (or *ATXN3*), is located on chromosome 14. The gene product, ataxin-3, has an unknown function. The defect involves repeats of the trinucleotide sequence CAG, and the number of repeats is related to the severity of the disease and age at onset. It has been suggested that this repeat may be responsible for inducing apoptosis, or programmed cell death.

HEENT/AIRWAY: Bulging eyes, limited eye movement, nystagmus, external ophthalmoplegia. Eventual swallowing difficulties.

NEUROMUSCULAR: Parkinson-like features. Loss of leg reflexes, ataxia, dystonia, cerebellar tremors, Babinski sign, spasticity. Facial and lingual fasciculations, other muscle fasciculations. Muscle atrophy. Can develop dementia. Can have peripheral nerve involvement.

OTHER: Diabetes mellitus.

MISCELLANEOUS: This disease is named for the family in which it was first described. Although that family was from the Azores, the syndrome has subsequently been described in other populations, including the Japanese, possibly because of the early Portuguese influence in Japan. This disease has also been reported in a Yemenite Jewish family. Interestingly, the family name was Yoseph.

Apparently, nucleic acid base triplet repeats are also the etiology of other diseases, including Friedreich ataxia, fragile X syndrome, and spinocerebellar ataxia type I.

ANESTHETIC CONSIDERATIONS
Diabetes mellitus is common, and patients should be evaluated preoperatively for evidence of diabetes. Because of their bulging eyes, patients must receive meticulous perioperative eye care to avoid corneal injury. Succinylcholine is contraindicated in patients with significant muscle atrophy, secondary to the risk of hyperkalemia. Swallowing difficulties can increase the risk of aspiration.

Bibliography:
1. Rosenberg RN. DNA triplet repeats and neurologic disease. *N Engl J Med* 1996;335:1222–1224.
2. Barbeau A, Roy M, Cunha L, et al. The natural history of Machado-Joseph disease: an analysis of 138 personally examined cases. *Can J Neurol Sci* 1984;11:510–525.

Joubert Syndrome

SYNONYM: Joubert-Boltshauser syndrome

MIM #: 213300

This autosomal recessive disorder is similar to Dandy-Walker malformation because there is agenesis of the cerebellar vermis. It can be differentiated from Dandy-Walker malformation on computed tomography scan by the presence of normal cerebellar hemispheres in Joubert syndrome, and the presence of cerebellar hypoplasia in Dandy-Walker malformation. Most patients die by the age of 4 years. It is genetically heterogeneous. Defects in at least four distinct genes can result in the syndrome, and the phenotype is variable.

HEENT/AIRWAY: Jerky eye movements. Oculomotor apraxia. Often associated with congenital retinal blindness. Chorioretinal and optic nerve colobomas. Low-set ears. Upturned nose. Can be associated with high-arched palate, large protruding tongue, and micrognathia. Uncommon tumors of the tongue. Can have laryngomalacia. Can have short neck.

CHEST: Infants often present with episodic panting. Can have dysregulated neonatal breathing with periods of hyperpnea and apnea.

NEUROMUSCULAR: Agenesis or hypoplasia of the cerebellar vermis with cystic malformation of the brainstem. Other brainstem malformations. Ataxia, tremor, hypotonia, global developmental delay, central apnea. Occipital meningoencephalocele. Behavioral abnormalities such as hyperactivity, aggressiveness, and self-mutilation. "Molar tooth sign" on MRI, secondary to dysplasia of the isthmic segment of the brain stem.

GI/GU: Can have hepatic fibrosis. Can have renal cysts.

MISCELLANEOUS: Marie Joubert was just a resident when she first described this syndrome.

ANESTHETIC CONSIDERATIONS

When meeting the patient before surgery, be sensitive to the possibility that they are likely to have visual loss. Patients are sensitive to the respiratory depressant effects of opioids. Postoperatively, patients should be observed closely for adequacy of ventilation. Episodic panting is common, so postoperative hyperventilation can be central and not necessarily indicative of pain.

Bibliography:
1. Vodopich DJ, Gordon GJ. Anesthetic management in Joubert syndrome. *Paediatr Anaesth* 2004;14:871–873.
2. Habre W, Sims C, D'Souza M. Anaesthetic management of children with Joubert syndrome. *Paediatr Anaesth* 1997;7:251–253.
3. Saraiva JM, Baraitser M. Joubert syndrome: a review. *Am J Med Genet* 1992;43:726–731.
4. Cantani A, Lucenti P, Ronzani G, et al. Joubert syndrome: review of the fifty-three cases so far published. *Ann Genet* 1990;33:96–98.
5. Matthews NC. Anaesthesia in an infant with Joubert's syndrome. *Anaesthesia* 1989;44:920–921.

Joubert-Boltshauser Syndrome

See Joubert syndrome

Juvenile Hyaline Fibromatosis

MIM #: 228600

This autosomal recessive disorder results in deposition of hyaline material in a variety of tissues, leading to fibromatosis. The disorder is due to abnormalities in the gene *CMG2* (or *ANTXR2*), which encodes capillary morphogenesis protein-2. The name ANTXR2 is indicative of the fact that the gene product is an anthrax toxin receptor.

HEENT/AIRWAY: Gingival fibromatosis and hypertrophy. There can be deposits at the commissures of the lips, and mouth opening can be limited.

CHEST: There can be tracheal deposits.

CARDIOVASCULAR: There can be deposits in the heart.

NEUROMUSCULAR: Normal intelligence.

ORTHOPEDIC: Painful joint contractures. Osteolytic and osteoclastic long bone lesions, osteolysis of the terminal digits. Nodules of finger tips.

GI/GU: Perianal granulomas.

OTHER: Multiple, large, slow-growing subcutaneous nodules, primarily on the head and neck and on the hands, which are often the presenting sign. There is a high recurrence rate after wide surgical excision. The nodules frequently become infected, usually with a strain of *Staphylococcus*. Serious infections can lead to death. Thyroid and adrenal deposits have been described. Sclerodermaform and atrophic skin changes.

MISCELLANEOUS: When first described in 1873 and 1903, it was described as familial "molluscum fibrosum."

ANESTHETIC CONSIDERATIONS

Direct laryngoscopy and tracheal intubation can be exceedingly difficult secondary to oral and tracheal involvement as well as contractures of the temporomandibular joint and cervical spine. Oral disease worsens as the patient ages. A laryngeal mask has been used successfully (4). A single patient has been described who had succinylcholine resistance despite normal plasma cholinesterase activity and normal neuromuscular function (3). Response to nondepolarizing muscle relaxants is apparently normal.

Bibliography:
1. Mutlu NM, Kirdemir P, Göğüş N. Juvenile hyaline fibromatosis [Letter]. *Paediatr Anaesth* 2004;14:798–799.
2. Keser G, Karabulut B, Oksel F, et al. Two siblings with juvenile hyaline fibromatosis: case reports and review of the literature. *Clin Rheumatol* 1999;18:248–252.
3. Baraka AS. Succinylcholine resistance in a patient with juvenile hyaline fibromatosis. *Anesthesiology* 1997;87:1250–1252.
4. Norman B, Soni N, Madden N. Anaesthesia and juvenile hyaline fibromatosis. *Br J Anaesth* 1996;76:163–166.

Juvenile Macular Degeneration

See Stargardt disease

Juvenile Spinal Muscle Atrophy

See Kugelberg-Welander disease

K

Kabuki Syndrome

MIM #: 147920

This possibly autosomal dominant syndrome is recognized by characteristic facial features that include long palpebral fissures and eversion of the lower eyelids. The responsible gene and gene product are not known.

HEENT/AIRWAY: Long palpebral fissures, eversion of the lateral part of the lower eyelids, arched eyebrows, ptosis, strabismus, epicanthal folds, coloboma. Prominent ears, recurrent otitis media. Short nasal septum, depressed nasal tip. Broad philtrum. Abnormal dentition. Cleft palate.

CHEST: Rib anomalies. Can have pectus excavatum. Can have diaphragmatic eventration. Early thelarche in girls.

CARDIOVASCULAR: Cardiac defects are common, most commonly coarctation of the aorta, atrial septal defect, and ventricular septal defect. Right bundle branch block can also be seen.

NEUROMUSCULAR: Mild to moderate mental retardation. Hypotonia. Can have seizures.

ORTHOPEDIC: Short stature. Short digits, brachydactyly, cutaneous syndactyly. Dermatoglyphic abnormalities, nail hypoplasia. Scoliosis, vertebral anomalies. Hyperextensible joints. Dislocated hips.

GI/GU: Can have umbilical hernia, inguinal hernias, imperforate anus. Can have cryptorchidism, renal anomalies. Can have uteropelvic junction obstruction.

OTHER: Café au lait spots. Can be obese. Can be hirsute. Can have congenital hypothyroidism. Can have increased susceptibility to infections, probably based on an abnormal immunoglobulin response.

MISCELLANEOUS: Called Kabuki syndrome because of the similarity in the facial appearance between the affected people and the makeup of actors in Kabuki, a traditional Japanese theatrical form.

ANESTHETIC CONSIDERATIONS
Dental anomalies should be documented preoperatively. Patients with hyperextensible joints need to be positioned carefully. Patients with congenital cardiac disease will need perioperative antibiotic prophylaxis as indicated. Chronic use of anticonvulsant medications can alter the metabolism of some anesthetic drugs.

Bibliography:
1. Adam MP, Hudgins L. Kabuki syndrome: a review. *Clin Genet* 2005;67:209–219.
2. Wessels MW, Brooks AS, Hoogeboom J, et al. Kabuki syndrome: a review study of three hundred patients. *Clin Dysmorphol* 2002;11:95–102.
3. Kawame H, Hannibal MC, Hudgins L, et al. Phenotypic spectrum and management issues in Kabuki syndrome. *J Pediatr* 1999;134:480–485.

Kallmann Syndrome

MIM #: 308700, 147950, 244200

The clinical hallmarks of this syndrome are hypogonadotropic hypogonadism, midline intracranial anomalies and anosmia (inability to smell). X-linked (*KAL1* gene), autosomal dominant [fibroblast growth factor receptor-1 (*FGFR1*) gene], and autosomal recessive (*KAL3* gene) transmission have all been reported. The product of the X-linked *KAL* gene, termed anosmin-1, is synthesized by neural cells, and is involved in the migration of gonadotropin releasing hormone neurons and olfactory neurons to the hypothalamus. Patients can have findings of additional X-linked disorders, as the syndrome can be related to X chromosome deletions.

HEENT/AIRWAY: Hypotelorism. Sensorineural hearing loss. Anosmia, female carriers of the X-linked form have partial or complete anosmia. Choanal atresia. High-arched palate, cleft lip or palate.

CHEST: Gynecomastia.

CARDIOVASCULAR: Rarely can be associated with congenital cardiac defects.

NEUROMUSCULAR: Can have mental retardation. Agenesis of the olfactory lobes. Other midline intracranial anomalies. Mirror movements of the hands (bimanual synkinesia), cerebellar ataxia.

ORTHOPEDIC: In rare cases can be associated with short stature. Pes cavus.

GI/GU: Hypogonadism, due to a deficiency of hypothalamic gonadotropin-releasing hormone. Becomes apparent with the failure to develop secondary sex characteristics at puberty. Cryptorchidism. Can have unilateral or bilateral renal agenesis.

MISCELLANEOUS: Kallmann's opposition to Nazi racial doctrines led to his being banned from publishing in the medical literature and from speaking at medical meetings.

ANESTHETIC CONSIDERATIONS

When meeting the patient before surgery, confirm whether they have hearing loss. Endocrinologic dysfunction appears to be limited to gonadotropin. The presence of choanal atresia precludes a nasal airway, nasal intubation, or a nasogastric tube.

Bibliography:

1. Hermanussen M, Sippell WG. Heterogeneity of Kallmann's syndrome. *Clin Genet* 1985;28:106–111.

Kanner Syndrome

See Autism

Kanzaki Disease

Included in Schindler disease

Kartagener Syndrome

SYNONYM: Immotile cilia syndrome

MIM #: 244400

This autosomal recessive syndrome is characterized by situs inversus, chronic sinusitis, bronchiectasis, and male sterility. Kartagener syndrome is a subtype of the more generalized immotile cilia syndrome. The disorder is genetically diverse and the underlying defect is the absence of ciliary dynein arms, which renders the cilia immotile. Immotile cilia cause functional failure of the respiratory epithelium, leading to chronic sinusitis, chronic respiratory tract infection, and bronchiectasis. Immotile cilia also cause male sterility because sperm are rendered immobile. Immotile cilia in embryonic epithelial tissues may be the cause of situs inversus.

HEENT/AIRWAY: Can have corneal abnormalities. Frontal sinus may not develop, poor aeration of mastoid cells. Rhinitis, nasal polyps, chronic sinusitis. Olfactory incompetence. Chronic otitis media. Conductive hearing loss can develop.

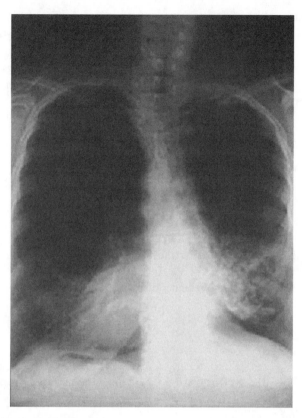

Kartagener syndrome. This adult man with Kartagener syndrome has situs inversus (note heart, stomach bubble and liver on the "incorrect" side and note the vertical angle of the left mainstem bronchus) and bronchiectasis. (Courtesy of Dr. David Jones, Department of Surgery, University of Virginia Health System.)

CHEST: Chronic cough with thick, tenacious sputum. Chronic respiratory tract infections, bronchiectasis. Bronchiectasis may necessitate partial lung resection.

CARDIOVASCULAR: Dextrocardia as part of situs inversus. However, there is not a significantly increased incidence of cardiac septation defects as is seen in isolated dextrocardia. The electrocardiogram with complete situs inversus is a mirror image of normal. Chronic bronchiectasis can result in cor pulmonale.

NEUROMUSCULAR: Chronic headaches (the ependyma of the brain is ciliated epithelium). Can have hydrocephalus. Can have a history of depression, schizophrenia.

GI/GU: Can have asplenia. Male sterility. Women may have decreased fertility.

OTHER: Situs inversus. May have low levels of IgA and abnormal neutrophil chemotaxis, but no increased incidence of infections other than respiratory tract infections.

MISCELLANEOUS: Manes Kartagener was born in Czechoslovakia, but practiced in Geneva. He reported the syndrome

29 years after Siewert. In affected families approximately half the affected individuals have situs inversus. Presumably chance determines the laterality.

ANESTHETIC CONSIDERATIONS
Patients have thick, tenacious sputum. Humidification of inspiratory gases is beneficial. Good perioperative chest physiotherapy is necessary. The increased incidence of sinusitis and otitis media is a relative contraindication for nasotracheal intubation. Anticholinergics decrease the volume of pulmonary secretions but not their chemical consistency—they are not thicker. Thus, anticholinergics are not contraindicated.

In the presence of situs inversus, an endotracheal tube placed too deeply will likely enter the left mainstem bronchus rather than the right mainstem bronchus. A left-sided, double-lumen endobronchial tube may occlude the proximal take-off of the left upper lobe bronchus. The origin of the upper lobe bronchus is more distal in the right lung. A left-sided tube can be rotated to the right and placed in the right mainstem bronchus, and vice versa for a right-sided tube (3). Cannulation of the left internal jugular vein is analogous to cannulation of the right internal jugular vein in normal patients. The electrocardiogram is a mirror image of normal, and leads should be placed accordingly. Defibrillator paddles should be placed in a mirror-image fashion over the right chest. Parturients should have right, rather than left, uterine displacement.

Bibliography:
1. Mathew PJ, Sadera GS, Sharafuddin S, et al. Anaesthetic considerations in Kartagener's syndrome—a case report. *Acta Anaesthesiol Scand* 2004;48:518–520.
2. Sahajananda H, Sanjay OP, Thomas J, et al. General anaesthesia for lobectomy in an 8-year-old child with Kartagener's syndrome. *Paediatr Anaesth* 2003;13:714–717.
3. Habibi A, Brodsky JB. Choice of double-lumen tube in Kartagener's syndrome [Letter]. *J Cardiothorac Vasc Anesth* 1997;6:810.
4. Tkebuchava T, von Segesser LK, Niederhauser U, et al. Cardiac surgery for Kartagener syndrome. *Pediatr Cardiol* 1997;18:72–73.
5. Losa M, Ghelfi D, Hof E, et al. Kartagener syndrome: an uncommon cause of neonatal respiratory distress? *Eur J Pediatr* 1995;154:236–238.
6. Ho AM, Friedland MJ. Kartagener's syndrome: anesthetic considerations. *Anesthesiology* 1992;77:386–388.

Kasabach-Merritt Syndrome

MIM #: 141000

This syndrome occurs when apparent capillary hemangiomas cause platelet trapping and a consumptive coagulopathy. Development of this syndrome is typically associated with rapid enlargement of the apparent hemangioma. Although this syndrome has been described as generically somewhat similar to hemangiomas, the histology of the lesions is not that of true hemangiomas (2), and is now described as kaposiform hemangioendotheliomas. In about 50% of the cases, this syndrome is present at birth, and unlike infantile hemangiomas has a predilection for the proximal extremities and trunk. Involvement of the head and face are rare. The tumor tends to be very difficult to treat medically, surgically, or by interventional radiologic techniques.

CARDIOVASCULAR: High-output cardiac failure, worsened by anemia.

ORTHOPEDIC: Can infiltrate muscle and bone.

GI/GU: Retroperitoneal hemangiomas with possible direct visceral spread.

OTHER: Microangiopathic hemolytic anemia with thrombocytopenia. Full-blown disseminated intravascular coagulation with hemorrhage may develop. Coagulopathies in adults with (the obsolete term) cavernous hemangioma are due to stasis which initiates the generation of thrombin and local clot formation, but the platelet count is minimally depressed (50–$150,000/mm^3$). Children with kaposiform hemangioendothelioma have platelet counts in the range of 3 to $60,000/mm^3$ due to platelet trapping within the tumor. There can also be red cell sequestration within the tumor. The peripheral blood smear does not show microangiopathic hemolytic changes. Severe hemorrhage is uncommon and chronic low platelet levels are generally well-tolerated.

ANESTHETIC CONSIDERATIONS
Patients may need perioperative red blood cell, platelet, or fresh frozen plasma transfusions. Transfused platelets have a shortened half-life of 1 to 24 hours due to consumption within the tumor. Tumor size can increase after platelet transfusion.

Bibliography:
1. Mulliken JB, Anupindi S, Ezekowitz RAB, et al. Case 13–2004: a newborn girl with a large cutaneous lesion, thrombocytopenia, and anemia. *N Engl J Med* 2004;350:1764–1775.
2. Enjolras O, Mazoyer E, Frieden IJ. Infants with Kasabach-Merritt syndrome do not have "true" hemangiomas. *J Pediatr* 1997;130:631–640.
3. Larsen EC, Zinkham WH, Eggleston JC, et al. Kasabach-Merritt syndrome: therapeutic considerations. *Pediatrics* 1987;79:971–980.

Kaufman-Mckusick Syndrome

See McKusick-Kaufman syndrome

Kearns-Sayre Syndrome

SYNONYM: Ophthalmoplegia-plus

MIM #: 530000

This sporadically occurring, but occasionally familial, mitochondrial myopathy is characterized by progressive external ophthalmoplegia, pigmented retinal degeneration, and atrioventricular conduction defects. Onset is before 20 years of age, usually in the pre-teen years. Light microscopy of the muscle often shows "ragged red" fibers, which represent abnormal, enlarged mitochondria and excess lipid. A deletion in the mitochondrial genome has been documented in many, but not all, patients and the disorder can be due to abnormalities in the mitochondrial leucine transfer ribonucleic acid (tRNA).

HEENT/AIRWAY: Abnormal retinal pigmentation associated with external ophthalmoplegia, ptosis, visual loss. Sensorineural hearing loss. Weakness can involve the pharyngeal muscles.

CHEST: There can be a depressed respiratory drive.

CARDIOVASCULAR: Heart block (second- or third-degree atrioventricular block, bundle branch block, or fascicular block) usually in the third decade of life, often presenting as Stokes-Adams attack or sudden death. Congestive cardiomyopathy can develop.

NEUROMUSCULAR: Can have cerebellar dysfunction with ataxia. Can have cranial nerve involvement. Can have weakness of bulbar and limb girdle muscles. Myopathy with proximal limb weakness. Seizures, dementia.

GI/GU: Fanconi syndrome (see earlier) can develop.

ORTHOPEDIC: Short stature. Kyphoscoliosis. Pes cavus.

OTHER: Hirsutism. Decreased 17-ketosteroid and 11-hydroxycorticoid excretion. A variety of defects in the respiratory chain and oxidative phosphorylation result in elevated serum lactate during exercise. Hyperglycemia and fatal hyperosmolar coma have been reported after steroid therapy.

ANESTHETIC CONSIDERATIONS

Stress, such as seen with surgery or infection, can increase the demand for adenosine triphosphate production to levels above which the patient can produce. Acidosis should be corrected preoperatively if possible. Patients with excessive lactic acidemia should not receive Ringer's lactate. Postoperative clinical deterioration has been reported (4).

Bulbar involvement and weakness of the pharyngeal muscles increase the perioperative aspiration risk. Second- or third-degree atrioventricular block, bundle branch block, or fascicular block are common. A temporary pacemaker should be available. Patients can have a cardiomyopathy.

Patients with Kearns-Sayre syndrome may be particularly sensitive to induction agents (11). Patients with mitochondrial myopathies may be more sensitive to mivacurium (5), curare (12), rocuronium (3), atracurium (3) and succinylcholine (14), although one report did not find increased sensitivity to succinylcholine or pancuronium (13). It is reasonable to avoid succinylcholine in patients with a significant myopathy because of the risk of an exaggerated hyperkalemic response. Nondepolarizing neuromuscular blockers should be given incrementally and with appropriate monitoring. Opioids or other drugs inhibiting respiratory drive should be used with caution, because increased central responsiveness

has been suggested (10). The issue of the relationship between the mitochondrial myopathies and malignant hyperthermia is not clear, but an association is unlikely.

Bibliography:

1. Hara K, Sata T, Shigematsu A. Anesthetic management for cardioverter-defibrillator implantation in a patient with Kearns-Sayre syndrome. *J Clin Anesth* 2004;16:539–541.
2. DiMauro S, Schon EA. Mitochondrial respiratory-chain diseases. *N Engl J Med* 2003;348:2656–2668.
3. Finsterer J, Stratil U, Bittner R, et al. Increased sensitivity to rocuronium and atracurium in mitochondrial myopathy. *Can J Anaesth* 1998;45:781–784.
4. Casta A, Quackenbush EJ, Houck CS, et al. Perioperative white matter degeneration and death in a patient with a defect in mitochondrial oxidative phosphorylation. *Anesthesiology* 1997;87:420–425.
5. Naguib M, el Dawlatly AA, Ashour M, et al. Sensitivity to mivacurium in a patient with mitochondrial myopathy. *Anesthesiology* 1996;84:1506–1509.
6. Kitoh T, Mizuno K, Otagiri T. Anesthetic management for a patient with Kearns-Sayre syndrome. *Anesth Analg* 1995;80:1240–1242.
7. Pivalizza EG, Ando KJ, Sweeney MS. Kearns-Sayre syndrome and cardiac anesthesia. *J Cardiothorac Vasc Anesth* 1995;9:189–191.
8. Lauwers MH, van Lersberghe C, Camu F. Inhalation anaesthesia and the Kearns-Sayre syndrome. *Anaesthesia* 1994;49:876–878.
9. Estes R, Ginsburg B, Bloch EC. Anaesthesia and the Kearns-Sayre syndrome. *Paediatr Anaesth* 1993;3:307–311.
10. Barohn RJ, Clayton T, Zarife S, et al. Recurrent respiratory insufficiency and depressed ventilatory drive complicating mitochondria myopathies. *Neurology* 1990;40:103–106.
11. James RH. Induction agent sensitivity and ophthalmoplegia plus [Letter]. *Anaesthesia* 1986;41:216.
12. Robertson JA. Ocular muscular dystrophy: a cause of curare sensitivity. *Anaesthesia* 1984;3:251–253.
13. D'Ambra MN, Dedrick D, Savarese JJ. Kearns-Sayre syndrome and pancuronium-succinylcholine-induced neuromuscular blockade. *Anesthesiology* 1979;51:343–345.
14. Lessell S, Kuwabara T, Feldman RG. Myopathy and succinylcholine sensitivity. *Am J Ophthalmol* 1969;68:789–796.

Kenny Syndrome

SYNONYM: Kenny-Caffey syndrome

MIM #: 127000, 244460

Both autosomal dominant and autosomal recessive forms of this syndrome exist. The autosomal recessive form is due to mutations in the gene *TBCE*, which encodes tubulin-specific chaperone E. Chaperones are a group of proteins which aid in proper protein folding. This syndrome is distinguished by proportional dwarfism.

HEENT/AIRWAY: Macrocephaly, delayed closure of the anterior fontanelle, absence of the diploic space of the skull. Dysmorphic ("birdlike") facies. Ophthalmologic abnormalities with hypertelorism, hyperopia, corneal and retinal calcifications, papilledema, and cataracts. Mandibular hypoplasia. Dental caries.

CHEST: Long thin clavicles and ribs. There is a single case report of the Mournier-Kuhn syndrome (tracheobronchomegaly and communicating paratracheal cysts) in an adult patient with Kenny syndrome.

NEUROMUSCULAR: Normal intelligence. Hypocalcemic seizures. Calcification of the basal ganglia.

ORTHOPEDIC: Proportional dwarfism of prenatal onset. Delayed bone age, cortical thickening of the tubular bones.

OTHER: Episodic hypocalcemia, presumably due to transient hypoparathyroidism. Hypophosphatemia, low calcitonin levels. Anemia.

MISCELLANEOUS: First described by Kenny. Caffey, a famous name in pediatric radiology, described the radiologic features a year later.

ANESTHETIC CONSIDERATIONS

Serum calcium and phosphorus levels should be evaluated, and may need to be corrected preoperatively. Mandibular hypoplasia may make direct laryngoscopy and tracheal intubation difficult. A laryngeal mask has been used successfully (1).

Bibliography:
1. Janke EL, Fletcher JE, Lewis IH, et al. Anaesthetic management of the Kenny-Caffey syndrome using the laryngeal mask. *Paediatr Anaesth* 1996;6:235–238.
2. Fanconi S, Fischer JA, Wieland P, et al. Kenny syndrome: evidence for idiopathic hypoparathyroidism in two patients and for abnormal parathyroid hormone in one. *J Pediatr* 1986;109:469–475.

Kenny-Caffey Syndrome

See Kenny syndrome

Ketotic Hyperglycinemia

See Propionic acidemia

Ketothiolase Deficiency

See Beta-ketothiolase deficiency

KID Syndrome

See Senter syndrome

King Syndrome

SYNONYM: King-Denborough syndrome

MIM #: 145600

This syndrome is characterized by Noonan-like features (see Noonan syndrome, later), congenital myopathy and susceptibility to malignant hyperthermia. Most reported cases are sporadic, but an autosomal dominant mode of inheritance is possible. It has been suggested that King syndrome represents a phenotype that can result from several different slowly progressive congenital myopathies (5, 6), and may simply be a synonym for malignant hyperthermia susceptibility (see later).

HEENT/AIRWAY: Unusual facies, suggestive of Noonan syndrome—ptosis, strabismus, low-set ears, malar hypoplasia, cleft or high-arched palate, crowded teeth. No hypertelorism or epicanthal folds as seen in Noonan syndrome. May have mild micrognathia. No webbed neck as seen in Noonan syndrome.

CHEST: Pectus carinatum or excavatum. May have thoracic kyphoscoliosis. May have restrictive lung disease. Progressive myopathy may lead to respiratory failure. May have diaphragmatic eventration.

CARDIOVASCULAR: No cardiac defects that are characteristic of Noonan syndrome. One report of dilated ventricles, aorta and pulmonary artery.

NEUROMUSCULAR: Congenital myopathy, which is slowly progressive. May have mild mental retardation. May have tethered spinal cord.

ORTHOPEDIC: Short stature. May have kyphoscoliosis, lumbar lordosis. Shoulder and patellar dislocation. Pes cavus.

GI/GU: Cryptorchidism.

OTHER: Susceptible to the development of malignant hyperthermia. May have elevated creatine kinase. No coagulation abnormalities as seen in Noonan syndrome.

ANESTHETIC CONSIDERATIONS

Patients are susceptible to the development of malignant hyperthermia, and must receive a nontriggering general anesthetic, neuraxial block or peripheral nerve block. (For more information see malignant hyperthermia susceptibility, later.) Succinylcholine is contraindicated in these patients with slowly progressive myopathy because of the risk of an exaggerated hyperkalemic response. Patients with advanced myopathy are at risk for perioperative respiratory compromise. Epidural analgesia has been utilized successfully for labor.

Bibliography:
1. Habib AS, Millar S, Deballi P, et al. Anesthetic management of a ventilator-dependent parturient with the King-Denborough syndrome. *Can J Anaesth* 2003;50:589–592.
2. Abel DE, Grotegut CA. King syndrome in pregnancy. *Obstet Gynecol* 2003;101:1146–1149.
3. Iwatsubo T, Yoshikawa M, Karashima Y, et al. Anesthetic management of the King-Denborough syndrome [Japanese]. *Masui* 2001;50:390–393.

4. Kinouchi K, Okawa M, Fukumitsu K, et al. Two pediatric cases of malignant hyperthermia caused by sevoflurane [Japanese]. *Masui* 2001;50: 1232–1235.
5. Graham GE, Silver K, Arlet V, et al. King syndrome: Further clinical variability and review of the literature. *Am J Med Genet* 1998;78: 254–259.
6. Chitayat D, Hodgkinson KA, Ginsburg O, et al. King syndrome: A genetically heterogenous phenotype due to congenital myopathies. *Am J Med Genet* 1992;43:954–956.
7. Isaacs H, Badenhorst ME. Dominantly inherited malignant hyperthermia (MH) in the King-Denborough syndrome. *Muscle Nerve* 1992;15:740–742.
8. Stewart CR, Kahler SG, Gilchrist JM. Congenital myopathy with cleft palate and increased susceptibility to malignant hyperthermia: King syndrome? *Pediatr Neurol* 1988;4:371–374.
9. Steenson AJ, Torkelson RD. King's syndrome with malignant hyperthermia: potential outpatient risks. *Am J Dis Child* 1987;141:271–273.

King-Denborough Syndrome

See King syndrome

Kinky Hair Syndrome

See Menkes kinky hair syndrome

Kleeblattschaedel

SYNONYM: Cloverleaf skull. (Includes scaphocephaly, dolichocephaly, brachycephaly, plagiocephaly, acrocephaly, turricephaly, trigonocephaly, and bathrocephaly)

MIM #: 148800

This deformity of the skull can occur in isolation or as part of a larger dysmorphic complex such as Carpenter, Crouzon, or Pfeiffer syndrome. It is due to congenital craniosynostosis (the premature closure of a skull suture) of multiple cranial sutures combined with hydrocephalus,

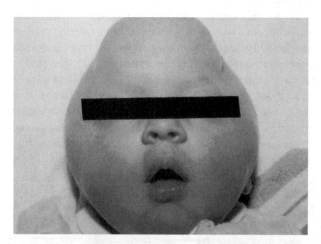

Kleeblattschaedel. An infant with kleeblattschaedel deformity of the skull. (Courtesy of Dr. K. Lin and the Craniofacial Anomalies Clinic, University of Virginia Health System.)

and results in a pattern of vertical and inferolateral skull growth, resulting in a cloverleaf-shaped (trilobular) skull. Although a single family with apparent autosomal dominant transmission has been described, the entity appears to be sporadic. Children require extensive craniofacial surgery, and may require multiple surgeries.

There are many patterns of craniosynostosis. All of the craniosynostoses can occur in isolation or as part of a syndrome complex. Sagittal synostosis prevents lateral skull growth, resulting in **scaphocephaly** (boat-shaped cranium) or **dolichocephaly** (long, narrow cranium). This can be seen in association with Marfan syndrome, Russell-Silver syndrome, and trisomy 18. Coronal synostosis prevents anteroposterior skull growth, resulting in **brachycephaly** (broad cranium). This can be seen in association with Down syndrome and Zellweger syndrome. Unilateral coronal synostosis results in **plagiocephaly** (slanted cranium). Coronal and lambdoid synostosis results in **acrocephaly** or **turricephaly,** where the cranium is pointed or tower shaped. This pattern is seen with the acrocephalosyndactyly syndromes. Metopic synostosis results in **trigonocephaly** (triangular cranium). Trigonocephaly can be associated with some of the chromosomal deletion syndromes and with C syndrome. Excessive bone formation at the lambdoid suture causes a step-like posterior projection of the skull, called **bathrocephaly** (step cranium).

HEENT/AIRWAY: Craniosynostosis of the coronal and lambdoid sutures results in cloverleaf (trilobular) skull. Can have severe exophthalmos. Can have other facial anomalies.

NEUROMUSCULAR: Hydrocephalus. Otherwise, there is rarely an abnormality of the central nervous system.

ORTHOPEDIC: Ankylosis of the elbow. Can have long bone anomalies.

ANESTHETIC CONSIDERATIONS
Precautions against increased intracranial pressure need to be taken in patients with significant hydrocephalus. Patients with exophthalmos need meticulous intraoperative eye care to avoid corneal abrasions. Patients with associated syndromes may have anesthetic implications specific to that syndrome.

Bibliography:
1. Sabry MZ, Wornom IL III, Ward JD. Results of cranial vault reshaping. *Ann Plast Surg* 2001;47:119–125.
2. Resnick DK, Pollack IF, Albright AL. Surgical management of the cloverleaf skull deformity. *Pediatr Neurosurg* 1995;22:29–37.
3. Frank LM, Mason MA, Magee WP, et al. The kleeblattschadel deformity: neurologic outcome with early treatment. *Pediatr Neurol* 1985;1:379–381.

Klein-Waardenburg Syndrome

Included in Waardenburg syndrome

Klinefelter Syndrome

SYNONYM: XXY syndrome. (Includes XXXY, XXXXY, and XXYY syndromes)

MIM #: None

Klinefelter syndrome is an anomaly of the sex chromosomes in which the patient has a 47,XXY karyotype. Klinefelter syndrome is the most common cause of male hypogonadism and infertility. Affected individuals are also often mildly mentally retarded and may exhibit behavioral problems. There is significant phenotypic variability. Karyotypes **XXXY, XXXXY,** and **XXYY** exhibit features of Klinefelter syndrome to varying degrees, and so are included here. XXXY, XXXXY, and XXYY patients are more likely to be mentally retarded than XXY patients. XXXY patients can also have growth deficiency, radioulnar synostosis at the elbow, and congenital heart disease.

CHEST: Chronic bronchitis is relatively common.

CARDIOVASCULAR: XXXY patients can have congenital heart disease.

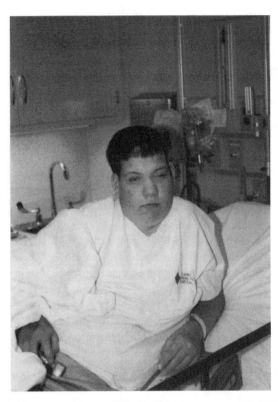

Klinefelter syndrome. FIG. 2. This teenager with XXXXY syndrome became physically violent in the preoperative holding area and refused oral premedication. After a long talk with him, induction of anesthesia was uneventful.

NEUROMUSCULAR: Most have mild mental retardation (especially the XXXY, XXXXY, and XXYY variants). Verbal performance is usually close to or within the normal range. Patients frequently exhibit behavioral problems, including aggressive behavior, poor judgment, and boastfulness. Can have an intention tremor.

ORTHOPEDIC: Relatively tall, slim stature, with long extremities. Scoliosis can develop during adolescence. Clinodactyly. XXXY patients can be short and have radioulnar synostosis at the elbow.

GI/GU: Hypogenitalism and hypogonadism (small penis and testes, inadequate testosterone production, inadequate virilization) appear at the time of puberty. Infertility. Can have cryptorchidism, hypospadias.

OTHER: Gynecomastia. Extragonadal malignant germ cell tumors, and increased incidence of breast cancer. Increased risk for development of diabetes mellitus. Despite the relatively benign clinical implications, approximately half of all cases are lost prenatally.

ANESTHETIC CONSIDERATIONS

Behavioral problems may make the smooth induction of anesthesia difficult. Patients may require a lot of preoperative effort and attention, and may benefit from premedication.

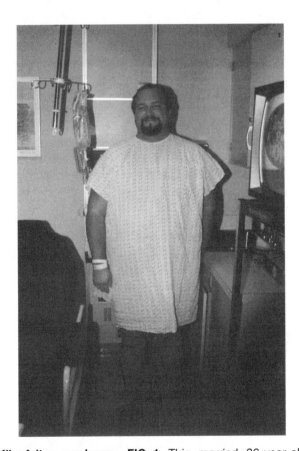

Klinefelter syndrome. FIG. 1. This married 36-year-old man receives chronic testosterone injections. He has had liposuction for gynecomastia and later developed breast cancer.

Bibliography:
1. Lanfranco F, Kamischke A, Zitzmann M, et al. Klinefelter's syndrome. *Lancet* 2004;364:273–283.
2. Visootsak J, Aylstock M, Graham JM Jr. Klinefelter syndrome and its variants: an update and review for the primary pediatrician. *Clin Pediatr* 2001;40:639–651.
3. Smyth CM, Bremner WJ. Klinefelter syndrome. *Arch Intern Med* 1998;158:1309–1314.
4. Rovet J, Netley C, Keenan M, et al. The psychoeducational profile of boys with Klinefelter syndrome. *J Learn Disabil* 1996;29:180–196.

Klippel-Feil Sequence

MIM #: 148900

This sometimes autosomal dominant but usually sporadically occurring disorder is characterized by a short neck, a low posterior hairline, and limited mobility of the cervical spine. It has been suggested that Klippel-Feil sequence, Moebius sequence, and Poland sequence (see later for both), all of which can occur in various combinations in the same patient, might represent anomalies from the intrauterine disruption of the subclavian or vertebral arteries, or one of their branches. Therefore, some suggest that these be called the subclavian artery supply disruption syndromes.

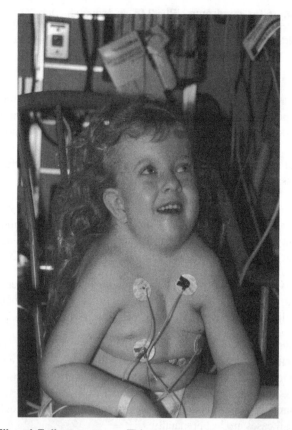

Klippel-Feil sequence. This young girl with Klippel-Feil sequence required home oxygen for obstructive sleep apnea and required a tonsillectomy. She has profound sensorineural hearing loss and absent neck flexion or extension. At 4 years of age laryngoscopy and intubation were reported as only moderately difficult.

HEENT/AIRWAY: Skull malformations can occur. May have facial asymmetry. Low posterior hairline. Can have sensorineural or conductive hearing loss. Can have cleft lip. Can have micrognathia. Webbed neck. Can have primary and permanent oligodontia. Torticollis. Malformed laryngeal cartilage with voice abnormalities can occur.

CHEST: Thoracic outlet syndrome has been reported.

CARDIOVASCULAR: Can have a congenital cardiac anomaly, particularly ventricular septal defect.

NEUROMUSCULAR: Hypermobility (though less common than limited mobility) of the upper cervical spine can be associated with neurologic impairment. Neurologic sequelae include paraplegia, hemiplegia, cranial or cervical nerve palsies. Syncope has been induced by sudden neck rotation. Can be associated with neural tube defects. May have posterior fossa dermoid cysts. A child with vertebral artery dissection has been reported.

ORTHOPEDIC: Limited mobility of the cervical spine secondary to vertebral fusion, hemivertebrae, or other vertebral defects. Atlantooccipital fusion. Increased susceptibility to cervical osteoarthritis and trauma. Scoliosis. May have winged scapulae (Sprengel deformity). Can have thoracic or lumbar vertebral anomalies. Can have sacral agenesis. It is thought that patients with hypermobility of the upper cervical spine are at risk for neurologic sequelae, whereas those with limited mobility in the lower cervical spine are more at risk for development of degenerative disease (8).

GI/GU: May have genitourinary or renal anomalies.

MISCELLANEOUS: Maurice Klippel was described in his obituary as a "philosopher, poet, historian and one of the most prominent masters of French medicine."

ANESTHETIC CONSIDERATIONS
Limited mobility of the cervical spine makes laryngoscopy and intubation extremely difficult. Since cervical fusion is progressive, a previous uncomplicated tracheal intubation does not assure repeated easy success (4). An unstable cervical spine raises the possibility of neurologic insult with head manipulation and positioning. Consider preoperative lateral flexion-extension radiographs of the cervical spine to identify patients with cervical spine instability. A laryngeal mask airway (LMA) has been used successfully (2,3,5). Consider fiberoptic intubation as an alternative to direct laryngoscopy because it requires significantly less head manipulation. Access to the central veins via the neck veins or subclavian veins may be problematic. High lumbar or thoracic epidural access should not be exceptionally problematic (5). Patients with congenital cardiac defects should receive perioperative antibiotic prophylaxis as indicated.

Bibliography:

1. Sehata H, Kohase H, Takahashi M, et al. Tracheal intubation using a new CCD camera-equipped device: a report of two cases with a difficult intubation. *Acta Anaesthesiol Scand* 2005;49:1218–1220.
2. Manivel S, Prasad R, Jacobi R. Anesthetic management of a child with Klippel-Feil syndrome in the radiology suite [Letter]. *Paediatr Anaesth* 2005;15:171–172.
3. Nargozian C. The airway in patients with craniofacial abnormalities. *Paediatr Anaesth* 2004;14:53–59.
4. Farid IS, Omar OA, Insler SR. Multiple anesthetic challenges in a patient with Klippel-Feil syndrome undergoing cardiac surgery. *J Cardiothorac Vasc Anesth* 2003;17:502–505.
5. O'Connor PJ, Moysa GL, Finucane BT. Thoracic epidural anesthesia for bilateral reduction mammoplasty in a patient with Klippel-Feil syndrome. *Anesth Analg* 2001;92:514–516.
6. Dresner MR, Maclean AR. Anaesthesia for Caesarean section in a patient with Klippel-Feil syndrome. *Anaesthesia* 1995;50:807–809.
7. Clarke RA, Davis PJ, Tonkin J. Klippel-Feil syndrome associated with malformed larynx: case report. *Ann Otol Rhinol Laryngol* 1994;103:201–207.
8. Pizzutillo PD, Woods M, Nicholson L, et al. Risk factors in Klippel-Feil syndrome. *Spine* 1994;19:2110–2116.
9. Daum RE, Jones DJ. Fibreoptic intubation in Klippel-Feil syndrome. *Anaesthesia* 1988;43:18–21.
10. Burns AM, Dorje P, Lawes EG, et al. Anaesthetic management of caesarean section for a mother with pre-eclampsia, the Klippel-Feil syndrome and congenital hydrocephalus. *Br J Anaesth* 1988;61:350–354.
11. Dresner MR, Maclean AR. Anaesthesia for caesarean section in a patient with Klippel-Feil syndrome. The use of a microspinal catheter. *Anaesthesia* 1988;61:350–354.
12. Naguib M, Farag H, Ibrahim AE. Anaesthetic considerations in Klippel-Feil syndrome. *Can Anaesth Soc J* 1986;33:66–70.

Klippel-Trenaunay Syndrome

See Klippel-Trenaunay-Weber syndrome

Klippel-Trenaunay-Weber Syndrome

SYNONYM: Klippel-Trenaunay syndrome

MIM #: 149000

This syndrome involves asymmetric extremity hypertrophy and various vascular abnormalities, including varicose veins, hemangiomas, arteriovenous fistulae, and phlebectasia. The syndrome occurs sporadically. At least some cases are due to mutations in the gene *VG5Q*, which encodes an angiogenic factor. Clinically, this syndrome often resembles Sturge-Weber syndrome (see later).

HEENT/AIRWAY: Asymmetric facial hypertrophy. Can have microcephaly or macrocephaly. Glaucoma, cataracts, Marcus Gunn pupil.

CHEST: Pectus excavatum. Intrathoracic hematomas, pleural hemangiomas. Risk of pulmonary thromboembolism from the deep venous malformations.

CARDIOVASCULAR: In rare cases, large arteriovenous fistulae lead to high-output congestive heart failure. Postural hypotension can occur with the filling of a massively dilated venous bed. Inferior vena cava may be absent.

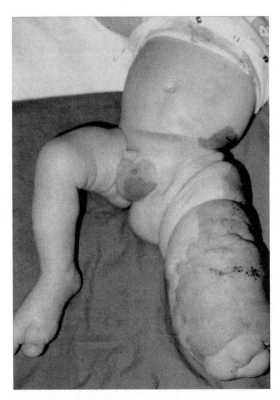

Klippel-Trenaunay-Weber syndrome. Severely involved lower extremity in a young child with Klippel-Trenaunay-Weber syndrome. (Courtesy of Dr. Kenneth E. Greer, Department of Dermatology, University of Virginia Health System.)

NEUROMUSCULAR: Epidural hemangiomas, which can bleed. Spinal cord arteriovenous malformations, which can rupture. Intracranial hemangiomas or calcifications. Patients with facial hemangiomas can have seizures or mental retardation. Otherwise, intelligence is normal.

ORTHOPEDIC: Asymmetric extremity hypertrophy—can be bony and soft tissue hypertrophy or massive enlargement from vascular lesions. The latter may require amputation. The most common site for involvement is the leg. Digits can be large or small, and there can be polydactyly. Can have kyphoscoliosis. Arthritis may develop.

GI/GU: Visceral or pelvic hemangiomas. Rupture of hemangiomas can cause gastrointestinal or urinary tract bleeding or menorrhagia.

OTHER: Vascular abnormalities occur most commonly in the legs, buttocks, and abdomen. Vascular abnormalities are also usually asymmetric. Increased risk of chronic disseminated intravascular coagulation (Kasabach-Merritt syndrome, see earlier). Thrombophlebitis. Cutis marmorata.

MISCELLANEOUS: Weber described the occurrence of arteriovenous fistulae with this syndrome, and sometimes the name Klippel-Trenaunay-Weber syndrome is used when arteriovenous fistulae are a feature of the syndrome, whereas

Klippel-Trenaunay syndrome is used when arteriovenous fistulae are not present.

Maurice Klippel was described in his obituary as a "philosopher, poet, historian and one of the most prominent masters of French medicine." F. Parkes Weber was a British physician who had an interest in rare disorders and uncommon syndromes. Weber's father came from Germany to Britain (where he became physician to Queen Victoria), and Weber continued to pronounce his last name with the "W" pronounced as the Germanic "V." He had an encyclopedic knowledge of rare disorders. It is said that when, at a meeting of the Royal Society of Medicine, he first announced that he had not heard of a certain syndrome, such cheers and applause broke out from the audience that the meeting had to be abandoned. He wrote a total of 1,200 medical papers.

ANESTHETIC CONSIDERATIONS

Expanding hemangiomas can result in Kasabach-Merritt syndrome (see earlier), with thrombocytopenia and consumptive coagulopathy. Surgical injury to hemangiomas or fistulae can result in excessive intraoperative bleeding. Blood for intraoperative transfusion should be available. These vessels also have abnormal autoregulation, so perioperative blood pressure must be carefully controlled.

Because of the risk of bleeding from epidural hemangiomas and spinal cord arteriovenous malformations, regional anesthesia is relatively contraindicated (7). However, it has been undertaken after a magnetic resonance imaging evaluation of the lumbosacral spine and back (2, 6). Consumptive coagulopathy should be excluded prior to attempting regional techniques. One patient experienced severe pain in an affected leg coincident with the onset of the sympathectomy following epidural anesthesia, which resolved with the onset of the sensory blockade (3).

Limb involvement can limit peripheral venous access. Excessive venous pulsations can result in erroneously low pulse oximetry readings if the probe is placed on an affected limb. Peripheral nerve stimulators should not be placed on an involved extremity. Cardiac function should be evaluated preoperatively for evidence of high-output failure. Excision of veins for coronary artery bypass grafting should be avoided in favor of arterial conduits if at all possible.

Bibliography:

1. El Oakley R, Al Aseedi A, Aitizazuddin S, et al. Coronary artery bypass graft surgery in a patient with atypical Klippel-Trenaunay syndrome. *J Cardiothorac Vasc Anesth* 2000;14:66–67.
2. Dobbs P, Caunt A, Alderson TJ. Epidural analgesia in an obstetric patient with Klippel-Trenaunay syndrome. *Br J Anaesth* 1999;82:144–146.
3. Collier C. More on Klippel-Trenaunay syndrome [Letter]. *Anaesth Intensive Care* 1999;26:599.
4. Ezri T, Szmuk P, Pansky A. Anaesthetic management for Klippel-Trenaunay-Weber syndrome [Letter]. *Paediatr Anaesth* 1996;6:81.
5. Samuel M, Spitz L. Klippel-Trenaunay syndrome: clinical features, complications and management in children. *Br J Surg* 1995;82:757–761.
6. Gaiser RR, Cheek TG, Gutsche BB. Major conduction anesthesia in a patient with Klippel-Trenaunay syndrome. *J Clin Anesth* 1993;7:316–319.
7. de Leon-Casasola OA, Lema MJ. Anesthesia for patients with Sturge-Weber disease and Klippel-Trenaunay syndrome. *J Clin Anesth* 1991;3:409–413.
8. Gloviczki P, Stanson AW, Stickler GB. et al. Klippel-Trenaunay syndrome: the risks and benefits of vascular interventions. *Surgery* 1991;110:469–479.

Kniest Dysplasia

See Kniest syndrome

Kniest Syndrome

SYNONYM: Kniest dysplasia; Metatropic dysplasia, type II; Pseudometatrophic dysplasia

MIM #: 156550

This autosomal dominant disorder is characterized by progressive short-trunk dwarfism, short limbs, flat facies, and limited joint mobility. The clinical features are similar to metatropic dysplasia, type I (also known as metatropic dwarfism, see later), except that inheritance is autosomal dominant. Kniest syndrome is caused by a mutation in the *COL2A1* gene, which leads to abnormal type II collagen. Abnormal type II collagen leads to soft cartilage that has a "Swiss cheese" appearance on microscopic examination, secondary to multiple lacunae. Mutations in the *COL2A1* gene are also responsible for achondrogenesis, spondyloepiphyseal dysplasia congenita, and Stickler syndrome.

HEENT/AIRWAY: Macrocephaly. Flat facies. Prominent eyes, myopia, cataracts, vitreoretinal degeneration, retinal detachment. Flat nasal bridge. Cleft palate. Recurrent otitis media related to cleft palate can cause hearing loss. Can have micrognathia. Tracheomalacia.

CHEST: Increased anteroposterior diameter of the chest.

NEUROMUSCULAR: Intelligence is normal.

ORTHOPEDIC: Short stature. Short trunk secondary to marked lumbar lordosis and kyphoscoliosis. Atlantooccipital instability. Short limbs. Limited joint mobility. Flexion contractures of major joints. Premature arthritis. Small pelvis.

GI/GU: Umbilical hernia, inguinal hernias.

MISCELLANEOUS: Described by Kniest when he was a chief resident in pediatrics.

ANESTHETIC CONSIDERATIONS

Despite the child-size stature, patients have intelligence that is normal for their chronologic age. Tracheomalacia may be severe enough to cause perioperative respiratory distress. Patients must be carefully positioned secondary to limited joint mobility. There are no reports of cervical spine injury during laryngoscopy in patients with atlantooccipital instability.

Bibliography:
1. Spranger J, Winterpacht A, Zobel B. The type II collagenopathies: a spectrum of chondrodysplasias. *Eur J Pediatr* 1994;153:56–65.
2. Berkowitz I, Raja SBender K, et al. Dwarfs: pathophysiology and anesthetic implications. *Anesthesiology* 1990;73:739–759.

Kok Disease

See Stiff-baby syndrome

Kostmann Disease

MIM #: 202700

This autosomal recessive neonatal immune deficiency syndrome is marked by neutropenia. The bone marrow shows normal granulocyte precursors, and the disease is thought to be due to arrested neutrophil development. Death often occurs during infancy. Treatment is with granulocyte-colony stimulating factor (G-CSF) or bone marrow transplantation.

HEENT: Otitis media. Periodontal disease.

CHEST: Upper and lower respiratory tract infections. Pneumonia.

GI/GU: Mild hepatosplenomegaly. Neonatal omphalitis.

OTHER: Overwhelming (and fatal) bacterial infections develop during infancy. There can also be eosinophilia and thrombocytosis. Increased risk for acute monocytic leukemia and myelodysplasia.

ANESTHETIC CONSIDERATIONS
Meticulous aseptic technique and appropriate perioperative antibiotics are imperative.

Bibliography:
1. Zeidler C, Welte K. Kostmann syndrome and severe congenital neutropenia. *Sem Hematol* 2002;39:82–88.
2. Zeidler C, Boxer L, Dale DC. Management of Kostmann syndrome in the G-CSF era. *Br J Haematol* 2000;109:490–495.
3. Calhoun DA, Christensen RD. The occurrence of Kostmann syndrome in preterm neonates. *Pediatrics* 1997;99:259–261.

Kozlowski Spondylometaphyseal Dysplasia

See Spondylometaphyseal dysplasia

Krabbe Disease

SYNONYM: Cerebroside lipidosis; Galactocerebrosidase deficiency; Globoid-cell leukodystrophy

MIM #: 245200

All the leukodystrophies involve defective formation of myelin. This autosomal recessive leukodystrophy is caused by a deficiency of galactocerebrosidase (galactosylceramidase). Galactocerebrosidase splits the galactocerebroside into ceramide and galactose. Galactocerebroside is a sphingoglycolipid containing sphingosine, fatty acid, and galactose, and is found almost entirely within the myelin sheath. This disease is characterized by loss of myelin and oligodendroglia. It is thought that the accumulation of psychosine, also a metabolic substrate for this enzyme, is responsible for the destruction of the oligodendroglia by inducing apoptosis. Globoid cells (mesodermal macrophages containing undigested galactocerebroside) are seen in the white matter. Because myelination begins just before birth in human beings, patients often exhibit a relatively normal neonatal course, which is then followed by deterioration. This disease is typically devastating and fatal in the first 2 years. However, improved diagnostic techniques have identified older patients with milder disease, and there is a subset of patients with juvenile and even adult onset disease. There is no specific therapy. Bone marrow or banked umbilical cord stem cell transplantation has recently been shown to reverse or prevent the central nervous system deterioration, as microglia are derived from hematopoietic stem cells. Survival is markedly improved if transplantation occurs when patients are still asymptomatic.

The other leukodystrophies include adrenoleukodystrophy, metachromatic leukodystrophy, Canavan disease, Pelizaeus-Merzbacher disease, and Alexander disease.

HEENT/AIRWAY: Blindness, slow pupillary reflexes. Protruding ears, hearing loss. Copious oral secretions.

CHEST: Respiratory failure eventually develops in most patients.

NEUROMUSCULAR: Profound mental and motor deterioration. Early hypertonicity. Prominent pyramidal tract signs. Severe demyelination. Peripheral neuropathy. Seizures, choreoathetosis. Irritability, hypersensitivity to external stimuli, and hypertonicity progressing to weakness, hypotonia, and flaccidity. Eventual decerebration, which can on occasions persist for several years.

GI/GU: Increased incidence of gastroesophageal reflux. Recurrent vomiting and feeding difficulty.

OTHER: Episodic fever.

MISCELLANEOUS: Knud Krabbe was an exceptional Danish neurologist. He spoke Greek by the age of 3 years, and he published his first scientific paper at age 10.

ANESTHETIC CONSIDERATIONS
Patients are at increased risk for perioperative aspiration because of copious secretions, poor airway tone, and gastroesophageal reflux. Consideration should be given to anticholinergic premedication to dry oral secretions.

Careful intraoperative positioning and padding is important in patients with poor nutrition. Chronic use of anticonvulsant medications can alter the metabolism of some anesthetic drugs, requiring more frequent dosing. Anticonvulsant medications should be continued through the perioperative period. A parenteral form of anticonvulsant medication may need to be substituted while patients are unable to take oral medications. Phenothiazines, butyrophenones, and other dopaminergic blockers should be avoided because they can exacerbate movement disorders. Ondansetron may be an appropriate antiemetic because it does not have anti-dopaminergic effects. Increased risk from succinylcholine has not been reported, but it is not unreasonable to avoid it in patients with profound muscle disease. Because of copious oral secretions and airway hypotonia, patients should be observed closely for postoperative ventilatory adequacy.

Bibliography:

1. Escolar ML, Poe MD, Provenzale JM, et al. Transplantation of umbilical-cord blood in babies with infantile Krabbe's disease. *N Engl J Med* 2005;352:2069–2081.
2. Krivit W, Shapiro EG, Peters C, et al. Hematopoietic stem-cell transplantation in globoid-cell leukodystrophy. *N Engl J Med* 1998;338:1119–1126.
3. Aicardi J. The inherited leukodystrophies: a clinical overview. *J Inherit Metab Dis* 1993;16:733–743.
4. Tobias JD. Anaesthetic considerations for the child with leukodystrophy. *Can J Anaesth* 1992;39:394–397.

Kugelberg-Welander Disease

SYNONYM: Spinal muscular atrophy III; Juvenile spinal muscle atrophy

MIM #: 253400, 158600

This usually autosomal recessive disease of the anterior horn cells involves a defect in the gene *SMN1* (survival of motor neuron 1), which appears to have a role in RNA processing. This is the same gene that is responsible for spinal muscular atrophy I (Werdnig-Hoffmann disease, see later), which is the most severe form, and spinal muscular atrophy II, which is an intermediate form. The three forms are likely allelic. Autosomal dominant forms of Kugelberg-Welander disease have also been described. This lower motor neuron disease usually has its onset in childhood, with an expected survival into adulthood. In fact, life expectancy is normal. Boys are often more severely affected than their female siblings. Kugelberg-Welander disease may initially be misdiagnosed as limb-girdle muscular dystrophy (see later) because muscle weakness and atrophy often begin with the proximal limb muscles.

CHEST: Decreased pulmonary function with recurrent respiratory infections. Disordered breathing during sleep.

NEUROMUSCULAR: Lower motor neuron disease without sensory loss. Muscle weakness and atrophy beginning with the proximal limb muscles, especially the hip girdle. Later, muscle weakness involves the distal musculature. There can be pseudohypertrophy of the calf muscles (appearing hypertrophied in comparison to the atrophied thigh muscles). Facial and bulbar involvement is rare. The electromyogram shows evidence of denervation and reinnervation, with fibrillations, fasciculations and large-amplitude polyphasic potentials.

ORTHOPEDIC: Kyphoscoliosis and contractures late in the disease.

OTHER: Abdominal weakness in affected women may necessitate an instrumented delivery or cesarean section.

MISCELLANEOUS: In 1964, Lisa Welander became the first female professor of neurology in Sweden.

ANESTHETIC CONSIDERATIONS
Succinylcholine is contraindicated in this disease of lower motor neurons because of the risk of exaggerated hyperkalemia. Nondepolarizing muscle relaxants should be used sparingly, if at all, and titrated to effect. Patients may require protracted postoperative ventilation. Kyphoscoliosis may make regional techniques difficult, although they are not contraindicated.

Bibliography:

1. McLoughlin L, Bhagvat P. Anaesthesia for caesarean section in spinal muscular atrophy type III. *Int J Obstet Anesth* 2004;13:192–195.
2. Buettner AU. Anaesthesia for a Caesarean section in a patient with spinal muscular atrophy. *Anaesth Intensive Care* 2003;31:92–94.
3. Veen A, Molenbuur B, Richardson FJ. Epidural anaesthesia in a child with possible spinal muscle atrophy. *Paediatr Anaesth* 2002;12:556–558.
4. Weston LA, DiFazio C. Labor analgesia and anesthesia in a patient with spinal muscular atrophy and vocal cord paralysis: a rare and unusual case report. *Reg Anesth* 1996;21:350–354.
5. Samaha FJ, Buncher CR, Russman BS, et al. Pulmonary function in spinal muscular atrophy. *J Child Neurol* 1994;9:326–329.
6. Litman RS, Voisone R. Obstetric anaesthesia and spinal cord injury [Letter]. *Can J Anaesth* 1992;39:1117.

L

Lacrimoauriculodentodigital Syndrome

See Levy-Hollister syndrome

LADD Syndrome

See Levy-Hollister syndrome

Landouzy-Dejerine Disease

See Facioscapulohumeral muscular dystrophy

Langer Mesomelic Dysplasia

MIM #: 249700

This syndrome is distinguished by mesomelic dwarfism, aplastic or severely hypoplastic fibulae, and mandibular hypoplasia. This syndrome is the homozygous form of the autosomal dominant disorder known as Leri-Weill dyschondrosteosis (see later). Both are due to a deletion or mutation in the gene *SHOX*. Although this gene is located on the X chromosome, it is said to be pseudoautosomal. Langer mesomelic dysplasia is associated with more severe involvement of the forearms and lower legs and more striking mesomelic dwarfism than is the autosomal dominant form. The homozygous form also has the additional feature of mandibular hypoplasia.

HEENT/AIRWAY: Hypoplastic mandible.

NEUROMUSCULAR: Normal intelligence.

ORTHOPEDIC: Mesomelic dwarfism. Hypoplastic and bowed radius. Aplastic or severely hypoplastic ulna. Aplastic or severely hypoplastic fibulae. Hypoplastic and bowed tibia. No other skeletal abnormalities.

ANESTHETIC CONSIDERATIONS
It should be kept in mind that despite the significant orthopedic disability, patients are of normal intelligence. Direct laryngoscopy and tracheal intubation may be more difficult secondary to mandibular hypoplasia. Severe mesomelic dwarfism makes peripheral intravenous access more difficult.

Bibliography:
1. Berkowitz I, Raja S, Bender K. et al. Dwarfs: pathophysiology and anesthetic implications. *Anesthesiology* 1990;73:739–759.
2. Kunze J, Klemm T. Mesomelic dysplasia, type Langer: a homozygous state for dyschondrosteosis. *Eur J Pediatr* 1980;134:269–272.

Langer-Giedion Syndrome

SYNONYM: Trichorhinophalangeal syndrome, type II

MIM #: 150230

This usually sporadic syndrome is characterized by mental retardation, multiple bony exostoses, cone-shaped epiphyses, characteristic facies with a bulbous nose, and redundant skin in infancy. The facies of Langer-Giedion syndrome resemble those of trichorhinophalangeal syndrome, type I, but the Langer-Giedion syndrome also involves mental retardation, multiple exostoses, and redundant skin. Different-sized deletions on the long arm of chromosome 8 are responsible for both the Langer-Giedion syndrome and trichorhinophalangeal syndrome, type I. The Langer-Giedion syndrome involves deletion of a greater amount of genetic material, involving functional loss of the genes *TRPS1* and *EXT1*.

HEENT/AIRWAY: Microcephaly. Deep-set eyes, heavy eyebrows, exotropia, coloboma. Large, protruding ears. Hearing loss. Bulbous nose with broad nasal bridge. Long, prominent philtrum, thin upper lip. Abnormal dentition. Micrognathia.

CHEST: Recurrent upper respiratory tract infections.

CARDIOVASCULAR: May have congenital cardiac defects.

NEUROMUSCULAR: Variable mental retardation. Speech delay. Hypotonia in infancy. Electroencephalographic abnormalities or seizures may develop.

ORTHOPEDIC: Mild growth deficiency. Multiple bony exostoses, particularly of the long bones. Single report of a large cervical exostotic osteochondroma causing cord compression and quadraparesis. Multiple exostoses affect bone growth and increase the risk of fracture. Cone-shaped epiphyses. Syndactyly. Hypoplastic nails. Winged scapulae. Hyperextensible joints. Vertebral defects. Scoliosis.

GI/GU: May have umbilical hernia, inguinal hernias. May have cryptorchidism, cloacal anomalies. May have ureteral reflux.

OTHER: Loose, redundant skin in infancy. Fine, sparse scalp hair. Maculopapular nevi on the head, neck, upper trunk and limbs. May have hypochromatic anemia.

ANESTHETIC CONSIDERATIONS
Consider obtaining a preoperative hematocrit because of the possibility of hypochromic anemia. Recurrent upper respiratory tract infections are common, and may lead to cancellation of elective cases. Direct laryngoscopy and endotracheal intubation may be difficult secondary to micrognathia, particularly in infancy. Abnormal dentition may be more easily injured during laryngoscopy. Patients must be carefully positioned intraoperatively secondary to hyperextensible joints and the increased risk of bony fracture. Patients with congenital cardiac defects require perioperative antibiotic prophylaxis as indicated.

Bibliography:
1. Buhler EM, Buhler UK, Beutler C, et al. A final word on the tricho-rhino-phalangeal syndromes. *Clin Genet* 1987;31:273–275.
2. Langer LO, Krassikoff N, Laxova R, et al. The tricho-rhino-phalangeal syndrome with exostosis (or Langer-Giedion syndrome): four additional patients without mental retardation and a review of the literature. *Am J Med Genet* 1984;19:81–111.

Langer-Saldino Achondrogenesis

Included in Achondrogenesis

Langerhans Cell Histiocytosis

Previously called Histiocytosis-X
(Includes Eosinophilic granuloma, Hand-Schüller-Christian disease, and Letterer-Siwe disease)

MIM #: 604856

This relatively new term includes three entities that were previously included under the designation "histiocytosis-X." In increasing order of severity, these entities are **eosinophilic granuloma, Hand-Schüller-Christian disease,** and **Letterer-Siwe disease.** They are all caused by a proliferation of a specific type of histiocyte, the Langerhans cell. These are not malignant diseases but rather manifestations of immune dysregulation. The proliferation of these normal cells affects the function of a variety of organs. It is suggested that the disease be characterized specifically by the degree and number of organ systems involved, rather than by the names used previously. Originally, **eosinophilic granuloma** referred to solitary, circumscribed, nonprogressive skull lesions, sometimes associated with eosinophilia. **Hand-Schüller-Christian disease** referred to a triad of exophthalmos, bony defects, and diabetes insipidus. **Letterer-Siwe disease** referred to acute disseminated histiocytosis with cutaneous, mucosal, and bony lesions.

HEENT/AIRWAY: Solitary or multiple circumscribed skull lesions. Orbital lesions may cause proptosis. Hearing loss may develop. Lesions of the mastoid or petrous portion of the temporal bone can lead to chronic ear drainage that mimics chronic draining otitis media. Lesions of the mandible and maxilla can cause displacement, loosening or loss of teeth.

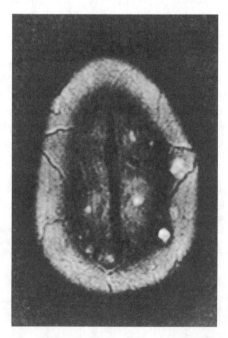

Langerhans cell histiocytosis. FIG. 1. Intracranial lesions.

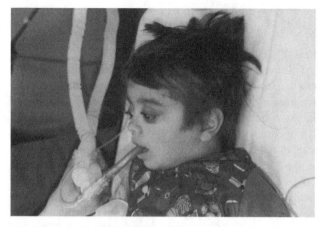

Langerhans cell histiocytosis. FIG. 2. This 6-year-old with Langerhans cell histiocytosis has exophthalmos, diabetes insipidus, skull lesions, splenomegaly, and a scaly rash. She also has seizures and temperature instability from hypothalamic involvement.

CHEST: Pulmonary involvement with cough, dyspnea, cyanosis and pleural effusions. Infiltrative nodules, interstitial pneumonitis. Lung cysts, which can rupture and cause a pneumothorax. Respiratory failure in severe cases.

CARDIOVASCULAR: Involvement of pericardial fat can result in constrictive pericarditis.

NEUROMUSCULAR: Lesions at the base of the skull place pressure on the pituitary, sometimes leading to hypopituitarism. Myalgias. Degenerative central nervous system lesions.

ORTHOPEDIC: Growth retardation. Lesions in a variety of bones, including the femur, pelvis, and vertebral bodies, with pathologic fractures. Arthralgias.

GI/GU: Hepatic dysfunction with hypoalbuminemia, hyperbilirubinemia, hepatosplenomegaly, and ascites. Pancreatic infiltration. Abdominal pain from mesenteric involvement. Retroperitoneal involvement may affect adrenal function.

OTHER: Lymphadenopathy. Skin rash, which looks like "cradle cap" (greasy, scaly, and crusted), and may be tender. Pancytopenia with decreased absolute neutrophil count. Recurrent fever. Infiltration of the thyroid may cause hypothyroidism. May have hypopituitarism, diabetes insipidus, hyperprolactinemia, hypogonadism, panhypopituitarism.

MISCELLANEOUS: The Langerhans cell was described by Paul Langerhans when he was a medical student (1868). Because of its dendritic character, he thought it was part of the nervous system.

Artur Schüller escaped from Vienna in 1938 shortly before the Nazis arrived. His two sons were not so lucky, and ultimately died in concentration camps.

ANESTHETIC CONSIDERATIONS

Patients should be evaluated preoperatively for evidence of hypopituitarism. Patients who are on steroids should receive perioperative stress doses of steroids. Patients may have pancytopenia, and the hematocrit and the platelet count should be evaluated preoperatively. Dental abnormalities, including the presence of loose teeth, should be evaluated and documented preoperatively. Low airway pressures or spontaneous ventilation should be maintained intraoperatively in patients known to have lung cysts. Hepatic dysfunction may affect the binding and metabolism of certain anesthetic drugs. Edema secondary to hypoalbuminemia may make vascular access challenging. Recurrent fevers may be mistaken for postoperative infection.

Bibliography:

1. Broscheit J, Eichelbroenner O, Greim C, et al. Anesthetic management of a patient with histiocytosis X and pulmonary complications during Caesarean section. *Eur J Anaesthesiol* 2004;21:919–921.
2. Donadieu J, Rolon M-A, Thomas C, et al. Endocrine involvement in pediatric-onset Langerhans' cell histiocytosis: a population-based study. *J Pediatr* 2004;144:344–350.
3. Matsumoto K, Yoshitake S, Noguchi T. Anesthesia management for a patient with pulmonary eosinophilic granuloma associated with bilateral pneumothorax—general anesthesia with positive pressure ventilation [Japanese]. *Masui* 1997;46:1483–1486.
4. Egeler RM, D'Angio GJ. Langerhans cell histiocytosis. *J Pediatr* 1995;127:1–11.

Laron Dwarfism

MIM #: 262500, 245590

This autosomal recessive dwarfing disorder is due to a mutation in the gene encoding the growth hormone receptor (type I disease), or a defect in the postreceptor signaling mechanism that at least in some instances is due to a mutation in the *STAT5B* gene (type II disease). Patients with this disorder are resistant to the effects of growth hormone. Treatment with insulin-like growth factor-1 has been used experimentally.

HEENT/AIRWAY: Small face. Occasional blue sclerae. High-pitched voice.

NEUROMUSCULAR: Intelligence is usually normal.

ORTHOPEDIC: Proportionate short stature. More pronounced decrement in body size than in head size, resulting in childlike body proportions in adults. Delayed bone age. Limited extension of elbow. Degenerative hip disease.

OTHER: Growth hormone resistance. Failure to generate somatomedin in response to growth hormone. Delayed menses.

ANESTHETIC CONSIDERATIONS

Recall that despite their short stature, patients have intelligence that is normal for their chronologic age, and they must be treated in an age-appropriate manner. Might require a smaller-than-expected endotracheal tube if sized for age.

Bibliography:

1. David A, Metherell LA, Clark AJ, et al. Diagnostic and therapeutic advances in growth hormone insensitivity. *Endocrinol Metab Clin North Am* 2005;34:581–595.
2. Laron Z. Laron syndrome (primary growth hormone resistance or insensitivity): the personal experience 1958–2003. *J Clin Endocrinol Metab* 2004;89:1031–1044.
3. Parks JS, Brown MR, Faase ME. The spectrum of growth-hormone insensitivity. *J Pediatr* 1997;131:S45–S50.
4. Carel JC, Chaussain JL, Chatelain P, et al. Growth hormone insensitivity syndrome (Laron syndrome): main characteristics and effects of IGF1 treatment. *Diabetes Metab* 1996;22:251–256.
5. Laron Z. Prismatic cases: laron syndrome (primary growth hormone resistance) from patient to laboratory to patient. *J Clin Endocrinol Metab* 1995;80:1526–1531.

Larsen Syndrome

MIM #: 150250, 245600

This dysmorphic syndrome is both genetically and phenotypically variable. It is characterized by flat facies and multiple joint dislocations. Both autosomal dominant and autosomal recessive inheritance have been documented. Autosomal dominant Larsen syndrome is caused by a mutation in the gene *FLNB*.

HEENT/AIRWAY: Flat facies with prominent forehead. Hypertelorism. Conductive or sensorineural hearing loss. Depressed nasal bridge. Cleft palate. Mobile, infolding arytenoid cartilage. Subglottic stenosis. Laryngomalacia, tracheomalacia.

CHEST: Tracheomalacia, bronchomalacia. May have restrictive lung disease or chronic respiratory infections secondary to thoracic kyphoscoliosis. May have pectus excavatum. Rare pulmonary hypoplasia.

CARDIOVASCULAR: A variety of cardiac defects have been reported, including atrial septal defect, ventricular septal defect, mitral valve prolapse, aortic dilatation, and aortic valvular insufficiency.

NEUROMUSCULAR: Cervical spine instability or cervical kyphosis may cause symptomatic spinal cord impingement. Hydrocephalus. May have developmental delay.

ORTHOPEDIC: Short stature. Multiple joint dislocations, particularly at the elbows, wrists, hips, and knees. Long, cylindrical fingers, spatulate thumbs, hypoplastic fingernails. Short terminal phalanges cause pseudoclubbing. Accessory carpal bones. Vertebral anomalies, including segmentation defects, hypoplastic vertebrae, wedged vertebrae, spina bifida. Abnormal cervical vertebrae may lead to cervical spine instability. Kyphoscoliosis. Osteoarthritis. Clubfoot deformity. Double ossification center of the calcaneus—may be diagnostic for this syndrome.

GI/GU: May have cryptorchidism.

OTHER: May have poor wound healing.

ANESTHETIC CONSIDERATIONS

Patients should be evaluated preoperatively for cervical spine instability. Care should be taken during positioning for laryngoscopy secondary to the potential for cervical subluxation. Laryngoscopy should be performed with axial traction due to the possibility of an unstable cervical spine. Complications associated with intubation can be minimized or avoided with the use of a laryngeal mask airway (LMA), which requires little or no neck extension during airway access (2). Prior cervical fusion may make intubation difficult. Spinal cord myelopathy from impingement on the cervical cord may produce distal muscle disuse atrophy and a risk of hyperkalemia with succinylcholine administration.

The larynx may be difficult to visualize because of mobile, infolding arytenoid cartilages. Patients with subglottic stenosis may require a smaller-than-expected endotracheal tube. Tracheomalacia or subglottic stenosis may be so severe as to warrant a tracheostomy. However, abnormalities of the trachea may extend beyond the tracheostomy tube and continue to cause symptoms. Postextubation airway problems due to tracheomalacia are possible.

Patients with restrictive lung disease may be at increased risk for postoperative pulmonary complications. On rare occasions patients have pulmonary hypoplasia, which is usually lethal in the neonatal period. Patients with hydrocephalus may have elevated intracranial pressure, and measures should be taken to avoid further increases in intracranial pressure. Patients with congenital cardiac defects require perioperative antibiotic prophylaxis as indicated.

Bibliography:

1. Critchley LAH, Chan L. General anaesthesia in a child with Larsen syndrome. *Anaesth Intensive Care* 2003;31:217–220.
2. Malik P, Choudhry DK. Larsen syndrome and its anaesthetic considerations. *Paediatr Anaesth* 2002;12:632–636.
3. Michel TC, Rosenberg AL, Polley LS. Obstetric anesthetic management of a parturient with Larsen syndrome and short stature. *Anesth Analg* 2001;92:1266–1267.
4. Tobias JD. Anesthetic implications of Larsen syndrome. *J Clin Anesth* 1996;8:255–257.
5. Lauder GR, Sumner E. Larsen's syndrome: anaesthetic implications. Six case reports. *Paediatr Anaesth* 1995;5:133–138.
6. Le Marec B, Chapuis M, Treguier C, et al. A case of Larsen syndrome with severe cervical malformations. *Genet Couns* 1994;5:179–181.
7. Stevenson GW, Hall SC, Palmieri J. Anesthetic considerations for patients with Larsen syndrome. *Anesthesiology* 1991;75:142–144.

Laryngoonychocutaneous Syndrome

SYNONYM: LOGIC syndrome

MIM #: 245660

This autosomal recessive disease results in ulcerations and granuloma formation in a variety of epidermal tissues, particularly the larynx, the nails and the skin. It is due to a mutation in the gene *LAMA3*, located on the long arm of chromosome 18. This syndrome may represent a subtype of junctional epidermolysis bullosa. In somewhat of a stretch for an acronym, it has been suggested that this syndrome be called LOGIC syndrome, for **L**aryngeal and **O**cular **G**ranulation **I**n **C**hildren from the Indian subcontinent, because it has been described exclusively in Punjabi populations.

HEENT/AIRWAY: Skin lesions of the face. Conjunctival scarring. Blisters that heal with scarring may occur in the mouth. Deformed teeth with hypoplastic enamel. Vocal cord thickening with or without nodules, hoarse cry and voice. Laryngeal obstruction can be fatal.

OTHER: The skin and mucosal surfaces are sensitive to trauma. There are dystrophic changes of the nails with chronic bleeding, crusted lesions that heal with scarring. There is a risk of intercurrent infection.

MISCELLANEOUS: The 2:1 male-to-female ratio has been ascribed to the increased tendency of poor families in the areas in which this was first described to take only male children in for medical treatment.

ANESTHETIC CONSIDERATIONS

Lesions on the vocal cords may cause significant airway obstruction. Spontaneous ventilation without the use of muscle relaxants has been recommended when laryngeal lesions are present (2). Dental abnormalities should be documented before surgery. The skin and mucosal surfaces are sensitive to trauma, so these patients must be carefully positioned and padded.

Bibliography:

1. Phillips RJ, Atherton DJ, Gibbs M, et al. Laryngo-onycho-cutaneous syndrome: an inherited epithelial defect. *Arch Dis Child* 1994;70:319–326.
2. Hodges UM, Lloyd-Thomas A. Anaesthesia for airway obstruction in laryngo-onycho-cutaneous syndrome. *Anaesthesia* 1993;48:503–506.

Laurence-Moon Syndrome

MIM #: 245800

This autosomal recessive disorder is similar to, but possibly distinct from, that described by Bardet and Biedl (see earlier, Bardet-Biedl syndrome). It is characterized by mental retardation, retinal dystrophy, hypogenitalism, and spastic paraplegia. Unlike the patients described by Bardet and Biedl, the patients described by Laurence and Moon had spastic paraplegia, and did not have obesity or polydactyly. The two syndromes have sometimes been recognized as distinct, and have sometimes not. Thus the literature contains many references to both the Laurence-Moon-Biedl syndrome and the Laurence-Moon-Biedl-Bardet syndrome.

HEENT/AIRWAY: Pigmentary retinopathy, with visual loss. May have bifid epiglottis. May have dental abnormalities.

NEUROMUSCULAR: Mental retardation, behavioral problems. Spastic paraplegia.

ORTHOPEDIC: No polydactyly.

GI/GU: Hypogenitalism, hypogonadism without apparent structural or functional pituitary abnormality.

OTHER: No obesity. May have speech disorder.

MISCELLANEOUS: Laurence was a British ophthalmologist and Moon was his student. Moon later practiced in Philadelphia.

ANESTHETIC CONSIDERATIONS
Mental retardation, behavioral problems, and speech disorders may make the smooth induction of anesthesia a challenge. Succinylcholine may be contraindicated in patients with severe spastic paraplegia, secondary to the risk of hyperkalemia.

Bibliography:
1. Urben SL, Baugh RF. Otolaryngologic features of Laurence-Moon-Bardet-Biedl syndrome. *Otolaryngol Head Neck Surg* 1999;120:571–574.
2. Farag TI, Teebi AS. Bardet-Biedl and Laurence-Moon syndromes in a mixed Arab population. *Clin Genet* 1988;33:78–82.
3. Whitaker MD, Scheithauer BW, Kovacs KT, et al. The pituitary gland in the Laurence-Moon syndrome. *Mayo Clin Proc* 1987;62:216–222.
4. Schachat AP, Maumenee IH. The Bardet-Biedl syndrome and related disorders. *Arch Ophthalmol* 1982;100:285–288.

LCAD Deficiency

See Long-chain acyl-CoA dehydrogenase deficiency

Leber Congenital Amaurosis

Note: This disorder is distinct from Leber hereditary optic atrophy (see later).

MIM #: 204000, 204100
Autosomal recessive defects in at least two separate genes can produce this disorder. Type I disease is due to a defect in the gene encoding retinal guanylyl cyclase (*GUCY2D*), with at least six different loci described. It may be that some of these cases are also caused by a defect in the gene for guanylyl cyclase activating proteins, which are required for the activation of retinal guanylyl cyclase. Type II disease is due to a defect in the gene encoding retinal pigment epithelium (*RPE65*). It is sometimes termed "congenital absence of the rods and cones."

HEENT/AIRWAY: Early vision loss with nystagmus, photophobia. Pigmentary retinopathy that may resemble retinitis pigmentosa. Keratoconus. Infants may poke at their eyes (the digitoocular sign of Franceschetti). May have hearing loss.

NEUROMUSCULAR: Mental retardation, neuropsychiatric problems, hypoplastic cerebellar vermis may be found in type II disease.

ORTHOPEDIC: Growth retardation.

GI/GU: Hepatomegaly.

MISCELLANEOUS: This disease may be due to a defect in one of two distinct genes. Thus, a family has been reported in which both parents had the disease, but they had normal children because each parent had a defect in a different gene. A variant of Leber congenital amaurosis in Briard puppies has been cured and sight restored by gene therapy.

Theodor Leber pronounced his name "Layber," and was the founder of scientific ophthalmology. He had wanted to be a chemist, but was told by Professor Bunsen that there were already too many chemists, so he chose medicine as an alternative.

ANESTHETIC CONSIDERATIONS
Infants with photophobia may be extremely sensitive to the bright lights in operating rooms. Efforts should be made to minimize their discomfort.

Bibliography:
1. Koenekoop RK. An overview of Leber congenital amaurosis: a model to understand human retinal development. *Surv Ophthalmol* 2004;49:379–398.
2. Hanein S, Perrault I, Gerber S, et al. Leber congenital amaurosis: comprehensive survey of the genetic heterogeneity, refinement of the clinical definition, and genotype-phenotype correlations as a strategy for molecular diagnosis. *Hum Mutat* 2004;23:306–317.

Leber Hereditary Optic Atrophy

Note: This disorder is distinct from Leber congenital amaurosis (see earlier).

MIM #: 535000
This disease is due to an abnormality in mitochondrial DNA. Clinical findings are typically limited to optic nerve disease with visual loss, although at least one form results in a spectrum of findings. At least 18 separate missense mutations in mitochondrial DNA can result in this syndrome. However, three mutations are responsible for over 90% of the cases. Although the onset is usually in adulthood, this disorder has been diagnosed as early as 1 year of age. It is likely that the defect(s) occur in the respiratory chain, particularly in complexes III, IV, or V (see earlier, complex III, IV, or V deficiency). The disease may manifest a latent phase, an acute phase, and a chronic phase. It may be confused with multiple sclerosis.

As a mitochondrial DNA defect, this disorder is maternally transmitted. There appears to be increased clinical severity in male patients.

HEENT/AIRWAY: Subacute, painless loss of central vision with a central scotoma. Vascular changes in the fundus, with peripapillary telangiectasis, microangiopathy, disk pseudopapilledema, and vascular tortuousity. The degree of visual loss is variable, and in part depends on the specific mutation.

CARDIOVASCULAR: Conduction defects, including Wolff-Parkinson-White and Lown-Ganong-Levine syndromes, and long QT syndrome (see later for all) have been reported in one family.

NEUROMUSCULAR: Headaches. Posterior column and corticospinal tract involvement with tremor, ataxia, dystonia, sensory neuropathy, and extrapyramidal rigidity. Seizures on rare occasions, cerebral edema. Depression.

OTHER: Lactic acidosis. Death in childhood.

MISCELLANEOUS: Theodor Leber pronounced his name "Layber," and was the founder of scientific ophthalmology. He had wanted to be a chemist, but was told by Professor Bunsen that there were already too many chemists, so he chose medicine as an alternative.

ANESTHETIC CONSIDERATIONS

There are no recent reports of anesthesia for patients with this disease. It might seem reasonable, however, given the clinical experience with other mitochondrial diseases, to avoid succinylcholine. Adequate perioperative glucose should be ensured to minimize the need for anaerobic metabolism. Some patients with mitochondrial diseases have been shown to have abnormal respiratory drive (5), so narcotics and other respiratory depressants should be used with care. A baseline electrocardiogram should exclude cardiac conduction abnormalities. Cyanide can inhibit the electron transport chain. It has been suggested that there may be an inability to handle cyanide adequately in this and related diseases, and for this reason nitroprusside should be used with caution or avoided (6).

Bibliography:

1. Kerrison JB. Latent, acute, and chronic Leber's hereditary optic neuropathy. *Ophthalmology* 2005;112:1–2.
2. DiMauro S, Schon EA. Mitochondrial respiratory-chain diseases. *N Engl J Med* 2003;348:2656–2668.
3. Man PY, Turnbull DM, Chinnery PF. Leber hereditary optic neuropathy. *J Med Genet* 2002;39:162–169.
4. Keyes MA, Van de Wiele B, Stead SW. Mitochondrial myopathies: an unusual cause of myotonia in infants and children. *Paediatr Anaesth* 1996;6:329–335.
5. Barohn RJ, Clayton T, Zarife S, et al. Recurrent respiratory insufficiency and depressed ventilatory drive complicating mitochondrial myopathies. *Neurology* 1990;40:103–106.
6. Davies DW, Kadar D, Steward DJ, et al. A sudden death associated with the use of sodium nitroprusside for induction of hypotension during anaesthesia. *Can Anaesth Soc J* 1975;22:547–552.

Legg-Calvé-Perthes Disease

MIM #: 150600

This disorder is fairly common, and is characterized by ischemic or avascular necrosis and resorption of the proximal femoral epiphysis. It has also been called coxa plana. The onset is during childhood, and boys are affected four times as often as girls, although in familial cases the sex ratio approximates 1:1. Approximately 15% of cases are bilateral. Treatment consists of bracing or surgical osteotomy. Although apparently autosomal dominant cases have been reported, most cases are sporadic. The cause is unknown, although it has been suggested that it may be related to thrombophilia or hypofibrinolysis (which can be familial). It has also been suggested that low levels of proteins C or S, which render the patient hyperthrombotic, could increase the risk of development of the disease.

ORTHOPEDIC: Avascular necrosis of the proximal femoral epiphysis. Short stature. Patients limp, but often have minimal pain.

MISCELLANEOUS: This disease was not fully differentiated from the much more common tuberculous bone and joint disease until after the development of radiography. Calvé described this disease after examining the radiographs of 500 children purported to have tuberculosis of the hip joints. Ten of the children turned out to have avascular necrosis of the proximal femoral epiphysis.

During the German campaign in China in the early 1900s, the German army surgeon Georg Perthes experimented with the (then) new technology of radiography by taking radiographs of the feet of Chinese women, which had been bound in the traditional manner.

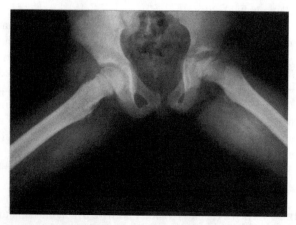

Legg-Calvé-Perthes disease. Note the avascular necrosis of the head of the left femur.

ANESTHETIC CONSIDERATIONS

There are no specific anesthetic considerations.

Bibliography:

1. Levin C, Zalman L, Shalev S, et al. Legg-Calve-Perthes disease, protein C deficiency, and beta-thalassemia major: report of two cases. *J Pediatr Orthop* 2000;20:129–131.
2. Wall EJ. Legg-Calve-Perthes' disease. *Curr Opin Pediatr* 1999;11:76–79.
3. Gruppo R, Glueck CJ, Wall E, et al. Legg-Perthes disease in three siblings, two heterozygous and one homozygous for the factor V Leiden mutation. *J Pediatr* 1998;132:885–888.
4. Foster BK. Pediatric hip and pelvis disorders. *Curr Opin Pediatr* 1993;5:356–362.

Leigh Disease

MIM #: 256000, 266150

This disease is characterized by gray matter degeneration and focal brainstem necrosis. The disease has been linked primarily to deficiencies of mitochondrial complexes, but has also been associated with other abnormalities such as pyruvate carboxylase deficiency. It appears that defects in a variety of genes involved in energy metabolism, in particular the mitochondrial genes, can cause this clinical phenotype. The clinical course of Leigh disease is marked by remissions and acute exacerbations. Patients may be receiving dichloroacetate, thiamine and riboflavin.

HEENT/AIRWAY: External ophthalmoplegia, abnormal eye movements, sluggish pupils, blindness.

CHEST: Wheezing, gasping, aspiration pneumonia. Cheyne-Stokes respirations, hypoventilation, central apnea, respiratory failure. Respiratory status may be acutely worsened by surgery, general anesthesia, or intercurrent illness.

CARDIOVASCULAR: Hypertrophic cardiomyopathy.

NEUROMUSCULAR: Gray matter degeneration and focal brainstem necrosis. Symmetric lesions are often found in the walls of the third ventricle and in the brainstem. Variable clinical manifestations include developmental delay, hypotonia, seizures, weakness, tremor, ataxia, absent deep tendon reflexes, and a Babinski sign.

ORTHOPEDIC: Growth retardation.

OTHER: Increased serum lactate, impaired gluconeogenesis.

MISCELLANEOUS: Denis Leigh pronounced his name "Lee," not "Lay."

ANESTHETIC CONSIDERATIONS

Stress, as with surgery or infection, can increase demands for adenosine triphosphate production to levels above the production ability of the patient. Elective surgery should be postponed for fever or other intercurrent illness. Acidosis should be corrected preoperatively, and patients with excessive lactic acidemia should not receive lactated Ringer's solution. Prolonged preoperative fasts should be avoided, adequate glucose should be supplied perioperatively, and blood glucose appropriately monitored. These patients warrant close postoperative observation because they may have abnormal responses to hypoxia and hypercarbia, in addition to muscle weakness. Postoperative clinical deterioration has been reported (8), and one patient's magnetic resonance imaging was consistent with activation of her underlying disease. Patients may be at increased risk for aspiration. Chronic use of anticonvulsant medications may alter the metabolism of some anesthetic drugs.

Although barbiturates and volatile anesthetics can inhibit mitochondrial respiration, induction of anesthesia with thiopental has been used without complication (13). Succinylcholine should be used with caution in patients with evidence of a myopathy because of the risk of exaggerated hyperkalemia. There is a report of a single patient with an unspecified mitochondrial myopathy who exhibited increased sensitivity to rocuronium and atracurium (6). Although there are no clinical reports, it is reasonable to avoid the use of nitroprusside because cyanide can inhibit the electron transport chain. There is a report of three patients in whom general anesthesia precipitated respiratory failure, leading to death (10). All three had preoperative respiratory findings. In one, the diagnosis of Leigh syndrome had not yet been made. Acute respiratory compromise has also been reported in two children after receiving chloral hydrate for a radiologic procedure (11). Both had had apnea and gagging before the procedure. Many children with mitochondrial diseases have abnormal respiratory control (3,4,12), suggesting that narcotics and other respiratory depressants be used with care. In addition, patients with Leigh disease may have a cardiomyopathy.

It has been suggested that postoperative pain management in patients with Leigh disease can be difficult, and parenteral or oral clonazepam has been used successfully. The relationship between the mitochondrial myopathies and malignant hyperthermia is not clear, but an association is unlikely.

Bibliography:

1. Gozal D, Goldin E, Shafran-Tikva S, et al. Leigh syndrome: Anesthetic management in complicated endoscopic procedures. *Paediatr Anaesth* 2006;16:38–42.
2. Ellis Z, Bloomer C. Outpatient anesthesia for oral surgery in a juvenile with Leigh disease. *Anesth Prog* 2005;52:70–73.
3. Shear T, Tobias JD. Anesthetic implications of Leigh's syndrome. *Paediatr Anaesth* 2004;14:792–797.
4. DiMauro S, Schon EA. Mitochondrial respiratory-chain diseases. *N Engl J Med* 2003;348:2656–2668.
5. Cooper MA, Fox R. Anesthesia for corrective spinal surgery in a patient with Leigh's disease. *Anesth Analg* 2003;97:1539–1541.
6. Finsterer J, Stratil U, Bittner R, et al. Increased sensitivity to rocuronium and atracurium in mitochondrial myopathy. *Can J Anaesth* 1998;45:781–784.

7. Shenkman Z, Krichevski I, Elpeleg ON, et al. Anaesthetic management of a patient with Leigh syndrome. *Can J Anaesth* 1997;44:1091–1095.
8. Casta A, Quackenbush EJ, Houck CS, et al. Perioperative white matter degeneration and death in a patient with a defect in mitochondrial oxidative phosphorylation. *Anesthesiology* 1997;87:420–425.
9. Keyes MA, Van de Wiele B, Stead SW. Mitochondrial myopathies: an unusual cause of myotonia in infants and children. *Paediatr Anaesth* 1996;6:329–335.
10. Grattan-Smith PJ, Shield LK, Hopkins IJ, et al. Acute respiratory failure precipitated by general anesthesia in Leigh syndrome. *J Child Neurol* 1990;5:137–141.
11. Greenberg SB, Faerber EN. Respiratory insufficiency following chloral hydrate sedation in two children with Leigh disease. *Pediatr Radiol* 1990;20:287–288.
12. Barohn RJ, Clayton T, Zarife S, et al. Recurrent respiratory insufficiency and depressed ventilatory drive complicating mitochondrial myopathies. *Neurology* 1990;40:103–106.
13. Ward DS. Anesthesia for a child with Leigh syndrome. *Anesthesiology* 1981;55:80–81.

Lennox-Gastaut Syndrome

MIM #: None

Lennox-Gastaut syndrome is a severe seizure disorder of childhood. The seizures are difficult to control and the syndrome is often associated with developmental and mental retardation. Apparently it is not genetically transmitted, and there is no one single known etiologic process or causative event.

NEUROMUSCULAR: Early childhood seizures of multiple types [tonic, tonic-clonic, atonic, akinetic (drop attacks), myoclonic, and absence]. These seizures are often preceded by infantile spasms ("salaam seizures"). The electroencephalogram is abnormal. Mental and motor function, which may have been normal before the onset of seizures, deteriorate. The seizures may be refractory to common anticonvulsant medications, and most patients are on multiple medications. The anticonvulsant drug lamotrigine has been shown to have activity against the generalized seizure component (2). Patients may be on a ketogenic diet.

MISCELLANEOUS: Salaam seizures, which usually carry a poor prognosis, are so named because during the seizure the child's arms come up to the head, which is flexed downward along with the trunk, mimicking a "salaam" gesture.

Lennox-Gastaut syndrome was featured in the *The Spirit Catches You and You Fall Down*, written by journalist Anne Fadiman and published in 1997. This is the (true) story of the tremendous medical and cultural clashes that occurred between American medical providers and a Hmong family whose youngest child had Lennox-Gastaut syndrome.

ANESTHETIC CONSIDERATIONS

Chronic use of anticonvulsant medications may alter the metabolism of some anesthetic drugs.

Bibliography:
1. Markand ON. Lennox-Gastaut syndrome (childhood epileptic encephalopathy). *J Clin Neurophysiol* 2003;20:426–441.
2. Motte J, Trevathan E, Arvidsson JFV, et al. Lamotrigine for generalized seizures associated with the Lennox-Gastaut syndrome. *N Engl J Med* 1997;337:1807–1812.

Lenz-Majewski Hyperostosis Syndrome

MIM #: 151050

This sporadic disorder is characterized by short stature, hyperostosis, symphalangism, and skin hypoplasia. Those affected die in infancy or childhood, and have been described as looking somewhat like patients with progeria.

HEENT/AIRWAY: Macrocephaly, prominent forehead. Late closure of large fontanelles. Hypertelorism, nasolacrimal duct obstruction. Large ears. Choanal stenosis or atresia, which may cause respiratory insufficiency. Dysplastic dental enamel. May have facial palsy. May have cleft palate. May have micrognathia.

CHEST: Broad, thick ribs and clavicles cause thoracic immobility. Recurrent pneumonia is common.

NEUROMUSCULAR: Mental retardation. May have cerebral atrophy. May have agenesis of the corpus callosum. May have hydrocephalus.

ORTHOPEDIC: Short stature. Hyperostosis of skull and diaphyses. Delayed bone age. Proximal symphalangism. Hypoplastic or absent middle phalanges. Cutaneous syndactyly. Hyperextensible joints. May have flexion contractures at elbows and knees.

GI/GU: Inguinal hernias. Cryptorchidism, hypospadias.

OTHER: Cutis laxa, sparse hair in infancy. Skin becomes hypoplastic with prominent cutaneous veins.

ANESTHETIC CONSIDERATIONS

Choanal stenosis or atresia may cause respiratory insufficiency, and precludes the use of a nasal airway or a nasogastric tube. Recurrent pneumonia may cause chronic lung disease and place patients at increased risk of postoperative respiratory complications. Patients must be carefully positioned and padded because of hyperextensible joints, flexion contractures at the elbows and knees, and hypoplastic skin.

Bibliography:
1. Wattanasirichaigoon D, Visudtibhan A, Jaovisidha S, et al. Expanding the phenotypic spectrum of Lenz-Majewski syndrome: facial palsy, cleft palate and hydrocephalus. *Clin Dysmorphol* 2004;13:137–142.
2. Majewski F. Lenz-Majewski hyperostotic dwarfism: reexamination of the original patient. *Am J Med Genet* 2000;93:335–338.
3. Chrzanowska KH, Fryns JP, Krajewska-Walasek M, et al. Skeletal dysplasia syndrome with progeroid appearance, characteristic facial and limb anomalies, multiple synostoses, and distinct skeletal changes: a variant example of the Lenz-Majewski syndrome. *Am J Med Genet* 1989;32:470–474.

LEOPARD Syndrome

SYNONYM: Multiple lentigines syndrome

MIM #: 151100

This autosomal dominant syndrome consists of **L**entigines (multiple), **E**lectrocardiographic conduction abnormalities, **O**cular hypertelorism, **P**ulmonic stenosis, **A**bnormal genitalia, **R**etardation of growth, and **D**eafness. Lentigines are large freckles. LEOPARD syndrome is thought to be due to a primary abnormality in neural crest cells. There is marked variability in the clinical expression of this syndrome. Some patients may even fail to exhibit the characteristic lentigines. The syndrome is due to mutations in the gene *PTPN11*, which encodes a protein-tyrosine phosphatase. Mutations in this gene are also responsible for approximately half of the cases of Noonan syndrome (see later); thus these two syndromes are allelic.

HEENT/AIRWAY: Hypertelorism. Protruding ears. Sensorineural deafness. May have dental abnormalities. May have cleft palate, prognathism. Tooth abnormalities.

CHEST: Pectus excavatum or carinatum. Restrictive lung disease with pulmonary arterial hypertension from scoliosis has been reported.

CARDIOVASCULAR: Cardiac conduction abnormalities, with variable types of conduction block. Abnormal P waves. Pulmonic stenosis—the pulmonic valve may be dysplastic. Hypertrophic obstructive cardiomyopathy, which has also been reported to involve the right ventricle. Subaortic stenosis, mitral valve involvement, and a left atrial myxoma have also been reported.

NEUROMUSCULAR: May have mental retardation.

ORTHOPEDIC: Growth deficiency. Winged scapulae. May have kyphoscoliosis.

GI/GU: Cryptorchidism, hypospadias. May have renal agenesis or hypoplasia.

OTHER: Multiple lentigines of the skin, particularly on the neck and trunk. The number of lentigines can increase with age. Lentigines are macules similar to freckles, but unlike freckles are not restricted to sun-exposed areas. They are dark brown to black, and round to oval.

MISCELLANEOUS: The multiple spotting of the skin by lentigines led Gorlin to formulate the mnemonic LEOPARD syndrome as an aid to recalling the features of the multiple lentigines syndrome.

ANESTHETIC CONSIDERATIONS

Provisions should be made for communication with patients who are deaf. Baseline renal function should be assessed. Patients warrant a preoperative cardiac evaluation. Given the incidence of obstructive cardiomyopathy, which can be asymptomatic, preoperative screening echocardiography could be considered. Cardiac conduction abnormalities are also common. Patients with valvular heart disease require perioperative antibiotic prophylaxis as indicated.

Bibliography:
1. Hagspiel KD, Candinas RC, Hagspiel HJ, et al. LEOPARD syndrome: cardiac imaging findings. *AJR Am J Roentgenol* 2005;184:S21–S24.
2. Torres J, Russo P, Tobias JD. Anaesthetic implications of LEOPARD syndrome. *Paediatr Anaesth* 2004;14:352–356.
3. Rodrigo MRC, Cheng CH, Tai YT, et al. "Leopard" syndrome. *Anaesthesia* 1990;45:30–33.

Leprechaunism

SYNONYM: Donohue syndrome

MIM #: 246200

This autosomal recessive disorder is characterized by severe growth deficiency, hyperplasia of the islets of Langerhans, and a deficiency of subcutaneous fat. There is usually severe failure to thrive, recurrent infection, and death during infancy. The syndrome is caused by a mutation of the insulin receptor gene (*INSR*), which is located on the short arm of chromosome 19. Abnormal insulin receptors result in severe insulin resistance, islet cell hyperplasia, hyperinsulinemia, hyperglycemia, and growth deficiency.

HEENT/AIRWAY: Elfin-like facies with prominent eyes, large ears, wide nostrils, and thick lips. Gingival hyperplasia.

CARDIOVASCULAR: May have myocardial hypertrophy.

NEUROMUSCULAR: Mental and motor retardation.

ORTHOPEDIC: Intrauterine and postnatal growth deficiency with marked deficiency of subcutaneous fat and decreased muscle mass. Relatively large hands and feet. Delayed osseous maturation.

GI/GU: Relatively large abdomen. Large penis or clitoris. Breast hyperplasia.

OTHER: Multiple endocrinologic abnormalities, including hyperplasia of the islets of Langerhans, Leydig cell hyperplasia, hyperinsulinemia, hyperglycemia, and precocious puberty. Hirsutism. Hyperkeratosis. Nail dysplasia. Wrinkled, loose skin.

MISCELLANEOUS: Originally called "dysendocrinism" by Donohue, it was later renamed "leprechaunism" (because of the elfin-like facies) by Donohue and Uchida.

ANESTHETIC CONSIDERATIONS

Patients may have a variety of endocrinologic abnormalities. Although usually hyperglycemic secondary to lack of response to insulin, patients may become hypoglycemic during a fast. Perioperative glucose monitoring is essential.

Bibliography:

1. Ozbey H, Ozbey N, Tunnessen WW. Picture of the month. Leprechaunism. *Arch Pediatr Adolesc Med* 1998;152:1031–1032.
2. Taylor SI, Cama A, Accili D, et al. Mutations in the insulin receptor. *Endocr Rev* 1992;13:566–595.
3. Cantani A, Ziruolo MG, Tacconi ML. A rare polydysmorphic syndrome: leprechaunism—review of forty-nine cases reported in the literature. *Ann Genet* 1987;30:221–227.
4. Bier DM, Schedewie H, Larner J, et al. Glucose kinetics in leprechaunism: accelerated fasting due to insulin resistance. *J Clin Endocrinol Metab* 1980;51:988–994.

Leri-Weill Dyschondrosteosis

SYNONYM: Dyschondrosteosis

MIM #: 127300

This autosomal dominant syndrome is distinguished by mesomelic dwarfism, short, bowed forearms, and radial deviation of the hands secondary to shortening of the distal radius. Patients may also have short lower extremities. The homozygous form of this disorder is known as Langer mesomelic dysplasia (see earlier). This disorder is usually caused by mutations in the gene *SHOX* (short stature homeobox). This gene is located on the X chromosome, but is said to be pseudoautosomal. Female patients are more severely affected. There is a recent report of a Leri-Weill dyschondrosteosis phenotype associated with a pseudoautosomal deletion that does not involve the *SHOX* gene.

NEUROMUSCULAR: Normal intelligence.

ORTHOPEDIC: Mesomelic dwarfism, with variable short stature. Short forearms. Bowed radius. Dorsal dislocation of distal ulna. Radial deviation of the hands at the wrist (Madelung deformity) secondary to shortening of the distal radius. May have partial dislocation of the ulna at the wrist or elbow, with limitation of joint mobility at the wrist or elbow. May have short lower extremities, with tibiofibular disproportion.

ANESTHETIC CONSIDERATIONS
Radial arterial access might be difficult. Patients should be addressed in a manner appropriate to their chronologic age and not their height age. Positioning may be complicated by restricted elbow and wrist movement.

Bibliography:

1. Cakir M, Kalyoncu M, Odemis E, et al. A rare cause of short stature: Leri Weill dyschondrosteosis. *Genet Couns* 2003;14:215–220.
2. Roubicek M, Arriazu MC, Isaac G. SHOX deficiency phenotypes. *J Clin Endocrinol Metab* 2003;88:4004.

Lesch-Nyhan Syndrome

MIM #: 300322

Lesch-Nyhan syndrome is an X-linked recessive disease caused by a mutation in the gene that encodes hypoxanthine

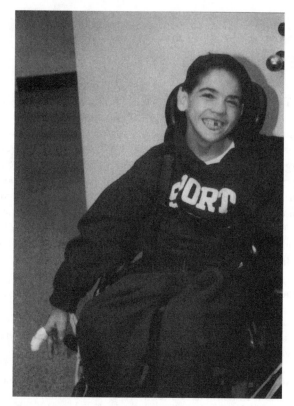

Lesch-Nyhan syndrome. This 21-year-old man with Lesch-Nyhan syndrome recognizes when he has an uncontrollable self-mutilating urge and his parents give him chloral hydrate. Although not well seen here, his lips have been extensively chewed. Note the bandage on his finger, and that his hands are tied to the wheelchair as a restraint.

phosphoribosyltransferase. This enzyme is involved in the salvage of the purines hypoxanthine and guanine. There are a variety of different mutations in the gene for this enzyme that may result in the clinical syndrome. Some patients may have a partial deficit in enzyme activity and manifest less than the full syndrome. The hallmark clinical findings are developmental delay, motor abnormalities, and self-mutilation.

HEENT/AIRWAY: May have sequelae of perioral self-mutilation. Dysarthria.

CHEST: Risk of recurrent aspiration from athetoid dysphagia.

NEUROMUSCULAR: Mental retardation. Dysarthria makes intelligence testing difficult, and patients may have less impairment than is immediately obvious. Developmental delay followed by pyramidal and extrapyramidal tract signs. Early hypotonia followed by development of hypertonia and spasticity. Cerebellar ataxia in some. Choreoathetosis, spasticity, dystonia. Self-mutilatory behavior, with head banging as a common manifestation. Other behavior problems, including aggression.

ORTHOPEDIC: Gouty arthritis. Self-mutilation of fingers and hands.

GI/GU: Hyperuricemia with renal stones. Hyperuricemia can be controlled by inhibition of xanthine oxidase (e.g., with allopurinol).

OTHER: There is diminished monoamine oxidase activity. There is diminished adrenergic response to stress. Megaloblastic anemia. Abnormal B-cell lymphocyte proliferation or function. Overwhelming infection may be a cause of death.

MISCELLANEOUS: Lesch was only a medical student (at Johns Hopkins) when he and Nyhan described this disease in 1964.

ANESTHETIC CONSIDERATIONS

Spastic musculoskeletal malformations may make intravenous access and positioning difficult. Although there are multiple metabolic abnormalities, routine anesthetic techniques have been used successfully (4). Patients have tolerated propofol sedation for noninvasive radiologic procedures (3), despite the fact that propofol may increase urinary uric acid excretion (2). This may be a consideration for prolonged cases using propofol for anesthesia or sedation. Abnormal monoamine oxidase activity and abnormal adrenergic pressor responses suggest that exogenous catecholamines should be used with care.

Bibliography:
1. McCarthy G. Medical diagnosis, management and treatment of Lesch Nyhan disease. *Nucleosides Nucleotides Nucleic Acids* 2004;23: 1147–1152.
2. Miyazawa N, Takeda J, Izawa H. Does propofol change uric acid metabolism? *Anesth Analg* 1998;86:S486.
3. Williams KS, Hankerson JG, Ernst M, et al. Use of propofol anesthesia during outpatient radiographic imaging studies in patients with Lesch-Nyhan syndrome. *J Clin Anesth* 1997;9:61–65.
4. Larson LO, Wilkins RG. Anesthesia and the Lesch-Nyhan syndrome. *Anesthesiology* 1985;63:197–199.

Letterer-Siwe Disease

Included in Langerhans cell histiocytosis

Levy-Hollister Syndrome

SYNONYM: Lacrimoauriculodentodigital syndrome; LADD syndrome

MIM #: 149730

This autosomal dominant syndrome is characterized by lacrimal gland and duct abnormalities, external ear anomalies, dental hypoplasia, and digital anomalies. There is wide variability in clinical expression. Most patients have persistent dry mouth secondary to decreased salivation, and are prone to development of severe dental caries. The responsible gene and gene product are not known.

HEENT/AIRWAY: Nasolacrimal duct obstruction, hypoplasia or aplasia of lacrimal glands. Chronic dacryocystitis. Small, simple, cup-shaped ears. Conductive or sensorineural hearing loss. May have cleft lip/palate. Dental hypoplasia, enamel dysplasia. Severe dental caries often develop. Parotid gland hypoplasia or aplasia.

CHEST: Rare pulmonary vascular and alveolar malformations. Rare unilateral diaphragmatic nerve palsy.

CARDIOVASCULAR: May have QT prolongation.

ORTHOPEDIC: Digital anomalies, including digitalization of the thumb, duplication of the distal phalanx of the thumb, triphalangeal thumb, digital bone and soft tissue hypoplasia, thenar muscle hypoplasia, polydactyly, syndactyly, clinodactyly. May have shortening of radius and ulna, or absent radius.

GI/GU: May have hypospadias, cystic ovarian disease. May have renal disease.

ANESTHETIC CONSIDERATIONS

Patients have absent or decreased tear production, and are prone to chronic dacryocystitis. Meticulous intraoperative eye care is imperative to avoid exacerbation of symptoms and corneal abrasions. Dental abnormalities should be documented preoperatively. Patients with severe dental caries may be at risk of intraoperative tooth loss. Recall that patients may have hearing loss. Hypoplasia or absence of the radius may make intravenous or intraarterial access more difficult. At least one patient has been noted to have QT prolongation (2).

Bibliography:
1. Lehotay M, Kunkel M, Wehrbein H. Lacrimo-auriculo-dento-digital syndrome. Case report, review of the literature, and clinical spectrum. *J Orofac Orthop* 2004;65:425–432.
2. Onrat E, Kaya D, Onrat ST. Lacrimo-auriculo-dento-digital syndrome with QT prolongation. *Acta Cardiol* 2003;58:567–570.
3. Heinz GW, Bateman JB, Barrett DJ, et al. Ocular manifestations of the lacrimo-auriculo-dento-digital syndrome. *Am J Ophthalmol* 1993;115:243–248.

Li-Fraumeni Syndrome

MIM #: 151623

Originally described as an autosomal dominant cause of childhood sarcomas, this syndrome is also responsible for an excess of a variety of other cancers, including breast cancer, brain tumors, osteosarcoma, leukemia, and adrenocortical carcinoma. It is due to a mutation in the tumor suppressor gene *TP53,* which encodes the p53 protein. The p53 protein is thought to be involved in some as yet unclear way in cell regulation. It is undetectable or present in very low levels in resting cells, but is present in a wide variety of proliferating or transformed cells. It has structural and functional similarities to the *MYC* family of oncogenes. Multiple primary tumors frequently occur in this syndrome. More than 50% of the patients with the gene would be expected to have cancer by the age of 30 years, and 90% by age 70.

OTHER: The long list of tumors for which these patients are at risk includes rhabdomyosarcoma, soft tissue sarcomas, breast cancer, brain tumors, osteosarcoma, leukemia, adrenocortical carcinoma, lymphocytic or histiocytic lymphoma, lung adenocarcinoma, melanoma, gonadal germ cell tumors, prostate carcinoma, and pancreatic carcinoma.

ANESTHETIC CONSIDERATIONS
The anesthetic management is specific to the particular tumor present, the type and amount of chemotherapy the patient has received, and the proposed surgery.

Bibliography:
1. Varley JM. Germline TP53 mutations and Li-Fraumeni syndrome. *Hum Mutat* 2003;21:313–320.
2. Olivier M, Goldgar DE, Sodha N, et al. Li-Fraumeni and related syndromes: correlation between tumor type, family structure, and TP53 genotype. *Cancer Res* 2003;63:6643–6650.
3. Birch JM, Alston RD, McNally RJQ, et al. Relative frequency and morphology of cancers in carriers of germline TP53 mutations. *Oncogene* 2001;20:4621–4628.

Liddle Syndrome

SYNONYM: Pseudohyperaldosteronism (pseudoaldosteronism)

MIM #: 177200

Liddle syndrome is an autosomal dominant cause of heritable hypertension that is caused by a defect in the beta or gamma subunit of the epithelial sodium channel *SCNN1,* leading to constitutive activation of the epithelial sodium channel in the collecting tubule luminal memberane with unregulated sodium resorption in the distal renal tubule. Patients are hypertensive and have a hypokalemic metabolic alkalosis that is not secondary to hyperaldosteronism. The metabolic defects are completely reversible with renal transplantation.

CARDIOVASCULAR: Hypertension.

GI/GU: Late renal failure.

OTHER: Hypokalemic metabolic alkalosis, hypoaldosteronism, decreased serum renin and angiotensin.

MISCELLANEOUS: Dr. Grant Liddle was the chair of Medicine at Vanderbilt University.

ANESTHETIC CONSIDERATIONS
Patients are likely to be hypertensive. Serum electrolytes, particularly potassium and bicarbonate, should be evaluated preoperatively. Spironolactone is ineffective in correcting the metabolic alterations, but amiloride or triamterene with dietary sodium restriction is helpful.

Bibliography:
1. Lang F, Capasso G, Schwab M, et al. Renal tubular transport and the genetic basis of hypertensive disease. *Clin Exp Nephrol* 2005;9:91–99.
2. Warnock DG. Liddle syndrome: genetics and mechanisms of Na$^+$ channel defects. *Am J Med Sci* 2001;322:302–307.
3. Scheinman SJ, Guay-Woodford LM, Thakker RV, et al. Genetic disorders of renal electrolyte transport. *N Engl J Med* 1999;340:1177–1187.

Limb-Girdle Muscular Dystrophy

MIM #: 159000, 253600

Limb-girdle muscular dystrophy can be inherited in an autosomal dominant fashion (type 1) or in an autosomal recessive fashion (type 2). A variety of muscle-related proteins can be defective in this disorder. Patients may have a mutation in the gene encoding myotilin (type 1A) or a mutation in the gene encoding the proteolytic enzyme calpain-3 (type 2A). Other causes include mutations in the gene encoding lamin A/C, mutations in the gene encoding the skeletal muscle protein dysferlin, and mutations in the sarcoglycan genes. The disorder is marked by muscle weakness, particularly in the pelvis and legs.

HEENT/AIRWAY: Nasal speech. Late facial weakness.

CHEST: Respiratory muscle weakness can lead to recurrent respiratory tract infections. Scoliosis can cause restrictive lung disease.

CARDIOVASCULAR: Atrioventricular conduction disorders, symptomatic bradyarrhythmias. Dilated cardiomyopathy is uncommon.

NEUROMUSCULAR: Myopathy with muscle weakness, legs often weaker than arms. In type 2 disease the muscle weakness is first evident in the pelvis or, less frequently, the shoulder girdle. Serum creatine kinase is usually moderately or markedly increased, but can be normal.

ORTHOPEDIC: Scoliosis. Late joint contractures.

ANESTHETIC CONSIDERATIONS
Cardiac conduction disorders are common, and the baseline cardiac rhythm should be determined. Patients are at increased risk for development of perioperative respiratory complications, secondary to respiratory muscle weakness. Succinylcholine is contraindicated in patients with a myopathy because of the risk of an exaggerated hyperkalemic response. Malignant hyperthermia has not been reported in association with this disease.

Bibliography:

1. Zatz M, Starling A. Calpains and disease. *N Engl J Med* 2005;352: 2413–2423.
2. Angelini C. Limb-girdle muscular dystrophies: heterogeneity of clinical phenotypes and pathogenetic mechanisms. *Acta Myol* 2004;23:130–136.
3. Duggan DJ, Gorospe JR, Fanin M, et al. Mutations in the sarcoglycan genes in patients with myopathy. *N Engl J Med* 1997;336:618–624.
4. van Ommen GJ. A foundation for limb-girdle muscular dystrophy. *Nat Med* 1995;1:412–414.
5. Ekblad U, Kanto J. Pregnancy outcome in an extremely small woman with muscular dystrophy and respiratory insufficiency. *Acta Anaesthesiol Scand* 1993;37:228–230.

Linear Sebaceous Nevus Syndrome

See Nevus sebaceus of Jadassohn

Lip Pit–Cleft Lip Syndrome

See van der Woude syndrome

Lipodystrophy

Synonym: Berardinelli lipodystrophy; Seip syndrome

MIM #: 269700, 608594

This autosomal recessive disease is one of generalized lipodystrophy and insulin-resistant diabetes mellitus. There is an inability to store energy as fat, and patients have elevated basal metabolic rates. It is caused by a mutation in the *AGPAT2* gene (type 1 lipodystrophy) or a mutation in the gene encoding seipin (type 2 lipodystrophy).

Heent/Airway: Triangular facies. Corneal opacities.

Cardiovascular: Peripheral pulmonic stenosis has been reported.

Neuromuscular: Diabetic neuropathy. Muscular hypertrophy.

Orthopedic: Long bone sclerosis or angiomatosis.

Gi/Gu: Hepatomegaly, cirrhosis, portal hypertension. Diabetic nephropathy. Polycystic ovaries. Sexual precocity.

Other: Marked lack of adipose tissue. Hyperlipidemia, hypercholesterolemia, insulin-resistant diabetes mellitus. Acanthosis nigricans. Abnormal hypothalamic or pituitary function. Hyperpigmentation. Hypertrichosis with curly scalp hair.

Anesthetic Considerations
Patients with diabetes may have an autonomic neuropathy. Significantly diminished body fat may make intraoperative temperature maintenance difficult. Serum glucose levels should be followed perioperatively, and adequate glucose should be supplied to avoid hypoglycemia. Hepatic failure may affect the binding and metabolism of some anesthetic drugs.

Bibliography:

1. Garg A. Acquired and inherited lipodystrophies. *N Engl J Med* 2004;350:1220–1234.
2. Agarwal AK, Simha V, Oral EA, et al. Phenotypic and genetic heterogeneity in congenital generalized lipodystrophy. *J Clin Endocrinol Metab* 2003;88:4840–4847.
3. Uzun O, Blackburn MEC, Gibbs JL. Congenital total lipodystrophy and peripheral pulmonary artery stenosis. *Arch Dis Child* 1997;76:456–457.

Lipoid Proteinosis

Synonym: Urbach-Wiethe disease

MIM #: 247100

Lipoid proteinosis is an autosomal recessive disease involving the skin and blood vessels. The primary manifestations are early hoarseness and an unusual skin rash. This disorder is caused by a mutation in the *ECM1* gene located on the long arm of chromosome 1.

Heent/Airway: Skin lesions resembling acne, particularly along the borders of the eyelids. Drusen-like lesions of the fundus. An immobile, woody tongue from infiltration of the tongue and frenulum may cause problems with swallowing and mouth opening. Hoarseness at an early age is the most common finding. Laryngeal mucosal involvement causes decreased mucous production. There is progressive narrowing of the upper respiratory tract.

Cardiovascular: There is deposition of hyaline material in arterial and capillary vessel walls

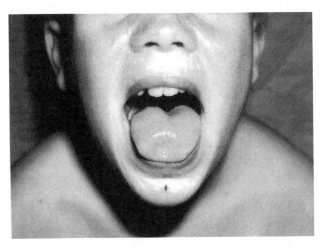

Lipoid proteinosis. The tongue of this patient with lipoid proteinosis has limited mobility. This is its maximal protrusion.

NEUROMUSCULAR: Intracranial calcifications and possibly seizures. Paranoia and rage attacks have been reported.

OTHER: There is deposition of hyaline material in the skin. There may be hyperkeratosis and scarring in areas of skin trauma.

ANESTHETIC CONSIDERATIONS

Limitations in mouth opening and infiltration of the soft tissues of the tongue and larynx may make laryngoscopy and tracheal intubation difficult. Because of laryngeal involvement, patients may require a smaller-than-expected endotracheal tube. An impaired gag reflex may increase the risk of aspiration associated with laryngoscopy. Antisialagogues are best avoided because of the secretory defect of the larynx. Chronic use of anticonvulsant medications may affect the metabolism of some anesthetic drugs.

Bibliography:
1. Nanda A, Alsaleh QA, Al-Sabah H, et al. Lipoid proteinosis: report of four siblings and brief review of the literature. *Pediatr Dermatol* 2001;18:21–26.
2. Kelly JE, Simpson MT, Jonathan D, et al. Lipoid proteinosis: Urbach-Wiethe disease. *Br J Anaesth* 1989;63:609–611.

Lipoprotein Lipase Deficiency

MIM #: 238600

This autosomal recessive disease is usually caused by abnormalities in the gene encoding the enzyme lipoprotein lipase (LPL). There are multiple alleles. The disease may also be the result of a deficiency in the activator of lipoprotein lipase, apolipoprotein C-II. Patients exhibit massive chylomicronemia on a normal diet. This resolves after several days of a fat-free diet. The disease is marked by xanthomas and recurrent abdominal pain.

HEENT/AIRWAY: Lipemia retinalis.

CARDIOVASCULAR: May develop premature atherosclerotic peripheral vascular and coronary artery disease.

GI/GU: Attacks of abdominal pain, nausea, and vomiting. Pancreatitis. Hepatosplenomegaly, bile duct stenosis, jaundice.

OTHER: Eruptive xanthomas. Hypercholesterolemia, hyperlipidemia.

ANESTHETIC CONSIDERATIONS

Patients may have atherosclerotic cardiovascular disease (2,3). Episodes of abdominal pain may mimic a "surgical abdomen."

Bibliography:
1. Mead JR, Irvine SA, Ramji DP. Lipoprotein lipase: structure, function, regulation, and role in disease. *J Mol Med* 2002;80:753–769.
2. Nordestgaard BG, Abildgaard S, Wittrup HH, et al. Heterozygous lipoprotein lipase deficiency: frequency in the general population, effect on plasma lipid levels, and risk of ischemic heart disease. *Circulation* 1997;96:1737–1744.
3. Benlian P, De Gennes JL, Foubert L, et al. Premature atherosclerosis in patients with familial chylomicronemia caused by mutations in the lipoprotein lipase gene. *N Engl J Med* 1996;335:848–854.

Lissencephaly Syndrome

See Miller-Dieker syndrome

Liver Phosphorylase Deficiency

See Hers disease

LOGIC Syndrome

See Laryngoonychocutaneous syndrome

Long-Chain Acyl-CoA Dehydrogenase Deficiency

SYNONYM: Hydroxyacyl-CoA dehydrogenase deficiency; Hydroxydicarboxilic acidemia; LCAD deficiency

MIM #: 201460

This autosomal recessive disease involves defects in the gene for long-chain acyl-CoA dehydrogenase (LCAD), which plays a role in the first step of mitochondrial oxidation of fatty acids. This defect prevents the use of adipose or dietary long-chain (C8-18) fatty acids for energy production or hepatic ketone formation. Short- and medium-chain fatty acids are metabolized normally. LCAD activity is found in mitochondrial trifunctional protein (see later, mitochondrial trifunctional protein deficiency). Defects in LCAD can be isolated or found in association with defects in the two other LCAD proteins, enoyl-CoA hydratase, and 3-ketoacyl-CoA thiolase. A patient with LCAD deficiency has been reported with hypoparathyroidism, a characteristic of mitochondrial trifunctional protein deficiency. The primary clinical manifestation of this disease is hypoglycemia.

Fatty acids are oxidized in the mitochondria. After mobilization from adipose tissue, they are taken up by the liver and other tissues, and converted to acyl-CoA esters in the cytoplasm. They enter mitochondria as carnitine esters, and become reesterified as acyl-CoA esters. Beta-oxidation results in the liberation of electrons. As beta-oxidation proceeds, the acyl chain is gradually shortened, and this first step in the oxidation process is catalyzed by acyl-CoA dehydrogenases with differing, but overlapping, chain-length specificities. These are very-long-chain, long-chain, medium-chain, and short-chain acyl-CoA dehydrogenases.

Although the classic presenting finding is hypoketonemic hypoglycemia with fasting or a mild illness, presenting signs are often nonspecific, making rapid diagnosis problematic.

HEENT/AIRWAY: Retinopathy.

CARDIOVASCULAR: Cardiomegaly and possibly cardiomyopathy. Cardiorespiratory arrest.

NEUROMUSCULAR: Hypotonia. Recurrent muscle cramps with elevated serum creatinine kinase levels. Peripheral neuropathy.

GI/GU: Hepatomegaly. Liver disease with cholestasis.

OTHER: Fasting hypoglycemia without ketonemia. Lactic acidemia during episodes of metabolic decompensation. There is secondary carnitine deficiency of unclear etiology. A patient with hypoparathyroidism has been described.

MISCELLANEOUS: Presence of this abnormality in a fetus can cause acute fatty liver of pregnancy or HELLP syndrome in the mother. Presumably, abnormal fetal metabolites overwhelm the ability of the heterozygote mother's mitochondria to oxidize them.

ANESTHETIC CONSIDERATIONS

The patient's cardiac status should be evaluated before surgery for the presence of a cardiomyopathy. Serum glucose levels should be monitored perioperatively, and adequate glucose should be supplied perioperatively. Extensive perioperative fasting should be avoided.

Bibliography:

1. Olpin SE, Clark S, Andresen BS, et al. Biochemical, clinical and molecular findings in LCHAD and general mitochondrial trifunctional protein deficiency. *J Inherit Metab Dis* 2005;28:533–544.
2. den Boer ME, Wanders RJ, Morris AA, et al. Long-chain 3-hydroxyacyl-CoA dehydrogenase deficiency: clinical presentation and follow-up of 50 patients. *Pediatrics* 2002;109:99–104.
3. Ibdah JA, Bennett MJ, Rinaldo P, et al. A fetal fatty-acid oxidation disorder as a cause of liver disease in pregnant women. *N Engl J Med* 1999;340:1723–1731.
4. Tyni T, Rapola J, Palotie A, et al. Hypoparathyroidism in a patient with long-chain 3-hydroxyacyl-coenzyme A dehydrogenase deficiency. *J Pediatr* 1997;131:766–768.

Long QT Syndrome

SYNONYM: Prolonged QT syndrome (includes Jervell-Lange-Nielson syndrome, Romano-Ward syndrome and Andersen syndrome)

MIM #: 192500 and 220400 (LQTS 1), 152427 (LQTS 2), 603830 (LQTS 3), 600919 (LQTS 4), 176261 (LQTS 5), 603796 (LQTS 6), 170390 (LQTS 7)

Long QT syndrome is a cardiac disorder which leads to an increase in cardiac arrhythmogenicity. Mutations in genes encoding the cardiac ion channels lead to a prolongation of ventricular repolarization, often evidenced by a prolonged QT interval on the electrocardiogram. However, up to 40% of patients with long QT syndrome do not manifest a prolonged QT interval on the electrocardiogram, and remain undiagnosed until they become symptomatic. Long QT syndrome may present as syncope, seizures, or sudden death. Patients are predisposed to develop polymorphic ventricular tachycardia (*torsade de pointes*), which results in syncope or seizure-like activity if it ceases spontaneously, or sudden death if it degenerates into ventricular fibrillation. Triggers include physical activity, anxiety, and stress, and therefore include surgery and anesthesia. In 1957, **Jervell and Lange-Nielson** described an autosomal recessive form of long QT syndrome associated with congenital nerve deafness, and later **Romano and Ward** independently described a much more common autosomal dominant form that is not associated with deafness. Heterozygotes with Jervell-Lange-Nielson syndrome have a prolonged QT interval without deafness (15). Congenital long QT syndrome is due to one of several mutations in a variety of genes. Long QT syndrome 1 (LQTS 1), accounting for approximately 42% of the patients, is due to a mutation of the *KCNQ1* gene, which encodes part of the cardiac slow delayed rectifier potassium channel (I_{Ks}), and is also found in the inner ear. Long QT syndrome 2 (LQTS 2), accounting for approximately 45% of patients, is due to a mutation of the *HERG* gene, which encodes the channel carrying the rapid delayed rectifier current. Long QT syndrome 3 (LQTS 3), which accounts for approximately 5% of patients, is due to a mutation of the *SCN5A* gene, which encodes a sodium channel. Long QT syndrome 4 (LQTS 4) is due to a defect in the ankyrin-B gene. Long QT syndrome 5 (LQTS 5), accounting for approximately 3% of patients, has been ascribed to the gene *KCNE1* which encodes I_{Ks}, a potassium channel subunit that regulates both *KCNQ1* and *HERG*, and can cause both clinical syndromes. Long QT syndrome 6 (LQTS 6), accounting for about 2% of patients, is due to a mutation in the gene *KCNE2*, another regulatory gene involved with the rapid delayed rectifier (with *HERG*) and with the slow rectifier (with *KCNQ1*); and long QT syndrome 7 (LQTS 7), which is due to abnormalities in the gene *KCNJ2*, coding for the inward rectifier potassium current. LQTS 7, which is also known as **Andersen syndrome**, is very rare and produces a skeletal and a cardiac muscle phenotype. It has several distinctive dysmorphic features, including hypertelorism, ptosis, low set ears, cleft palate and micrognathia.

The age of onset of symptoms in long QT syndrome varies by genotype, ranging from infancy to adulthood, but in most cases occurs sometime during childhood or adolescence. The clinical consequences of cardiac events also vary by genotype. The risk of cardiac events is highest in patients with LQTS 1 and LQTS 2, whereas the highest percentage of lethal cardiac events occurs in patients with LQTS 3 (13).

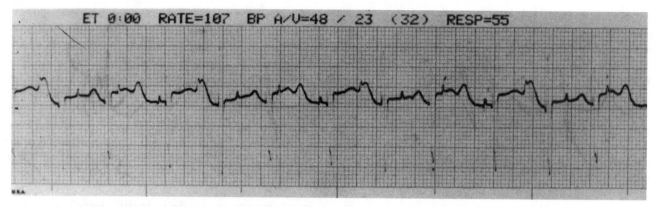

ET 0:00 RATE=107 BP A/V=48 / 23 (32) RESP=55

Long QT syndrome. This electrocardiogram is from a newborn boy in whom an arrhythmia was noticed. In addition to prolongation of the QT interval, there is also 4:3 Wenckebach second degree block. His mother and maternal grandmother had been treated for a "seizure disorder" with anticonvulsants, and both died suddenly (the mother died shortly before the diagnosis was made in her infant.)

HEENT/AIRWAY: Congenital nerve deafness with Jervell-Lange-Nielson syndrome. Low set ears, hypertelorism, and hypoplastic mandible with Andersen syndrome.

CARDIOVASCULAR: Prolonged QTc interval (QT interval corrected for heart rate), usually defined as >440 millisecond. Can cause sudden death due to ventricular tachyarrhythmia, classically *torsade de pointes*. Untreated symptomatic patients have a 5% to 20% annual risk of a syncopal episode and 50% of them have an approximate 10-year survival rate. If treated, the 10-year mortality can be reduced to 3% to 4%. Therapies have included beta antagonists, cardiac pacing, and left stellate ganglion ablation (see later). Current therapy includes beta-blockers and an implantable defibrillator with pacing capability (to counteract the bradycardic effects of beta blockade). The effect of beta-blockers is indirect, through the autonomic nervous system. By themselves, they actually increase the QT interval. The incidence of syncopal episodes decreases with age. Patients with Andersen syndrome may have associated congenital cardiac defects and a particularly high incidence of sudden death (16, 18).

NEUROMUSCULAR: Potassium sensitive periodic paralysis in Andersen syndrome.

ORTHOPEDIC: Syndactyly, short stature, scoliosis and clinodactyly with Andersen syndrome.

OTHER: The postpartum period is associated with a significantly increased risk of cardiac events.

MISCELLANEOUS: The first reported case of long QT syndrome may have been that of a deaf girl in 1856 who reportedly died suddenly while being admonished at school. Jervell was one person, Lange-Nielson was another. *HERG*, the gene involved in LQTS 2, is the human homologue of the *ether-a-go-go* gene, a potassium channel gene originally described in *Drosophila*, which was so named because it results in abnormal movements on exposure to ether.

ANESTHETIC CONSIDERATIONS

Patients with long QT syndrome are at risk of developing ventricular tachyarrhythmias perioperatively, particularly *torsade de pointes*. Unfortunately there is no definitive perioperative standard of care for these patients. Beta blockade therapy can reduce, but not eliminate, the risk of malignant tachyarrhythmias. Cardiac medications should be continued perioperatively. Patients should be receiving beta blockade therapy, and the adequacy of beta blockade should be evaluated. Hypocalcemia, hypomagnesemia, and hypokalemia can all prolong the QT interval and should be corrected prior to surgery and averted intraoperatively. Pretreatment with magnesium, even in normomagnesemic patients, has been suggested (6). A left stellate ganglion block with local anesthetic has been experimented with in the past to shorten the QT interval and decrease the risk of ventricular tachyarrhythmias perioperatively. Unfortunately this approach has not proven beneficial in most patients, and is now reserved for patients refractory to all other interventions (6). Implanted defibrillators should have the defibrillator function disabled immediately prior to surgery, with the concurrent placement of cutaneous defibrillator pads. An external defibrillator and appropriate resuscitation drugs should always be available. Patients should have continuous electrocardiographic monitoring throughout surgery and well into the recovery period, possibly for a full 24 hours after the completion of surgery (6). Adequate premedication and good control of postoperative pain are important. Maintenance of a quiet environment perioperatively is also important, as auditory stimuli can trigger tachyarrhythmias.

Light anesthesia, hypoxemia, hypocarbia, and hypercarbia should be avoided. Hypothermia prolongs the QT interval, and should be avoided. Periods of brief stimulation, such as laryngoscopy and tracheal intubation or extubation, can be covered with the addition of a short acting beta blocker or opioid. Intraoperative esmolol has been reported to have been beneficial in a child (23). The Valsalva maneuver can increase the QT interval, and should be avoided. Extubation should be considered while the patient is still deeply anesthetized, or, if done at a lighter plane, after the additional beta blockade, because ventricular fibrillation has developed during emergence (21). Placement of a central line could be considered, as it would facilitate transvenous pacing, should that become necessary. Drugs like phenothiazines and erythromycin that can prolong the QT interval should be avoided. The list of drugs which have been shown to potentially lengthen the QT interval continues to grow and includes many drugs encountered in everyday anesthetic practice, such as lidocaine, ondansetron, droperidol, chlorpromazine, haloperidol, and tamoxifen. The QT is also prolonged by class Ia (e.g., quinidine, procainamide), class II (e.g., sotalol), and class III (e.g., amiodarone) antiarrhythmics. Surgical infiltration of local anesthetic with epinephrine has resulted in intraoperative *torsade de pointes* (22). Consider using local anesthesia without epinephrine when performing local and regional blocks (2).

Because of the sensitization of the myocardium to catecholamines by halothane, other volatile anesthetics have been suggested as better choices. Halothane, enflurane, isoflurane, and sevoflurane have all been shown to prolong the QT interval in healthy humans, which may or may not be predictive of their effect in patients with long QT syndrome. All four volatile agents have a record of use in both eventful and uneventful anesthestics in patients with long QT syndrome. Experience with desflurane has not yet been reported. Isoflurane has shortened the QT interval in patients with long QT syndrome (26, 27), and thiopental has had no effect (26). However, an opposing study arrived at the conclusion that halothane shortened the QT interval in normal patients, whereas isoflurane prolonged it (19). Sevoflurane has been shown to prolong the QT interval in a patient with long QT syndrome; however, ventricular arrhythmias did not occur except during periods of intense stimulation and increased sympathetic tone (14). In another patient with long QT syndrome, sevoflurane precipitated *torsade de pointes* intraoperatively, which resolved when the anesthetic was changed to propofol. Because of its sympathomimetic properties, ketamine should be avoided in patients with long QT syndrome. Thiopental prolongs the QT interval in healthy humans (2). Propofol causes less QT prolongation than does thiopentone in normal humans (24). Propofol has also been shown to reverse sevoflurane induced QT prolongation (10). Succinylcholine and other nondepolarizing relaxants have been used without complications, even though succinylcholine prolongs the QTc. Because of the tachycardia associated with pancuronium, other nondepolarizing muscle relaxants have been suggested as better choices. Vecuronium may be the best choice, as it lacks significant autonomic side effects. Atropine and glycopyrrolate both prolong QT interval in healthy humans, and reversal of muscle relaxant has been associated with ventricular fibrillation (11). Midazolam has no effect on the QTc (6). Narcotics have been used in patients with long QT syndrome without adverse effects (2). Spinal and epidural anesthesia have been used successfully for Cesarean section (4, 5, 20, 25).

Treatment of intraoperative *torsade de pointes* includes electrical cardioversion if the patient is hemodynamically compromised. Even normomagnesemic patients should receive magnesium (30 mg/kg loading dose, followed by 2 to 4 mg/minute and monitoring of serum levels). Other treatment options include intravenous amiodarone, correction of any electrolyte abnormalities (particularly potassium, magnesium, and calcium), beta blockade, nicorandil for LQTS 2 (12), and increasing the heart rate (which decreases the QT interval). The heart rate may be increased by using atrial pacing (overdrive pacing) or intravenous isoproterenol.

Patients with Andersen syndrome (LQTS 7) have dysmorphic facial features which may lead to difficulty with intubation. In patients with Andersen syndrome, succinylcholine should be avoided because of the risk of a hyperkalemic response (3).

Bibliography:

1. Saussine M, Massad I, Raczka F, et al. Torsade de pointes during sevoflurane anesthesia in a child with congenital long QT syndrome. *Paediatr Anaesth* 2006;16:63–65.
2. Kies SJ, Pabelick CM, Hurley HA, et al. Anesthesia for patients with congenital long QT syndrome. *Anesthesiology* 2005;102:204–210.
3. Young DA. Anesthesia for the child with Andersen syndrome. *Paediatr Anaesth* 2005;15:1019–1020.
4. Al-Refai A, Gunka V, Douglas J. Spinal anesthesia for Cesarean section in a parturient with long QT syndrome. *Can J Anaesth* 2004;51:993–996.
5. Kameyama E, Ito Y, Ito J, et al. Anesthetic management of caesarean section in a patient with asymptomatic idiopathic prolonged QT interval syndrome [Japanese]. *Masui* 2004;53:1167–1169.
6. Booker PD, Whyte SD, Ladusans EJ. Long QT syndrome and anaesthesia. *Br J Anaesth* 2003;90:349–366.
7. Katz RI, Quijano I, Barcelon N, et al. Ventricular tachycardia during general anesthesia in a patient with congenital long QT syndrome. *Can J Anaesth* 2003;50:398–403.
8. Wisely NA, Shipton EA. Long QT syndrome and anaesthesia. *Eur J Anaesth* 2002;19:853–859.
9. Das SN, Kiran U, Saxena N. Perioperative management of long QT syndrome in a child with congenital heart disease. *Acta Anaesthesiol Scand* 2002;46:221–223.
10. Kleinsasser A, Loeckinger A, Lindner KH, et al. Reversing sevoflurane-associated Q-Tc prolongation by changing to propofol. *Anaesthesia* 2001;56:248–250.
11. Pleym H, Bathen J, Spigset O, et al. Ventricular fibrillation related to reversal of the neuromuscular blockade in a patient with long QT syndrome. *Acta Anaesthesiol Scand* 1999;43:352–355.
12. Saitoh K, Suzuki H, Hirabayashi Y, et al. Nicorandil successfully abolished intraoperative torsade de pointes. *Anesthesiology* 1998;88:1669–1671.
13. Zareba W, Moss AJ, Schwartz PJ, et al. Influence of genotype on the clinical course of the long-QT syndrome. International long-QT syndrome registry research group. *N Engl J Med* 1998;339:960–965.
14. Gallagher JD, Weindling SN, Anderson G, et al. Effects of sevoflurane on QT interval in a patient with congenital long QT syndrome. *Anesthesiology* 1998;89:1569–1573.
15. Duggal P, Vesely MR, Wattanasirichaigoon D, et al. Mutation of the gene for IsK associated with both Jervell and Lange-Nielson and Romano-Ward forms of long-QT syndrome. *Circulation* 1998;97:142–146.

16. Heard CM, Fletcher JE. Perioperative considerations in a newly described subtype of congenital long QT syndrome. *Paediatr Anaesth* 1998;8:93–94.
17. Splawski I, Timothy KW, Vincent GM, et al. Molecular basis of the long-QT syndrome associated with deafness. *N Engl J Med* 1997;336:1562–1567.
18. Joseph-Reynolds AM, Auden SM, Sobczyzk WL. Perioperative considerations in a newly described subtype of congenital long QT syndrome. *Paediatr Anaesth* 1997;7:237–241.
19. Michaloudis D, Fraisakis O, Lefaki I, et al. Anaesthesia and the QT interval in humans: the effects of isoflurane and halothane. *Anaesthesia* 1996;51:219–224.
20. Ganta R, Roberts C, Elwood RJ, et al. Epidural anesthesia for cesarean section in a patient with Romano-Ward syndrome. *Anesth Analg* 1995;81:425–426.
21. Holland JJ. Cardiac arrest under anaesthesia in a child with previously undiagnosed Jervell and Lange-Nielson syndrome. *Anaesthesia* 1993;48:149–151.
22. Richardson MG, Roark GL, Helfaer MA. Intraoperative epinephrine-induced torsades de pointes in a child with long QT syndrome. *Anesthesiology* 1992;76:647–649.
23. Dunn CM, Gunter JB, Quattromani A, et al. Esmolol in the anaesthetic management of a boy with Romano-Ward syndrome. *Paediatr Anaesth* 1991;1:129–132.
24. McConachie I, Keaveny JP, Healy TE, et al. Effect of anaesthesia on the QT interval. *Br J Anaesth* 1989;63:558–560.
25. Ryan H. Anaesthesia for caesarean section in a patient with Jervell, Lange-Nielsen syndrome. *Can J Anaesth* 1988;35:422–424.
26. Wilton NC, Hantler CB. Congenital long QT syndrome: changes in QT interval during anesthesia with thiopental, vecuronium, fentanyl, and isoflurane. *Anesth Analg* 1987;66:357–360.
27. Carlock FJ, Brown M, Brown EM. Isoflurane anaesthesia for a patient with long Q-T syndrome. *Can Anaesth Soc J* 1984;31:83–85.

Louis-Bar Syndrome

See Ataxia—telangiectasia

Lowe Syndrome

SYNONYM: Oculocerebrorenal syndrome

MIM #: 309000

The hallmarks of this X-linked disorder are hydrophthalmia, cataracts, mental retardation, vitamin D-resistant rickets, aminoaciduria, and reduced ammonia production by the kidney. This syndrome is caused by a defect in the *OCRL1* gene. The gene product is a lipid phosphatase that controls levels of a critical cellular metabolite, phosphatidylinositol 4,5-bisphosphate-5-phosphatase, which is localized in a trans-Golgi network involved in actin polymerization.

HEENT/AIRWAY: Hydrophthalmia, cataracts, lens opacities, corneal scarring, enophthalmos, nystagmus. Dental cysts, enamel hypoplasia.

NEUROMUSCULAR: Mild to moderate mental retardation. Hypotonia, intention tremor. Behavioral problems including stereotypical behavior, stubbornness, and temper tantrums.

ORTHOPEDIC: Vitamin D-resistant rickets. Scoliosis, kyphosis, platyspondyly. Genu valgum. Subcutaneous nodules on fingers.

GI/GU: Cryptorchidism. Renal failure, renal tubular acidosis, aminoaciduria, proteinuria, carnitine wasting, phosphaturia with hypophosphatemia. Can develop Fanconi syndrome (see earlier).

OTHER: Failure to thrive.

ANESTHETIC CONSIDERATIONS

Serum electrolytes, ionized calcium levels, and acid–base status should be evaluated preoperatively. Patients may be receiving chronic bicarbonate therapy. Chronic stable hypokalemia is usually well tolerated, but the risk of perioperative arrhythmia exists. Hyperventilation and hyperglycemia can both further decrease blood potassium levels, and should be avoided. If the patients are acidotic, they may be more sensitive to opioids, as more opioids will exist in the nonionized state, facilitating penetration into the brain. Renal dysfunction has implications for the titration of perioperative fluids and for the choice of anesthetic drugs. Rachitic extremities must be carefully positioned. Patients can have elevated intraocular pressure, hence positions or interventions which elevate intraocular pressure should be avoided if possible.

Bibliography:
1. Saricaodlu F, Demirtas F, Aypar Ü. Preoperative and perioperative management of a patient with Lowe syndrome diagnosed to have Fanconi's syndrome [Letter]. *Paediatr Anaesth* 2004;14:530–531.
2. Charnas LR, Bernardini I, Rader D, et al. Clinical and laboratory findings in the oculocerebrorenal syndrome of Lowe, with special reference to growth and renal function. *N Engl J Med* 1991;324:1318–1325.

Lown-Ganong-Levine Syndrome

MIM #: 108950

This electrophysiologic syndrome is closely related to Wolff-Parkinson-White syndrome (WPW). In WPW, Kent fibers bypass the atrioventricular (AV) node to enter the ventricular myocardium directly, accounting for the short PR interval (the normal AV nodal delay is bypassed) and the initial slow upstroke of the QRS, because of the initial cell-to-cell transmission of the electrical impulse, until the normally conducted impulse finally gets through the AV node and depolarizes the ventricles rapidly by way of the His-Purkinje system. In Lown-Ganong-Levine syndrome, James fibers, which are analogous to Kent fibers, bypass the AV node, but insert into the His bundle. As a consequence, the PR interval is short, but there is no delta wave because the sequence of ventricular depolarization is normal. The presence of James fibers sets up a potential reentry circuit with the possibility of development of paroxysmal supraventricular tachycardia, just as in WPW.

CARDIOVASCULAR: Risk of atrial tachyarrhythmias.

ANESTHETIC CONSIDERATIONS

Episodes of reentrant tachycardia may be induced by sympathetic stimulation, and therefore good preoperative sedation would seem reasonable. Drugs used to terminate tachycardia (adenosine or beta blockers) may exacerbate reactive airway disease. Beta$_2$ agonists such as albuterol should not induce arrhythmias.

Perioperative increases in vagal tone, such as from drugs or gagging, may inhibit normal antegrade conduction through the AV node, and unmask conduction down the bypass tract with preexcitation (short PR interval) suddenly visible.

Verapamil and digoxin (without quinidine) are contraindicated for the treatment of atrial flutter or fibrillation in these patients because they may accelerate the rate of conduction through the bypass tract and induce ventricular fibrillation. Concurrent verapamil and propranolol (and possibly other combinations of calcium channel and beta blockers) may cause significant bradycardia. Chronic therapy with amiodarone may cause hypothyroidism or pulmonary fibrosis.

Isoflurane has been used without apparent problems during electrophysiologic mapping or radiofrequency catheter ablation in patients with the related Wolff-Parkinson-White syndrome (see later).

Bibliography:
1. Eichholz A, Whiting RB, Artal R. Lown-Ganong-Levine syndrome in pregnancy. *Obstet Gynecol* 2003;102:1393–1395.
2. Vidaillet HJ, Pressley JC, Henke E, et al. Familial occurrence of accessory atrioventricular pathways (preexcitation syndrome). *N Engl J Med* 1987;317:65–69.

Lysinuric Protein Intolerance

SYNONYM: Dibasic amino aciduria type 2

MIM #: 222700

This autosomal recessive disease is the result of a disorder in the transport of lysine as well as the other cationic amino acids arginine and ornithine. It is due to a mutation in the gene *SLC7A7*, which encodes an amino acid transporter. Urinary clearance and excretion of these amino acids is increased, and intestinal absorption is decreased. The intestinal defect has been localized to the antiluminal epithelial surface. The effects on lysine are most pronounced. Symptoms usually develop when infants stop breastfeeding. Patients learn to avoid a high-protein diet. Treatment is by protein restriction and oral citrulline supplementation.

CHEST: Interstitial pneumonitis, which is of unclear origin and may be severe or even fatal. Patients may have dyspnea, cough and rarely hemoptysis or pulmonary hemorrhage. Histologically, the process looks like alveolar proteinosis. A child has been reported who received a lung transplant for pulmonary alveolar proteinosis, which then recurred 18 months later in the transplanted lung. The interstitial pneumonitis may be steroid responsive.

NEUROMUSCULAR: Episodes of stupor and asterixis. Coma with high-protein diets. Most patients have normal intelligence, but there may be mild to moderate retardation. Hypotonia. Force feeding a high-protein diet has resulted in an isoelectric electroencephalogram.

ORTHOPEDIC: Short stature. Osteopenia with bone fragility.

GI/GU: Diarrhea, malabsorption. Episodes of nausea and vomiting. Hepatosplenomegaly, cirrhosis. Immune complex glomerulopathy, renal failure.

OTHER: Protein intolerance, failure to thrive, hyperammonemia (from ornithine insufficient to support ornithine transcarbamylase), low blood urea nitrogen. May be pancytopenic. May be hypertriglyceridemic. Sparse hair. Pregnancies highly increase the risk of hemorrhage and toxemia, but infants of mothers with the disease are unaffected. May exhibit intermittent hemophagocytic lymphohistiocytosis—defined as fever, hepatosplenomegaly, hypofibrinogenemia, hypertriglyceridemia, and pancytopenia, with hemophagocytosis occurring in bone marrow, spleen, or lymph nodes.

MISCELLANEOUS: Patients have been misdiagnosed as having celiac disease.

ANESTHETIC CONSIDERATIONS

The patient's pulmonary and renal function should be evaluated carefully preoperatively. Blood urea nitrogen may be a poor indicator of renal function. May be pancytopenic. A low-protein diet should be continued perioperatively. Patients with interstitial pneumonitis may be taking steroids, and will therefore require perioperative stress doses of steroids.

Bibliography:
1. Palacin M, Bertran J, Chillaron J, et al. Lysinuric protein intolerance: mechanisms of pathophysiology. *Mol Genet Metab* 2004;81: S27–S37.
2. Duval M, Fenneteau O, Doireau V, et al. Intermittent hemophagocytic lymphohistiocytosis is a regular feature of lysinuric protein intolerance. *J Pediatr* 1999;134:236–239.
3. Parto K, Kallajoki M, Aho H, et al. Pulmonary alveolar proteinosis and glomerulonephritis in lysinuric protein intolerance: case reports and autopsy findings of four pediatric patients. *Hum Pathol* 1994;25: 400–407.

M

Machado-Joseph Disease

See Joseph disease

MADD

See Glutaric aciduria type II

Maffucci Syndrome

Included in Ollier disease

Majewski Type Short Rib-Polydactyly Syndrome

See Short rib-polydactyly syndrome

Malignant Atrophic Papulosis

SYNONYM: Degos disease

MIM #: 602248

This multisystem vasculitis affects primarily the skin, gastrointestinal tract, and central nervous system. The etiology of this disease is not known, although familial cases have been reported. Boys are more frequently affected than girls, with a ratio of 3:1. The disease is sometimes limited to the skin. Systemic involvement may indicate severe and even fatal disease.

HEENT/AIRWAY: Avascular patches on the conjunctivae. May have avascular involvement of sclerae, choroid, retina, or optic nerve.

CHEST: Pleuritis with pleural effusions.

CARDIOVASCULAR: Constrictive pericarditis. Myocardial infarctions have been reported.

NEUROMUSCULAR: Central nervous system infarcts or hemorrhages.

GI/GU: Gastrointestinal lesions may result in bowel infarction and perforation.

OTHER: Skin lesions are marked by a wedge-shaped area of necrosis extending from the epidermis through the dermis. There are multiple atrophic skin papules with an atrophic white center surrounded by a telangiectatic border.

ANESTHETIC CONSIDERATIONS

Pleural and pericardial disease should be excluded preoperatively if possible. Patients may require urgent surgery for bowel perforation, and can be quite ill at the time of surgery.

Bibliography:

1. Scheinfeld N. Degos disease is probably a distinct entity: a review of clinical and laboratory evidence [Letter]. *J Am Acad Dermatol* 2005;52:375–376.
2. Amato C, Ferri R, Elia M, et al. Nervous system involvement in Degos disease. *AJNR Am J Neuroradiol* 2005;26:646–649.
3. High WA, Aranda J, Patel SB, et al. Is Degos disease a clinical and histological end point rather than a specific disease? *J Am Acad Dermatol* 2004;50:895–899.
4. Torrelo A, Sevilla J, Mediero IG, et al. Malignant atrophic papulosis in an infant. *Br J Dermatol* 2002;146:916–918.
5. Chave TA, Varma S, Patel GK, et al. Malignant atrophic papulosis (Degos disease): clinicopathological correlations. *J Eur Acad Dermatol Venereol* 2001;15:43–45.
6. Katz SK, Mudd LJ, Roenigk HH. Malignant atrophic papulosis (Degos disease) involving three generations of a family. *J Am Acad Dermatol* 1997;37:480–484.

Malignant Hyperthermia Susceptibility

MIM #: 145600

Malignant hyperthermia is a potentially lethal disorder of skeletal muscle. In humans, susceptibility to malignant hyperthermia is inherited in an autosomal dominant fashion. Malignant hyperthermia manifests as a hypermetabolic response to volatile inhalational anesthetic agents and/or succinylcholine, characterized by increased oxygen consumption, increased carbon dioxide production, and rhabdomyolysis. Clinical signs of the hypermetabolic state include elevated end-tidal carbon dioxide, tachypnea, tachycardia, acidosis, hyperkalemia, muscle rigidity, myoglobinuria, and hyperpyrexia (usually a late finding). Children appear to be at greater risk for developing malignant hyperthermia than adults. Malignant hyperthermia can occur at anytime during an anesthetic, and can even present postoperatively (usually in the postanesthesia care unit). Interestingly, the reaction does not always occur in susceptible individuals. Malignant hyperthermia is caused by an abnormal elevation of intracellular calcium secondary to an increase in the release of calcium from the sarcoplasmic reticulum. This increased release of calcium is due to a mutation in the gene encoding for the ryanodine receptor (*RYR1*), which is embedded in the sarcoplasmic reticulum and is responsible for regulating calcium transport. There are at least 30 different mutations of *RYR1* associated with malignant hyperthermia susceptibility. Patients with central core disease or King-Denborough syndrome (see earlier) are likely to be malignant hyperthermia susceptible.

The caffeine-halothane contracture test has been the gold standard for diagnosing malignant hyperthermia susceptibility for several decades. This test involves extracting a piece of skeletal muscle from the patient's thigh, exposing it *in vitro* to the ryanodine receptor agonists halothane and caffeine, and measuring the degree of muscle contraction. Muscle tissue from patients who are susceptible to malignant hyperthermia typically shows an excessive degree of contraction. Development of a genetic screen for malignant hyperthermia susceptibility has been the focus of considerable research. The number of *RYR1* mutations associated with malignant hyperthermia susceptibility have made genetic testing for this disorder challenging. In some families a specific mutation can be found to correlate with susceptibility to malignant hyperthermia, and in those families a genetic test can be used in place of the muscle biopsy. If the same mutation is found, then the patient is considered to be susceptible to malignant hyperthermia. If the mutation is not identified, susceptibility to malignant hyperthermia CANNOT be ruled out.

Initially the mortality rate associated with malignant hyperthermia was 70%, but with the advent of dantrolene and advances in supportive care the mortality rate is now less than 5% in developed countries. Dantrolene works by directly inhibiting the ryanodine receptor and preventing further calcium release.

MISCELLANEOUS: Malignant hyperthermia was first described in 1962 by Denborough and Lovell who identified a family in Australia in which 10 of the 38 people who had been administered a general anesthesia had died.

ANESTHETIC CONSIDERATIONS
Patients known to be susceptible to malignant hyperthermia must receive a nontriggering general anesthetic, neuraxial block or peripheral nerve block. If an anesthetic machine is used it should either be "malignant hyperthermia dedicated" or adequately flushed with oxygen. Administration of prophylactic dantrolene is not necessary in these patients. The treatment of malignant hyperthermia includes immediate discontinuation of triggering agents, hyperventilation with 100% oxygen, administration of dantrolene in doses of 2.5 mg/kg up to 10 mg/kg, active cooling, and appropriate treatment of hyperkalemia (hyperventilation, bicarbonate, calcium, glucose and insulin, epinephrine). Calcium channel blockers should not be used with dantrolene, as this may exacerbate hyperkalemia. Patients should be monitored closely for 48 to 72 hours after the initiation of the treatment, with particular vigilance for adequate urine output, the development of myoglobinuria or renal failure, or the development of a coagulopathy. Relapse may occur in 25% of the patients within 24 hours of the initial administration of dantrolene; so dantrolene should be continued in the postoperative period (1 mg/kg intravenously or orally every 6 hours until the patient's vital signs have stabilized in the normal range). In 1981 the Malignant Hyperthermia Association of the United States (MHAUS) established a hotline which can be accessed for medical consultation 24 hours a day 7 days a week by calling 1 (800) MH HYPER [1 (800) 644–9737], or (315) 464–7079 from outside of the United States. The MHAUS website can be visited at www.mhaus.org.

Bibliography:
1. Litman RS, Rosenberg H. Malignant hyperthermia: update on susceptibility testing. *JAMA* 2005;293:2918–2924.
2. Robinson RL, Anetseder MJ, Brancadoro V, et al. Recent advances in the diagnosis of malignant hyperthermia susceptibility: how confident can we be of genetic testing? *Eur J Hum Genet* 2003;11:342–348.
3. Hoenemann CW, Halene-Holtgraeve TB, Booke M, et al. Delayed onset of malignant hyperthermia in desflurane anesthesia. *Anesth Analg* 2003;96:165–167.
4. Rosenberg H, Antognini JF, Muldoon S. Testing for malignant hyperthermia. *Anesthesiology* 2002;96:232–237.
5. Ruffert H, Olthoff DDeutrich C, et al. Current aspects of the diagnosis of malignant hyperthermia. *Anaesthesist* 2002;51:904–913.
6. Rosenbaum HK, Miller JD. Malignant hyperthermia and myotonic disorders. *Anesthesiol Clin North America* 2002;20:623–664.
7. Monnier N, Krivosic-Horber R, Payen JF, et al. Presence of two different genetic traits in malignant hyperthermia families: implication for genetic analysis, diagnosis, and incidence of malignant hyperthermia susceptibility. *Anesthesiology* 2002;97:1067–1074.
8. Anetseder M, Hager M, Muller CR, et al. Diagnosis of susceptibility to malignant hyperthermia by use of a metabolic test. *Lancet* 2002;359:1579–1580.
9. Tobin JR, Jason DR, Challa VR, et al. Malignant hyperthermia and apparent heat stroke. *JAMA* 2001;286:168–169.
10. Urwyler A, Deufel T, McCarthy T, et al. Guidelines for molecular genetic detection of susceptibility to malignant hyperthermia. *Br J Anaesth* 2001;86:283–287.
11. Sambuughin N, Sei Y, Gallagher KL, et al. North American malignant hyperthermia population: screening of the ryanodine receptor gene and identification of novel mutations. *Anesthesiology* 2001;95:594–599.
12. Jurkat-Rott K, McCarthy T, Lehmann-Horn F. Genetics and pathogenesis of malignant hyperthermia. *Muscle Nerve* 2000;23:4–17.
13. Short JA, Cooper CM. Suspected recurrence of malignant hyperthermia after post-extubation shivering in the intensive care unit, 18 h after tonsillectomy. *Br J Anaesth* 1999;82:945–947.
14. Larach MG, Localio AR, Allen GC, et al. A clinical grading scale to predict malignant hyperthermia susceptibility. *Anesthesiology* 1994;80:771–779.

Mandibulofacial Dysostosis

See Treacher Collins syndrome

Mannosidosis

SYNONYM: Alpha-mannosidosis

MIM #: 248500

This autosomal recessive lysosomal storage disease is due to a mutation in the gene encoding lysosomal alpha-mannosidase. There is a severe, infantile form (type I) which is fatal in childhood, and a less severe juvenile or adult form (type II) with progressive neurological deterioration. As a lysosomal storage disease, the phenotype resembles that of Hurler syndrome.

HEENT/AIRWAY: Large head with thick calvarium. Coarse features. Low anterior hairline. Thick eyebrows. Lens opacification. Flat nose. Macroglossia, widely-spaced teeth, gingival hypertrophy. Prognathism. Deafness.

CHEST: Recurrent respiratory tract infections. Pectus carinatum.

NEUROMUSCULAR: Hypotonia. Mental retardation. Dilated cerebral ventricles.

ORTHOPEDIC: Lumbar gibbus, big hands and feet, dysostosis multiplex, bowed femurs. Spondylosis. Spondylolisthesis of L5 on S1.

GI/GU: Mild hepatosplenomegaly. Recurrent vomiting.

OTHER: Tall stature. Pancytopenia, storage cells in marrow. Immunoglobulin deficiency. Susceptibility to infections. Antiplatelet and antineutrophil antibodies. Low haptoglobin.

MISCELLANEOUS: Alpha-mannosidosis has been described in cattle, cats, and guinea pigs. Hematopoietic stem cell transplantation has ameliorated the disease in human beings.

ANESTHETIC CONSIDERATIONS

Although specific anesthetic implications have not been published, it would seem that given the phenotypic similarity with Hurler syndrome, similar concerns apply. These include difficult face mask fit, and difficult laryngoscopy and intubation which may worsen with age.

Bibliography:
1. Gutschalk A, Harting I, Cantz M, et al. Adult alpha-mannosidosis: clinical progression in the absence of demyelination. *Neurology* 2004;63:1744–1746.
2. Grewal SS, Shapiro EG, Krivit W, et al. Effective treatment of α-mannosidosis by allogeneic hematopoietic stem cell transplantation. *J Pediatr* 2004;144:569–573.

Maple Syrup Urine Disease

MIM #: 248600

This is an autosomal recessive disease whose well known name is derived from the odor imparted to the urine by the increased concentration of a metabolite, the keto acid of isoleucine (alpha-keto-beta-methylvaleric acid). Maple syrup urine disease can be caused by several defects in the mitochondrial multienzyme complex, branched-chain alpha-keto acid dehydrogenase. This enzyme is required for the catabolism of branched-chain amino acids. Routine neonatal screening has improved the clinical outcome because early diagnosis allows for early dietary modification. Today it is rare to come across an untreated, and therefore clinically unmodified, patient. A variety of clinical subtypes, varying in the timing of onset and severity of symptoms, have been described. The classic type presents at several days of age. Other subtypes are intermittent, with symptomatic episodes triggered by stress (surgery included), intercurrent illness, or acute increases in dietary protein, as is typical of many metabolic diseases. Some subtypes are responsive to therapy with thiamine.

HEENT/AIRWAY: Ptosis and ophthalmoplegia if untreated.

NEUROMUSCULAR: In the classic form, lethargy and poor feeding rapidly progress to apnea and coma. Severe psychomotor developmental delay if untreated. Intermittent subtypes may have intermittent ataxia, irritability, and progressive lethargy. Cerebral edema has been described in older patients. Patients with an intermittent type are usually normal between episodes.

GI/GU: Episodic pancreatitis.

OTHER: Hypoglycemia if untreated. Metabolic acidosis. Failure to thrive.

MISCELLANEOUS: This syndrome was first described by Menkes (of Menkes kinky hair syndrome). The abnormal, sweet smell may not be present in the urine for the first few months. It is first noticed in the cerumen, probably because of the lipophilic nature of the involved organic acids.

A case of pseudo-maple syrup urine disease has been reported in a young infant who was given herbal tea made from fenugreek seeds with a resultant abnormal odor similar to that of maple syrup urine. Evaluation showed the presence of sotolone which is responsible for the peculiar smell in the maple syrup urine disease, as also in the fenugreek seeds and the child's urine.

ANESTHETIC CONSIDERATIONS

Patients may become hypoglycemic, so prolonged perioperative fasting should be avoided; intravenous fluids containing glucose should be used, and serum glucose levels should be monitored. Additional caloric sources should include intravenous fat emulsion to minimize the glucose load. The patient's special diet should be reinstituted postoperatively as soon as is practicable. High levels of keto acids can result in metabolic acidosis. An orogastric tube or throat packs should be placed if the surgery has the potential to cause oral or intestinal bleeding because blood aspirated into the gastrointestinal tract after oral or nasal surgery might present an excessive protein load and trigger an acute decompensation. Patients should be observed closely postoperatively for evidence of symptomatic worsening.

Overhydration may exacerbate cerebral edema. It has been suggested that hypertonic glucose may exacerbate this condition because of increases in CO_2 production and norepinephrine secretion.

FIGURE: See **Appendix D**

Bibliography:
1. Harris RA, Joshi M, Jeoung NH, et al. Overview of the molecular and biochemical basis of branched-chain amino acid catabolism. *J Nutr* 2005;135:S1527–S1530.
2. Kahraman S, Ercan M, Akkus O, et al. Anaesthetic management in maple syrup urine disease. *Anaesthesia* 1996;51:575–578.
3. Delaney A, Gal TJ. Hazards of anesthesia and operation in maple-syrup-urine disease. *Anesthesiology* 1976;44:83–86.

Marden-Walker Syndrome

MIM #: 248700

This autosomal recessive disorder is characterized by blepharophimosis, immobile facies, micrognathia, multiple joint contractures, and mental retardation. Many patients die in infancy. The responsible gene and the gene product are not known.

HEENT/AIRWAY: Microcephaly. Large anterior fontanelle. Immobile facies. Blepharophimosis, strabismus. Small mouth. High-arched palate or cleft palate. Micrognathia. May have short frenulum. May have short neck.

CHEST: Pectus excavatum or carinatum. Rare pulmonary hypoplasia.

CARDIOVASCULAR: May have congenital cardiac defect.

NEUROMUSCULAR: Severe mental retardation. Aggressive behavior and hyperactivity in patients as they approach puberty. Hypotonia. May have electroencephalographic abnormalities, seizures. May have agenesis of the corpus callosum, Dandy-Walker malformation, hydrocephalus. May have hypoplastic cerebellum, inferior vermis, or brainstem.

ORTHOPEDIC: Severe growth deficiency. Multiple joint contractures. Kyphoscoliosis. Camptodactyly, arachnodactyly. Clubfoot deformity.

GI/GU: Inguinal hernias, pyloric stenosis. Cryptorchidism, hypospadias, micropenis. Rare renal hypoplasia.

OTHER: Zollinger-Ellison syndrome has been reported. May have pilonidal sinus.

ANESTHETIC CONSIDERATIONS

Direct laryngoscopy and tracheal intubation may be difficult secondary to micrognathia and short neck. Patients are at risk for perioperative aspiration. Patients must be carefully positioned perioperatively because of multiple joint contractures. Patients with hydrocephalus may have elevated intracranial pressure, and perioperative measures should be taken to avoid further elevation in pressure. Patients with congenital cardiac defects need perioperative prophylactic antibiotics as indicated.

Bibliography:

1. Ozbek S, Saglam H, Ozdamar E. Marden-Walker syndrome with some additional anomalies. *Pediatr Int* 2005;47:92–94.
2. Orrico A, Galli L, Zappella M, et al. Additional case of Marden-Walker syndrome: support for the autosomal-recessive inheritance and refinement of phenotype in a surviving patient. *J Child Neurol* 2001;16:150–153.
3. Garavelli L, Donadio A, Banchini G, et al. Marden-Walker syndrome: case report, nosologic discussion and aspects of counseling. *Genet Couns* 2000;11:111–118.
4. Ozkinay F, Ozyurek AR, Bakiler AR, et al. A case of Marden-Walker syndrome with Dandy-Walker malformation. *Clin Genet* 1995;47:221–223.

Marfan Syndrome

MIM #: 154700

This autosomal dominant disease has widespread manifestations in both skeletal and connective tissue. Prominent characteristics include optic lens dislocation, aortic

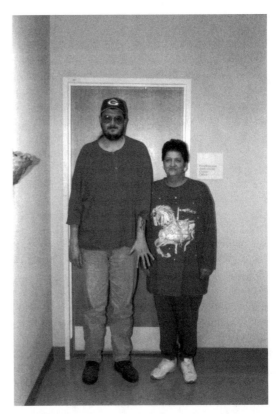

Marfan syndrome. FIG. 1. This 6′ 7″ (201 cm) 27-year-old man was seen the day before surgery for repair of a detached retina, and is pictured with his mother. Six months previously, he had had a dislocated lens repaired. His father (6′ 8″), also with Marfan syndrome, died at 25 years of age from an aortic dissection. At the time this patient was seen in the preoperative evaluation center, he was noted to have new T-wave inversions that were not present 6 months previously. Echocardiography showed that he also had mitral valve prolapse with insufficiency and a slightly dilated ascending aorta. Three years later he required urgent surgery for an aortic dissection.

dissection, mitral valve prolapse, a tall, asthenic build, arachnodactyly, joint laxity, and scoliosis. There is a high degree of penetrance but incomplete expressivity, so there is much individual variation. Approximately 15% of the cases are sporadic. The disease is due to a defect in the gene fibrillin-1. Fibrillin is the major element of extracellular microfibrils in the elastic as well as the nonelastic connective tissues.

HEENT/AIRWAY: Dolichocephaly. Long, narrow facies with a high-arched palate and crowded teeth. Lens dislocation is very common, and can result in cataract formation. The globe is elongated and patients tend to be myopic and have increased risk of retinal detachment. Risk of glaucoma, even at a young age. Rare tracheomalacia.

CHEST: Pectus excavatum, less commonly pectus carinatum. Even patients without scoliosis or other spine deformity can have lower-than-predicted forced vital capacity,

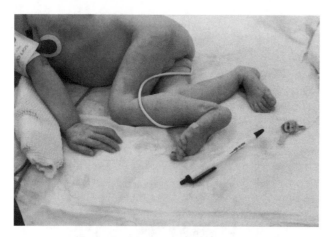

Marfan syndrome. FIG. 2. Long fingers and toes are already apparent in this 6-month-old with Marfan syndrome.

presumably due to earlier airway closure from inadequate small airway elastic tissue. Emphysema and bronchogenic cysts can develop. Pulmonary blebs with spontaneous pneumothoraces are relatively common. Obstructive sleep apnea (possibly secondary to pharyngeal laxity).

CARDIOVASCULAR: Aortic or pulmonary artery dilatation, aortic dissection, aortic insufficiency, mitral prolapse with insufficiency. The most common type of aortic dissection is DeBakey type 2 (ascending aorta proximal to the innominate artery). The histologic change in the aorta is cystic medial necrosis. Elective root replacement has much lower operative mortality than emergency repair of aortic dissection. Valvar and vascular findings may be present at birth. Echocardiography can demonstrate mitral valve prolapse in over 80% of patients.

In coronary arteries, including those supplying the sinus and atrioventricular nodes, medial necrosis can develop that can progress to luminal narrowing.

Marfan disease can present in the neonatal period and neonates, if they experience major problems, tend to have mitral insufficiency rather than aortic insufficiency as the primary manifestation.

NEUROMUSCULAR: Widened lumbosacral canal. Spinal arachnoid cysts or dural ectasia (widened lumbosacral dural sac).

ORTHOPEDIC: Tall with an arm span greater than the height. Winged scapula. Ulnar deviation of the metacarpophalangeal joints, and arachnodactyly (long fingers). Recurrent dislocations due to joint laxity. Scoliosis, sometimes at multiple locations along the spine. (Thoracic scoliosis is almost always convex to the right.) Kyphosis. Congenital contractures. Flat feet.

GI/GU: Increased incidence of inguinal, umbilical, and femoral hernias.

OTHER: Skin striae.

MISCELLANEOUS: It has been suggested that the 5-year-old girl described by Marfan in 1896 actually had contractural arachnodactyly [Beals contractural arachnodactyly (see earlier), which is due to a defect in the gene fibrillin-2]. Achard may have reported the first true case of Marfan syndrome in 1902. The aneurysms of the ascending aorta were first described by Helen Taussig (and coauthors). Marfan syndrome is phenotypically similar to homocystinuria. Interestingly, the optic lens dislocates down in homocystinuria, and up in Marfan syndrome.

Bernard J. A. Marfan held the first chair in pediatrics in Paris early in the 20th century. Although he did not use the term "arachnodactyly" in his 1896 report (Achard did so in a report 6 years later), the term probably derives from Marfan's use of the phrase *pattes d'araignee* ("spider legs") in his original report.

Abraham Lincoln and Nicolò Paganini are hypothesized to have had Marfan syndrome.

ANESTHETIC CONSIDERATIONS

Hypertension should be avoided in these patients who are at risk of aortic dissection. Preoperative echocardiography should be considered so as to exclude cardiac or aortic pathology. Patients may be on beta-blocker therapy. A patient has been reported who had acute, intraoperative coronary artery obstruction (presumably not a coronary air embolus) (8). Patients should receive appropriate perioperative antibiotic prophylaxis when indicated, most commonly for mitral valve prolapse with insufficiency.

These patients are at increased risk of pneumothoraces, which must be kept in mind when using positive pressure ventilation. Midtracheal obstruction has been reported after Harrington rod placement (10, 14), and secondary to unexpected tracheomalacia after the induction of general anesthesia (4).

Patients must be carefully positioned to avoid joint dislocations secondary to joint laxity. Although there is a possibility of temporomandibular joint dysfunction, this has not been reported to cause difficulty with laryngoscopy.

These patients may require larger-than-normal doses of spinal or epidural anesthetics because of their increased length. In addition, inadequate spread of spinal anesthesia has been reported, presumably due to increased cerebrospinal fluid volume due to dural ectasia (2). Both regional and general anesthesia have been used successfully in parturients (5, 6, 9, 11, 12).

Bibliography:

1. Ioscovich A, Elstein D. Images in Anesthesia: Transesophageal echocardiography during Cesarean section in a Marfan patient with aortic dissection. *Can J Anaesth* 2005;52:737–738.
2. Lacassie HJ, Millar S, Leithe LG, et al. Dural ectasia: a likely cause of inadequate spinal anaesthesia in two parturients with Marfan syndrome. *Br J Anaesth* 2005;94:500–504.
3. Kuczkowski KM. Labor analgesia for the parturient with an uncommon disorder: a common dilemma in the delivery suite. *Obstet Gynecol Surv* 2003;58:800–803.

4. Oh AY, Kim YH, Kim BK, et al. Unexpected tracheomalacia in Marfan syndrome during general anesthesia for correction of scoliosis. *Anesth Analg* 2002;95:331–332.

5. Handa F, Ohnishi Y, Takauchi Y, et al. Anesthetic management of parturients with Marfan syndrome [Japanese]. *Masui* 2001;50:399–404.

6. Brar HB. Anaesthetic management of a caesarean section in a patient with Marfan's syndrome and aortic dissection. *Anaesth Intensive Care* 2001;29:67–70.

7. Gott VL, Greene PS, Alejo DE, et al. Replacement of the aortic root in patients with Marfan's syndrome. *N Engl J Med* 1999;340:1307–1313.

8. Pizov R, Kaplan L, Floman Y, et al. Temporary right coronary flow disruption during instrumented correction of the spine. *Anesthesiology* 1997;86:1210–1211.

9. Tritapepe L, Voci P, Pinto G, et al. Anaesthesia for caesarean section in a Marfan patient with recurrent aortic dissection. *Can J Anaesth* 1996;43:1153–1155.

10. Kai Y, Yamaoka A, Irita K, et al. Transient tracheal obstruction during surgical correction of scoliosis in a patient with Marfan's syndrome [Japanese]. *Masui* 1995;44:868–873.

11. Gordon CF, Johnson MD. Anesthetic management of the pregnant patient with Marfan syndrome. *J Clin Anesth* 1994;5:248–251.

12. Pinosky ML, Hopkins RA, Pinckert TL, et al. Anesthesia for simultaneous cesarean section and acute aortic dissection repair in a patient with Marfan's syndrome. *J Cardiothorac Vasc Anesth* 1994;8:451–454.

13. Wells DG, Podolakin W. Anaesthesia and Marfan's syndrome: case report. *Can J Anaesth* 1987;34:311–314.

14. Mesrobian RB, Epps JL. Midtracheal obstruction after Harrington rod placement in a patient with Marfan's syndrome. *Anesth Analg* 1986;65:411–413.

15. Verghese C. Anaesthesia in Marfan's syndrome. *Anaesthesia* 1984;39:917–922.

Marinesco-Sjögren Syndrome

MIM #: 248800

This is an autosomal recessive disorder whose primary manifestations are cerebellar ataxia, congenital cataracts, and retarded mental and physical development. This disorder is caused by a mutation in the gene *SIL1*, which encodes a nucleotide exchange factor for the heat-shock protein 70 (HSP70) chaperone HSPA5. Hypergonadotropic hypogonadism is often associated with Marinesco-Sjögren syndrome. The two genes may be linked, or this may be a further manifestation of Marinesco-Sjögren syndrome.

HEENT/AIRWAY: Microcephaly, congenital cataracts, nystagmus, strabismus. Dysarthria.

CHEST: Pectus carinatum.

NEUROMUSCULAR: Retarded mental and physical development. Cerebellar cortical atrophy with vacuolated Purkinje cells. Cerebellar ataxia, spasticity. Hypotonia, progressive muscle weakness and atrophy, myopathy.

ORTHOPEDIC: Short stature. Kyphosis, scoliosis, contractures. Short metacarpals and metatarsals. Coxa valga, cubitus valgus, pes planus.

MISCELLANEOUS: An early name for this disorder was "hereditary oligophrenic cerebellolental degeneration." The syndrome was first described in the Hungarian literature a quarter century before Marinesco's report.

ANESTHETIC CONSIDERATIONS
Succinylcholine should be avoided in patients with significant myopathy secondary to the risk of exaggerated hyperkalemia. Kyphoscoliosis and contractures may complicate intraoperative positioning. Severe muscle weakness combined with severe kyphoscoliosis increases the risk of postoperative pulmonary complications, and patients should be monitored closely in the postanesthesia care unit.

Bibliography:

1. Anttonen AK, Mahjneh I, Hamalainen RH, et al. The gene disrupted in Marinesco-Sjögren syndrome encodes SIL1, an HSPA5 cochaperone. *Nat Genet* 2005;37:1309–1311.

2. Tachi N, Nagata N, Wakai S, et al. Congenital muscular dystrophy in Marinesco-Sjögren syndrome. *Pediatr Neurol* 1991;7:296–298.

3. Superneau DW, Wertelecki W, Zellweger H, et al. Myopathy in Marinesco-Sjögren syndrome. *Eur Neurol* 1987;26:8–16.

Maroteaux-Lamy Syndrome

SYNONYM: Mucopolysaccharidosis VI

MIM #: 253200

This autosomal recessive mucopolysaccharidosis is due to a defect in the gene for the lysosomal enzyme arylsulfatase B. It is characterized by prominent bone and eye findings with usually normal intelligence. There are both mild and severe forms.

HEENT/AIRWAY: The face is usually mildly involved, but some patients may have the coarse facies characteristic of Hurler syndrome. Corneal clouding. Recurrent middle ear infections.

CHEST: Pectus carinatum. A deformed chest may be present at birth. Recurrent upper respiratory tract infections. Sleep apnea. Patients with a mucopolysaccharidosis are susceptible to pulmonary hemorrhage after bone marrow transplantation.

CARDIOVASCULAR: Aortic valve calcification, with possible mitral involvement. Heart failure is the most common cause of death, usually in the second or third decade of life.

NEUROMUSCULAR: Intelligence is usually normal. Spinal compression from dural thickening is common, particularly in adults with milder disease. The compression is usually cervical, and its onset may be insidious. Communicating hydrocephalus has occurred with lumbar stenosis.

ORTHOPEDIC: Growth can be normal for the first few years and then virtually stops. Skeletal changes are similar to those seen in Hurler syndrome (see earlier). There is hypoplasia of the hip acetabulae and small, flared iliac wings. There

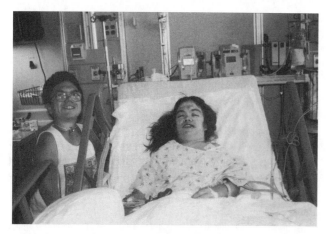

Maroteaux-Lamy syndrome. This 23-year-old woman with Maroteaux-Lamy syndrome is pictured with her 26-year-old sister who also has the syndrome. The patient could not be intubated orally and nasal intubation was extremely difficult. Her sister, who has had a cervical spine fusion in the past, has required an emergency tracheostomy.

is hypoplasia of the L1-2 vertebral bodies and prominent lumbar kyphosis. There is proximal femoral dysplasia and irregular diaphyseal distention of the tubular bones. Storage of polysaccharide in ligaments causes contractures of joints. Restriction in mobility of the hips, knees, and elbows results in these children assuming a crouched stance. Involvement of the wrists and hands causes carpal tunnel syndrome or a claw hand.

GI/GU: Umbilical and inguinal hernias. Hepatosplenomegaly with hypersplenism.

OTHER: "Tight" skin with mild hirsutism. Anemia and thrombocytopenia secondary to hypersplenism. Inclusions seen in white blood cells.

ANESTHETIC CONSIDERATIONS

Laryngoscopy and tracheal intubation may be extremely difficult. Intubation may become increasingly difficult with age. An oropharyngeal airway may worsen airway obstruction by pushing down a long, high epiglottis over the larynx. A nasopharyngeal airway may help, but on occasions advancement is difficult because of mucopolysaccharide deposits. The laryngeal mask airway has been used successfully in patients with mucopolysaccharidoses (2). Patients should be closely observed postoperatively for the development of airway obstruction. There may be postoperative respiratory compromise, and postobstructive pulmonary edema has been reported (1).

A thorough preoperative cardiac evaluation is indicated because heart failure is the most common cause of death. The hematocrit and platelet count should be evaluated preoperatively in patients with a history of hypersplenism. Severe contractures may make vascular access more difficult

to obtain. Patients must be carefully positioned secondary to contractures.

Bibliography:
1. Walker RWM, Colovic V, Robinson DN, et al. Postobstructive pulmonary oedema during anaesthesia in children with mucopolysaccharidoses. *Paediatr Anaesth* 2003;13:441–447.
2. Walker RWM, Allen DL, Rothera MR. A fibreoptic intubation technique for children with mucopolysaccharidoses using the laryngeal mask airway. *Paediatr Anaesth* 1997;7:421–426.
3. Moores C, Rogers JG, McKenzie IM, et al. Anaesthesia for children with mucopolysaccharidoses. *Anaesth Intensive Care* 1996;24:459–463.
4. Walker RWM, Darowski M, Morris P. Anaesthesia and mucopolysaccharidoses: a review of airway problems in children. *Anaesthesia* 1994;49:1078–1084.
5. Diaz JH, Belani K. Perioperative management of children with mucopolysaccharidoses. *Anesth Analg* 1993;77:1261–1270.
6. Mahoney A, Soni N, Vellodi A. Anaesthesia and the mucopolysaccharidoses: a review of patients treated by bone marrow transplantation. *Paediatr Anaesth* 1992;2:317–324.
7. Sjögren P, Pedersen T, Steinmetz H. Mucopolysaccharidoses and anaesthetic risks. *Acta Anaesthesiol Scand* 1987;31:214–218.
8. King DH, Jones RM, Barrett MB. Anaesthetic considerations in the mucopolysaccharidoses. *Anaesthesia* 1984;39:126–131.
9. Baines D, Kenneally J. Anaesthetic management of the mucopolysaccharidoses: a fifteen-year experience in a children's hospital. *Anaesth Intensive Care* 1983;11:198–202.
10. Kempthorne PM, Brown TCK. Anaesthesia and the mucopolysaccharidoses: a survey of techniques and problems. *Anaesth Intensive Care* 1983;11:203–207.

Marshall Syndrome

MIM #: 154780

This autosomal dominant syndrome involves cataracts, sensorineural deafness, and a very small nose. It is caused by a mutation in the gene *COL11A1* which is located on the short arm of chromosome 1. There is wide variability in clinical expression.

HEENT/AIRWAY: Thick calvarium, absent frontal sinuses, flat midface. Shallow orbit with prominent eyes, hypertelorism. Cataracts, lens dislocation, myopia, esotropia, glaucoma, retinal detachment. Sensorineural deafness. Short nose with flat nasal bridge, upturned tip, and anteverted nares. Prominent upper incisors. May have dental dysplasia. May have cleft palate.

NEUROMUSCULAR: May have mental deficiency. Falx, tentorial, and meningeal calcifications.

ORTHOPEDIC: Short stature. Vertebral epiphyseal abnormalities of a wide variety and varying degree.

OTHER: May have ectodermal dysplasia.

ANESTHETIC CONSIDERATIONS

When talking with patients, remember that they may have sensorineural hearing loss. Dental abnormalities should be documented preoperatively. Patients should be carefully positioned and padded perioperatively secondary to ectodermal dysplasia.

Bibliography:

1. Shanske AL, Bogdanow A, Shprintzen RJ, et al. The Marshall syndrome: report of a new family and review of the literature. *Am J Med Genet* 1997;70:52–57.
2. Stratton RF, Lee B, Ramirez F. Marshall syndrome. *Am J Med Genet* 1991;41:35–38.

Marshall-Smith Syndrome

MIM #: 602535

This syndrome of unknown etiology has as its most marked feature accelerated growth and maturation. One affected person reportedly had a wristbone age of 3 to 4 years by the age of 4 weeks. Most patients die before the age of 2 years.

HEENT/AIRWAY: Prominent forehead. Shallow orbits with prominent eyes, bluish sclerae. May have abnormal ears, hearing loss. Upturned nose, flat nasal bridge. Hypoplastic mandibular ramus. Dental anomalies. May have choanal atresia or stenosis, rudimentary epiglottis, abnormal larynx, laryngomalacia.

CHEST: Tracheomalacia. Pneumonia, atelectasis, and aspiration are common. Patients with severe lung disease may have pulmonary hypertension. Childhood death from pulmonary infections is common.

CARDIOVASCULAR: May develop pulmonary arterial hypertension secondary to chronic airway obstruction.

NEUROMUSCULAR: Mental retardation, developmental delay. Hypotonia. May have cerebral atrophy, absent corpus callosum. Severe spinal stenosis at the craniocervical junction may cause dysfunction of the lower medulla, leading to apnea.

ORTHOPEDIC: Markedly accelerated skeletal maturation. Broad proximal and middle phalanges with narrow distal phalanges. May have craniocervical instability. Scoliosis. May have sacrococcygeal hypersegmentation. May have osteopenia and/or bony fragility.

GI/GU: Umbilical hernia. Occasional omphalocele.

OTHER: Failure to thrive in terms of weight. Hypertrichosis. May have immunologic defects.

ANESTHETIC CONSIDERATIONS
Patients should be evaluated preoperatively for evidence of craniocervical instability. Dental abnormalities should be documented preoperatively. Laryngoscopy may be extremely difficult due to abnormal pharyngeal anatomy. Patients may have perioperative respiratory distress secondary to choanal atresia or stenosis, abnormal larynx, or laryngomalacia. Difficult mask ventilation following thiopentone which became impossible after administration of succinylcholine has been reported. Ketamine with spontaneous ventilation

was used successfully for a later laryngoscopy (2). The authors suggest that intubation be performed without the use of muscle relaxants. Prolonged use of a nasopharyngeal airway to maintain airway patency and for use during induction of an inhalational anesthetic has been reported (3). The presence of choanal atresia precludes the use of a nasal airway or a nasogastric tube. Patients are at risk of perioperative apnea, particularly if there is dysfunction of the lower medulla. Patients with significant lung disease may have pulmonary hypertension. Patients are at risk of perioperative aspiration. Abnormal sacrococcygeal anatomy might make caudal anesthesia technically difficult. Patients with osteopenia and/or bony fragility require careful perioperative handling and positioning.

Bibliography:

1. Adam MP, Hennekam RC, Keppen LD, et al. Marshall-Smith syndrome: natural history and evidence of an osteochondrodysplasia with connective tissue abnormalities. *Am J Med Genet A* 2005;137:117–124.
2. Antila H, Laitio T, Aantaa R, et al. Difficult airway in a patient with Marshall-Smith syndrome. *Paediatr Anaesth* 1998;8:425–428.
3. Dernedde G, Pendeville Ph, Veyckemans F, et al. Anaesthetic management of a child with Marshall-Smith syndrome. *Can J Anaesth* 1998;45:660–663.
4. Cullen A, Clarke TA, O'Dwyer TP. The Marshall-Smith syndrome: a review of the laryngeal complications. *Eur J Pediatr* 1997;156:463–464.

Martin-Bell Syndrome

See Fragile X syndrome

MASA Syndrome

SYNONYM: X-linked hydrocephalus syndrome

MIM #: 303350

This syndrome of hydrocephalus associated with aqueductal stenosis is inherited in an X-linked recessive fashion. The acronym MASA stands for **M**ental retardation, **A**phasia, **S**huffling gait, and **A**dducted thumbs. Female carriers may have mild mental retardation or minimally adducted thumbs. This syndrome is caused by a mutation in the gene for the neural L 1 cell adhesion molecule (*L1CAM*).

HEENT/AIRWAY: Macrocephaly. May have facial asymmetry.

NEUROMUSCULAR: Hydrocephalus associated with aqueductal stenosis is present *in utero,* and may be severe enough to necessitate delivery by cesarean section. Mental retardation. Aphasia. Shuffling gait secondary to spasticity of the lower extremities. May have spastic paraplegia. Hyperactive deep tendon reflexes in the lower extremities.

ORTHOPEDIC: Adducted thumbs (thumb flexed over the palms) secondary to hypoplastic or absent extensor pollicis longus or brevis muscles. Small stature. Rounded shoulders with internally rotated arms. Lumbar lordosis.

ANESTHETIC CONSIDERATIONS
Precautions against increases in intracranial pressure are needed in patients with severe hydrocephalus. Succinylcholine may be contraindicated in patients with spastic paraplegia because of the risk of exaggerated hyperkalemia.

Bibliography:
1. Weller S, Gartner J. Genetic and clinical aspects of X-linked hydrocephalus (L1 disease): Mutations in the L1CAM gene. *Hum Mutat* 2001;18:1–12.
2. Kaepernick L, Legius E, Higgins J, et al. Clinical aspects of the MASA syndrome in a large family, including expressing females. *Clin Genet* 1994;45:181–185.
3. Fryns JP, Schrander-Stumpel C, de Die-Smulders C, et al. MASA syndrome: delineation of the clinical spectrum at prepubertal age. *Am J Med Genet* 1992;43:402–407.

Maternal PKU Syndrome

SYNONYM: Fetal hyperphenylalaninemia syndrome

MIM #: None

This syndrome is due to the teratogenic effects of elevated serum phenylalanine levels in women with phenylketonuria (PKU). Only relatively recently have women with treated PKU reached childbearing age, and therefore the maternal PKU syndrome was not recognized until recently. The affected offspring exhibit microcephaly, mental retardation, growth deficiency, and a variety of structural defects. Elevated levels of phenylalanine in the first trimester cause abnormalities of organogenesis. Thereafter, elevated levels of phenylalanine cause abnormalities of myelination and organ maturation. These children are not at risk of having PKU unless their fathers also have a PKU gene.

HEENT/AIRWAY: Microcephaly. Round facies. Epicanthal folds, short palpebral fissures, strabismus. Small, upturned nose. Long, simple philtrum with thin upper lip. May have cleft lip or palate. Mandibular hypoplasia.

CARDIOVASCULAR: May have congenital heart disease, particularly ventricular septal defect and tetralogy of Fallot.

NEUROMUSCULAR: Mental retardation, which is not progressive because newborns are able to regulate their phenylalanine levels. Hypertonicity. May exhibit hyperactivity.

ORTHOPEDIC: Intrauterine and postnatal growth retardation. May have cervical and sacral spine anomalies. Pigeon-toed gait.

GI/GU: May have esophageal atresia.

MISCELLANEOUS: Adverse effects on the fetus can be correlated with maternal serum levels of phenylalanine, and timely and adequate dietary restriction of phenylalanine during pregnancy may provide protection to the fetus during organ development and may maximize the offspring's intellectual potential.

ANESTHETIC CONSIDERATIONS
Mental deficiency or hyperactivity may make the smooth induction of anesthesia a challenge. Direct laryngoscopy and tracheal intubation may be difficult secondary to mandibular hypoplasia. Patients with congenital heart disease need perioperative prophylactic antibiotics as indicated.

Bibliography:
1. Lee PJ, Ridout D, Walter JH, et al. Maternal phenylketonuria: report from the United Kingdom Registry 1978–97. *Arch Dis Child* 2005;90:143–146.
2. Koch R, Hanley W, Levy H, et al. The maternal phenylketonuria international study: 1984–2002. *Pediatrics* 2003;112:1523–1529.
3. Waisbren SE, Azen C. Cognitive and behavioral development in maternal phenylketonuria offspring. *Pediatrics* 2003;112:1544–1547.
4. Levy HL, Guldberg P, Guttler F. Congenital heart disease in maternal phenylketonuria: report from the Maternal PKU Collaborative Study. *Pediatr Res* 2001;49:636–642.

Mayer-Rokitansky-Kuster Syndrome

See Rokitansky-Kuster-Hauser syndrome

May-Hegglin Anomaly

Inluded in Fechtner syndrome

MCAD Deficiency

See Medium-chain acyl-CoA dehydrogenase deficiency

McArdle Syndrome

SYNONYM: Glycogen storage disease type V; Muscle phosphorylase deficiency

MIM #: 232600

This autosomal recessive glycogen storage disease is due to the absence of muscle phosphorylase, which results in the inability to convert glycogen to lactate in muscle, with consequent accumulation of glycogen and the development of a myopathy. For unclear reasons, young children are usually asymptomatic. Boys are more frequently affected, which some suggest is a reflection of the fact that boys are required to exercise their muscles more, and so are more likely to become symptomatic. Patients require no specific therapy.

CARDIOVASCULAR: The heart is usually unaffected, although rare incidences of conduction block have been reported.

NEUROMUSCULAR: Muscle pain, easy fatigability. Stiffness, pain, or cramps with moderate exertion. Symptoms disappear rapidly with rest. In some patients a "second wind" can develop, presumably from increased blood flow to the muscle, delivering fatty acids that can be used as an energy source, and also possibly due to the recruitment of more motor units. Among older patients muscle wasting may occur, particularly in the upper extremities. Patients can usually perform moderate exercise on level ground for prolonged periods.

GI/GU: The liver is normal. Many patients have myoglobinuria after intense exercise. On rare occasions this has caused renal impairment. Uterine muscle is apparently normal.

OTHER: Hypoglycemia is not a typical feature. There is a fall in serum lactate levels with exercise. Blood creatine kinase levels are elevated at rest and may be significantly elevated after exercise. Glucose or glucagon may provide temporary improvement in symptoms.

MISCELLANEOUS: This was the first hereditary myopathy shown to be caused by an enzyme defect. The first patient described by McArdle was 30 years of age at the time.

ANESTHETIC CONSIDERATIONS

Because glycogen cannot be used as an energy source for muscle, it has been suggested that patients receive perioperative infusions of glucose. Oral sucrose has been shown to improve exercise tolerance, and presumably would also help perioperative muscle strength and limit rhabdomyolysis. Succinylcholine may be contraindicated in patients with a myopathy because of the risk of exaggerated hyperkalemia. Because muscle destruction is thought to be secondary to repeated ischemic episodes, prolonged use of tourniquets (as for a Bier block or for minimizing blood loss in extremity surgery) should be limited. Muscle destruction may be associated with rhabdomyolysis, myoglobinuria and acute renal failure. Although several patients have had a positive *in vitro* contracture test, there have been no reports of malignant hyperthermia in the literature (1). The heart is usually unaffected, although rare incidences of conduction block have been reported.

FIGURE: See **Appendix E**

Bibliography:

1. Bollig G, Mohr S, Raeder J. McArdle disease and anaesthesia: Case reports. Review of potential problems and association with malignant hyperthermia. *Acta Anaesthesiol Scand* 2005;49:1077–1083.
2. Vissing J, Haller RG. The effect of oral sucrose on exercise tolerance in patients with McArdle disease. *N Engl J Med* 2003;349:2503–2509.
3. Lobato EB, Janelle GM, Urdaneta F, et al. Noncardiogenic pulmonary edema and rhabdomyolsis after protamine administration in a patient with unrecognized McArdle disease. *Anesthesiology* 1999;91:303–305.
4. Tzabar Y, Ross DG. Vecuronium and McArdle disease [Letter]. *Anaesthesia* 1990;45:697.
5. Samuels TA, Coleman P. McArdle disease and caesarean section [Letter]. *Anaesthesia* 1988;43:161–162.
6. Rajah A, Bell CF. Atracurium and McArdle disease [Letter]. *Anaesthesia* 1986;41:93.
7. Coleman P. McArdle disease: problems of anaesthetic management for caesarean section. *Anaesthesia* 1984;39:784–787.

McCune-Albright Syndrome

SYNONYM: Osteitis fibrosa cystica; Polyostotic fibrous dysplasia; Albright syndrome

Note: This is a distinct entity from Albright hereditary osteodystrophy (see later, Pseudohypoparathyroidism).

MIM #: 174800

This is a disease of irregularly shaped café au lait spots, precocious puberty, and fibrous dysplasia of bone. It occurs in both sexes and may be associated with excessive hormone production by other glands. Inheritance may be autosomal dominant lethal, with viability occurring only when the genetic defect occurs in the mosaic state. The disease is caused by defects in the gene *GNAS1* (encoding guanine nucleotide-binding protein, alpha-stimulating polypeptide). This protein, commonly abbreviated $G_{s\alpha}$, is the stimulatory G protein, and is involved in numerous adenylyl cyclase-mediated intracellular functions. Affected tissues have gsp mutations, which encode substitutions on the arginine finger of the protein, which is that portion which engages the G protein-coupled receptor. The genetic defect here apparently makes this protein constitutively active (i.e., always active). Similar changes have been found in some hormone secreting pituitary tumors and thyroid tumors. Because the mutation is not present in areas of normal skin, this likely represents mosaicism from postzygotic somatic cell mutation and mosaicism. As such, there tends to be variation from patient to patient.

HEENT/AIRWAY: May have fibrous dysplasia of skull and facial bones. Blindness and deafness from bony impingement on cranial foramina.

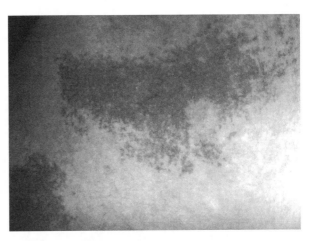

McCune-Albright syndrome. "Coast of Maine" skin lesion in McCune-Albright syndrome.

CARDIOVASCULAR: Increased incidence of arrhythmias and sudden death in infancy.

ORTHOPEDIC: Fibrous dysplasia of multiple bones. Involvement is typically asymmetric. Pathologic fractures, bone deformity, pseudarthroses. There may be malignant transformation of bone lesions.

GI/GU: Testicular microlithiasis.

OTHER: Asymmetric, irregularly shaped café au lait spots. These may stop abruptly at the midline and are due to the mimicking of the normal effects of melanocyte-stimulating hormone. Precocious puberty, thyrotoxicosis, pituitary gigantism or acromegaly, and Cushing syndrome from hyperadrenalism. Gynecomastia.

MISCELLANEOUS: Skin lesions are described as "coast of Maine" for their irregular border (the smoother, but superficially similar lesions of neurofibromatosis are termed "coast of California").

Donovan McCune was a pediatrician at Columbia University. Fuller Albright, the Boston physician, is the father figure of endocrinology. This is the same Albright of Albright hereditary osteodystrophy. He also described vitamin D-resistant rickets (once known as Albright-Butler-Bloomberg system). Albright suffered from early-onset Parkinson disease. In 1946, Albright lamented that Parkinson disease "does not belong to my special medical interests, or else I am certain I would have solved it long ago."

ANESTHETIC CONSIDERATIONS
Cushingoid patients with a buffalo hump may be difficult to position for intubation. Cushingoid patients may have fragile veins. Excessive growth hormone may result in a larger-than-normal larynx and the need for a somewhat larger-than-normal endotracheal tube. The larynx may be difficult to visualize in patients with acromegaly. Bone fragility requires careful patient positioning.

Bibliography:
1. Bullmann V, Waurick R, Rodl R, et al. Corrective osteotomy of the humerus using perivascular axillary anesthesia according to Weber in a patient suffering from McCune-Albright syndrome. *Anaesthesist* 2005;54:889–894.
2. Bhansali A, Sharma BS, Sreenivasulu P, et al. Acromegaly with fibrous dysplasia: McCune-Albright Syndrome—clinical studies in 3 cases and brief review of literature. *Endocr J* 2003;50:793–799.
3. Bolger WE, Ross AT. McCune-Albright syndrome: a case report and review of the literature. *Int J Pediatr Otorhinolaryngol* 2002;65:69–74.
4. Farfel Z, Bourne HR, Iiri T. The expanding spectrum of G protein diseases. *N Engl J Med* 1999;340:1012–1020.
5. Langer RA, Yook warning, Capan LM. Anesthetic considerations in McCune-Albright syndrome: case report with literature review. *Anesth Analg* 1995;80:1236–1239.

McKusick-Kaufman Syndrome

SYNONYM: Kaufman-McKusick syndrome

MIM #: 236700

The hallmarks of this syndrome are hydrometrocolpos and postaxial polydactyly. It is caused by a mutation in a gene located on the short arm of chromosome 20, which encodes a protein that is similar to members of the chaperonin family. Mutations in the same gene can also cause Bardet-Biedl syndrome (see earlier).

HEENT/AIRWAY: May have complete tracheal ring. May have tracheomalacia.

CHEST: A large pelvic mass may extend cephalad enough to displace the diaphragm.

CARDIOVASCULAR: May have congenital heart disease.

ORTHOPEDIC: Postaxial polydactyly.

GI/GU: May have Hirschsprung disease. May have imperforate anus. Hydrometrocolpos beginning in the fetus due to a transverse vaginal membrane or vaginal atresia. Hypospadias, prominent scrotal raphae, and micropenis in males. Undescended testes. The large pelvic mass can obstruct the urinary tract resulting in hydroureter or hydronephrosis.

OTHER: Can develop fetal hydrops due to caval compression and lymphatic obstruction from the pelvic mass.

MISCELLANEOUS: Because of diagnostic overlap in infancy, children should be evaluated later for possible development of additional manifestations of Bardet-Biedl syndrome.

ANESTHETIC CONSIDERATIONS
Mechanical ventilation is probably preferred to spontaneous ventilation in young infants with large masses. Nitrous oxide will increase bowel distension, potentially further displacing the diaphragm and decreasing the functional residual capacity. Baseline renal function should be evaluated in the presence of hydronephrosis.

Bibliography:
1. Tekin I, Ok G, Genc A, et al. Anaesthetic management in McKusick-Kaufman syndrome. *Paediatr Anaesth* 2003;13:167–170.
2. Slavotinek AM, Biesecker LG. Phenotypic overlap of McKusick-Kaufman syndrome with Bardet-Biedl syndrome: a literature review. *Am J Med Genet* 2000;95:208–215.

Meadow Syndrome

See Münchausen syndrome by proxy

Meckel Syndrome

See Meckel-Gruber syndrome

Meckel-Gruber Syndrome

SYNONYM: Meckel syndrome; Dysencephalia splanchnocystica

MIM #: 249000

This autosomal recessive syndrome includes occipital encephalocele, polydactyly, polycystic kidney disease, and bile duct anomalies. Patients usually die in the perinatal period. Renal failure is a contributing factor in most deaths. A gene for Meckel-Gruber syndrome has been mapped to the long arm of chromosome 17. However, there is evidence to suggest genetic heterogeneity, which has long been suspected on the basis of wide phenotypic variability.

HEENT/AIRWAY: Microcephaly, sloping forehead. Microphthalmia, coloboma of the iris. External ear anomalies. Cleft lip or palate. May have neonatal teeth. Micrognathia. Short neck, sometimes with webbing. May have cleft epiglottis.

CHEST: May have pulmonary hypoplasia.

CARDIOVASCULAR: Congenital cardiac defects include atrial septal defect, ventricular septal defect, patent ductus arteriosus, coarctation of the aorta, and pulmonary stenosis.

NEUROMUSCULAR: Occipital encephalocele. Holoprosencephaly. Anencephaly. Cortical hypoplasia. Agenesis of the corpus callosum. Hydrocephalus. Seizures. May have Arnold-Chiari malformation. May have Dandy-Walker malformation. Absent optic nerve, olfactory tracts.

ORTHOPEDIC: Polydactyly, usually postaxial. Syndactyly, clinodactyly. Clubfoot deformity. May have simian crease, bowed limbs.

GI/GU: Bile duct anomalies, including bile duct proliferation, bile duct dilatation, and portal fibrosis. May have omphalocele, intestinal malrotation, imperforate anus. May have accessory spleens, adrenal hypoplasia. Polycystic kidney disease. Cryptorchidism. Ureteral or urethral anomalies.

MISCELLANEOUS: The oldest account of this syndrome may date to 1684, with the description of "a monstrous child" whose features are suggestive of Meckel-Gruber syndrome. Meckel's detailed description of the syndrome appeared in 1822. Johann Friedreich Meckel the Younger was an early 19th century German physician who was a founder of the field of embryology. Johann Friedreich the Elder, his grandfather, was a professor of anatomy and surgical obstetrics. Meckel the Younger also described Meckel diverticulum.

ANESTHETIC CONSIDERATIONS
Laryngoscopy and tracheal intubation may be difficult secondary to micrognathia and a short neck. Patients may

have neonatal teeth (teeth present at birth), which can easily be dislodged during laryngoscopy. Renal disease has implications for the titration of perioperative fluids and for the choice of perioperative medications, avoiding or adjusting the dose of renally excreted drugs. Careful perioperative positioning is required secondary to the presence of an occipital encephalocele. Patients with hydrocephalus may have elevated intracranial pressure, and precautions should be taken to avoid further elevations in pressure. Chronic use of anticonvulsant medications alters the metabolism of some anesthetic drugs. Patients with congenital heart disease should receive perioperative antibiotic prophylaxis as indicated.

Bibliography:
1. Cincinnati P, Neri ME, Valentini A. Dandy-Walker anomaly in Meckel-Gruber syndrome. *Clin Dysmorphol* 2000;9:35–38.
2. Paavola P, Salonen R, Baumer A, et al. Clinical and genetic heterogeneity in Meckel syndrome. *Hum Genet* 1997;101:88–92.
3. Wright C, Healicon R, English C, et al. Meckel syndrome: what are the minimum diagnostic criteria? *J Med Genet* 1994;31:482–485.

Median Cleft Face Syndrome

SYNONYM: Frontonasal dysplasia sequence

MIM #: 136760

This syndrome of unknown etiology involves a primary defect in midline facial development that results in midline facial clefting. The clinical severity is highly variable. The abnormalities are confined to the head and face. This syndrome may be due to errors in early fetal development, and may not be genetically based. Frontonasal dysplasia may also occur as one feature of a multiple malformation syndrome.

HEENT/AIRWAY: May have anterior cranium bifidum occultum (midline bony defect). Widow's peak. Marked hypertelorism. Lateral displacement of the inner canthi. May have optic anomalies. May have low-set ears, conductive hearing loss. Broad nasal root with variable clefting of the nose—from an abnormality confined to the tip to widely separated nares. May have notching of the alae nasi. May have cleft lip.

CARDIOVASCULAR: Has been associated with tetralogy of Fallot.

NEUROMUSCULAR: Intelligence is usually normal.

ANESTHETIC CONSIDERATIONS
Except in patients with associated tetralogy of Fallot, there are no specific anesthetic considerations with this syndrome.

Bibliography:
1. Mohammed SN, Swan MC, Wall SA, et al. Monozygotic twins discordant for frontonasal malformation. *Am J Med Genet* 2004;130A:384–388.

2. De Moor MMA, Baruch R, Human DG. Frontonasal dysplasia associated with tetralogy of Fallot. *J Med Genet* 1987;24:107–109.
3. Marquez X, Roxas RS. Induction of anesthesia in infant with frontonasal dysplasia and meningoencephalocele: a case report. *Anesth Analg* 1977;56:736–738.

Medium-Chain Acyl-CoA Dehydrogenase Deficiency

SYNONYM: MCAD deficiency

MIM #: 201450

This autosomal recessive disorder of the gene encoding medium-chain acyl-CoA dehydrogenase (MCAD) presents with an intermittent Reye syndrome-like picture. MCAD is one of several acyl-CoA dehydrogenases, which are mitochondrial enzymes that are required for beta-oxidation of fatty acids. Deficiencies in any of the acyl-CoA dehydrogenases will cause clinical symptoms. MCAD deficiency is the most common of these. It occurs most commonly in Northern Europeans. Symptomatic episodes are often precipitated by intercurrent viral infections. Compound heterozygotes (carrying two different mutations) often have a more benign course.

Fatty acids are oxidized in mitochondria. After mobilization from adipose tissue, they are taken up by the liver and other tissues, and converted to acyl-CoA esters in the cytoplasm. They enter mitochondria as carnitine esters and become reesterified as acyl-CoA esters. Beta-oxidation results in the liberation of electrons. As beta-oxidation proceeds, the acyl chain is gradually shortened, and this first step in the oxidation process is catalyzed by acyl-CoA dehydrogenases with differing, but overlapping, chain-length specificities. These are very-long-chain, long-chain, medium-chain, and short-chain acyl-CoA dehydrogenases.

NEUROMUSCULAR: Lethargy and coma during acute episodes.

GI/GU: Peripheral lobular fatty changes.

OTHER: Intermittent hypoglycemia, hyperammonemia, metabolic acidosis, impaired ketogenesis with hypoketotic hypoglycemia, secondary carnitine deficiency. Carnitine therapy is not uniformly beneficial. In fact, treatment with carnitine may be ineffective and possibly dangerous.

ANESTHETIC CONSIDERATIONS

Prolonged perioperative fasting should be avoided. Serum glucose levels should be monitored, and patients will likely need perioperative glucose supplementation.

Bibliography:
1. Wang SY, Kannan S, Shay D, et al. Anesthetic considerations for a patient with compound heterozygous medium-chain acyl-CoA dehydrogenase deficiency. *Anesth Analg* 2002;94:1595–1597.

2. Grice AS, Peck TE. Multiple acyl-CoA dehydrogenase deficiency: a rare cause of acidosis with an increased anion gap. *Br J Anaesth* 2001;86:437–441.
3. Zschocke J, Schulze A, Lindner M, et al. Molecular and functional characterization of mild MCAD deficiency. *Hum Genet* 2001;108:404–408.
4. Iafolla AK, Thompson RJ, Roe CR. Medium-chain acyl-coenzyme A dehydrogenase deficiency: clinical course in 120 affected children. *J Pediatr* 1994;124:409–405.

MELAS Syndrome

MIM #: 540000

MELAS syndrome is a mitochondrial disease, related to Kearns-Sayre syndrome, MERRF (myoclonic epilepsy with ragged red fibers) and others. MELAS stands for **M**itochondrial myopathy, **E**ncephalopathy, **L**actic **A**cidosis, and **S**troke-like episodes. It is caused by a deficiency in oxidative phosphorylation in the mitochondria. Many patients have deficiency in NADH-cytochrome c reductase (complex I). The disease has been ascribed to a mutation of the mitochondrial transfer RNA (*leu-UUR*) gene. Because this is a mitochondrial disease, transmission is maternal. Because of the varying distribution of mitochondria, in most cases there is only a single family member with the disease, but other family members can have single features of the syndrome. Onset is late in childhood. Treatment with coenzyme Q10 is helpful. MELAS syndrome is in the differential diagnosis of most strokes in childhood.

HEENT/AIRWAY: Cataracts, blindness, pigmentary retinopathy, ophthalmoplegia. Progressive sensorineural hearing loss.

CHEST: Respiratory failure is the most common cause of death.

CARDIOVASCULAR: Cardiomyopathy, Wolff-Parkinson-White syndrome (see later).

NEUROMUSCULAR: Diffuse spongy degeneration and focal encephalomalacia with focal infarcts, cortical or cerebellar atrophy, or basal ganglia calcification on computed tomography scan. Stroke-like episodes, including sudden onset of hemiparesis, hemianopsia, or cortical blindness. Strokes are very focal, asymmetric, and do not follow a specific vascular territory. Seizures. Headaches. Dementia. Myoclonus, peripheral neuropathy. Myopathy, with muscle weakness and poor exercise tolerance. Reduced muscle mass. Muscle biopsies show "ragged red" fibers, which represent a proliferation of mitochondria.

ORTHOPEDIC: Short stature.

GI/GU: Episodic vomiting. Nephropathy.

OTHER: Metabolic acidosis, worse with fasting. Thin habitus, hirsutism, purpura.

ANESTHETIC CONSIDERATIONS

Patients who are blind and deaf benefit from the presence of a family member or translator during induction of anesthesia. A baseline electrocardiogram should exclude cardiac conduction abnormalities. There may be excessive perioperative heat loss in these very thin patients. Protracted preoperative fasts should be avoided and adequate perioperative glucose should be ensured to minimize the need for anaerobic metabolism. It is unclear if episodic emesis correlates with gastroesophageal reflux and intraoperative aspiration risk (2). Patients with mitochondrial myopathies may be more sensitive to mivacurium (8), curare (12), rocuronium (6), atracurium (6) and succinylcholine (13), although one report did not find increased sensitivity to succinylcholine or pancuronium (14), and there is even one report of resistance to cisatracurium (1). Although use of succinylcholine has been reported, the use of this drug in a myopathic patient is better avoided if possible because of the risk of exaggerated hyperkalemia. Some patients with mitochondrial disease may have abnormal respiratory control (11), suggesting that narcotics and other respiratory depressants be used with care, although excessive respiratory depression from sedatives and opioids has not been reported in this syndrome. Treatment with anticonvulsant medications may alter the metabolism of some anesthetic drugs. The issue of the relationship between the mitochondrial myopathies and malignant hyperthermia is not clear, but an association seems unlikely. Spinal anesthesia has been used successfully. Wolff-Parkinson-White syndrome carries with it the risk of the development of paroxysmal supraventricular tachycardia.

Treatment with anticoagulants and antiplatelet drugs is probably not helpful in preventing strokes.

Bibliography:

1. Aouad MT, Gerges FJ, Baraka AS. Resistance to cisatracurium in a patient with MELAS syndrome. *Paediatr Anaesth* 2005;15:1124–1127.
2. Bolton P, Peutrell J, Zuberi S, et al. Anaesthesia for an adolescent with mitochondrial encephalopathy-lactic acidosis-stroke-like episodes syndrome. *Paediatr Anaesth* 2003;13:453–456.
3. DiMauro S, Schon EA. Mitochondrial respiratory-chain diseases. *N Engl J Med* 2003;348:2656–2668.
4. Hsiao PN, Cheng YJ, Tseng HC, et al. Spinal anesthesia in MELAS syndrome: a case with mitochondrial myopathy, encephalopathy, lactic acidosis and stroke-like episodes. *Acta Anaesthesiol Sin* 2000;38:107–110.
5. Dashe JF, Boyer PJ. Case records of the Massachusetts General Hospital. Weekly clinicopathological exercises. Case 39-1998. *N Engl J Med* 1998;339:1914–1923.
6. Finsterer J, Stratil U, Bittner R, et al. Increased sensitivity to rocuronium and atracurium in mitochondrial myopathy. *Can J Anaesth* 1998;45:781–784.
7. Thompson VA, Wahr JA. Anesthetic considerations in patients presenting with mitochondrial myopathy, encephalopathy, lactic acidosis, and stroke-like episodes (MELAS) syndrome. *Anesth Analg* 1997;85:1404–1406.
8. Naguib M, el Dawlatly AA, Ashour M, et al. Sensitivity to mivacurium in a patient with mitochondrial myopathy. *Anesthesiology* 1996;84:1506–1509.
9. Keyes MA, Van de Wiele BV, Stead SW. Mitochondrial myopathies: an unusual cause of hypotonia in infants and children. *Paediatr Anaesth* 1996;6:329–335.
10. Ciafaloni E, Ricci E, Shanske S, et al. MELAS: clinical features, biochemistry, and molecular genetics. *Ann Neurol* 1992;31:391–398.
11. Barohn RJ, Clayton T, Zarife S, et al. Recurrent respiratory insufficiency and depressed ventilatory drive complicating mitochondrial myopathies. *Neurology* 1990;40:103–106.
12. Robetson JA. Ocular muscular dystrophy: a cause of curare sensitivity. *Anaesthesia* 1984;3:251–253.
13. Maslow AM, Lisbon A. Anesthetic considerations in patients with mitochondrial dysfunction. *Anesth Analg* 1983;76:884–886.
14. D'Ambra MN, Dedrick D, Savarese JJ. Kearns-Sayre syndrome and pancuronium-succinylcholine-induced neuromuscular blockade. *Anesthesiology* 1979;51:343–345.
15. Lessell S, Kuwabara T, Feldman RG. Myopathy and succinylcholine sensitivity. *Am J Ophthalmol* 1969;68:789–796.

Melkersson Syndrome

See Melkersson-Rosenthal syndrome

Melkersson-Rosenthal Syndrome

SYNONYM: Melkersson syndrome

MIM #: 155900

This autosomal dominant syndrome results in episodic swelling of the face and relapsing peripheral facial palsy. With time the episodes take longer to resolve, and eventually there is chronic facial weakness and swollen, disfigured lips.

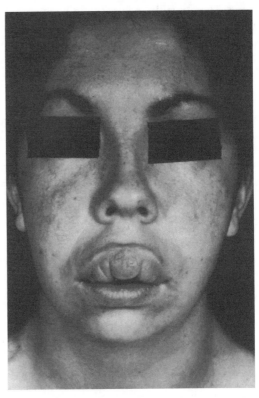

Melkersson-Rosenthal syndrome. FIG. 1. Chronic swelling of the lips in a patient with Melkersson-Rosenthal syndrome. (Courtesy of Dr. Kenneth E. Greer, Department of Dermatology, University of Virginia Health System.)

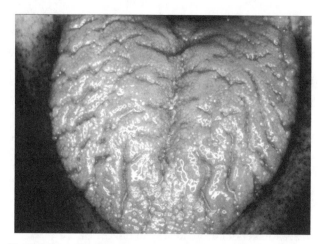

Melkersson-Rosenthal syndrome. FIG. 2. Fissured tongue of a patient with Melkersson-Rosenthal syndrome. (Courtesy of Dr. Kenneth E. Greer, Department of Dermatology, University of Virginia Health System.)

The responsible gene has not been identified, but is thought to be on chromosome 9. There is no effective therapy.

HEENT/AIRWAY: Chronic facial swelling, which may be limited to the lips. Relapsing peripheral facial palsy, clinically identical to Bell palsy. Fissured ("scrotal") tongue. May have eyelid edema. There may be swelling, erythema, or painful erosions of the gingiva, buccal mucosa, palate, or tongue. There may be noncaseating granulomas in the edematous tissue. There may be visual disturbances during exacerbations. Possibly reduced lacrimation and salivation.

CHEST: Acute episodes may be accompanied by exacerbations of asthma.

NEUROMUSCULAR: Recurrent facial nerve palsy. Exacerbations may be accompanied by migraines.

OTHER: Exacerbations may be accompanied by fever. Two cases of Melkersson-Rosenthal syndrome in association with Ehlers-Danlos syndrome have been reported.

ANESTHETIC CONSIDERATIONS
Significant oral and laryngeal swelling during acute exacerbations may compromise laryngoscopy and tracheal intubation (3). Patients may require endotracheal intubation until the episode of swelling resolves.

Bibliography:
1. Ziem PE, Pfrommer C, Goerdt S, et al. Melkersson-Rosenthal syndrome in childhood: a challenge in differential diagnosis and treatment. *Br J Dermatol* 2000;143:860–863.
2. Cockerham KP, Hidayat AA, Cockerham GC, et al. Melkersson-Rosenthal syndrome: new clinicopathologic findings in four cases. *Arch Ophthalmol* 2000;118:227–232.
3. Rogers RS. Melkersson-Rosenthal syndrome and orofacial granulomatosis. *Dermatol Clin* 1996;14:371–379.
4. Jayamaha JEL. Respiratory obstruction in a patient with Melkersson-Rosenthal syndrome. *Anesth Analg* 1993;77:395–397.

Melnick-Fraser Syndrome

SYNONYM: BOR syndrome; Branchiootorenal syndrome

MIM #: 113650

This autosomal dominant syndrome has as its main features branchial arch abnormalities, hearing loss, and renal disease. The disorder is due to a mutation in the gene *EYA1*. This gene is the human homologue of the *Drosophila* gene "eyes absent." The role of this gene and its gene product is not known, but it is expressed in all areas of the developing inner ear, and in the metanephric cells of the early developing kidney. There is variability in the expression of this syndrome, so any patient in whom hearing loss develops in childhood should be carefully examined for evidence of branchial arch abnormalities and renal disease. Often the syndrome is not diagnosed until after the onset of hearing loss.

HEENT/AIRWAY: Branchial arch abnormalities, including preauricular pits and branchial fistulas or cysts. Hearing loss—conductive or sensorineural. May have cholesteatoma. Cup-shaped external ear. Middle or inner ear abnormalities, particularly cochlear hypoplasia. Lacrimal duct stenosis. Occasional deep overbite, cleft palate. Occasional facial paralysis.

GI/GU: Renal dysplasia. A small percentage have renal agenesis or renal failure. Anomalies of the renal collecting system.

ANESTHETIC CONSIDERATIONS
Recognize that some patients with this syndrome are profoundly deaf. A severe overbite may make laryngoscopy

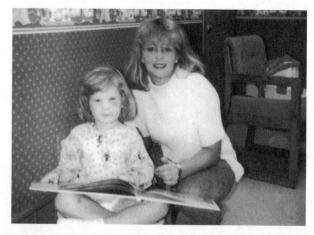

Melnick-Fraser syndrome. This 4-year-old girl is about to have surgical repair of her stenosed left nasolacrimal duct. She is hearing impaired and uses hearing aids. In addition, she has cup-shaped ears, a preauricular pit, a small branchial arch cyst, and small kidneys with normal renal function. Her mother also has the syndrome and has also required treatment of nasolacrimal duct stenosis.

more difficult. Renal disease has implications for the titration of perioperative fluid and the choice of perioperative drugs.

Bibliography:

1. Chang EH, Menezes M, Meyer NC, et al. Branchio-oto-renal syndrome: the mutation spectrum in EYA1 and its phenotypic consequences. *Hum Mutat* 2004;23:582–589.
2. Rodriguez Soriano J. Branchio-oto-renal syndrome. *J Nephrol* 2003;16: 603–605.
3. Chen A, Francis M, Ni L, et al. Phenotypic manifestations of branchiootorenal syndrome. *Am J Med Genet* 1995;58:365–370.

Melnick-Needles Syndrome

MIM #: 309350

This X-linked dominant syndrome is distinguished by a small face with exophthalmos, bowing of the extremities, and ribbon-like ribs. It is caused by mutations in the gene encoding filamin A. Most of those affected are female, and there is evidence of greater severity and early lethality in male patients.

HEENT/AIRWAY: Small face, prominent forehead, late-closing fontanelles, delayed paranasal sinus development, sclerosis of the skull base. Exophthalmos, hypertelorism, down-slanting palpebral fissures, glaucoma. Large ears. Broad nasal bridge and tip, anteverted nares. Malaligned teeth, gingival hypertrophy. May have high-arched palate or cleft palate. Micrognathia. May have hoarse voice.

CHEST: Small thoracic cage with irregular, ribbon-like ribs. Short clavicles with narrow shoulders. Pectus excavatum. Recurrent respiratory tract infections are common. Patients with severe lung disease may have pulmonary hypertension.

CARDIOVASCULAR: May have mitral or tricuspid valve prolapse.

NEUROMUSCULAR: May have hypotonia, motor delay.

ORTHOPEDIC: May have short stature. Short upper limbs. Bowing of the humerus, radius, ulna, and tibia. May have abnormal gait secondary to bowing. Metaphyseal flaring of long bones. Short distal phalanges with cone-shaped epiphyses. Clubfoot deformity. Iliac flaring. Kyphoscoliosis. May have dislocated hip, osteoarthritis of back and hip.

GI/GU: May have ureteral obstruction and hydronephrosis.

OTHER: Small pelvis in affected women may necessitate delivery by cesarean section.

ANESTHETIC CONSIDERATIONS

Direct laryngoscopy and tracheal intubation may be difficult in patients with significant micrognathia. There is an increased risk of postoperative respiratory complications in these patients with small thoracic cages and irregular, ribbon-like ribs. Patients with severe lung disease may have pulmonary hypertension. Short clavicles may make placement of a subclavian venous catheter more difficult. Consider preoperative evaluation of renal function in patients with a history of renal abnormalities which predispose to renal insufficiency.

Bibliography:

1. Kristiansen M, Knudsen GP, Soyland A, et al. Phenotypic variation in Melnick-Needles syndrome is not reflected in X inactivation patterns from blood or buccal smear. *Am J Med Genet* 2002;108:120–127.
2. Neou P, Kyrkanides S, Gioureli E, et al. Melnick-Needles syndrome in a mother and her son. *Genet Couns* 1996;7:123–129.

Menkes Kinky Hair Syndrome

SYNONYM: Kinky hair syndrome

MIM #: 309400

This X-linked recessive disorder is due to an abnormality in the gene encoding copper-transporting adenosine triphosphatase, alpha polypeptide (*ATP7A*). Abnormal copper transport results in low serum levels of copper and ceruloplasmin. A variety of enzymes requiring copper as a cofactor are affected, including tyrosinase, monoamine oxidase, lysyl oxidase, and cytochrome c oxidase. The manifestations of this disorder are due to deficiencies in these enzymes. The syndrome derives its name from the characteristic kinky hair of patients with this syndrome. Patients also have progressive cerebral deterioration and seizures, with death occurring by 3 years of age. Female carriers may have subtle manifestations of the disorder. The occipital horn syndrome, formerly known as X-linked Ehlers-Danlos syndrome, is caused by a mutation in the same gene.

HEENT/AIRWAY: May have microcephaly or brachycephaly. Fat cheeks.

CARDIOVASCULAR: Vascular elongation and tortuousity, aneurysms, capillary fragility secondary to lysyl oxidase deficiency.

NEUROMUSCULAR: Progressive cerebral and cerebellar degeneration, beginning at 1 to 2 months of age. Focal gliosis. Hypertonia. Seizures, often difficult to control. Eventual decerebration. May have occipital horns (wedge-shaped calcifications within the tendinous insertions of the trapezius and sternocleidomastoid muscles to the occipital bone).

ORTHOPEDIC: Growth retardation. Skeletal demineralization due to ascorbate oxidase deficiency (similar to lesions of scurvy). May have fractures.

GI/GU: May have gastroesophageal reflux. May have gastric polyps and gastrointestinal bleeding. Small testes. Bladder diverticula.

OTHER: Depigmentation of the hair and skin secondary to tyrosinase deficiency, abnormal (kinky) hair secondary to monoamine oxidase deficiency, abnormal collagen function secondary to lysyl oxidase deficiency, and hypothermia secondary to cytochrome c oxidase deficiency. Hair is sparse, stubby, and depigmented. Microscopically, hair shafts are twisted, of varying diameter, and have regularly spaced shaft fractures.

MISCELLANEOUS: John Menkes was also the first to describe maple syrup urine disease.

ANESTHETIC CONSIDERATIONS

A child was reported in whom bulky pharyngeal tissue, hypotonic pharyngeal muscles, and possibly abnormal neural control of oropharyngeal muscles conspired to cause airway obstruction and difficult laryngoscopy and tracheal intubation (3). Patients may have gastroesophageal reflux and are at increased risk of aspiration. Capillary fragility is a relative contraindication to regional techniques. Capillary fragility might increase the risk of intraoperative bleeding, but this has not been documented. Patients are prone to development of perioperative hypothermia. Anticonvulsant drugs should be continued perioperatively, and alternatives given parenterally, if required. Chronic use of anticonvulsant medications may alter the metabolism of anesthetic drugs, requiring more frequent dosing.

Bibliography:

1. Gerard-Blanluet M, Birk-Moller L, Caubel I, et al. Early development of occipital horns in a classical Menkes patient. *Am J Med Genet* 2004;130A:211–213.
2. Tumer Z, Horn N. Menkes disease: recent advances and new aspects. *J Med Genet* 1997;34:265–274.
3. Kazim R, Weisberg R, Sun LS. Upper airway obstruction and Menkes syndrome. *Anesth Analg* 1993;77:856–857.
4. Kaler SG, Westman JA, Bernes S, et al. Gastrointestinal hemorrhage associated with gastric polyps in Menkes disease. *J Pediatr* 1993;122:93–95.
5. Tobias JD. Anaesthetic considerations in the child with Menkes' syndrome. *Can J Anaesth* 1992;39:712–715.

MERRF Syndrome

MIM #: 545000

Myoclonus **E**pilepsy with **R**agged **R**ed **F**ibers is due to a defect in one or more mitochondrial genes. Eighty to ninety percent of the cases are due to a defect in the gene encoding mitochondrial lysine transfer ribonucleic acid (tRNA). A specific mutation in mitochondrial DNA causes multiple deficiencies in the complexes of the respiratory chain, particularly complexes I and IV (see earlier). This syndrome is associated with "ragged red" fibers in muscle biopsy specimens, which represent a proliferation of mitochondria and excess lipid.

HEENT/AIRWAY: Sensorineural hearing loss.

NEUROMUSCULAR: Myoclonus epilepsy, ataxia, spasticity, intention tremor. Myopathy with muscle weakness. Optic atrophy. Degenerative changes in the cerebrum, cerebellum, and spinal cord.

OTHER: Elevated serum pyruvate or lactate. Elevated serum alanine.

ANESTHETIC CONSIDERATIONS

It is important to be sensitive to the fact that patients may have hearing loss. Stress, such as seen with surgery or infection, may increase demands for adenosine triphosphate production to levels above that which the patient can produce. Acidosis should be corrected preoperatively, and patients with excessive lactic acidemia should not receive Ringer's lactate. Protracted preoperative fasting should be avoided. Postoperative clinical deterioration in patients with a mitochondrial myopathy has been reported (6). Patients with mitochondrial myopathies may be more sensitive to succinylcholine (13), curare (11), mivacurium (7), rocuronium and atracurium (5), although one report did not find increased sensitivity to succinylcholine or pancuronium (12). The use of succinylcholine is better avoided in this myopathy, secondary to the risk of exaggerated hyperkalemia. Some patients with mitochondrial disease have abnormal control of respiration, suggesting that narcotics and other respiratory depressants be used with care. Chronic use of anticonvulsant medication affects the metabolism of some anesthetic drugs. The relationship between the mitochondrial myopathies and malignant hyperthermia is unclear, but an association is unlikely (1).

Bibliography:

1. Vilela H, García-Fernández J, Parodi E, et al. Anesthetic management of a patient with MERRF syndrome. *Paediatr Anaesth* 2005;15:77–79.
2. Shahwan A, Farrell M, Delanty N. Progressive myoclonic epilepsies: a review of genetic and therapeutic aspects. *Lancet Neurol* 2005;4:239–248.
3. DiMauro S, Schon EA. Mitochondrial respiratory-chain diseases. *N Engl J Med* 2003;348:2656–2668A.
4. DiMauro S, Hirano M, Kaufmann P, et al. Clinical features and genetics of myoclonic epilepsy with ragged red fibers. *Adv Neurol* 2002;89:217–229.
5. Finsterer J, Stratil UBittner R, et al. Increased sensitivity to rocuronium and atracurium in mitochondrial myopathy. *Can J Anaesth* 1998;45:781–784.
6. Casta A, Quackenbush EJ, Houck CS, et al. Perioperative white matter degeneration and death in a patient with a defect in mitochondrial oxidative phosphorylation. *Anesthesiology* 1997;87:420–425.
7. Naguib M, el Dawlatly AA, Ashour M, et al. Sensitivity to mivacurium in a patient with mitochondrial myopathy. *Anesthesiology* 1996;84:1506–1509A.
8. Keyes MA, Van de Wiele BV, Stead SW. Mitochondrial myopathies: an unusual cause of hypotonia in infants and children. *Paediatr Anaesth* 1996;6:329–335A.
9. Bindoff LA, Desnuelle C, Birch-Machin MA, et al. Multiple defects of the mitochondrial respiratory chain in a mitochondrial encephalopathy (MERRF): a clinical, biochemical and molecular study. *J Neurol Sci* 1991;102:17–24.
10. Barohn RJ, Clayton T, Zarife S, et al. Recurrent respiratory insufficiency and depressed ventilatory drive complicating mitochondrial myopathies. *Neurology* 1990;40:103–106A.

11. Robertson JA. Ocular muscular dystrophy: a cause of curare sensitivity. *Anaesthesia* 1984;3:251–253.
12. D'Ambra MN, Dedrick D, Savarese H. Kearns-Sayre syndrome and pancuronium-sucinylcholine-induced neuromuscular blockade. *Anesthesiology* 1979;51:343–345.
13. Lessell S, Kuwabara T, Feldman RG. Myopathy and succinylcholine sensitivity. *Am J Ophthalmol* 1969;68:789–796A.

Metachromatic Leukodystrophy

MIM #: 250100

Metachromatic leukodystrophy is an autosomal recessive disease due to the absence of arylsulfatase A, the lysosomal enzyme responsible for the degradation of sulfatide, an important constituent of myelin. There is accumulation of sulfatide (galactosyl and, to a lesser extent, lactosyl) in both neural and non-neural tissues, which can be identified as metachromatic granules. Metachromatic leukodystrophy is the most common of the leukodystrophies. Infantile, juvenile, and adult forms have been described, but they really represent a clinical spectrum rather than distinct entities. Patients with juvenile-type disease have been described who have normal arylsulfatase, but who have an autosomal recessive defect in the gene encoding sphingolipid activator protein-1 (*SAP-1*).

HEENT/AIRWAY: Optic atrophy. Copious oral secretions.

NEUROMUSCULAR: There is regression of neurologic development with loss of motor skills, gait disturbances, ataxia, hypotonia, Babinski sign, seizures, choreoathetosis. Torsion spasms of the neck, spine, and limbs. There is a loss of deep tendon reflexes. Eventual spastic quadriparesis. Loss of mental development. The adult form may include dementia and psychotic thought processes.

GI/GU: Increased incidence of gastroesophageal reflux. Megacolon. Gallbladder dysfunction. Sulfatide deposition can also be seen in the kidney, but without renal dysfunction.

OTHER: Associated with intermittent fever and abdominal pain.

MISCELLANEOUS: One of the leukodystrophies, the others of which are adrenoleukodystrophy, Krabbe disease, Canavan disease, Pelizaeus-Merzbacher disease, and Alexander disease. Leukodystrophies involve defective formation of myelin. Metachromatic staining of the central nervous system was first described by Alzheimer. Sulfatides received their name because they contain sulfur.

ANESTHETIC CONSIDERATIONS
Patients are at risk of perioperative aspiration secondary to poor airway tone, copious oral secretions, and an increased incidence of gastroesophageal reflux (1). Consideration should be given to anticholinergic premedication to dry oral secretions. Careful intraoperative positioning and padding is important in these patients with poor nutrition. Hypertonia resolves with muscle relaxants. Phenothiazines, butyrophenones, and other dopaminergic blockers should be avoided because they may exacerbate movement disorders. Ondansetron should be safe as an antiemetic because it does not have antidopaminergic effects. Anticonvulsant medications need to be continued and may alter metabolism of anesthetic drugs, requiring more frequent dosing. Risk of exaggerated hyperkalemia from succinylcholine use has not been demonstrated, but it is reasonable to avoid succinylcholine in patients with chronic disabling diseases involving muscle disuse. Copious oral secretions and airway hypotonia make close postoperative observation important.

Bibliography:
1. Hernández-Palazón J. Anaesthetic management in children with metachromatic leukodystrophy. *Paediatr Anaesth* 2003;13:733–734.
2. Berger J, Moser HW, Forss-Petter S. Leukodystrophies: recent developments in genetics, molecular biology, pathogenesis and treatment. *Curr Opin Neurol* 2001;14:305–312.
3. Malde AD, Naik LD, Pantvaidya SH, et al. An unusual presentation in a patient with metachromatic leukodystrophy. *Anaesthesia* 1997;52:690–694.
4. Tobias JD. Anaesthetic considerations for the child with leukodystrophy. *Can J Anaesth* 1992;39:394–397.

Metaphyseal Chondrodysplasia, Jansen Type

SYNONYM: Metaphyseal dysplasia, Jansen type

MIM #: 156400

There are many types of metaphyseal chondrodysplasia—see also McKusick type (cartilage-hair hypoplasia syndrome), Pyle type, Schmid type, Shwachman syndrome, and Spahr type [not included in this text (*MIM #* 250400)]. The Jansen type of metaphyseal chondrodysplasia is inherited in an autosomal dominant fashion, with most cases representing fresh mutations. It is characterized by severe short stature and significant joint dysfunction. It is caused by a mutation in the parathyroid hormone receptor resulting in constitutive activity of the cyclic adenosine monophosphate (cAMP) signaling pathway.

HEENT/AIRWAY: Cranial bone sclerosis, wide cranial sutures. Small face, prominent eyes and supraorbital ridge. May have hearing loss. High-arched palate. Micrognathia. May have choanal stenosis.

CHEST: Small thorax. Thoracic kyphoscoliosis. Abnormal ribs, with a tendency to fracture.

NEUROMUSCULAR: Intelligence is normal.

ORTHOPEDIC: Severe short stature. Enlarged, dysfunctional joints with flexion contractures, particularly at knees and hips. Short distal phalanges. Irregular and disorganized metaphyses, with normal-appearing epiphyses. Waddling gait. Evidence of increased bone resorption without sufficient compensatory bone formation.

OTHER: Hypercalcemia, hypercalciuria.

ANESTHETIC CONSIDERATIONS

Direct laryngoscopy and tracheal intubation may be difficult secondary to micrognathia. Choanal stenosis, if present, may preclude the use of a nasal airway or a nasogastric tube. There is an increased risk of perioperative respiratory complications because of thoracic cage abnormalities. Asphyxiating thoracic dysplasia, as in Jeune syndrome (see earlier), has been described. Patients must be carefully positioned secondary to severe joint dysfunction. Patients are hypercalcemic. Adequate urine output should be maintained secondary to hypercalciuria.

Bibliography:

1. Calvi LM, Schipani E. The PTH/PTHrP receptor in Jansen's metaphyseal chondrodysplasia. *J Endocrinol Invest* 2000;23:545–554.
2. Kruse K, Schutz C. Calcium metabolism in the Jansen type of metaphyseal dysplasia. *Eur J Pediatr* 1993;152:912–915.
3. Berkowitz I, Raja S, Bender K, et al. Dwarfs: pathophysiology and anesthetic implications. *Anesthesiology* 1990;73:739–759.
4. Charrow J, Poznanski AK. The Jansen type of metaphyseal chondrodysplasia: confirmation of dominant inheritance and review of radiographic manifestations in the newborn and adult. *Am J Med Genet* 1984;18:321–327.

Metaphyseal Chondrodysplasia, McKusick Type

See Cartilage-hair hypoplasia syndrome

Metaphyseal Chondrodysplasia, Schmid Type

SYNONYM: Metaphyseal dysplasia, Schmid type

MIM #: 156500

There are many types of metaphyseal chondrodysplasia—see also Jansen type, McKusick type (cartilage-hair hypoplasia syndrome), Pyle type, Shwachman syndrome, and Spahr type [not included in this text (*MIM #* 250400)]. The Schmid type of metaphyseal chondrodysplasia is inherited in an autosomal dominant fashion with variable expression. It is characterized by moderate short stature, bowed legs, and a waddling gait. The orthopedic abnormalities tend to improve over time. Schmid-type metaphyseal chondrodysplasia is caused by a mutation in the gene for type X collagen (*COL10A1*).

CHEST: Lower rib cage mildly flared anteriorly.

NEUROMUSCULAR: Intelligence is normal.

ORTHOPEDIC: Moderate short stature. Bowed legs. Enlarged capital femoral epiphyses. Coxa vara. Waddling gait. Irregular metaphyses, with normal-appearing epiphyses. Metaphyseal cupping of the proximal phalanges and metacarpals. No vertebral abnormalities.

ANESTHETIC CONSIDERATIONS

Patients must be carefully positioned secondary to orthopedic abnormalities.

Bibliography:

1. Makitie O, Susic M, Ward L, et al. Schmid type of metaphyseal chondrodysplasia and COL10A1 mutations—findings in 10 patients. *Am J Med Genet* 2005;137A:241–248.
2. Berkowitz I, Raja S, Bender K, et al. Dwarfs: pathophysiology and anesthetic implications. *Anesthesiology* 1990;73:739–759A.
3. Lachman RS, Rimoin DL, Spranger J. Metaphyseal chondrodysplasia: Schmid type: clinical and radiographic delineation with review of the literature. *Pediatr Radiol* 1988;18:93–102.

Metaphyseal Dysplasia, Jansen Type

See Metaphyseal chondrodysplasia, Jansen type

Metaphyseal Dysplasia, Mckusick Type

See Cartilage-hair hypoplasia syndrome

Metaphyseal Dysplasia, Pyle Type

See Pyle metaphyseal dysplasia

Metaphyseal Dysplasia, Schmid Type

See Metaphyseal chondrodysplasia, Schmid type

Metatropic Dwarfism

SYNONYM: Metatropic dysplasia, type I

MIM #: 250600

This genetically heterogeneous disorder is characterized by progressive short-trunk dwarfism, short limbs, small thorax, odontoid hypoplasia and metaphyseal flaring. There are likely three genetic types of metatropic dwarfism: a nonlethal autosomal recessive form, a nonlethal autosomal dominant form, and a lethal autosomal recessive form. Many features of this disorder are similar to Kniest syndrome (see earlier; also known as metatropic dysplasia, type II).

HEENT/AIRWAY: Macrocephaly. Short neck. May have overgrowth of cartilage in the trachea.

CHEST: Small thorax with short ribs, thoracic kyphoscoliosis. May have severe restrictive lung disease. May have sleep apnea.

NEUROMUSCULAR: May have cervical cord compression secondary to atlantoaxial instability. May have ventriculomegaly.

ORTHOPEDIC: Short-trunk dwarfism develops secondary to severe kyphoscoliosis. Odontoid hypoplasia with atlantoaxial instability may lead to cord compression, quadriplegia and death. Short limbs with metaphyseal flaring (long bones appear dumbbell shaped). Large joints with limited joint mobility, particularly at knees and hips. Small pelvis.

OTHER: Small pelvis in affected women may necessitate delivery by cesarean section.

MISCELLANEOUS: "Metatropic" derives from the Greek for "different shape," referring to the changing body proportions with age as the kyphoscoliosis progresses. These patients may be misdiagnosed with achondroplasia at birth, and with Morquio syndrome when older.

ANESTHETIC CONSIDERATIONS

May have atlantoaxial instability. Direct laryngoscopy may be difficult in patients with a short neck, particularly if there is limited neck mobility secondary to C1-2 fusion done for atlantoaxial instability. Neck flexion may occlude the airway. Might require a smaller-than-expected endotracheal tube if sized for age. Patients must be carefully positioned secondary to limited joint mobility.

Bibliography:
1. Genevieve D, Le Merrer M, Munnich A, et al. Long-term follow-up in a patient with metatropic dysplasia. *Am J Med Genet* 2005;135:342–343.
2. Berkowitz I, Raja S, Bender K, et al. Dwarfs: pathophysiology and anesthetic implications. *Anesthesiology* 1990;73:739–759B.
3. Shohat M, Lachman R, Rimoin DL. Odontoid hypoplasia with vertebral cervical subluxation and ventriculomegaly in metatropic dysplasia. *J Pediatr* 1989;114:239–243.
4. Beck M, Roubicek M, Rogers JG, et al. Heterogeneity of metatropic dysplasia. *Eur J Pediatr* 1983;140:231–237.

Metatropic Dysplasia, Type I

See Metatropic dwarfism

Metatropic Dysplasia, Type II

See Kniest syndrome

Methemoglobinemia

SYNONYM: Congenital methemoglobinemia

MIM #: 250800, 250790

Methemoglobin is hemoglobin in which the iron has not been reduced from its ferric (Fe^{3+}) state to its ferrous (Fe^{2+}) state. Methemoglobin cannot bind molecular oxygen. Methemoglobin in low levels (less than 1% of total hemoglobin) is normally formed in the red blood cells. There is an intracellular mechanism responsible for maintaining normal levels of reduced hemoglobin, which is normally well in excess of the rate of hemoglobin oxidation. The classic reductase is located solely in the red blood cells. A more severe and even lethal disease is caused by a generalized reductase deficiency, which has major neurologic manifestations.

Methemoglobinemia results from one of three mechanisms. First, the normal cellular mechanisms can be overwhelmed by exogenous agents. This is particularly easy to happen in infants, whose red blood cells have approximately half the methemoglobin-reducing capability of adult red blood cells. For example, there was a case report of carrot juice inducing methemoglobinemia in an infant. Second, there can be a structurally abnormal hemoglobin. These are designated as the hemoglobins M (with the location of the place of discovery following as a subscript). The amino acid substitutions in the hemoglobins M form a covalent link with iron, stabilizing it in the oxidized (Fe^{3+}) state. These are transmitted in an autosomal dominant fashion. Defects in the alpha chain present with cyanosis from birth. Cyanosis develops at several months of age in patients with defects in the beta chain, coincident with the postnatal shift to synthesis of this chain. Third, there can be a defect in the cell's ability to reduce red blood cell iron, either NADH-dependent hemoglobin reductase (methemoglobin reductase, cytochrome b5 reductase), or cytochrome b5 itself. Cytochrome b5 is required as a cofactor for the functioning of methemoglobin reductase. These are transmitted in an autosomal recessive fashion.

Cyanosis develops at methemoglobin levels greater than 10% to 20%; headaches, fatigue, weakness, tachycardia, and dizziness at levels from about 30% to 40%; dyspnea and lethargy at about 40% to 50%; acidosis, hypoxia, seizures, and coma at levels of about 50% to 60%; and death at levels over about 70%.

HEENT/AIRWAY: Microcephaly and nystagmus in the generalized reductase defect only. Conjunctival cyanosis is present in patients with methemoglobinemia, but not in patients with cyanosis from poor oxygenation of blood. Apparently the conjunctival sac allows oxygenation of red blood cells from the air, which would not make any difference in patients with methemoglobinemia.

NEUROMUSCULAR: Variable mental retardation, opisthotonos, attacks of athetosis, and hypertonia in the generalized reductase defect only.

OTHER: Blood with over approximately 10% methemoglobin turns dark red or brownish on standing or on shaking with air. Methemoglobin is detectable by cooximeters.

MISCELLANEOUS: A variety of compounds can cause methemoglobin formation either directly or indirectly. Endogenous intracellular compounds that can produce methemoglobin include molecular oxygen, hydrogen peroxide and several free radicals. Toxic exogenous compounds include (but are not limited to) benzocaine, prilocaine, chloral hydrate, nitrites (which can be found in well water), nitrates, hydrazines, primaquine, chloroquine, sulfonamide, dapsone, phenacetin, and acetanilide.

The defect is common in both Navajo and Athabaskan Indians. Interestingly, the languages of both of these groups are also similar, suggesting a common origin.

ANESTHETIC CONSIDERATIONS

The color of these infants is not really the same as that of patients with cyanosis. It is more of a slate-grayish color, somewhat like that seen with venous suffusion. Arterial partial pressure of oxygen (pO_2) is otherwise appropriate for the fraction of inspired oxygen (FiO_2). Patients breathing supplemental oxygen are cyanotic appearing, but have a high arterial pO_2. Benzocaine, prilocaine (in EMLA cream, a eutectic mixture of local anesthetics), nitroglycerin, sulfonamides, and chloral hydrate can produce methemoglobin and should be avoided if possible. Exogenous agents in sufficient quantities can induce methemoglobinemia even in normal patients (patients without congenital methemoglobinemia), as, for instance, with the overuse of benzocaine when topicalizing the airway (6, 7).

Pulse oximeters (and oximetric pulmonary arterial catheters) do not reliably reflect hemoglobin oxygen saturation in the presence of methemoglobin (8). Methemoglobin increases light absorbance at both the wavelengths that are used by pulse oximeters to calculate oxygen saturation. The large increase in absorbance in both the numerator and denominator of the formula used to calculate oxygen saturation forces the ratio towards one. At a ratio of one, the oxygen saturation is calculated as 85%. Thus, methemoglobinemia forces a saturation approaching 85% independent of the pO_2 or true hemoglobin oxygen saturation.

The rate of methemoglobin reduction can be accelerated by a variety of agents, including methylene blue and ascorbic acid. The dose of methylene blue is 1 to 2 mg/kg intravenously (it comes as a 1%, or 10 mg/mL solution), or 2 mg/kg orally per day (100 to 300 mg in adults). It has been used prophylactically prior to surgery (1). Methylene blue does not work in patients with one of the hemoglobinopathies, or in patients who are also glucose-6-phosphate dehydrogenase deficient. Oral ascorbic acid (500 to 1,000 mg/day in an adult) also lowers methemoglobin levels, but has certain long-term side effects. Oral riboflavin (20 to 60 mg/day in adults) is also said to help.

Bibliography:

1. Baraka AS, Ayoub CM, Yazbek-Karam V, et al. Prophylactic methylene blue in a patient with congenital methemoglobinemia. *Can J Anaesth* 2005;52:258–261.
2. Sharma D, Pandia MP, Bithal PK. Anaesthetic management of Osler-Weber-Rendu syndrome with coexisting congenital methaemoglobinaemia. *Acta Anaesthesiol Scand* 2005;49:1391–1394.
3. Maurtua MA, Emmerling L, Ebrahim Z. Anesthetic management of a patient with congenital methemoglobinemia. *J Clin Anaesth* 2004;16:455–457.
4. Groeper K, Katcher K, Tobias JD. Anesthetic management of a patient with methemoglobinemia. *South Med J* 2003;96:504–509.
5. Baraka AS, Ayoub CM, Kaddoum RN, et al. Severe oxyhemoglobin desaturation during induction of anesthesia in a patient with congenital methemoglobinemia. *Anesthesiology* 2001;95:1296–1297.
6. Kern K, Langevin PB, Dunn BM. Methemoglobinemia after topical anesthesia with lidocaine and benzocaine for a difficult intubation. *J Clin Anaesth* 2000;12:167–172.
7. Ellis FD, Seiler JG, Palmore MM. Methemoglobinemia: a complication after fiberoptic orotracheal intubation with benzocaine spray: a case report. *J Bone Joint Surg Am* 1995;77:937–939.
8. Barker SJ, Tremper KK, Hyatt J. Effects of methemoglobinemia on pulse oximetry and mixed venous oximetry. *Anesthesiology* 1989;70:112–117.

Methylmalonic Acidemia

SYNONYM: Methylmalonic aciduria; Methylmalonyl-coenzyme A mutase deficiency

MIM #: 251000, 251100

This disorder is caused by defects in the activity of one of several enzymes, resulting in methylmalonic acidemia. Severe metabolic acidosis, ketosis, and hyperammonemia can develop at times of increased protein catabolism. There can be a defect in methylmalonyl-coenzyme A mutase (autosomal recessive), a defect in adenosylcobalamin synthesis causing impaired mutase function (and which may respond to pharmacologic doses of cyanocobalamin or adenosylcobalamin), or a defect in the function of both adenosylcobalamin synthesis and methylcobalamin-dependent N5-methyltetrahydrofolate methyltransferase. The latter causes methylmalonic acidemia and homocystinuria. In addition, there may be multiple alleles for each of these. Methylmalonyl-coenzyme A mutase converts propionyl-CoA to succinyl-CoA. In its absence its substrate is converted to methylmalonyl-CoA. This enzyme requires a B_{12}-dependent coenzyme (adenosylcobalamin) as a cofactor. Treatment includes a nonproprionate-producing amino acid diet with adequate carbohydrates and lipids as energy sources, continuous nighttime gastric feeding, L-carnitine supplementation to increase renal excretion of propionyl groups via propionyl-carnitine, supplemental vitamin B_{12} (in B_{12} responsive types), and ultimately liver transplantation. Hemodialysis is useful in the acute management of catabolic crises. Untreated, the mean age at death is 1.5 to 2 years.

CARDIOVASCULAR: May have cardiomyopathy.

NEUROMUSCULAR: Lethargy, hypotonia, dystonia, seizures. Occasional mental retardation. Rare progression to coma. Patients do not have the neurologic findings of cobalamin deficiency.

ORTHOPEDIC: Growth retardation. Osteoporosis with pathologic fractures.

GI/GU: Recurrent vomiting. Episodic pancreatitis. Hepatomegaly.

OTHER: Failure to thrive, hypoglycemia, metabolic acidosis, ketosis, and hyperammonemia. Neutropenia, thrombocytopenia. Patients do not have the hematologic findings of cobalamin deficiency.

MISCELLANEOUS: Patients may be receiving chronic oral citrate or bicarbonate to maintain a normal pH, and supplemental cobalamin. It has been suggested that therapy with intramuscular cyanocobalamin alone is inadequate for patients with methylmalonic acidemia and homocystinuria, and patients should be treated with hydroxocobalamin (3).

ANESTHETIC CONSIDERATIONS

All preoperative medications related to the disease should be continued perioperatively. Chronic use of anticonvulsant medications may alter the metabolism of some anesthetic drugs. Prolonged fasting must be avoided perioperatively. Abnormal diet in the days after the surgery can result in an exacerbation of acidosis (4). Intravenous fluids and dextrose should be used generously perioperatively to avoid hypovolemia and protein catabolism. An orogastric tube or throat packs should be placed if the surgery has the potential to cause oral or intestinal bleeding because the blood in the gastrointestinal tract provides a protein load that may trigger acute decompensation. The platelet count should be evaluated preoperatively to screen for thrombocytopenia. Intraoperative arterial blood gas tensions and measurements of electrolytes, glucose, and ammonia may be warranted to detect acidosis or hyperammonemia. Acute preoperative hemodialysis has been used. Nitrous oxide inhibits vitamin B_{12}-dependent enzymes, including adenosylcobalamin, and should probably be avoided in these patients. Patients must be carefully positioned secondary to osteoporosis. Postoperative metronidazole has been used to diminish production of propionate by gut flora (2).

FIGURE: See Appendix D

Bibliography:

1. Tanpaiboon P. Methylmalonic acidemia (MMA). *Mol Genet Metab* 2005;85:2–6.
2. Ho D, Harrison V, Street N. Anaesthesia for liver transplantation in a patient with methylmalonic acidaemia. *Paediatr Anaesth* 2000;10:215–218.
3. Andersson HC, Shapira E. Biochemical and clinical response to hydroxocobalamin versus cyanocobalamin treatment in patients with methylmalonic acidemia and homocystinuria (cblC). *J Pediatr* 1998;132:121–124.
4. Martin HB. Management of a patient with methylmalonic acidemia for prolonged surgery. *Am J Anesthesiol* 1997;24:145–148.
5. Sharar SR, Haberkern CM, Jack R, et al. Anesthetic management of a child with methylmalonyl-coenzyme A mutase deficiency. *Anesth Analg* 1991;73:499–501.

Methylmalonic Aciduria

See Methylmalonic acidemia

Methylmalonyl-Coenzyme A Mutase Deficiency

See Methylmalonic acidemia

Microgastria-Limb Reduction Complex

See Congenital microgastria-limb reduction complex

Microphthalmia-Linear Skin Defects Syndrome

SYNONYM: MIDAS syndrome

MIM #: 309801

This X-linked syndrome involves microphthalmia, sclerocornea, and focal linear dermal hypoplasia. The mnemonic MIDAS stands for **MI**crophthalmia, **D**ermal **A**plasia, and **S**clerocornea. Patients have severe visual impairment. All affected individuals are female, suggesting lethality in males. The gene and gene product are not known.

HEENT/AIRWAY: Microphthalmia. Sclerocornea. May also have anterior chamber defects, cataracts, iris coloboma, pigmentary retinopathy, glaucoma.

CHEST: Diaphragmatic hernia has been reported. May have costovertebral anomalies.

CARDIOVASCULAR: May have cardiomyopathy, cardiac conduction abnormality, atrial septal defect, ventricular septal defect, overriding aorta.

NEUROMUSCULAR: May have agenesis of the corpus callosum, absence of the septum pellucidum.

ORTHOPEDIC: Mild short stature.

GI/GU: May have anomalies of external or internal genitalia.

OTHER: Focal dermal hypoplasia or aplasia, usually linear, particularly affecting the head and neck. On rare occasions there may be herniation of adipose tissue through the defect.

ANESTHETIC CONSIDERATIONS

Patients must be carefully positioned and padded secondary to focal dermal hypoplasia. Patients may have cardiac conduction abnormalities. Patients with congenital cardiac defects require perioperative antibiotic prophylaxis as indicated.

Bibliography:

1. Morleo M, Pramparo T, Perone L, et al. Microphthalmia with linear skin defects (MLS) syndrome: clinical, cytogenetic, and molecular characterization of 11 cases. *Am J Med Genet* 2005;137:190–198.
2. Mucke J, Hoepffner W, Thamm B, et al. MIDAS syndrome (microphthalmia, dermal aplasia and sclerocornea): an autonomous entity with linear skin defects within the spectrum of focal hypoplasias. *Eur J Dermatol* 1995;5:197–203.

MIDAS Syndrome

See Microphthalmia-linear skin defects syndrome

Miller Syndrome

SYNONYM: Postaxial acrofacial dysostosis syndrome

MIM #: 263750

This autosomal recessive syndrome consists of craniofacial abnormalities somewhat similar to those of the Treacher Collins syndrome, plus postaxial upper and lower limb defects. The responsible gene and gene product are not known.

HEENT/AIRWAY: Malar hypoplasia. Absent superior orbital ridges, down-slanting palpebral fissures, eyelid coloboma, lower lid ectropion. Hypoplastic, low-set, cup-shaped ears. May have hearing loss. Cleft lip or palate. Micrognathia. May have choanal atresia. Ectropion and facial asymmetry may progress over time. Micrognathia may improve over time.

CHEST: May have pectus excavatum. May have rib anomalies. May have absent hemidiaphragm.

CARDIOVASCULAR: Congenital cardiac defects include atrial septal defects, ventricular septal defects, patent ductus arteriosus.

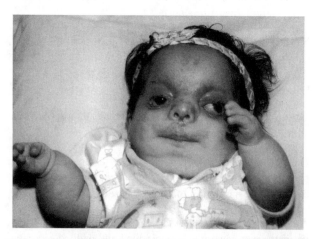

Miller syndrome. FIG. 1. This young girl has Miller syndrome. She was reported in the paper by Stevenson et al. Note tracheostomy, coloboma, absent fifth fingers, short forearms, and micrognathia.

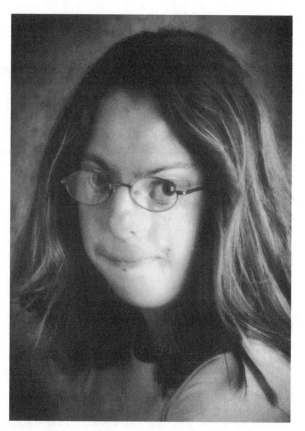

Miller syndrome. FIG. 2. The young girl in figure 1 at age 16.

NEUROMUSCULAR: Intelligence is usually normal.

ORTHOPEDIC: Postaxial upper and lower limb defects, including absent fifth digit of all four limbs. Forearm shortening, secondary to ulnar or radial hypoplasia. Syndactyly. Congenital hip dislocation.

GI/GU: Cryptorchidism. May have pyloric stenosis, malrotation, volvulus. May have renal anomaly.

OTHER: Accessory nipples.

MISCELLANEOUS: Previously known as Genee-Wiedemann syndrome. Nager syndrome (see later) also has Treacher Collins-like facies, but is distinguishable from Miller syndrome because it involves preaxial rather than postaxial upper limb defects.

ANESTHETIC CONSIDERATIONS
Malar hypoplasia may result in a poor mask fit. Direct laryngoscopy and tracheal intubation can be extremely difficult. Choanal atresia, if present, precludes the use of a nasal airway or nasogastric tube. Peripheral intravenous access may be difficult secondary to limb defects. Radial anomalies may make placement of a radial arterial catheter more difficult. The eyelids may not completely cover the eyes, which then need additional intraoperative protection.

Bibliography:

1. Neumann L, Pelz J, Kunze J. A new observation of two cases of acrofacial dysostosis type Genee-Wiedemann in a family—remarks on the mode of inheritance: report on two sibs. *Am J Med Genet* 1996;64:556–562.
2. Chrzanowska K, Fryns JP. Miller postaxial acrofacial dysostosis: the phenotypic changes with age. *Genet Couns* 1993;4:131–133.
3. Giannotti A, Digilio MC, Virgili Q, et al. Familial postaxial acrofacial dysostosis syndrome. *J Med Genet* 1992;29:752.
4. Stevenson GW, Hall SC, Bauer BS, et al. Anaesthetic management of Miller syndrome. *Can J Anaesth* 1991;38:1046–1049.
5. Richards M. Miller syndrome. *Anaesthesia* 1987;42:871–874.

Miller-Dieker Syndrome

SYNONYM: Lissencephaly syndrome

MIM #: 247200

This autosomal dominant or autosomal recessive disorder is caused by defects in several genes that are located on the short arm of chromosome 17. A defect in the gene *L1S1* is responsible for the lissencephaly. Defects in contiguous genes cause the other features of the Miller-Dieker syndrome, such as microcephaly, bitemporal narrowing, short nose with anteverted nares, micrognathia, and agenesis of the corpus callosum. There is evidence that the *L1S1* gene product is the human homolog of a subunit of bovine brain platelet-activating factor acetylhydrolase, which inactivates the platelet-activating factor in the bovine brain. The exact role of the *L1S1* gene product is not known, but it may be involved in a signal transduction pathway that is crucial for cerebral development.

HEENT/AIRWAY: Microcephaly, prominent forehead, bitemporal narrowing. Midline forehead furrowing, especially noticeable during crying. Hypertelorism. Up-slanted palpebral fissures, ptosis. Low-set and/or posteriorly rotated ears. Short nose with anteverted nares. Prominent philtrum. Thin, protuberant upper lip. Micrognathia. May have cleft palate.

CHEST: Recurrent aspiration pneumonia.

CARDIOVASCULAR: May have a cardiac defect such as atrial septal defect, ventricular septal defect, tetralogy of Fallot, pulmonic stenosis.

NEUROMUSCULAR: Lissencephaly—smooth brain surface (absent gyri) with incomplete development of the brain. Thickened cortex. Wide sylvian fissure apparent on computed tomography scan. Large ventricles. Absent corpus callosum. Midline calcifications. Severe mental retardation and severe developmental delay. Initial hypotonia progresses to opisthotonos, spasticity, decorticate and decerebrate posturing. Seizures. Occasional lipomeningocele with tethered cord.

ORTHOPEDIC: Transverse palmar crease. Clinodactyly, polydactyly. May have growth deficiency.

GI/GU: Dysphagia and gastroesophageal reflux are common. Cryptorchidism. Pilonidal sinus. May have omphalocele. May have renal dysplasia.

OTHER: Polyhydramnios. Failure to thrive.

MISCELLANEOUS: Dr. James Q. Miller was a respected and well-liked neurologist at the University of Virginia. He passed away recently.

ANESTHETIC CONSIDERATIONS
Severe mental retardation and severe developmental delay may make the smooth induction of anesthesia a challenge. Direct laryngoscopy and tracheal intubation may be difficult secondary to micrognathia. Gastroesophageal reflux is common, and patients are at increased risk of perioperative aspiration. Patients with recurrent aspiration pneumonia have chronic lung disease, and are more likely to experience postoperative respiratory complications. Chronic use of anticonvulsant medications alters the metabolism of some anesthetic drugs. Patients with congenital cardiac defects require perioperative antibiotic prophylaxis as indicated.

Bibliography:

1. Thomas MA, Duncan AM, Bardin C, et al. Lissencephaly with der(17)t(17;20)(p13.3;p12.2)mat. *Am J Med Genet A* 2004;124:292–295.
2. Tjoelker LW, Stafforini DM. Platelet-activating factor acetylhydrolases in health and disease. *Biochim Biophys Acta* 2000;1488:102–123.
3. Chitayat D, Toi A, Babul R, et al. Omphalocele in Miller-Dieker syndrome: expanding the phenotype. *Am J Med Genet* 1997;69:293–298.
4. Kohler A, Hain J, Muller U. Clinical and molecular genetic findings in five patients with Miller-Dieker syndrome. *Clin Genet* 1995;47:161–164.

Mitochondrial Trifunctional Protein Deficiency

MIM #: 609015

This protein catalyzes three steps in the beta-oxidation of fatty acids in mitochondria. The three enzyme activities are enoyl-CoA hydratase, 3-ketoacyl-CoA thiolase, and long-chain acyl-CoA dehydrogenase (LCAD) (see Long-chain acyl-CoA dehydrogenase deficiency, earlier). There may be defects in either the alpha or the beta subunits of the protein, with differing limitations in enzyme action. The alpha subunit contains the hydratase and LCAD activity, and the beta subunit contains the thiolase activity. In general, the clinical picture is worse than that of isolated LCAD deficiency. The disorder is inherited in an autosomal recessive fashion. It may present as sudden infant death, as a Reye-like syndrome, or more insidiously with hypotonia and cardiomyopathy. Mortality is often due to cardiac disease.

CARDIOVASCULAR: Cardiomyopathy, arrhythmias.

NEUROMUSCULAR: Decreased level of consciousness. Skeletal myopathy. Hypotonia.

GI/GU: Reye-like syndrome with abnormal liver function tests, recurrent myoglobinuria.

OTHER: Sudden unexplained death. Recurrent hypoglycemia with lactic acidosis. Older patients may exhibit recurrent myoglobinuria. Hypocalcemia sometimes with hypoparathyroidism has been described.

MISCELLANEOUS: Presence of this abnormality in a fetus can cause acute fatty liver of pregnancy or HELLP syndrome in the mother. Presumably, abnormal fetal metabolites overwhelm the ability of the heterozygote mother's mitochondria to oxidize them.

ANESTHETIC CONSIDERATIONS

Patients should be evaluated preoperatively for evidence of cardiomyopathy. Patients may require a glucose infusion perioperatively secondary to their predisposition to hypoglycemia. Succinylcholine may be contraindicated in patients with skeletal myopathy because of the risk of hyperkalemia.

Bibliography:

1. Olpin SE, Clark S, Andresen BS, et al. Biochemical, clinical and molecular findings in LCHAD and general mitochondrial trifunctional protein deficiency. *J Inherit Metab Dis* 2005;28:533–544.
2. Spierkerkoetter U, Khuchua Z, Yue Z, et al. The early-onset phenotype of mitochondrial trifunctional protein deficiency: a lethal disorder with multiple tissue involvement. *J Inherit Metab Dis* 2004;27:294–296.
3. Spiekerkoetter U, Sun B, Khuchua Z, et al. Molecular and phenotypic heterogeneity in mitochondrial trifunctional protein deficiency due to beta-subunit mutations. *Hum Mutat* 2003;21:598–607.
4. den Boer ME, Dionisi-Vici C, Chakrapani A, et al. Mitochondrial trifunctional protein deficiency: a severe fatty acid oxidation disorder with cardiac and neurologic involvement. *J Pediatr* 2003;142:684–689.
5. Ibdah JA, Bennett MJ, Rinaldo P, et al. A fetal fatty-acid oxidation disorder as a cause of liver disease in pregnant women. *N Engl J Med* 1999;340:1723–1731.
6. Tyni T, Rapola J, Palotie A, et al. Hypoparathyroidism in a patient with long-chain 3-hydroxyacyl-coenzyme A dehydrogenase deficiency. *J Pediatr* 1997;131:766–768.
7. Tyni T, Rapola J, Palotie A, et al. Hypoparathyroidism in a patient with long-chain 3-hydroxyacyl-coenzyme A dehydrogenase deficiency. *J Pediatr* 1997;131:766–768.

Moebius Sequence

MIM #: 157900

This sporadically occurring syndrome is characterized by masklike facies with congenital sixth and seventh cranial nerve palsies. Other cranial nerves also can be involved. The pathogenesis of Moebius sequence is related to absence, hypoplasia, or destruction of the cranial nerve nuclei, a peripheral nerve abnormality, or a myopathy. It has been suggested that Klippel-Feil sequence, Moebius sequence and Poland sequence, all of which can occur in various combinations in the same patient, may represent anomalies from an *in utero* disruption of the fetal subclavian or vertebral arteries. Moebius sequence, it appears, is usually the result of a focal *in utero* hypoxic/ischemic insult. However, Moebius sequence can be familial, and a gene responsible for at least some cases of Moebius sequence maps to the long arm of chromosome 13. In addition, Moebius syndrome has been reported as a complication of the maternal use of misoprostol as an unsuccessful abortifacient (5).

Plastic surgery has been offered to these children so that they are able to smile.

HEENT/AIRWAY: Masklike facies secondary to facial nerve palsy. Strabismus, ptosis. Prominent ears, which may be low set. May have hearing loss. May have cleft lip or palate. Microstomia, tethered tongue. Micrognathia. Speech difficulties.

CHEST: Weak swallow and poor cough result in recurrent aspiration. Patients may have idiopathic tachypnea.

CARDIOVASCULAR: May have a congenital cardiac defect.

NEUROMUSCULAR: Intelligence is usually normal. Cranial nerve palsies, especially cranial nerves VI and VII. May have other central nervous system anomalies. Peripheral neuropathy and autonomic dysfunction have been reported. Patients may have central hypoventilation.

ORTHOPEDIC: Frequently have clubfoot deformity. May have limb reduction defects, syndactyly, digital contractures. May have arthrogryposis. May have cervical spine anomalies.

GI/GU: Swallowing difficulties.

OTHER: Has been associated with hypogonadotrophic hypogonadism.

MISCELLANEOUS: Paul Moebius was a German neurologist in private practice. He gave up his teaching post after being told that he would not receive a professorial appointment. Moebius also described ophthalmic migraine. Both spellings, Moebius and Möbius, are used.

ANESTHETIC CONSIDERATIONS

Direct laryngoscopy and intubation of the trachea may be difficult secondary to oral/palatal abnormalities and micrognathia (1). A gum elastic bougie, Bellhouse laryngoscope (Belscope), and laryngeal mask have all been used successfully (6). Copious secretions and difficulty in swallowing may compromise the airway, and an antisialagogue may be helpful. Swallowing difficulties and a poor cough increase the risk of perioperative aspiration. Patients may have anomalies of the cervical spine, which should be assessed preoperatively.

Peripheral vascular access may be difficult secondary to extremity deficits. Patients may have a peripheral neuropathy, which must be taken into account before undertaking regional anesthesia. Facial (seventh) nerve palsy may result in an inability to close the eyes. The eyes must be protected perioperatively to avoid corneal abrasions. In addition, monitoring neuromuscular blockade through the facial nerve may be inaccurate. Recurrent apneic episodes have been described, suggesting that patients should be monitored closely postoperatively, particularly when narcotics are given. Patients with congenital cardiac defects should receive perioperative antibiotic prophylaxis as indicated.

Bibliography:
1. Ames WA, Shichor TM, Speakman M, et al. Anesthetic management of children with Moebius sequence. *Can J Anaesth* 2005;52:837–844.
2. Verzijl HT, Padberg GW, Zwarts MJ. The spectrum of Möbius syndrome: an electrophysiological study. *Brain* 2005;128:1728–1736.
3. Ha CY, Messieha ZS. Management of a patient with Möbius syndrome: a case report. *Spec Care Dentist* 2003;23:111–116.
4. Verzijl HT, van der Zwaag B, Cruysberg JR, et al. Möbius syndrome redefined: a syndrome of rhombencephalic maldevelopment. *Neurology* 2003;61:327–333.
5. Goldberg AB, Greenberg MB, Darney PD. Misoprostol and pregnancy. *N Engl J Med* 2001;344:38–47.
6. Ferguson S. Moebius syndrome: a review of the anaesthetic implications. *Paediatr Anaesth* 1996;6:51–56.
7. St. Charles S, DiMario FJ, Grunnet ML. Möbius sequence: further *in vivo* support for the subclavian artery supply disruption sequence. *Am J Med Genet* 1993;47:289–293.
8. Kumar D. Moebius syndrome. *J Med Genet* 1990;27:122–126.
9. Bouwes-Bavinck JN, Weaver DD. Subclavian artery supply disruption sequence: hypothesis of a vascular etiology for Poland, Klippel-Feil, and Möbius anomalies. *Am J Med Genet* 1986;23:903–218.
10. Krajcirik WJ, Azar I, Opperman S, et al. Anesthetic management of a patient with Moebius syndrome. *Anesth Analg* 1985;64:369–370.

Mohr Syndrome

SYNONYM: Oral-facial-digital syndrome, type II

MIM #: 252100

This autosomal recessive syndrome is characterized by conductive hearing loss, cleft tongue, and partial reduplication of the big toe. The gene and gene product are not known.

HEENT/AIRWAY: Cranium may contain wormian bones. Maxillary hypoplasia. Inner canthi are displaced laterally. Conductive hearing loss secondary to a defect of the incus. Flat nasal bridge, broad nasal tip. Partial midline cleft lip; may have cleft palate. Midline cleft tongue. Papilliform protuberances on tongue. Hyperplastic frenulum, may have multiple frenula. Mild mandibular hypoplasia.

CHEST: Tachypnea is common. May have pectus excavatum.

CARDIOVASCULAR: May have endocardial cushion defect.

NEUROMUSCULAR: Intelligence is usually normal. May have hydrocephalus, arachnoid cysts, hypotonia, seizures, apnea, Dandy-Walker abnormality, cerebellar atrophy.

ORTHOPEDIC: Mild short stature. Partial reduplication of the big toe. Short hands. Polydactyly (hands or feet), clinodactyly, or brachydactyly. Flared metaphyses. May have scoliosis.

GI/GU: May have hypoplastic genitalia.

MISCELLANEOUS: Otto Mohr was a distinguished Norwegian geneticist. He was the first to recognize the effects of radiation on chromosomes, and he also described the genetic basis of phenylketonuria. He was dismissed by the Nazis during the occupation of Norway in 1940 because of his opposition to their policy of eugenics, and was incarcerated in a concentration camp. After the war, he became the president of the University of Oslo. He has also authored several books on Norwegian painters and poets.

ANESTHETIC CONSIDERATIONS
The mild mandibular hypoplasia is not likely to affect the ease of direct laryngoscopy.

Bibliography:
1. Sakai N, Nakakita N, Yamazaki Y, et al. Oral-facial-digital syndrome type II (Mohr syndrome): clinical and genetic manifestations. *J Craniofac Surg* 2002;13:321–326.
2. Prpic I, Cekada S, Franulovic J. Mohr syndrome (oro-facial-digital syndrome II): a familial case with different phenotypic findings. *Clin Genet* 1995;48:304–307.
3. Reardon W, Harbord MG, Hall-Craggs MA, et al. Central nervous system malformations in Mohr syndrome. *J Med Genet* 1989;26:659–663.

Molybdenum Cofactor Deficiency

SYNONYM: Combined deficiency of sulfite oxidase, xanthine dehydrogenase, and aldehyde oxidase

MIM #: 252150

This autosomal recessive syndrome is caused by a mutation at one of the two steps in the formation of the molybdenum cofactor. This cofactor is required for the functioning of three enzymes: sulfite oxidase, xanthine dehydrogenase, and aldehyde oxidase. Findings are related to those caused by deficiencies in these enzymes. The most common presentation is intractable seizures in the neonatal period. The prognosis is very poor, and the disorder is usually fatal in infancy or early childhood. Sulfite oxidase converts sulfite (a metabolite of methionine and cysteine) to sulfate. Xanthine dehydrogenase catalyzes the hydroxylation of xanthine and hypoxanthine to uric acid. Aldehyde oxidase hydroxylates hypoxanthine into xanthine.

HEENT/AIRWAY: Can have acquired microcephaly. Narrow bifrontal diameter. Deep-set eyes. Dislocated lens. Lack of light response.

NEUROMUSCULAR: Profound mental retardation, seizures, spastic tetraparesis, brain atrophy, encephalopathy. Myoclonus. Opisthotonos. Axial hypotonia with peripheral hypertonia. Milder disease can present later, with loss of milestones. Central nervous system volume loss has resulted in a malformation that resembles the Dandy-Walker malformation.

GI/GU: Feeding difficulties. Urinary xanthine stones.

OTHER: May have absent serum homocysteine.

ANESTHETIC CONSIDERATIONS

Chronic use of anticonvulsant medications may alter the metabolism of some anesthetic drugs. Perioperative fluid administration must be adequate to maintain a diuresis and prevent further concentration of xanthine in the urine. Xanthine is more soluble at an alkaline pH. However, symptomatic xanthinuria has not been a problem in these young children with limited life expectancy. Methylxanthines such as theophylline and caffeine are not metabolized by xanthine oxidase, and are not contraindicated.

Bibliography:

1. Teksam O, Yurdakok M, Coskun T. Molybdenum cofactor deficiency presenting with severe metabolic acidosis and intracranial hemorrhage. *J Child Neurol* 2005;20:155–157.
2. Salman MS, Ackerley C, Senger C, et al. New insights into the neuropathogenesis of molybdenum cofactor deficiency. *Can J Neurol Sci* 2002;29:91–96.
3. Arslanoglu S, Yalaz M, Goksen D, et al. Molybdenum cofactor deficiency associated with Dandy-Walker complex. *Brain Dev* 2001;23:815–818.
4. Simmonds HA, Hoffmann GF, Perignon JL, et al. Diagnosis of molybdenum cofactor deficiency. *Lancet* 1999;353:675.

Morning Glory Syndrome

Included in Papillorenal syndrome

Morquio Syndrome

SYNONYM: Mucopolysaccharidosis IV

MIM #: 253000, 253010

This autosomal recessive mucopolysaccharidosis occurs in a severe form (type A) and a milder form (type B). The lysosomal enzyme defect does not allow the degradation of keratin sulfate in the cartilage, which then accumulates along with chondroitin-6-sulfate. Type A is due to an abnormality in the gene encoding *N*-acetylgalactosamine-6-sulfate sulfatase (galactose-6-sulfatase), and type B is due to an abnormality in the gene encoding beta-galactosidase, which is specific for keratin sulfate. Clinically, the two forms are similar. The major findings are skeletal.

HEENT/AIRWAY: Dense calvarium. There may be mild coarsening of the facial features. Mild corneal clouding. Progressive sensorineural or mixed hearing loss. Short, anteverted nose. Broad mouth with redundant pharyngeal mucosa. Macroglossia. Hypertrophied tonsils and adenoids. Enamel hypoplasia with pitting (type A only). The maxillary

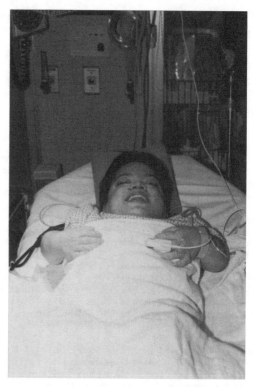

Morquio syndrome. FIG. 1. A pleasant and intelligent 20-year-old woman with Morquio syndrome.

anterior teeth are widely spaced. Short neck with limited movement. May have limited mouth opening due to the temporomandibular joint involvement.

CHEST: Pectus carinatum, rib flaring. Restrictive lung disease from kyphoscoliosis. May have obstructive sleep apnea. The most common cause of death has been respiratory

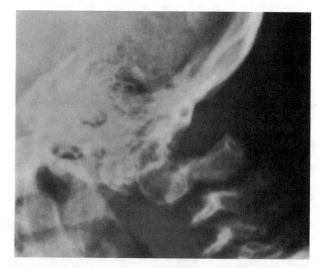

Morquio syndrome. FIG. 2. The same patient at 5 years of age, showing anterior dislocation of C1 on C2. She later had surgical fusion of her cervical spine.

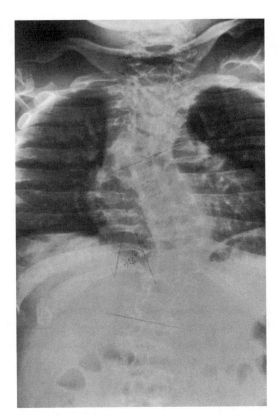

Morquio syndrome. FIG. 3. The same patient at age 13 showing severe scoliosis.

insufficiency from spine and chest deformity. Patients with mucopolysaccharidoses are susceptible to pulmonary hemorrhage after bone marrow transplantation.

CARDIOVASCULAR: Mitral and aortic valve involvement. Aortic insufficiency is relatively common late in the disease. Pulmonary hypertension may develop secondary to lung disease.

NEUROMUSCULAR: Normal intelligence. Atlantoaxial instability with subsequent myelopathy. Most patients require posterior cervical fusion.

ORTHOPEDIC: Short stature due to shortening of the trunk and neck. Shortening of the long bones leading to short, stubby hands. Flattening of the vertebral bodies (platyspondyly). High incidence of cervical spine instability with severe odontoid hypoplasia and atlantoaxial subluxation with risk of paraplegia. Genu valgum. Joint laxity and instability. Kyphoscoliosis, lumbar lordosis.

GI/GU: Hepatomegaly.

MISCELLANEOUS: This disorder was described separately in the same year (1929) by Morquio of Uruguay and Brailsford, a British radiologist. It has in the past been known as Morquio-Brailsford syndrome. Morquio was professor of pediatrics at the University of Montevideo (Uruguay). Conveniently, the chair was established by his family, and he was its second holder. Previously, Osler had misdiagnosed the disorder as cretinism (congenital hypothyroidism).

ANESTHETIC CONSIDERATIONS

These patients have a high incidence of cervical spine instability, particularly odontoid hypoplasia with atlantoaxial subluxation. The cervical spine should be evaluated preoperatively, and precautions should be taken to avoid compression of the cervical spinal cord during positioning or laryngoscopy. Direct laryngoscopy and tracheal intubation may be difficult, and become more and more difficult with age. Neck flexion may occlude the airway. The laryngeal mask airway has been used successfully in patients with mucopolysaccharidoses, as has fiberoptic intubation (4). Patients may require an endotracheal tube that is smaller than predicted. Patients must be carefully positioned intraoperatively secondary to joint laxity and instability. Patients with valvar heart disease need perioperative antibiotic prophylaxis as indicated. Although meningeal involvement has been noted, and scoliosis can occur, a (continuous) spinal technique has been used (3). Needless to say, care must be taken in positioning for a spinal or epidural block in the face of a potentially unstable cervical spine.

Bibliography:

1. Morgan KA, Rehman MA, Schwartz RE. Morquio syndrome and its anaesthetic considerations. *Paediatr Anaesth* 2002;12:641–644.
2. Bartz HJ, Wiesner L, Wappler F. Anaesthetic management of patients with mucopolysaccharidosis IV presenting for major orthopedic surgery. *Acta Anaesthesiol Scand* 1999;43:679–683.
3. Tobias JD. Anesthetic care for the child with Morquio syndrome: general *versus* regional anesthesia. *J Clin Anesth* 1999;11:242–246.
4. Walker RWM, Allen DL, Rothera MR. A fibreoptic intubation technique for children with mucopolysaccharidoses using the laryngeal mask airway. *Paediatr Anaesth* 1997;7:421–426A.
5. Moores C, Rogers JG, McKenzie IM, et al. Anaesthesia for children with mucopolysaccharidoses. *Anaesth Intensive Care* 1996;24:459–463A.
6. Walker RWM, Darowski M, Morris P. Anaesthesia and mucopolysaccharidoses: a review of airway problems in children. *Anaesthesia* 1994;49:1078–1084A.
7. Nott MR, Al Hajaj WH. Anaesthesia for urinary diversion with ileal conduit in a patient with Morquio-Brailsford syndrome. *Anaesth Intensive Care* 1993;21:879–884.
8. Diaz JH, Belani K. Perioperative management of children with mucopolysaccharidoses. *Anesth Analg* 1993;77:1261–1270A.
9. Mahoney A, Soni N, Vellodi A. Anaesthesia and the mucopolysaccharidoses: a review of patients treated by bone marrow transplantation. *Paediatr Anaesth* 1992;2:317–324A.
10. Berkowitz I, Raja S, Bender K, et al. Dwarfs: pathophysiology and anesthetic implications. *Anesthesiology* 1990;73:739–759C.
11. Herrick IA, Rhine EJ. The mucopolysaccharidoses and anaesthesia: a report of clinical experience. *Can J Anaesth* 1988;35:67–73.
12. Sjogren P, Pedersen T, Steinmetz H. Mucopolysaccharidoses and anaesthetic risks. *Acta Anaesthesiol Scand* 1987;31:214–218.
13. King DH, Jones RM, Barrett MB. Anaesthetic considerations in the mucopolysaccharidoses. *Anaesthesia* 1984;39:126–131A.
14. Baines D, Kenneally J. Anaesthetic management of the mucopolysaccharidoses: a fifteen-year experience in a children's hospital. *Anaesth Intensive Care* 1983;11:198–202.
15. Kempthorne PM, Brown TCK. Anaesthesia and the mucopolysaccharidoses: a survey of techniques and problems. *Anaesth Intensive Care* 1983;11:203–207A.

16. Jones AEP. Croley TE Morquio syndrome and anesthesia. *Anesthesiology* 1979;51:261–262.
17. Birkinshaw KJ. Anaesthesia in a patient with an unstable neck: Morquio syndrome. *Anaesthesia* 1975;30:46–49.

Moyamoya Syndrome

MIM #: 252350

Moyamoya syndrome involves progressive occlusion of the intracranial portion of the carotid artery, the middle cerebral artery and the anterior and posterior communicating arteries, with the subsequent development of profuse collateral flow at various levels (leptomeningeal, basal ganglia, and transdural). The telangiectatic collateral vessels produce a characteristic pattern on cerebral angiography (see figure). Cerebral blood flow is severely compromised in these patients, leading to cerebral ischemia. Children usually present before 5 years of age with headache, new onset seizures, transient ischemic attacks and/or hemiplegia. Frequent transient ischemic attacks and strokes lead to a progressive loss of neurologic functions. A high incidence of moyamoya disease is found in Asia, predominantly in Japan. This disorder occurs more frequently in females (female-to-male ratio of 3:2). Surgical revascularization procedures designed to enhance cerebral flow have met with variable (mostly poor) results.

Moyamoya syndrome exhibits genetic heterogeneity, with mapping to chromosomes 3p, 8q, and 17q. There are over 50 cases of Moyamoya syndrome associated with neurofibromatosis (see later), a disease which has also been mapped to chromosome 17q.

Moyamoya syndrome refers to the genetic form of this disorder. Moyamoya disease has been used to refer to the acquired occlusion of the vessels in the circle of Willis, and describes a characteristic pattern of reaction to intracerebral vascular injury. Adults with Moyamoya disease usually present with subarachnoid hemorrhage.

NEUROMUSCULAR: Headaches, seizures, cerebrovascular ischemia—transient ischemic attacks and strokes. Progressive loss of neurologic functions.

MISCELLANEOUS: Moyamoya is a Japanese word which means "something hazy, like a puff of cigarette smoke drifting in the air," often shortened to "puff of smoke," which is descriptive of the net-like image of blood vessels seen on the cerebral angiogram.

ANESTHETIC CONSIDERATIONS
Preoperatively the patient's neurologic history and current status should be assessed. Cerebral blood flow is severely compromised in these patients, and anesthetic management should be tailored to minimize the risk of a perioperative stroke. The affected cerebral vessels and collaterals are maximally dilated, and cerebrovascular responses to changes in the arterial gas tensions and the systemic blood pressure

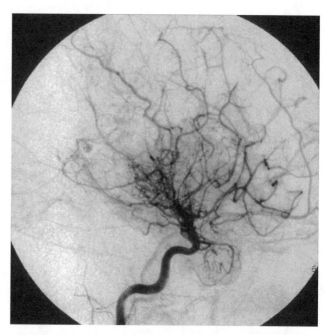

Moyamoya syndrome. Cerebral angiogram demonstrating the fine "puff of smoke" pattern.

can result in further ischemia. Cerebral vasodilators have been shown to lead to intracerebral steal. Cerebral blood flow and oxygen delivery must be maximized, which means that it is imperative to avoid hypoxemia, hypo- or hypercapnia, cerebral vasoconstriction, hypovolemia, hypotension, anemia and increases in blood viscosity. Attention should be given to minimizing the cerebral metabolic rate for oxygen. Inhalational anesthesia with isoflurane has been advocated for these patients because of the favorable cerebral blood flow/cerebral metabolic rate ratio. Total intravenous anesthesia techniques have also been used successfully (2, 5). Despite careful perioperative management, new neurologic deficits postoperatively are not uncommon, particularly after cerebral revascularization surgery. Hypocapnea secondary to crying has been implicated in the development of cerebral ischemia, so it would seem that adequate postoperative analgesia is critical (11). Because of the risk of hyperkalemia in patients with a history of stroke, succinylcholine should be used with caution.

Elective caesarean section has been advocated in the parturient to avoid increases in intracranial pressure with bearing down and hyperventilatory hypocapnea, which can lead to cerebral vasoconstriction. General anesthesia has been suggested as the anesthetic of choice because decreased systemic blood pressure after regional anesthesia may lead to decreased cerebral perfusion (9, 17), although regional techniques have also been used successfully (8, 15).

Bibliography:

1. Baykan N, Ozgen S, Ustalar ZS, et al. Moyamoya disease and anesthesia. *Paediatr Anaesth* 2005;15:1111–1115.

2. Adachi K, Yamamoto Y, Kameyama E, et al. Early postoperative complications in patients with Moyamoya disease—a comparison of inhaled anesthesia with total intravenous anesthesia (TIVA) [Japanese]. *Masui* 2005;54:653–657.
3. Nagashima M, Nagashima K, Endo A, et al. Anesthetic management for elective cesarean section due to placenta previa in a patient with Moyamoya disease [Japanese]. *Masui* 2002;51:1349–1351.
4. Williams DL, Martin IL, Gully RM. Intracerebral hemorrhage and Moyamoya disease in pregnancy. *Can J Anaesth* 2000;47:996–1000.
5. Khan-Ghori SN, Murshid WR, Samarkandi AH, et al. Use of propofol and sevoflurane in Moyamoya disease—case reports and literature review. *Middle East J Anesthesiol* 1999;15:73–83.
6. Sato K, Shirane RKato M, et al. Effect of inhalational anesthesia on cerebral circulation in Moyamoya disease. *J Neurosurg Anesthesiol* 1999;11:25–30.
7. Yusa T, Yamashiro K. Local cortical cerebral blood flow and response to carbon dioxide during anesthesia in patients with Moyamoya disease. *J Anesth* 1999;13:131–135.
8. Abouleish E, Wiggins M, Ali V. Combined spinal and epidural anesthesia for cesarean section in a parturient with Moyamoya disease. *Acta Anaesthesiol Scand* 1998;42:1120–1123.
9. Furuya A, Matsukawa T, Ozaki M, et al. Propofol anesthesia for cesarean section successfully managed in a patient with Moyamoya disease. *J Clin Anesth* 1998;10:242–245.
10. Sakamoto T, Kawaguchi M, Kurehara K, et al. Postoperative neurological deterioration following the revascularization surgery in children with Moyamoya disease. *J Neurosurg Anesthesiol* 1998;10:37–41.
11. Kansha M, Irita K, Takahashi S, et al.Anesthetic management of children with Moyamoya disease. *Clin Neurol Neurosurg* 1997;99:S110–S113.
12. Llorente de la Fuente A, Gimenez Garcia MC, Lopez Sanchez F. Regional anaesthesia in Moyamoya disease. *Br J Anaesth* 1997;78:478–479.
13. Sakamoto T, Kawaguchi M, Kurehara K, et al. Risk factors for neurologic deterioration after revascularization surgery in patients with Moyamoya disease. *Anesth Analg* 1997;85:1060–1065.
14. Wang N, Kuluz J, Barron M, et al. Cardiopulmonary bypass in a patient with Moyamoya disease. *Anesth Analg* 1997;84:1160–1163.
15. Kee WD, Gomersall CD. Extradural anaesthesia for caesarean section in a patient with Moyamoya disease. *Br J Anaesth* 1996;77:550–552.
16. Henderson MA, Irwin MG. Anaesthesia and Moyamoya disease. *Anaesth Intensive Care* 1995;23:503–506.
17. Venkatesh B, Taggart PC. Anaesthetic management of a patient with Moyamoya disease for Caesarean section. *Can J Anaesth* 1994;41:79–80.
18. Soriano SG, Sethna NF, Scott RM. Anesthetic management of children with Moyamoya syndrome. *Anesth Analg* 1993;77:1066–1070.

Muckle-Wells Syndrome

See Urticaria-deafness-amyloidosis syndrome

Mucolipidosis I

See Sialidosis

Mucolipidosis II

See I-cell disease

Mucolipidosis III

See Pseudo-Hurler syndrome

Mucolipidosis IV

MIM #: 252650

This autosomal recessive lysosomal storage disease results in deposits in almost every tissue in the body. It is caused by a mutation in the gene encoding mucolipin-1 (*MCOLN1*) located on the short arm of chromosome 19. A wide variety of gangliosides, phospholipids, and mucopolysaccharides are accumulated in the deposits. Primary manifestations include mental retardation, developmental delay, and eye defects.

Before the biochemistry of the mucolipidoses was understood, it was recognized that these patients had features of both the mucopolysaccharidoses and the sphingolipidoses, hence the name "mucolipidosis."

HEENT/AIRWAY: Normal facies. Corneal clouding from early infancy, retinal degeneration, decreased vision, myopia, puffy eyelids, strabismus, photophobia.

NEUROMUSCULAR: Psychomotor retardation, which is not progressive. Some patients may have improvement in language and motor skills with time, although most remain severely retarded. Hypotonia. Pyramidal tract signs.

ORTHOPEDIC: Normal.

GI/GU: No organomegaly.

MISCELLANEOUS: 80% of patients diagnosed with mucolipidosis IV are of Ashkenazi Jewish ancestry.

Geneological studies of the involved families (currently residing all over the world) indicate that the mucolipidosis IV mutation originated as recently as the 18th or 19th century in the region of northern Poland or Lithuania.

ANESTHETIC CONSIDERATIONS

Patients may have decreased vision, and patients with photophobia may be extremely sensitive to the bright lights in the operating room. Difficulty with direct laryngoscopy and tracheal intubation has not been reported with mucolipidosis IV, although it has been reported with mucolipidosis II, or I-cell disease (see earlier) (3). If the patient's tracheal wall is thickened by deposits, an endotracheal tube that is smaller than predicted may be required.

Bibliography:
1. Bach G. Mucolipidosis type IV. *Mol Genet Metab* 2001;73:197–203.
2. Raas-Rothschild A, Bargal R, DellaPergola S, et al. Mucolipidosis type IV: the origin of the disease in the Ashkenazi Jewish population. *Eur J Hum Genet* 1999;7:496–498.
3. Baines DB, Street N, Overton JH. Anaesthetic implications of mucolipidosis. *Paediatr Anaesth* 1993;3:303–306.
4. Chitayat D, Meunier CM, Hodgkinson KA, et al. Mucolipidosis type IV: clinical manifestations and natural history. *Am J Med Genet* 1991;41:313–318.

Mucopolysaccharidosis I H

See Hurler syndrome

Mucopolysaccharidosis I H/S

See Hurler-Scheie syndrome

Mucopolysaccharidosis I S

See Scheie syndrome

Mucopolysaccharidosis II

See Hunter syndrome

Mucopolysaccharidosis III

See Sanfilippo syndrome

Mucopolysaccharidosis IV

See Morquio syndrome

Mucopolysaccharidosis VI

See Maroteaux-Lamy syndrome

Mucopolysaccharidosis VII

See Sly syndrome

Mucoviscidosis

See Cystic fibrosis

Mulibrey Nanism Syndrome

SYNONYM: Perheentupa syndrome

MIM #: 253250

This autosomal recessive disorder is distinguished by short stature and pericardial constriction. The mnemonic MULIBREY stands for the organs that may be involved: **MU**scle, **LI**ver, **BR**ain, and **EY**es. 'Nanism' derives from the Greek word for "dwarf." The syndrome is caused by a mutation in the gene *TRIM37*, which encodes a peroxisomal protein. Most patients diagnosed with Mulibrey nanism have been Finnish.

HEENT/AIRWAY: Dolichocephaly. Long, shallow sella turcica, hypoplastic frontal or sphenoid sinuses. Triangular facies, frontal bossing. Abnormal retinal pigmentation with clusters of yellowish dots in the fundus. Dental anomalies, including crowded, hypoplastic teeth. High-pitched voice.

CARDIOVASCULAR: During infancy or childhood, a thick, adherent pericardium develops that leads to pericardial constriction and elevated central venous pressure. Many will need a pericardiectomy. Myocardial involvement (including myocardial hypertrophy and myocardial fibrosis) may lead to heart failure. Death from cardiac causes is not uncommon.

NEUROMUSCULAR: Muscular hypotonia. Hypoplastic corpus callosum.

ORTHOPEDIC: Short stature. Cystic fibrous dysplasia, especially of the tibia.

GI/GU: Hepatomegaly secondary to pericardial constriction. Post menarchal ovarian failure. Fibrothecoma (ovarian stromal tumor). Infertility in women.

OTHER: Nevus flammeus. Incomplete breast development. May have immunoglobulin deficiency.

ANESTHETIC CONSIDERATIONS
Patients may have visual abnormalities. Dental abnormalities should be documented preoperatively. Patients may have pericardial constriction with elevated central venous pressures and liver congestion. Myocardial involvement may contribute to congestive heart failure. Succinylcholine should be used with caution in patients with significant muscle involvement because of the risk of exaggerated hyperkalemia.

Bibliography:
1. Karlberg N, Jalanko H, Perheentupa J, et al. Mulibrey nanism: clinical features and diagnostic criteria. *J Med Genet* 2004;41:92–98.
2. Lipsanen-Nyman M, Perheentupa J, Rapola J, et al. Mulibrey heart disease: clinical manifestations, long-term course, and results of pericardiectomy in a series of 49 patients born before 1985. *Circulation* 2003;107:2810–2815.
3. Balg S, Stengel-Rutkowski S, Dohlemann C, et al. Mulibrey nanism. *Clin Dysmorphol* 1995;4:63–69.

Multiple Acyl-CoA Dehydrogenase Deficiency

See Glutaric aciduria II

Multiple Carboxylase Deficiency

See Biotinidase deficiency; Holocarboxylase synthetase deficiency

Multiple Epiphyseal Dysplasia

(Includes Fairbank and Ribbing types of multiple epiphyseal dysplasia)

MIM #: 132400, 226900

This usually autosomal dominant disorder is characterized by short stature, pain and stiffness in the hips and knees, and small, irregular epiphyses. There is extensive phenotypic variability, and multiple epiphyseal dysplasia has been subdivided into a more severe **Fairbank type** and a less severe **Ribbing type.** There is evidence of an autosomal recessive multiple epiphyseal dysplasia caused by a mutation in the *DTDST* gene. There is certainly genetic heterogeneity with this syndrome, even within types. A mutation in the gene for cartilage oligomeric matrix protein (*COMP*) has been identified in some people with multiple epiphyseal dysplasia, and excluded in others. Other genes implicated in multiple epiphyseal dysplasia include *COL9A1, COL9A2, COL9A3, MATN3,* and *DTDST.* Many patients have no identifiable mutations.

HEENT/AIRWAY: May have a round face.

ORTHOPEDIC: Short stature. Small, irregular epiphyses. Progressive joint pain and stiffness, especially of the hips and knees. Premature osteoarthritis, which may require joint replacement. May also have back pain. Short, stubby fingers. Brachydactyly. Hyperextensible fingers. May have symmetric shoulder involvement. Short femoral neck. Patellar dislocation. Abnormalities of the distal tibia. Waddling gait. Clubfoot deformity.

ANESTHETIC CONSIDERATIONS

Patients must be carefully positioned secondary to pain and stiffness in the hips, knees, and back. Older patients may have artificial joints secondary to premature osteoarthritis.

Bibliography:

1. Jakkula E, Makitie O, Czarny-Ratajczak M, et al. Mutations in the known genes are not the major cause of MED; distinctive phenotypic entities among patients with no identified mutations. *Eur J Hum Genet* 2005;13:292–301.
2. Chapman KL, Briggs MD, Mortier GR. Review: clinical variability and genetic heterogeneity in multiple epiphyseal dysplasia. *Pediatr Pathol Mol Med* 2003;22:53–75.
3. Ballhausen D, Bonafe L, Terhal P, et al. Recessive multiple epiphyseal dysplasia (rMED): phenotype delineation in eighteen homozygotes for DTDST mutation R279W [Letter]. *J Med Genet* 2003;40:65–71.
4. Deere M, Blanton SH, Scott CI, et al. Genetic heterogeneity in multiple epiphyseal dysplasia. *Am J Hum Genet* 1995;56:698–704.

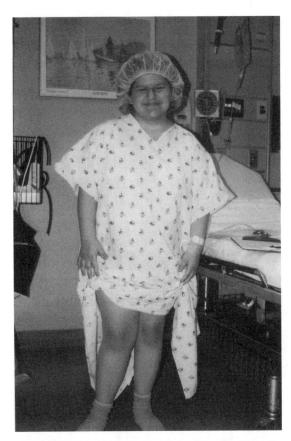

Multiple epiphyseal dysplasia. This 15-year-old with multiple epiphyseal dysplasia is only 4′ 10″ (127 cm) tall. Her mother is similarly short. She has short stubby fingers and involvement of multiple upper and lower extremity joints.

Multiple Exostoses Syndrome

SYNONYM: Diaphyseal aclasis

MIM #: 133700, 133701, 600209

This autosomal dominant syndrome is characterized by bony outgrowths of the cancellous bone between the diaphysis and the epiphysis that ultimately result in deformities of the extremities. The exostoses appear and expand during childhood and adolescence, but do not expand further during adulthood. Multiple exostoses syndrome is genetically heterogeneous. Genes have been mapped to chromosomes 8, 11, and 19. There is evidence that these genes have a tumor-suppressor function. Multiple exostoses can also occur in the Langer-Giedion syndrome (see earlier).

HEENT/AIRWAY: The cranium is usually not involved.

NEUROMUSCULAR: Compression of the spinal cord by exostoses has been reported. Compression of peripheral nerves by exostoses has been reported.

ORTHOPEDIC: Mild short stature. Multiple diaphyseal bony outgrowths, usually capped by cartilage, especially at the ends of long bones. Involved bone can be short or bowed. Deformity of the legs, forearms, and hands is most common. The knee is frequently involved. Overriding toes. Metacarpals can be short. Ribs and scapulae may be involved. May have enchondromas. Rare chondrosarcoma, osteosarcoma.

ANESTHETIC CONSIDERATIONS

The exostoses may compress peripheral nerves, causing a peripheral neuropathy. A complete neurologic examination should be performed before performing regional anesthesia. Patients need to be carefully positioned secondary to deformities of the extremities.

Bibliography:
1. Stieber JR, Dormans JP. Manifestations of hereditary multiple exostoses. *J Am Acad Orthop Surg* 2005;13:110–120.
2. Francannet C, Cohen-Tanugi A, Le Merrer M, et al. Genotype-phenotype correlation in hereditary multiple exostoses. *J Med Genet* 2001;38:430–434.
3. Quirini GE, Meyer JR, Herman M, et al. Osteochondroma of the thoracic spine: an unusual cause of spinal cord compression. *AJNR Am J Neuroradiol* 1996;17:961–964.

Multiple Lentigines Syndrome

See LEOPARD syndrome

Multiple Pterygium Syndrome

SYNONYM: Escobar syndrome; Pterygium syndrome

MIM #: 265000

This autosomal recessive disorder is characterized by multiple pterygia, camptodactyly, syndactyly, cleft palate, and severe micrognathia. The responsible gene and gene product for this probably autosomal recessive disorder are not currently known.

HEENT/AIRWAY: Hypertelorism, ptosis, inner canthal folds. Low-set ears. May have conductive hearing loss. Cannot open mouth widely, ankyloglossia (adhesion of the tongue to the palate). Syngnathia (intraoral webbing). Cleft palate. Severe micrognathia. Webbing of the neck.

CHEST: Severe kyphoscoliosis may lead to a restrictive lung disease and to problems such as dyspnea and recurrent pneumonia.

CARDIOVASCULAR: May have a cardiac defect.

NEUROMUSCULAR: Normal intelligence. May have hypotonia, muscular atrophy.

ORTHOPEDIC: Pterygia (webbing of the skin) across multiple joints, usually progressive, and may lead to fixed contractures of the joints. Camptodactyly. Syndactyly. Clubfeet,

rocker-bottom feet. Small stature. Scoliosis. Kyphosis. Vertebral fusion, usually cervical.

GI/GU: Cryptorchidism, hypospadias. Hypoplastic labia majora. May have diaphragmatic hernia.

ANESTHETIC CONSIDERATIONS

Oral, mandibular, and neck involvement limit mouth opening, position the tongue posteriorly, limit neck extension, and severely limit direct visualization of the larynx. The laryngeal mask airway has been used successfully (1, 2). Increasing rotation and flexion of the neck may make airway management more difficult as the patient grows older.

Patients may have a restrictive lung disease. Morbidity from respiratory disease is reportedly high (4). Patients must be carefully positioned secondary to pterygia and possible fixed joint contractures. Severe scoliosis, kyphosis, or vertebral fusion makes neuraxial anesthesia technically difficult. One poorly documented case, not in the anesthesia literature, suggested association with malignant hyperthermia, but this is very unlikely (5).

Bibliography:
1. Saif-Ur-Rehman Siddiqui M, Kymer P, Mayhew JF. Escobar syndrome [Letter]. *Paediatr Anaesth* 2004;14:799–800.
2. Kuzma Pi, Calkins MD, Kline MD, et al. The anesthetic management of patients with multiple pterygium syndrome. *Anesth Analg* 1996;83:430–432.
3. Spranger S, Spranger M, Meinck HM, et al. Two sisters with Escobar syndrome. *Am J Med Genet* 1995;57:425–428.
4. Ramer JC, Ladda RL. Demuth WW Multiple pterygium syndrome. An overview. *Am J Dis Child* 1988;142:794–798.
5. Robinson LK, O'Brien NC, Puckett MC, et al. Multiple pterygium syndrome: a case complicated by malignant hyperthermia. *Clin Genet* 1987;32:5–9.

Multiple Synostosis Syndrome

MIM #: 186500

This autosomal dominant syndrome consists of multiple synostoses, particularly of the digits (symphalangism) and carpal and tarsal bones. The synostoses are progressive. This disorder is due to a mutation in the gene encoding noggin (*NOG*), which is important to fetal limb growth and development. There is marked variability in clinical expression.

HEENT/AIRWAY: Narrow face. Strabismus. External ear anomalies, conductive hearing loss. Hypoplastic alae nasi, hypoplastic nasal septum. Short philtrum, thin upper lip. May have Klippel-Feil sequence (see earlier).

CHEST: Pectus excavatum.

NEUROMUSCULAR: May have mental retardation. May have stenosis of the cervical spinal canal.

ORTHOPEDIC: Multiple and progressive synostoses, involving digits (symphalangism), elbows, carpal bones, and tarsal bones. Hypoplasia of distal digits, nails. Cutaneous syndactyly, clinodactyly, brachydactyly. May have subluxation of the radial head. May have calcaneonavicular synostosis. Limited joint mobility at the shoulder, elbow, hip. Short feet. May have vertebral anomalies.

ANESTHETIC CONSIDERATIONS

Positioning may be difficult due to limited joint mobility.

Bibliography:
1. Edwards MJ, Rowe L, Petroff V. Herrmann multiple stenosis syndrome with neurological complications caused by spinal canal stenosis. *Am J Med Genet* 2000;95:118–122.
2. Poush JR. Distal symphalangism: a report of two families. *J Hered* 1991;82:233–238.
3. da-Silva EO, Filho SM, de Albuquerque SC. Multiple synostosis syndrome: study of a large Brazilian kindred. *Am J Med Genet* 1984;18:237–247.

Multisynostotic Osteodysgenesis

See Antley-Bixler syndrome

Münchausen Syndrome by Proxy

SYNONYM: Meadow syndrome

MIM #: None

Münchausen syndrome by proxy is an entity in the pediatric population that is analogous to the Münchausen syndrome in the adult population. In Münchausen syndrome by proxy, parents report or create fictitious medical problems in their children to gain medical attention. This type of child endangerment can be extremely difficult to diagnose. Children of both sexes and all ages are at risk, although it is most common in infants and young children. In most cases, the responsible parent is the mother. These parents often have some rudimentary medical training, appear to be extremely conscientious caregivers, and tend to form intense personal bonds with the medical personnel who are involved with their child's care. There are many ways in which Münchausen syndrome by proxy can present, the most common being vomiting, diarrhea, fever, bleeding (hematemesis, hematuria), seizures, and apnea. Münchausen syndrome by proxy should be considered in any patient who has repeated serious illnesses of unknown etiology, whose siblings have had a similar history, whose symptoms occur only in the presence of the parent, whose illness takes an atypical course, or whose illness fails to respond to the usual therapy. Little physical harm is done to the child if the parent merely fabricates the symptoms in the child, although these children are at risk of unnecessary diagnostic tests, many of which are invasive. More harm is done if the parent actually produces the symptoms in the child. This can be accomplished in a multitude of ways, most commonly through poisoning, suffocation, exsanguination,

introduction of exogenous blood into the GI tract or bladder, or inoculation with bacteria. The mortality rate from this syndrome may be as high as 10%.

MISCELLANEOUS: Born in Germany in 1720, Baron von Münchausen was notorious for his fictitious accounts of travel, adventure, and achievement. In the 1950s, his name became associated with the syndrome in which adults fabricate medical illness to gain medical attention. In 1977, Roy Meadow coined the phase 'Münchausen syndrome by proxy' in an article in *The Lancet* to describe how children could be victimized by this disorder. Meadow became an expert on the sudden infant death syndrome (SIDS) and was knighted in 1998 for "services to child health." However, in 2005 the British General Medical Council found Meadow guilty of "serious professional misconduct" for his expert testimony (which was subsequently found to be erroneous) in the trials of three women who were initially convicted (but later exonerated) of murdering their infant children.

ANESTHETIC CONSIDERATIONS

Occasionally, anesthesiologists or surgeons are in a position to suspect Münchausen syndrome by proxy, as when a child is repeatedly referred for diagnostic tests that are always normal. When such a diagnosis is suspected, the patient's primary care physician must be consulted. Extreme care must be taken in dealing with the parents, particularly in the perioperative setting (3). The management and treatment of Münchausen syndrome by proxy is difficult and lengthy, and involves multiple health care professionals as well as child protective services.

Bibliography:
1. Galvin HK, Newton AW, Vandeven AM. Update on Munchausen syndrome by proxy. *Curr Opin Pediatr* 2005;17:252–257.
2. Craft AW, Hall DM. Munchausen syndrome by proxy and sudden infant death. *Br Med J* 2004;328:1309–1312.
3. Watts J. Parental presence during induction of anaesthesia. *Anaesthesia* 1997;52:284.

MURCS Association

MIM #: 601076

This sporadically occurring disorder involves **MU**llerian duct aplasia, **R**enal aplasia, and **C**ervicothoracic **S**omite dysplasia.

HEENT/AIRWAY: May have facial asymmetry. May have external ear defects, hearing loss. May have cleft lip or palate, micrognathia.

CARDIOVASCULAR: A patient has been reported with tetralogy of Fallot.

NEUROMUSCULAR: Occipital encephalocele. Rare cerebellar cyst.

ORTHOPEDIC: Short stature. Cervicothoracic vertebral defects, including partial to complete cervical fusion. May have rib anomalies, winged scapula, absent radius, duplicated thumb.

GI/GU: Mullerian duct aplasia—absence of the proximal vagina and hypoplasia or absence of the uterus (the Rokitansky-Kuster-Hauser syndrome, see later). Renal aplasia. May have anal atresia.

ANESTHETIC CONSIDERATIONS
Micrognathia is usually mild, and is unlikely to interfere with the ease of direct laryngoscopy and intubation. Cervicothoracic vertebral defects, particularly cervical spine fusion, may make visualization of the larynx by direct laryngoscopy more difficult. Renal insufficiency affects perioperative fluid management and the choice of anesthetic drugs.

Bibliography:
1. Suri M, Brueton LA, Venkatraman N, et al. MURCS association with encephalocele: report of a second case. *Clin Dysmorphol* 2000;9:31–33.
2. Carranza-Lira S, Forbin K, Martinez-Chequer JC. Rokitansky syndrome and MURCS association–clinical features and basis for diagnosis. *Int J Fertil Womens Med* 1999;44:250–255.
3. Braun-Quentin C, Billes CBowing B, et al. MURCS association: case report and review. *J Med Genet* 1996;33:618–620.

Muscle Phosphofructokinase Deficiency

See Glycogen storage disease type VII

Muscle Phosphorylase Deficiency

See McArdle syndrome

Muscle–Eye–Brain Disease

MIM #: 253280
This autosomal recessive disorder affects the eyes, muscle, and brain. It is caused by a mutation in *O*-mannose beta-1,2-*N*-acetylglucosaminyltransferase (*POMGNT1*), which is important in the synthesis of *O*-mannosyl glycan. There are phenotypic similarities between this disorder and Walker-Warburg syndrome (see later), but they are nonetheless distinct syndromes caused by distinct chromosomal abnormalities. The Walker-Warburg phenotype tends to be more severe.

HEENT/AIRWAY: Glaucoma, cataracts, retinal hypoplasia, retinal detachment, congenital myopia, strabismus, nystagmus, centrally regulated abnormal eye movements, blindness. Temporomandibular joint contractures may limit mouth opening.

NEUROMUSCULAR: Severe mental retardation, seizures, myoclonic jerks. Surface abnormalities of the brain and cerebellum (lissencephaly, agyria, pachygyria, polymicrogyria). Absence of cortical lamination. Aqueductal stenosis. Hypotonia, weakness, and congenital muscular dystrophy with elevated creatine kinase levels. Creatine kinase levels do not correlate with the clinical severity, they tend to be highest in infancy and decline with age.

ORTHOPEDIC: Joint contractures may be present at birth.

GI/GU: Abnormal swallowing.

OTHER: Hypothermia, suggesting abnormal hypothalamic function has been reported (1).

ANESTHETIC CONSIDERATIONS
Temporomandibular joint contractures may limit mouth opening and make direct laryngoscopy difficult (3). Chronic use of anticonvulsant medications may alter the metabolism of some anesthetic drugs. Perioperative temperature regulation may be abnormal. Rhabdomyolysis and elevations of creatine kinase with the administration of succinylcholine have been reported, and succinylcholine is contraindicated (3, 4). Malignant hyperthermia has not been reported after halothane/succinylcholine anesthesia.

Bibliography:
1. Taniguchi K, Kobayashi K, Saito K, et al. Worldwide distribution and broader clinical spectrum of muscle-eye-brain disease. *Hum Mol Genet* 2003;12:527–534.
2. Cormand B, Pihko H, Bayes M, et al. Clinical and genetic distinction between Walker-Warburg syndrome and muscle-eye-brain disease. *Neurology* 2001;56:1059–1069.
3. Gropp A, Kern C, Frei FJ. Anaesthetic management of a child with muscle-eye-brain disease. *Paediatr Anaesth* 1994;4:197–200.
4. Karhunen U. Serum creatinine kinase levels after succinylcholine in children with "muscle, eye, and brain disease". *Can J Anaesth* 1988;35:90–92.

Muscular Dystrophy

See the specific type of muscular dystrophy: Becker muscular dystrophy, Duchenne muscular dystrophy, Emery-Dreifuss muscular dystrophy, Facioscapulohumeral muscular dystrophy, Limb-girdle muscular dystrophy.

Myositis Ossificans Progressiva

See Fibrodysplasia ossificans progressiva syndrome

Myotonia Congenita

SYNONYM: Thomsen disease

MIM #: 160800
Myotonia congenita is one of the myotonic syndromes. The most common of the myotonic syndromes is myotonic dystrophy (see later). Myotonia congenita is an autosomal

dominant form of myotonia that is due to a mutation in the *CLCN1* (skeletal muscle chloride channel) gene. The myotonia is related to lack of normal chloride influx during repolarization, which impairs the ability of the skeletal muscle voltage-gated chloride channels to maintain normal muscle excitability. Becker disease (see earlier), a recessive disorder, involves different mutations in the same gene. The disease presents in childhood without further progression, and is associated with normal life expectancy without significant handicap.

HEENT/AIRWAY: Blepharospasm (myotonia of the eyelids) may be symptomatic.

CARDIOVASCULAR: No cardiac involvement.

NEUROMUSCULAR: The hallmark finding, myotonia, refers to delayed relaxation of contracted muscle. Examples include the inability to release a handshake ("action myotonia"), or the sustained contraction caused by direct tapping or stimulation of a tendon reflex ("percussion myotonia"—best elicited by tapping the thenar eminence or finger extensors). In myotonia congenita, unlike in myotonic dystrophy, the myotonia worsens after rest and improves after exercise (the "warm-up phenomenon"). In myotonia congenita (unlike in myotonic dystrophy), the myotonia worsens with cold. All muscle groups are affected. There may be muscle hypertrophy.

MISCELLANEOUS: First described by Dr. A. J. T. Thomsen, a Danish physician practicing in Germany, in himself and his family. In 1876, when Dr. Thomsen was 61 years old, his youngest son, who was affected by the disease, was accused of trying to avoid military service. Thomsen reacted by writing his definitive account, in which he traced the disease back to his maternal great-grandmother.

ANESTHETIC CONSIDERATIONS

Anesthetic or surgical manipulations may induce myotonic contractions, as can cold and shivering. Even pain from the intravenous injection of propofol may cause myotonic contractions. These patients may have abnormal drug reactions.

Neither regional anesthesia nor muscle relaxants prevent or reverse myotonic contractions. Drugs that have been used to attenuate the contractions are quinine, procainamide, phenytoin, volatile anesthetics, and steroids. When all else fails, direct infiltration of the muscle with a local anesthetic has been recommended. Succinylcholine can induce sustained contraction of chest wall muscles, making positive-pressure ventilation difficult even in the intubated patient (see figure, myotonic dystrophy, later). A case has been reported of a 32-year-old woman who displayed profound generalized muscle spasms which precluded mouth opening and adequate ventilation following succinylcholine administration. This was the first significant manifestation of her disease (3). Response to nondepolarizing muscle relaxants is normal in myotonia congenita, but nondepolarizing muscle relaxants will not counteract myotonic contractions which have already been provoked. Anticholinesterase drugs used to reverse nondepolarizing muscle relaxants can precipitate myotonia, and the use of shorter acting muscle relaxants that do not require reversal has been suggested. An association with susceptibility to malignant hyperthermia has been suggested, although the exact relationship is unclear (2,4,5,7,8). The muscle rigidity that routinely follows succinylcholine administration in patients with myotonia may confuse the question of malignant hyperthermia susceptibility.

Bibliography:
1. Colding-Jorgensen E. Phenotypic variability in myotonia congenita. *Muscle Nerve* 2005;32:19–34.
2. Veyckemans F. Muscular chanellopathies and hypermetabolic reactions [Letter]. *Acta Anaesthesiol Scand* 2005;49:124–125.
3. Farbu E, Softerland E, Bindoff LA. Anaesthetic complications associated with myotonia congenital: case study and comparison with other myotonic disorders. *Acta Anaesthesiol Scand* 2003;47:630–634.
4. Rosenbaum HK, Miller JD. Malignant hyperthermia and myotonic disorders. *Anesthesiol Clin North America* 2002;20:623–664A.
5. Russell SH, Hirsch NP. Anaesthesia and myotonia. *Br J Anaesth* 1994;72:210–216.
6. Ptacek LJ, Johnson KJ, Griggs RC. Genetics and physiology of the myotonic muscle disorders. *N Engl J Med* 1993;328:482–489.
7. Haberer JP, Fabre F, Rose E. Malignant hyperthermia and myotonia congenita (Thomsen disease). *Anaesthesia* 1989;44:166.
8. Heiman-Patterson T, Martino C, Rosenberg H, et al. Malignant hyperthermia in myotonia congenita. *Neurology* 1988;38:810–812.

Myotonic Dystrophy

SYNONYM: Steinert disease. (Includes congenital myotonic dystrophy)

MIM #: 160900

Myotonic dystrophy is the most common of the myotonic syndromes. Unlike the other myotonias, myotonic dystrophy is a multisystem disease. And, unlike most of the other myotonias, it is associated with dystrophy of the muscles. Children who are symptomatic from infancy typically have more severe disease in adulthood than those whose symptoms do not appear until later in childhood. Patients who have been symptomatic since infancy are often considered to have a clinically distinguishable disease, referred to as **congenital myotonic dystrophy.**

The molecular defect in myotonic dystrophy is the amplification of a GCT nucleotide triplet upstream from the gene for the protein myotonic dystrophy protein kinase. This kinase normally limits the intracellular sodium current. Dysfunction of the protein kinase results in a larger sodium current and altered muscle excitability. This is potentially the etiology of sudden (presumably tachyarrhythmic) death. Myotonic dystrophy is inherited in an autosomal dominant fashion. Interestingly, although it is autosomal dominant, symptomatic infants are more likely to have inherited this disease from their mother. Each successive generation inheriting the disease has an increased number of GCT triplets, and therefore increased severity of the disease.

Succinylcholine (mg/kg)

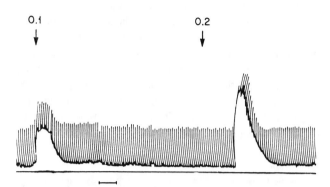

Myotonic dystrophy. The evoked thumb adductor response to succinylcholine in a myotonic patient. The upward shift in the baseline tension represents the contracture. (From Mitchell MM, Ali HN, Savarese JJ. Myotonia and neuromuscular blocking agents. *Anesthesiology* 1978;49:44–48 with permission.)

Newborns with symptomatic myotonic dystrophy may be dependent on a mechanical ventilator. Prolonged neonatal mechanical ventilation was previously thought to be uniformly fatal, but two recent survivors have been reported.

HEENT/AIRWAY: Premature frontal baldness, muscle wasting leading to hollowed cheeks and temporal fossae. Facial weakness leads to an "expressionless" face. Extraocular muscle involvement is a consistent finding. Cataracts. Neonates with congenital myotonic dystrophy can have facial diplegia with a tent-shaped mouth.

CHEST: Bulbar weakness may lead to recurrent aspiration pneumonia. Involvement of the diaphragm and intercostal muscles may lead to a poor cough and alveolar hypoventilation. Patients may have central or obstructive sleep apnea. Neonates with congenital myotonic dystrophy may have profound weakness of respiratory muscles, requiring mechanical ventilation.

CARDIOVASCULAR: Cardiac symptoms may be the presenting feature. Ninety percent of the patients have conduction abnormalities; first-degree heart block and intraventricular conduction delays are the most common. Patients may have left axis deviation and ST-T wave changes. Sudden death has been associated with the development of third-degree block, but also occurs in the presence of a functioning pacemaker, suggesting ventricular tachyarrhythmia. Inducible sustained ventricular tachycardia (in the electrophysiology laboratory) is due to bundle-branch reentry, which should be ablatable. Cardiac enlargement and interstitial fatty infiltration and fibrosis can occur. Impaired ventricular function is usually a late finding. There is an increased incidence of mitral valve prolapse. There is little correlation between the severity of the cardiac disease and the severity of the muscle disease.

NEUROMUSCULAR: The hallmark finding, myotonia, refers to delayed relaxation of contracted muscle. Examples include the inability to release a handshake ("action myotonia"), or the sustained contraction caused by direct tapping or stimulation of a tendon reflex ("percussion myotonia"–best elicited by tapping the thenar eminence or finger extensors). Facial, neck, and distal musculature is primarily involved, with the preservation of limb-girdle strength until late in the disease. In myotonic dystrophy, unlike in myotonia congenita, myotonia worsens after exercise. In some apparently unaffected siblings, myotonia can be detected only electromyographically. When made audible, the electromyogram sounds somewhat like being buzzed by a propeller-driven dive bomber. There may be mild mental retardation. Patients with congenital myotonic dystrophy are hypotonic at birth. Muscle tone and strength then improve over the first years of life, but there is an inexorable progression of the disease to the adult form during the first decade. Patients exhibit muscle wasting.

ORTHOPEDIC: Clubfoot deformity is common in young children with symptomatic disease. Neonates with congenital myotonic dystrophy may present with arthrogryposis.

GI/GU: Dysphagia, reduced peristalsis. Neonates with congenital myotonic dystrophy can have such poor sucking and swallowing that they require feeding through a nasogastric tube. Intestinal pseudoobstruction and spontaneous pneumoperitoneum have been reported. Gonadal atrophy or ovarian failure with infertility may occur.

OTHER: Associated with premature labor, uterine atony, and postpartum hemorrhage. Pregnancy may exacerbate muscle symptoms. May have abnormal insulin response to glucose. May have increased incidence of colloid goiters.

MISCELLANEOUS: "The production of muscle relaxation in a myotonic patient is one of the most difficult problems facing the anesthesiologist" (11). The incidence of this disease is particularly high in Quebec.

ANESTHETIC CONSIDERATIONS

Anesthetic or surgical manipulations may induce myotonic contractions, as can cold and shivering. The patient's body temperature should be maintained as close to normal as possible for this reason. Even pain from the intravenous injection of propofol may cause myotonic contractions (13).

Neither regional anesthesia nor muscle relaxants prevent or reverse myotonic contractions. Drugs that have been used to attenuate the contractions are quinine, procainamide, phenytoin, volatile anesthetics, and steroids. When all else fails, direct infiltration of the muscle with a local anesthetic has been recommended. Succinylcholine can induce sustained contraction of the chest wall muscles, making positive-pressure ventilation difficult even in the intubated patient (see figure). Succinylcholine may even cause tonic contractions in infants with congenital myotonic dystrophy in whom clinically apparent myotonia has not yet developed (24). Because of dystrophic muscle changes, it is possible that in advanced cases succinylcholine might result in an exaggerated hyperkalemic response—another reason to avoid the drug. This disease has not been associated with malignant hyperthermia.

Responses to nondepolarizing muscle relaxants have generally been reported as normal, although sensitivity to vecuronium has been described (2). Anticholinesterase drugs used for reversing nondepolarizing muscle relaxants can precipitate myotonia, hence the use of shorter acting muscle relaxants that do not require reversal has been suggested. Tracheal intubation can often be performed after an intravenous induction followed by the administration of a volatile anesthetic, without the use of muscle relaxants.

A baseline electrocardiogram should be examined because 90% of the patients have conduction abnormalities, usually first-degree heart block or intraventricular conduction delays. Patients may have ST-T wave changes that can be mistaken for ischemia. The development of a third-degree heart block has been associated with asystole. The patients may be at risk for ventricular tachyarrhythmias (3). Ventricular function usually remains normal until late in the disease. Patients with mitral valve prolapse and regurgitation require perioperative antibiotic prophylaxis as indicated.

These patients may have abnormal drug reactions. They appear more likely to experience apnea after the administration of a wide variety of intravenous anesthetics, including propofol, benzodiazepines, opioids, and barbiturates, although a primary propofol technique has been reported without complications. Preoperative sedation must be carefully titrated in a monitored setting. The patients also need to be observed closely postoperatively for signs of respiratory depression. There is a report of a patient experiencing severe respiratory depression after a small dose of epidural morphine (18). There are numerous potential possibilities for drug–drug interactions, as many of these patients are medicated with quinine, procainamide or phenytoin to attenuate the contractions. Procainamide, for example, can prolong nondepolarizing neuromuscular blockade (4).

These patients often have dysphagia and reduced peristalsis, and thus are at increased risk of perioperative aspiration (1,4,29). Weakness and atrophy of the respiratory muscles may cause postoperative respiratory complications in neonates as well as in adults. The response to nondepolarizing muscle relaxants is, however, normal. Even without significant respiratory muscle weakness, patients may have an inadequate cough, which predisposes to postoperative pulmonary complications.

Although epidural anesthesia has been used successfully (15), the associated shivering may precipitate myotonic contractions. Uterine atony may cause excessive postpartum hemorrhage.

Bibliography:

1. Jenkins JA, Facer EK. Anesthetic management of a patient with myotonic dystrophy for a Nissen fundoplication and gastrostomy. *Paediatr Anaesth* 2004;14:693–696.
2. Nishi M, Itoh H, Tsubokawa T, et al. Effective doses of vecuronium in a patient with myotonic dystrophy. *Anaesthesia* 2004;59:1216–1218.
3. Bassez G, Lazarus A, Desguerre I, et al. Severe cardiac arrhythmias in young patients with myotonic dystrophy type 1. *Neurology* 2004;63:1939–1941.
4. White RJ, Bass SP. Myotonic dystrophy and paediatric anaesthesia. *Paediatr Anaesth* 2003;13:94–102.
5. Colovic V, Walker RW. Myotonia dystrophica and spinal surgery. *Paediatr Anaesth* 2002;12:351–355.
6. Rosenbaum HK, Miller JD. Malignant hyperthermia and myotonic disorders. *Anesthesiol Clin North America* 2002;20:623–664B.
7. Imison AR. Anaesthesia and myotonia - an Australian experience. *Anaesth Intensive Care* 2001;29:34–37.
8. White RJ, Bass S. Anaesthetic management of a patient with myotonic dystrophy. *Paediatr Anaesth* 2001;11:494–497.
9. Bennun M, Goldstein B, Finkelstein Y, et al.Continuous propofol anaesthesia for patients with myotonic dystrophy. *Br J Anaesth* 2000;85:407–409.
10. Takahashi K, Nosaka S. Carbon dioxide narcosis caused by midazolam in a patient with myotonic dystrophy. *Anaesthesia* 2000;55:97.
11. Miller J, Rosenbaum H. Muscle diseases. In: Benumoff J, ed. *Anesthesia & uncommon diseases*, 4th ed. Philadelphia: WB Saunders, 1998:316–397.
12. Mathieu J, Allard P, Gobeil G. Anesthetic and surgical complications in 219 cases of myotonic dystrophy. *Neurology* 1997;49:1646–1650.
13. Kinney MAO, Harrison BA. Propofol-induced myotonia in myotonic dystrophy [Letter]. *Anesth Analg* 1996;83:665–666.
14. Campbell AM, Thompson N. Anaesthesia for caesarean section in a patient with myotonic dystrophy receiving warfarin therapy. *Can J Anaesth* 1995;42:409–414.
15. Tobias JD. Anaesthetic management of the child with myotonic dystrophy: epidural anaesthesia as an alternative to general anaesthesia. *Paediatr Anaesth* 1995;5:335–338.
16. Diefenbach C, Abel M, Buzello W. Vecuronium titration for muscle relaxation in myotonic dystrophy. *Paediatr Anaesth* 1994;4:133–135.
17. Russell SH, Hirsch NP. Anaesthesia and myotonia. *Br J Anaesth* 1994;72:210–216A.
18. Ogawa K, Iranami H, Yoshiyama T, et al. Severe respiratory depression after epidural morphine in a patient with myotonic dystrophy. *Can J Anaesth* 1993;40:968–970.
19. Walpole AR, Ross AW. Acute cord prolapse in an obstetric patient with myotonia dystrophica. *Anaesth Intensive Care* 1992;20:526–528.
20. Tanaka M, Tanaka Y. Cardiac anesthesia in a patient with myotonic dystrophy. *Anaesthesia* 1991;46:462–465.
21. Speedy H. Exaggerated physiological responses to propofol in myotonic dystrophy. *Br J Anaesth* 1990;64:110–112.
22. Blumgart CH, Hughes DG, Redfier N. Obstetric anaesthesia in dystrophia myotonica. *Anaesthesia* 1990;45:26–29.
23. White DA, Smyth DG. Continuous infusion of propofol in dystrophica myotonia. *Can J Anaesth* 1989;36:200–203.
24. Anderson BJ, Brown TCK. Anaesthesia for a child with congenital myotonic dystrophy. *Anaesth Intensive Care* 1989;17:351–354.
25. Anderson BJ, Brown TCK. Congenital myotonic dystrophy in children: a review of ten years' experience. *Anaesth Intensive Care* 1989;17:320–324.
26. Castano J, Pares N. Anaesthesia for major abdominal surgery in a patient with myotonia dystrophica. *Br J Anaesth* 1987;59:1629–1631.
27. Moore JK, Moore AR. Postoperative complications of dystrophia myotonica. *Anaesthesia* 1987;42:529–533.
28. Cope DK, Miller JN. Local and spinal anesthesia for cesarean section in a patient with myotonic dystrophy. *Anesth Analg* 1986;65:687–689.
29. Ishizawa Y, Yamaguchi H, Dohi S, et al. A serious complication due to gastrointestinal malfunction in a patient with myotonic dystrophy. *Anesth Analg* 1986;65:1066–1068.
30. Mitchell MM, Ali HN, Savarese JJ. Myotonia and neuromuscular blocking agents. *Anesthesiology* 1978;49:44–48.

Myotubular Myopathy

SYNONYM: Centronuclear myopathy

MIM #: 310400

This X-linked myopathy is due to mutations in the gene for myotubularin. Myotubularin is required for muscle cell differentiation. Histologically one sees a large number of centrally located nuclei in the myocytes, hence the synonym "centronuclear myopathy." This disease is usually fatal in infancy secondary to respiratory insufficiency. Prolonged survival often requires mechanical ventilation. Several families with X-linked disease with survival into adulthood have been reported. There are also autosomal recessive and dominant forms of this disease. The autosomal recessive form usually has an earlier onset than the autosomal dominant form. The disease is slowly progressive, and most patients are wheelchair bound or dead by the second or third decade of life. The autosomal dominant form is usually manifest by the third decade, and the progression is slower than with either the X-linked or autosomal recessive forms.

The other congenital myopathies are central core disease (see earlier), mini-core myopathy (not covered in this text) and nemaline rod myopathy (see later).

HEENT/AIRWAY: Large head circumference. External ophthalmoplegia. Ptosis. Can have high-arched palate. Micrognathia in the X-linked form.

CHEST: Neonatal respiratory distress. Respiratory failure from restrictive disease. Atrophic or thin diaphragm.

NEUROMUSCULAR: Profound hypotonia. Areflexia. Can develop seizures. Intellectual development is usually normal. May have difficulties in swallowing.

ORTHOPEDIC: Scoliosis.

GI/GU: Pyloric stenosis. Liver dysfunction. Gallstones. Renal stones or nephrocalcinosis. Cryptorchidism.

OTHER: Increased birth length. Polyhydramnios. Serum creatine kinase levels are usually normal or only mildly elevated.

MISCELLANEOUS: The name myotubular myopathy derives from the histological similarity of these diseased muscles to fetal myotubes. Some practitioners reserve the term "myotubular myopathy" for referring to the X-linked form, and use "centronuclear myopathy" for the autosomal forms.

ANESTHETIC CONSIDERATIONS
Patients with swallowing difficulties are at increased risk of perioperative aspiration. In view of a suspected case of malignant hyperthermia and the similarity of this disease to central core disease, it has been suggested that malignant hyperthermia precautions be observed (4,8). Succinylcholine should be avoided in this myopathy due to the risk of an excessive hyperkalemic response. Response to nondeplarizing muscle relaxants is probably normal, but they may not be required in this disease of markedly diminished muscle tone. Patients are at risk of perioperative respiratory failure.

Bibliography:

1. Schmid E, Johr M, Berger TM. X-linked myotubular myopathy: anesthetic management for muscle biopsy. *Paediatr Anaesth* 2006;16:218–220.
2. Pierson CR, Tomczak K, Agrawal P, et al. X-linked myotubular and centronuclear myopathies. *J Neuropathol Exp Neurol* 2005;64:555–564.
3. Costi D, Ven der Walt JH. General anesthesia in an infant with X-linked myotubular myopathy. *Paediatr Anaesth* 2004;14:964–968.
4. Tokarz A, Gaszynski T, Gaszynski W, et al. General anaesthesia with remifentanil and propofol for a patient with centronuclear (myotubular) myopathy. *Eur J Anaesthesiol* 2002;19:842–844.
5. Wallgren-Pettersson C. Nemaline and myotubular myopathies. *Semin Pediatr Neurol* 2002;9:132–144.
6. Breslin D, Reid JHayes A, et al.Anaesthesia in myotubular (centronuclear) myopathy. *Anaesthesia* 2000;55:471–474.
7. Herman GE, Finegold M, de Gouyon B, et al. Medical complications in long-term survivors with X-linked myotubular myopathy. *J Pediatr* 1999;134:206–214.
8. Gottschalk A, Heiman-Patterson T, deQuevedo R II, et al. General anesthesia for a patient with contronuclear (myotubular) myopathy. *Anesthesiology* 1998;89:1018–1020.

N

N-Acetylglutamate Synthetase Deficiency

SYNONYM: NAGS deficiency

MIM #: 237310

This autosomal recessive disorder is closely related to the urea cycle defects. The urea cycle degrades amino acids to urea, and defects in the urea cycle can lead to hyperammonemia. Symptoms of this disorder can be triggered by stress such as surgery or infection, or episodes of protein catabolism such as the involution of the postpartum uterus. Liver transplantation is curative.

N-acetylglutamate, an activator of carbamylphosphate synthetase, is synthesized in the liver by mitochondrial *N*-acetylglutamate synthetase (NAGS). Without *N*-acetylglutamate, carbamylphosphate synthetase cannot be activated. Carbamylphosphate synthetase deficiency (see earlier) is one of the urea cycle defects.

NEUROMUSCULAR: Hyperammonemic encephalopathy is clinically similar to hepatic encephalopathy, and is characterized by lethargy, agitation, and confusion with eventual coma and cerebral edema. Between acute episodes, mental status is normal, but there may be developmental delay or mental retardation.

OTHER: Episodes of hyperammonemia begin with anorexia and lethargy. Vomiting and headaches may be prominent.

ANESTHETIC CONSIDERATIONS

Patients should maintain high carbohydrate intake (and low protein intake) perioperatively. Intravenous fluids and dextrose should be used generously perioperatively to avoid hypovolemia and protein catabolism. An orogastric tube or throat packs should be placed if the surgery has the potential to cause oral or intestinal bleeding because blood in the gastrointestinal tract provides a protein load that may lead to the development of hyperammonemia. Acute metabolic encephalopathy can present after anesthesia.

FIGURES: See Appendix C

Bibliography:

1. Elpeleg O, Shaag A, Ben-Shalom E, et al. *N*-acetylglutamate synthase deficiency and the treatment of hyperammonemic encephalopathy. *Ann Neurol* 2002;52:845–849.
2. Urea Cycle Disorders Conference group. Consensus statement from a conference for the management of patients with urea cycle disorders. *J Pediatr* 2001;138:(S1-5).
3. Colombo JP. *N*-acetylglutamate synthetase (NAGS) deficiency. *Adv Exp Med Biol* 1994;368:135–143.
4. Schubiger G, Bachmann C, Barben P, et al. N-acetylglutamate synthetase deficiency: diagnosis, management and follow-up of a rare disorder of ammonia detoxication. *Eur J Pediatr* 1991;150:353–356.

NADH-Coenzyme Q Reductase Deficiency

See Complex I deficiency

NADH-Ubiquinone Oxidoreductase Deficiency

See Complex I deficiency

Nager Acrofacial Dysostosis Syndrome

See Nager syndrome

Nager Syndrome

SYNONYM: Nager acrofacial dysostosis syndrome

MIM #: 154400

This mandibulofacial dysostosis syndrome has craniofacial abnormalities that are similar to those of the Treacher Collins syndrome, conductive hearing loss and radial limb hypoplasia. Most cases of Nager syndrome have been sporadic, but there is some evidence for either autosomal dominant or autosomal recessive inheritance. Although genetic heterogeneity is likely, a gene responsible for this syndrome may reside on chromosome 9.

HEENT/AIRWAY: Characteristic facies with absent zygomatic arches and hypoplastic malar region. Down-slanting palpebral fissures, absent lower eyelashes, lower lid coloboma. Low-set, posteriorly rotated ears. Conductive hearing loss. Choanal atresia. Small mouth. Cleft palate, soft palate agenesis, velopharyngeal insufficiency. Micrognathia. Hypoplasia of the larynx or epiglottis.

CHEST: Neonates may experience respiratory distress secondary to micrognathia and palatal anomalies.

CARDIOVASCULAR: May have a congenital cardiac defect.

NEUROMUSCULAR: Intelligence is usually normal. May have hydrocephalus, agenesis of the corpus callosum, polymicrogyria.

ORTHOPEDIC: Short stature. Hypoplastic or aplastic radius. Radioulnar synostosis. Limited elbow extension. Hypoplastic or aplastic thumbs. Occasional syndactyly, clinodactyly, or camptodactyly. Shortened humerus. Clubfoot deformity. Dislocated hips. May have cervical vertebral anomalies, scoliosis.

GI/GU: May have Hirschsprung disease (see earlier). May have genitourinary anomalies.

MISCELLANEOUS: Mandibular hypoplasia is often worse than in Treacher Collins syndrome. Miller syndrome (see earlier) also has Treacher Collins-like facies, but is distinguishable from Nager syndrome because it involves postaxial rather than preaxial (radial) upper limb defects. In 2005, Gobbel and colleagues identified Nager syndrome in a fetus found in the Meckel anatomical collection at the University of Halle, Germany. The specimen dates to 1812, and is currently the earliest known example of Nager syndrome.

ANESTHETIC CONSIDERATIONS

Small mouth, micrognathia, and hypoplasia of the larynx make direct laryngoscopy and tracheal intubation very difficult or impossible. Urgent tracheostomy or retrograde intubation techniques have been required. Passage of an endotracheal tube through a laryngeal mask airway (LMA) has also been reported (2). The mouth may be too small to allow adequate surgical exposure to repair a palatal cleft (7). Choanal atresia precludes placement of a nasal airway, nasal intubation, or placement of a nasogastric tube. Peripheral vascular access may be difficult to obtain secondary to limb deformities. Radial anomalies may make placement of a radial arterial catheter more difficult. Patients with congenital cardiac defects require perioperative antibiotic prophylaxis as indicated.

Bibliography:

1. Groeper K, Johnson JO, Braddock SR, et al. Anaesthetic implications of Nager syndrome. *Paediatr Anaesth* 2002;12:365–368.

2. Pivalizza EG, McGraw-Wall BL, Khalil SN. Alternative approach to airway management in Nager syndrome [Letter]. *Can J Anaesth* 1997; 44:228.
3. Perkins JA, Sie KC, Milczuk H, et al. Airway management in children with craniofacial anomalies. *Cleft Palate Craniofac J* 1997;34:135–140.
4. Przybylo HJ, Stevenson GW, Vicari FA, et al. Retrograde fibreoptic intubation in a child with Nager syndrome. *Can J Anaesth* 1996;43:679–679.
5. Fryns JP, Bonhomme A, van den Berghe H. Nager acrofacialdysostosis: an adult male with severe neurological deficit. *Genet Couns* 1996;7: 147–151.
6. Friedman RA, Wood E, Pransky SM, et al. Nager acrofacial dysostosis: management of a difficult airway. *Int J Pediatr Otorhinolaryngol* 1996; 35:69–72.
7. Walker JS, Dorian RS, Marsh NJ. Anesthetic management of a child with Nager syndrome [Letter]. *Anesth Analg* 1994;79:1025–1026.

NAGS Deficiency

See *N*-acetylglutamate synthetase deficiency

Nail-Patella Syndrome

SYNONYM: Hereditary onychoosteodysplasia

MIM #: 161200

This autosomal dominant disorder is characterized by nail dysplasia, patellar hypoplasia, and dysplasia of other mesenchymal tissues. It is caused by a mutation in the gene for LIM-homeodomain protein (*LMX1B*). The nail-patella gene locus and the ABO blood group locus are closely linked on the long arm of chromosome 9.

HEENT/AIRWAY: Cloverleaf pigmentation of the inner margin of the iris. Sensorineural hearing loss. May have ptosis, microcornea, cataracts. May have cleft lip or palate.

NEUROMUSCULAR: May have mental deficiency, spina bifida. May have muscular aplasia. Occasional psychosis.

ORTHOPEDIC: Dysplastic nails. Hypoplastic or absent patella. Limited joint mobility, especially at the elbows. May have antecubital pterygia. Joint dislocations, especially the head of the radius. Posterior iliac spurs. Valgus deformity of femoral neck. Clubfoot deformity. Premature osteoarthritis. May have scoliosis.

GI/GU: Nephropathy similar to glomerulonephritis, with proteinuria, hematuria or casts. Renal insufficiency may develop by the late teens.

OTHER: May have polyarteritis-like vasculitis.

ANESTHETIC CONSIDERATIONS
Patients with renal insufficiency need careful titration of perioperative fluids and judicious use of renally excreted drugs. Proteinuria may lead to significant hypoalbuminemia. Patients must be carefully positioned, with attention to their limited joint mobility and tendency toward joint dislocation.

Bibliography:
1. Ogden JA, Cross GL, Guidera KJ, et al. Nail patella syndrome. A 55-year follow-up of the original description. *J Pediatr Orthop* 2002;11B: 333–338.
2. Bongers EM, Gubler MC, Knoers NV. Nail-patella syndrome. Overview on clinical and molecular findings. *Pediatr Nephrol* 2002;17:703–712.
3. Rizzo R, Pavone L, Micali G, et al. Familial bilateral pterygia with severe renal involvement in nail-patella syndrome. *Clin Genet* 1993;44:1–7.

NARP Syndrome

MIM #: 551500

This disorder is characterized by sensory **N**europathy, **A**taxia, and **R**etinitis **P**igmentosa. It is due to a specific point mutation in the segment of mitochondrial DNA encoding subunit 6 of mitochondrial adenosine triphosphatase. This is a component of complex V of the respiratory chain. The clinical severity in general parallels the relative amount of the mutant DNA, which may be unevenly distributed in the different tissues.

HEENT/AIRWAY: Retinitis pigmentosa with eventual blindness.

NEUROMUSCULAR: Sensory neuropathy, developmental delay, seizures, ataxia, dementia. Neurogenic muscle weakness without myopathy. Some reinnervation of muscle may occur.

ANESTHETIC CONSIDERATIONS
When meeting the patient before surgery, recall that he or she may have loss of vision. Chronic use of anticonvulsant medications may affect the metabolism of some anesthetic drugs. Although not reported, the small amount of denervation with collateral reinnervation described suggests that succinylcholine should be avoided. Although there are no clinical reports, it is reasonable to avoid the use of nitroprusside because cyanide can inhibit the electron transport chain. Although barbiturates and volatile anesthetics can inhibit mitochondrial respiration, induction of anesthesia with thiopental has been used without any complications in the related Leigh disease (see earlier).

Bibliography:
1. DiMauro S, Schon EA. Mitochondrial respiratory-chain diseases. *N Engl J Med* 2003;348:2656–2668.
2. Kerrison JB, Biousse V, Newman NJ. Retinopathy of NARP syndrome. *Arch Ophthalmol* 2000;118:298–299.
3. Ciccotelli KK, Prak EL, Muravchick S. An adult with inherited mitochondrial encephalomyopathy: report of a case. *Anesthesiology* 1997;87:1240–1242.

Nemaline Rod Myopathy

MIM #: 161800, 256030, 609284

This congenital myopathy is related to central core disease (see earlier) and the mitochondrial myopathies.

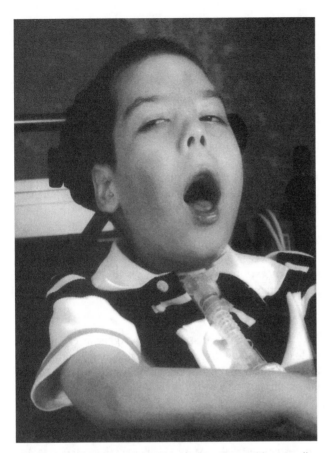

Nemaline rod myopathy. This young boy with nemaline rod myopathy has obvious myopathic facies and requires mechanical ventilation.

It is inherited autosomally, and displays clinical and genetic heterogeneity. There are several subtypes, which are clinically indistinguishable from each other. Type 1, which is autosomal dominant, is due to a defect in the gene for tropomyosin-3. Type 2, which is autosomal recessive, is due to a mutation in the gene encoding nebulin, another muscle protein. Type 3, which is apparently inherited in an autosomal dominant fashion, is caused by a mutation in the alpha-actin-1 gene. In all forms, the type I muscle fibers exhibit subsarcolemmal rod-like structures, which are presumably derived from Z-disk material. Some patients can have a moderate, non-progressive disease, and there can be clinical variability within a family.

The other congenital myopathies are central core disease (see earlier), mini-core myopathy (not covered in this text) and myotubular myopathy (see earlier).

HEENT/AIRWAY: The face is long with a high-arched palate. Malocclusion and micrognathia or prognathism are common.

CHEST: There can be involvement of the diaphragm and the intercostal muscles. Restrictive disease from kyphoscoliosis. Death is usually from respiratory failure. Pectus excavatum.

CARDIOVASCULAR: Although several children with congenital heart disease have been reported (4), it is not clear if this represents a part of the pathologic process or it is a chance occurrence. A small number of patients who have developed a cardiomyopathy have been reported.

NEUROMUSCULAR: Hypotonia, weak cry, and poor sucking in infancy. Delayed motor development. Truncal and proximal limbs are typically involved as in most myopathies, but distal limb, pharyngeal, and facial muscles can also become involved. Intelligence is usually normal.

ORTHOPEDIC: Kyphosis, scoliosis. Congenital hip dislocation, pes cavus.

GI/GU: Poor swallowing.

OTHER: Serum creatine kinase levels are usually normal. Sudden progression of the severity of the disease in late middle age has been reported.

MISCELLANEOUS: "Nema" is the Greek word for thread, descriptive of the subsarcolemmal rod-like structures that are seen histopathologically in this disease.

ANESTHETIC CONSIDERATIONS

The narrow face, micrognathia, and malocclusion may make direct laryngoscopy and tracheal intubation difficult. Preoperative pulmonary function testing may be used to evaluate the patient's pulmonary status at baseline. Patients should be evaluated for congenital heart disease and/or cardiomyopathy preoperatively. They may be at increased risk for aspiration. They are also at risk for postoperative respiratory complications. Severely affected patients may require postoperative ventilation. Postoperative pain with splinting may further impair pulmonary function. Successful spinal anesthesia in a neonate has been reported (2) but loss of intercostals muscle activity with a high level could be problematic.

The use of succinylcholine has been reported in a single case. There was delayed onset of relaxation and no excessive potassium release (6). Muscle relaxation is often not necessary in patients with significant muscle weakness, and in fact may be ill advised in patients with poor muscular reserve.

Malignant hyperthermia has not been described in patients with nemaline rod myopathy.

Bibliography:
1. Wallgren-Pettersson C. Nemaline and myotubular myopathies. *Semin Pediatr Neurol* 2002;9:132–144.
2. Shenkman Z, Sheffer O, Erez I, et al. Spinal anesthesia for gastrostomy in an infant with nemaline myopathy. *Anesth Analg* 2000;91:858–859.
3. Stackhouse R, Chelmow D, Dattel BJ. Anesthetic complications in a pregnant patient with nemaline myopathy. *Anesth Analg* 1994;79: 1195–1197.
4. Asai T, Fujise K, Uchida M. Anaesthesia for cardiac surgery in children with nemaline myopathy. *Anaesthesia* 1992;47:405–408.
5. Cunliffe M, Burrows FA. Anaesthetic implications of nemaline rod myopathy. *Can Anaesth Soc J* 1985;32:543–547.

6. Heard SO, Kaplan RF. Neuromuscular blockade in a patient with nemaline myopathy. *Anesthesiology* 1983;59:588–590.

Neonatal Progeroid Syndrome

SYNONYM: Wiedemann-Rautenstrauch syndrome

MIM #: 264090

Children with this autosomal recessive disorder present with progeroid features at birth (see Progeria later). The responsible gene and gene product are not known. Most patients die in infancy, however survival into the second decade has been reported.

HEENT/AIRWAY: Pseudohydrocephalus, macrocephaly, persistent anterior fontanelle, prominent scalp veins. Triangular face. Ectropion. Progressive beaking of nose. Dysphagia. High-pitched voice. May have neonatal teeth. Protruding chin.

CARDIOVASCULAR: May have congenital cardiac defects.

NEUROMUSCULAR: Mild to moderate psychomotor developmental delay.

ORTHOPEDIC: Osteopenia. Long slender bones. May develop scoliosis in adolescence.

GI/GU: Urinary reflux. Delayed onset of puberty.

OTHER: Prenatal growth deficiency, generalized lipodystrophy with absence of subcutaneous fat. Abnormal fat accumulation in flank, buttocks, and perineum. Sparse scalp hair, eyebrows, eyelashes. May have hyperinsulinemia and possibly insulin resistance. May have variable endocrine abnormalities.

ANESTHETIC CONSIDERATIONS
Unlike progeria, premature atherosclerotic cardiovascular disease has not been reported. Lack of subcutaneous fat may make a good mask fit difficult. Neonatal teeth (teeth present at birth) may be loose, and can be lost during laryngoscopy. Lack of subcutaneous fat may lead to perioperative hypothermia. A case of propofol infusion syndrome after six hours of propofol has been reported. Presumably this is related to abnormal lipid metabolism, although this patient had received propofol uneventfully before (1).

Bibliography:
1. Hermanns H, Lipfert P, Ladda S, et al. Propofol infusion syndrome during anaesthesia for scoliosis surgery in an adolescent with neonatal progeroid syndrome [Letter]. *Acta Anaesthesiol Scand* 2005;50:393–394.
2. Arboleda H, Arboleda G. Follow-up study of Wiedemann-Rautenstrauch syndrome: long-term survival and comparison with Rautenstrauch's patient "G". *Birth Defects Res A Clin Mol Teratol* 2005;73:562–568.
3. Pivnick EK, Angle B, Kaufman RA, et al. Neonatal progeroid (Wiedemann-Rautenstrauch) syndrome: report of five new cases and review. *Am J Med Genet* 2000;90:131–140.

Neu-Laxova Syndrome

MIM #: 256520

This autosomal recessive, early lethal syndrome is distinguished by microcephaly, characteristic facies with exophthalmos, lissencephaly, and syndactyly. Patients are stillborn or die in the neonatal period. The responsible gene and gene product are not currently known.

HEENT/AIRWAY: Microcephaly, sloping forehead. Characteristic canine facies with hypertelorism and exophthalmos. Absent eyelids, cataracts. Large ears. Flat nose. Round mouth with large lips. May have cleft lip or palate. Micrognathia. Short neck.

CARDIOVASCULAR: May have patent ductus arteriosus, patent foramen ovale, atrial septal defect, ventricular septal defect, transposition of the great vessels.

NEUROMUSCULAR: Lissencephaly. Agenesis of the corpus callosum, cortical hypoplasia, anencephaly, spina bifida, Dandy-Walker malformation, choroid plexus cysts. Muscular atrophy.

ORTHOPEDIC: Short limbs. Syndactyly. Calcaneovalgus. Joint contractures, pterygia. Poorly mineralized bones. Adipose hypertrophy. Marked subcutaneous edema.

GI/GU: Abnormal external genitalia, including cryptorchidism. May have renal agenesis.

OTHER: Thin skin with ichthyosis. Abnormal placenta. Intrauterine growth deficiency.

ANESTHETIC CONSIDERATIONS
This disorder is lethal early on, and there is rarely an indication for surgery. Intubation (also not indicated) may be difficult secondary to micrognathia, short neck, and marked edema.

Bibliography:
1. Manning MA, Cunniff CM, Colby CE, et al. Neu-Laxova syndrome: detailed prenatal diagnostic and post-mortem findings and literature review. *Am J Med Genet A* 2004;125:240–249.
2. Rouzbahani L. New manifestations in an infant with Neu Laxova syndrome [Letter]. *Am J Med Genet* 1995;56:239–240.

Neurocutaneous Melanosis

MIM #: 249400

This degenerative disorder is distinguished by skin and meningeal pigmentation, and central nervous system deterioration. Melanosis of the skin is apparent at birth. Central nervous system function may be normal at birth, but central nervous system deterioration usually results in death during early childhood. Neural or cutaneous malignant degeneration occurs in most patients. The pathogenesis is assumed to be related to a developmental aberration in the neural crest cells that ultimately form the skin and meninges.

NEUROMUSCULAR: Meninges are thick and pigmented, with focal accumulations of melanotic cells. The brain and spinal cord are involved. There is progressive deterioration of central nervous system function because of progressive pigmentation and thickening of the meninges. Mental retardation develops, as well as seizures, cranial nerve palsies, spinal cord compression, and psychosis. Hydrocephalus occurs secondary to blockage of cisternal pathways or obliteration of the arachnoid villi. There may be increased intracranial pressure. May have Dandy-Walker malformation. Meningeal melanomas eventually occur in most patients.

GI/GU: May have Meckel diverticulum. May have urinary tract anomalies, including ureteral malformations, unilateral renal cysts, renal agenesis.

OTHER: Large, pigmented nevus, usually on the trunk, or numerous smaller nevi are apparent at birth. Cutaneous nevi can become malignant.

ANESTHETIC CONSIDERATIONS

Patients with hydrocephalus and increased intracranial pressure warrant precautions to avoid further elevations in intracranial pressure. Patients may have symptomatic spinal cord compression. Patients with renal disease will need fluid and medications titrated carefully perioperatively. Chronic use of anticonvulsant medications may alter the metabolism of some anesthetic drugs.

Bibliography:
1. Plikaitis CM, David LR, Argenta LC. Neurocutaneous melanosis: clinical presentations. *J Craniofac Surg* 2005;16:921–925.
2. Burstein F, Seier H, Hudgins PA, et al. Neurocutaneous melanosis. *J Craniofac Surg* 2005;16:874–876.
3. Acosta FL, Binder DK, Barkovich AJ, et al. Neurocutaneous melanosis presenting with hydrocephalus. Case report and review of the literature. *J Neurosurg* 2005;102S:96–100.

Neurofibromatosis

SYNONYM: von Recklinghausen disease

MIM #: 162200, 101000

There are at least two types of neurofibromatosis (NF). NF-1 is the classic von Recklinghausen neurofibromatosis, and is seen in 85% of patients with NF. It is inherited in an autosomal dominant fashion, with a relatively high incidence of new mutations and significant clinical variability. Sporadic cases may arise from paternal germ cell mutations. NF-1 is characterized by cutaneous café au lait spots, peripheral and central nervous system neurofibromas, osseous

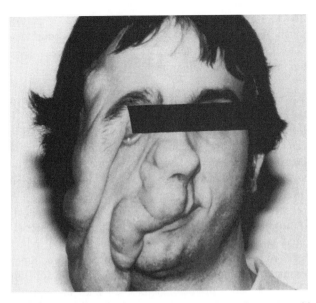

Neurofibromatosis. Severe cutaneous involvement with neurofibromatosis in a young man. (Courtesy of Dr. K. Lin and the Craniofacial Anomalies Clinic, University of Virginia Health System.)

abnormalities, and certain other tumors, particularly of the central nervous system. Pheochromocytomas may develop in adult patients. The gene responsible for NF-1 is located on the long arm of chromosome 17, and the gene product is called neurofibromin. Neurofibromin influences guanine nucleotide metabolism and the function of the ras oncoprotein. Presumably its effect on a tumor supressor gene modulates the development of the wide range of tumors which can be found in NF-1.

NF-2 ("central neurofibromatosis") lacks the peripheral and cutaneous manifestations of NF-1. It is characterized by bilateral schwannomas of the eighth cranial nerve, meningiomas of the brain, and schwannomas of the dorsal roots of the spinal cord. It is also inherited in an autosomal dominant fashion, and is linked to a gene on chromosome 22, clearly distinct from the gene that causes NF-1. The NF-2 gene product, called schwannomin, may have a tumor suppressor function. Some patients with NF have manifestations of Noonan syndrome (see later).

The expression of this disease is highly variable. Included in the following are the possible features of NF-1.

HEENT/AIRWAY: Macrocephaly. Dysplasia of the sphenoid wing. Hypertelorism. Lisch nodules (iris hamartomas), optic glioma possibly causing blindness, choroid hamartomas, glaucoma, cataracts. Sphenoid wing dysplasia may cause pulsating exophthalmos. Acoustic neuromas or bony deformity of the acoustic meatus may cause deafness. Airway obstruction from pharyngeal neurofibromas has been reported, but is rare. There can be laryngeal involvement, typically of the arytenoids and aryepiglottic folds. Large parapharyngeal tumors can also impinge upon the airway.

CHEST: Restrictive lung disease from kyphoscoliosis. Pulmonary fibrosis with pulmonary hypertension in adulthood. Pectus excavatum. Large posterior mediastinal masses can compress the trachea and bronchi.

CARDIOVASCULAR: An arterial vasculopathy affects typically the abdominal aorta or its branches, resulting in renovascular hypertension. The vasculopathy has recently been reported to affect the limb vasculature, causing limb hypoplasia (9). Hypertension secondary to pheochromocytoma may be intermittent or persistent. Death due to aneurysm rupture has been reported.

NEUROMUSCULAR: Neurofibromas of the cranial nerves, spinal cord, nerve roots, or peripheral nerves. Nodular plexiform neurofibromas may grow along the spinal columns, eventually eroding the spine and compressing the cord. Increased incidence of meningiomas, gliomas, and ependymomas. Pituitary or hypothalamic dysfunction. May have mental retardation, developmental delay, learning disabilities. May have seizures.

ORTHOPEDIC: Kyphoscoliosis (usually cervical and upper thoracic). An overlying hair whorl may precede the development of kyphoscoliosis (Ricardi sign). Cervical spine stiffness. Massive leg overgrowth, thinning of long bone cortex. Tibial pseudarthrosis is fairly specific to NF-1. Short stature. Pathologic fractures.

OTHER: The classic skin finding is café au lait spots. Commonly there is freckling in intertriginous regions, such as the axillae and inguinal area.

Pruritus may be associated with a rapidly growing neurofibroma. There are four types of neurofibromas:

1. Cutaneous: the most common.
2. Subcutaneous: may be tender.
3. Nodular plexiform: clusters of neurofibromas along proximal nerve roots and major nerves. These are noninfiltrating.
4. Diffuse plexiform: may have overlying hyperpigmentation. Infiltration of the surrounding tissue can cause disfigurement. These have the potential for malignant degeneration.

The list of tumors that can develop is long and includes meningioma, optic or other glioma, ependymoma, acoustic neuroma, hypothalamic tumors, schwannoma, neurofibrosarcoma, parathyroid adenoma, rhabdomyosarcoma, duodenal carcinoid, somatostatinoma, and pheochromocytoma. Although only 0.1% to 6% of patients with NF-1 will develop pheochromocytoma, up to 25% of patients with pheochromocytoma will have NF-1. NF has been associated with Moyamoya syndrome (see earlier).

Can develop endocrinopathies, including central precocious puberty or growth hormone deficiency. Pregnancy can initiate or exacerbate the growth of neurofibromas, and is associated with the development of pheochromocytoma. Pregnancy can also see worsening hypertension.

MISCELLANEOUS: This is one of the phakomatoses, or neurocutaneous disorders. Other phakomatoses include Sturge-Weber syndrome, tuberous sclerosis, von Hippel-Lindau syndrome and nevus sebaceus syndrome of Jadassohn. "Phakos" is Greek for a lentil or lens-shaped spot.

Friedreich von Recklinghausen was a German pathologist at the turn of the last century. He was an assistant to Virchow. The first clear description of the disorder was made by Robert W. Smith of the University of Dublin 33 years before von Recklinghausen's description in 1882. von Recklinghausen was the first to appreciate that the tumors had a neural origin.

It is now widely believed that Joseph Merrick (the "Elephant Man") probably had Proteus syndrome (see later) and not NF, as has been suggested in the past.

ANESTHETIC CONSIDERATIONS

Mask ventilation or tracheal intubation may be difficult because of neck stiffness, facial bone deformities, macroglossia, or tumors of the tongue or larynx (1, 8). A patient was reported in whom a large neurofibroma at the base of the tongue caused airway obstruction, requiring an emergency tracheostomy after the induction of anesthesia (14). Atlantoaxial dislocation has been reported, but is rare. Kyphoscoliosis may make supine positioning difficult.

Severe spinal deformity may cause restrictive lung disease. Hypertension is common in these patients, and has a variety of potential causes. Baseline hypertension should be evaluated preoperatively. In patients with sudden perioperative hypertension, the possibility of a pheochromocytoma should be considered.

Increased sensitivity to succinylcholine and nondepolarizing muscle relaxants has been reported in the past, but current thought is that these patients respond normally to neuromuscular blockers (6, 11). Chronic use of anticonvulsant medications may alter the metabolism of some anesthetic drugs.

Because of the high incidence of cord involvement, spinal or epidural techniques should be used only when neuroimaging has shown that there are no nearby cord lesions (3, 5).

Bibliography:

1. Moorthy SS, Radpour S, Weisberger EC. Anesthetic management of a patient with tracheal neurofibroma. *J Clin Anesth* 2005;17:290–292.
2. Alexianu D, Skolnick ET, Pinto AC, et al. Severe hypotension in the prone position in a child with neurofibromatosis, scoliosis and pectus excavatum presenting for posterior spinal fusion. *Anesth Analg* 2004; 98:334–335.
3. Sahin A, Aypar U. Spinal anesthesia in a patient with neurofibromatosis. *Anesth Analg* 2003;97:1855–1856.
4. Delgado JM, de la Matta Martin M. Anaesthetic implications of von Recklinghausen neurofibromatosis. *Paediatr Anaesth* 2002;12:374.
5. Esler MD, Durbridge J, Kirby S. Epidural haematoma after dural puncture in a parturient with neurofibromatosis. *Br J Anaesth* 2001;87: 932–934.
6. Hirsch NP, Murphy A, Radcliffe JJ. Neurofibramatosis: clinical presentations and anaesthetic implications. *Br J Anaesth* 2001;86:555–564.

7. Diaz JH. Perioperative management of children with congenital phakomatoses. *Paediatr Anaesth* 2000;10:121–128.
8. Wulf H, Brinkmann G, Rautenberg M. Management of the difficult airway. A case of failed fiberoptic intubation. *Acta Anaesthesiol Scand* 1997;41:1080–1082.
9. Zachos M, Parkin PC, Babyn PS. Neurofibromatosis type I vasculopathy associated with lower limb hypoplasia. *Pediatrics* 1997;100:395–398.
10. Gutmann DH, Aylsworth A, Carey JC, et al. The diagnostic evaluation and multidisciplinary management of neurofibromatosis 1 and neurofibromatosis 2. *JAMA* 1997;278:51–57.
11. Richardson MG, Setty GK, Rawoof SA. Responses to nondepolarizing neuromuscular blockers and succinylcholine in von Recklinghausen neurofibromatosis. *Anesth Analg* 1996;82:382–385.
12. Dounas M, Mercier FJ, Lhuissier C, et al. Epidural analgesia for labour in a parturient with neurofibromatosis. *Can J Anaesth* 1995;42:420–424.
13. Cohen MM. Understanding Proteus syndrome, unmasking the elephant man, and stemming elephant fever. *Neurofibromatosis* 1988;1:260–280.
14. Crozier C. Upper airway obstruction in neurofibromatosis. *Anaesthesia* 1987;42:1209–1211.

Nevoid Basal Cell Carcinoma Syndrome

See Basal cell nevus syndrome

Nevus Sebaceus of Jadassohn

SYNONYM: Linear sebaceous nevus syndrome; Epidermal nevus syndrome; Sebaceous nevus syndrome

MIM #: 163200

This neurocutaneous syndrome involves midfacial linear sebaceous nevi, seizures, and mental retardation. Some patients manifest sebaceous nevi without any neurologic signs. The genetic basis for this syndrome, if any, is unknown.

HEENT/AIRWAY: May have cranial asymmetry with hemimegalencephaly, facial asymmetry. Sphenoid abnormalities, abnormalities of the sella turcica. May have esotropia, colobomas of the eyes and eyelids, cleft palate, dental abnormalities.

CARDIOVASCULAR: Congenital cardiac lesions include patent ductus arteriosus, ventricular septal defect, coarctation of the aorta, hypoplastic left heart. May have cardiac arrhythmias. May have hypoplasia of the pulmonary artery.

NEUROMUSCULAR: Seizures, which are often difficult to control. Variable mental retardation. May have cortical hypoplasia, arachnoid cysts, hydrocephalus, hemiparesis, cranial nerve palsies, cortical blindness, intracerebral calcifications. May have cerebral hamartomas. Linear sebaceous nevi are more likely to be associated with the underlying central nervous system disorders.

ORTHOPEDIC: May have scoliosis, kyphosis. Abnormalities of the ulna, radial head, humerus, or fibula. May have polydactyly, syndactyly.

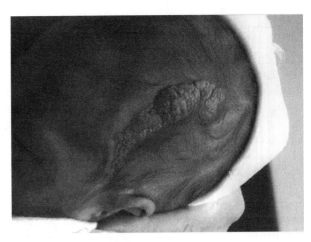

Nevus sebaceus of Jadassohn. A linear nevus on the scalp of an infant. (Courtesy of Dr. Ilona Frieden, Department of Dermatology, University of California, San Francisco.)

GI/GU: May have cryptorchidism. May have hypoplasia of the renal artery, renal hamartomas.

OTHER: Linear sebaceous nevi, especially in the midfacial region. Usually present at birth as raised, yellow, waxy lesions and may have periods of rapid growth. Over time, the lesions become hyperpigmented, hyperkeratotic, and verrucous. Malignant basal cell carcinoma may develop. There is an approximately 15 to 20% risk of malignant degeneration of the lesions.

Vitamin D-resistant rickets occasionally develops, which is responsive to calcitriol and phosphorus, or removal of the lesions. This form of rickets is a variant of tumor-induced osteomalacia.

MISCELLANEOUS: This is one of the phakomatoses, or neurocutaneous disorders. Other phakomatoses include neurofibromatosis, Sturge-Weber syndrome, tuberous sclerosis, and von Hippel-Lindau syndrome. "Phakos" is Greek for a lentil or lens-shaped spot.

ANESTHETIC CONSIDERATIONS

Dental abnormalities should be documented preoperatively. Asymmetric head and face may lead to difficult mask fit and/or difficult tracheal intubation (1). Chronic use of anticonvulsant medications may alter the metabolism of some anesthetic drugs. Patients with a congenital heart disease require perioperative antibiotic prophylaxis as indicated.

Bibliography:
1. Diaz JH. Perioperative management of infants with the naevus sebaceous syndrome of Jadassohn: report of two cases. *Paediatr Anaesth* 2000;10:669–673.
2. Diaz JH. Perioperative management of children with congenital phakomatoses. *Paediatr Anaesth* 2000;10:121–128.
3. van de Warrenburg BP, van Gulik S, Renier WO, et al. The linear naevus sebaceus syndrome. *Clin Neurol Neurosurg* 1998;100:126–132.
4. Carey DE, Drezner MK, Hamdan JA, et al. Hypophosphatemic rickets/osteomalacia in linear sebaceous nevus syndrome: a variant of tumor-induced osteomalacia. *J Pediatr* 1986;109:994–1000.

Niemann-Pick Disease

MIM #: 257200, 257220, 607616, 607625

Niemann-Pick disease is actually a group of diseases, the sphingomyelin-cholesterol lipidoses. Clinical manifestations are due to lipid storage, predominantly in the reticuloendothelial system, brain, and viscera. Large foam cells are found in the marrow and reticuloendothelial system.

These disorders are inherited in an autosomal recessive fashion, and have been classified into types. Type A (classic infantile form) and type B (visceral form) are due to a deficiency of sphingomyelinase, with accumulation of sphingomyelin and cholesterol. Type C (subacute or juvenile form) is due to a mutation in the *NPC1* gene (type C1) or the *NPC2* gene (type C2). Several other types have also been described. Type A has the most prominent neurologic findings.

HEENT/AIRWAY: Corneal opacification with brownish discoloration of the anterior lens capsule. Approximately half the cases have a cherry-red spot in the macular area.

CHEST: Pulmonary infiltration. Restrictive lung disease. Respiratory problems.

NEUROMUSCULAR: The classic disease, type A, has rapidly progressive central nervous system degeneration after approximately 1 year of age. Psychomotor delay and regression, seizures, behavioral changes, myoclonus, ataxia.

GI/GU: Hepatosplenomegaly, vomiting, diarrhea. Possible hypersplenism.

OTHER: Lipid-filled foam cells in the marrow, spleen, adrenals, brain, lymph nodes, and lung. Yellow-brown discoloration of the skin. Failure to thrive, recurrent fever.

Successful hematopoietic stem cell transplantation has been reported in at least three cases of type B disease.

MISCELLANEOUS: Niemann first described this disease, and thought it was a fulminant form of Gaucher disease. Thirteen years later, Pick, a pathologist, recognized this disease as a distinct entity. Despite having served with distinction in the German army during WWI, Pick was removed to the Theresienstadt concentration camp during WWII, where he died in 1944 at the age of 76 years.

ANESTHETIC CONSIDERATIONS

Patients usually accommodate a normal-sized endotracheal tube, rather than a tube that is smaller than predicted, as is the case in the closely related Gaucher disease. Moderate difficulty with intubation has been reported (1). Chronic use of anticonvulsant medications may affect the metabolism of some anesthetic drugs. Patients with pulmonary disease are at increased risk for postoperative respiratory complications, and should be closely observed during the postoperative period.

Bibliography:

1. Bujok LS, Bujok G, Knapik P. Niemann-Pick disease: a rare problem in anaesthesiological practice. *Paediatr Anaesth* 2002;12:806–808.
2. Minai OA, Sullivan EJ, Stoller JK. Pulmonary involvement in Niemann-Pick disease: case report and literature review. *Respir Med* 2000;94:1241–1251.
3. Kolodny EH. Niemann-Pick disease. *Curr Opin Hematol* 2000;7:48–52.
4. Mahoney A, Soni N, Vellodi A. Anaesthesia and the lipidoses: a review of patients treated by bone marrow transplantation. *Paediatr Anaesth* 1992;2:205–209.
5. Wark H, Gold P, Overton J. The airway of patients with a lipid storage disease. *Anaesth Intensive Care* 1984;12:343–344.

Nonketotic Hyperglycinemia

SYNONYM: Glycine encephalopathy

MIM #: 605899

This autosomal recessive disease involves a defect in the glycine cleavage enzyme system, a four-protein mitochondrial enzyme complex that metabolizes glycine to CO_2, ammonia and hydroxymethyltetrahydrofolic acid. The four proteins are known as P, H, T, and L. Defects, which lead to nonketotic hyperglycinemia, can arise in any of these four proteins. Glycine, an inhibitory neurotransmitter, is responsible for the clinical manifestations of this syndrome. Dextromethorphan and sodium benzoate have been used to treat this disease, and have resulted in transient improvement. Dextromethorphan is an antagonist of the glutamate NMDA receptor, of which glycine is an activator. Sodium benzoate complexes with glycine to form hippuric acid, which is excreted in the urine. Classically, the disease presents in the neonatal period with significant neurologic impairment, but there is variability in expression, and some patients are only mildly affected.

HEENT/AIRWAY: Microcephaly.

CHEST: Persistent hiccups. Prone to respiratory failure, and may become ventilator dependent.

CARDIOVASCULAR: May develop pulmonary hypertension.

NEUROMUSCULAR: Lethargy, weak cry, hypotonia, areflexia, and episodic myoclonic jerks in the newborn period, progressing to coma and apnea. May have hydrocephalus. Survivors have profound mental retardation, myoclonus, opisthotonos, hypertonicity, minimal cerebral development, and intractable seizures. Abnormal electroencephalogram (EEG) with burst suppression or hypsarrhythmia pattern. Absent corpus callosum.

OTHER: Nonketotic hyperglycinemia. Glycine is the only abnormally accumulated chemical, and glycine levels can be very high, particularly in the central nervous system.

ANESTHETIC CONSIDERATIONS

Ketamine is an NMDA receptor antagonist, and has been used to cause transient improvement in the EEG and clinical findings in a patient with nonketotic hyperglycinemia (4). Although these changes were not permanent, it suggests that ketamine might have a role in anesthetizing these patients. Benzodiazepines have proved particularly useful in the treatment of seizures in these patients because they compete for glycine receptors in the central nervous system.

Bibliography:

1. Applegarth DA, Toone JR. Glycine encephalopathy (nonketotic hyper-glycinaemia) : review and update. *J Inherit Metab Dis* 2004;27:417–422.
2. Cataltepe S, van Marter LJ, Kozakewich H, et al. Pulmonary hypertension associated with nonketotic hyperglycinaemia. *J Inherit Metab Dis* 2000;23:137–144.
3. Van Hove JLK, Kishnani PS, Demaerel P, et al. Acute hydrocephalus in nonketotic hyperglycinemia. *Neurology* 2000;54:754–756.
4. Ohya Y, Ochi N, Mizutani N, et al. Nonketotic hyperglycinemia: treatment with NMDA antagonist and consideration of neuropathogenesis. *Pediatr Neurol* 1991;7:65–68.

Noonan Syndrome

MIM #: 163950

This usually sporadic, but sometimes autosomal dominant, disorder is noted for its superficial similarities to Turner syndrome. People with Noonan syndrome exhibit short stature, characteristic facies, a webbed neck, pectus excavatum, cryptorchidism, pulmonic stenosis, and occasionally hearing loss and/or a bleeding diathesis. Unlike in Turner syndrome, patients with Noonan syndrome can be male or female. There is wide phenotypic variability. About half of the patients have familial disease (for an example, see later, under *Miscellaneous*) because of mutations in the gene *PTPN11*, which encodes the protein tyrosine phosphatase. LEOPARD syndrome (see earlier) is also caused by mutations in this gene, and these two syndromes are allelic. Some patients with neurofibromatosis (see earlier) have manifestations of Noonan syndrome.

HEENT/AIRWAY: Triangular facies. Low posterior hairline. Hypertelorism. High-arched eyebrows, downward-slanting palpebral fissures, epicanthal folds, ptosis, myopia, strabismus, nystagmus. Low-set ears with thickened helix. May have sensorineural hearing loss. Flattened midface, depressed nasal bridge. Wide mouth, full upper lip. High-arched palate. Dental malocclusion. Micrognathia. Short or webbed neck. May have posterior cervical cystic hygroma. Distinctive facial characteristics usually become less marked with age.

CHEST: Sternal deformities with shield chest and widely spaced nipples. Pectus excavatum or carinatum. May have thoracic kyphoscoliosis. Chest deformities may lead to decreased functional residual capacity or restrictive lung disease. Rare chylothorax.

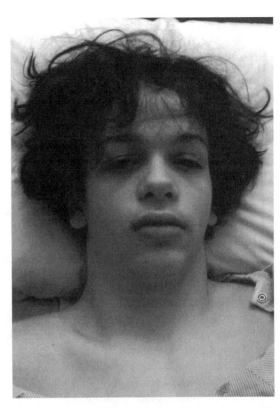

Noonan syndrome. This 14-year-old boy has a Turner phenotype (note the "webbed" neck). He has a history of coarctation of the aorta and aortic stenosis.

CARDIOVASCULAR: Unlike Turner syndrome, which is associated with left-sided cardiac lesions, patients with Noonan syndrome commonly have pulmonic stenosis. The valve is often dysplastic or thickened. There may be an associated septal defect. Patients often have hypertrophic obstructive cardiomyopathy [HOCM; also called idiopathic hypertrophic subaortic stenosis (IHSS)], which is sometimes nonobstructive and asymptomatic. Alternatively, patients may have generalized left ventricular hypertrophy. The electrocardiogram shows right axis deviation. Patent ductus arteriosus, aortic stenosis, and coarctation of the aorta have also been reported.

NEUROMUSCULAR: May have mental retardation, which is usually mild. A relatively narrow spinal canal contains a normal-sized spinal cord. May have Arnold-Chiari malformation. May have cerebral arteriovenous malformation.

ORTHOPEDIC: Short stature. Cubitus valgus. Abnormal vertebrae. May have kyphoscoliosis, lumbar lordosis. May have winged scapulae.

GI/GU: Cryptorchidism and decreased fertility in male patients. Male patients without cryptorchidism may be fertile. Female patients may have delayed menarche, but are fertile. May have renal dysfunction. May have hepatosplenomegaly. Infants may have poor feeding, gastric dysmotility, and gastroesophageal reflux.

OTHER: May have coagulation or platelet defects, including abnormalities in the intrinsic pathway, isolated factor XI deficiency, von Willebrand disease, thrombocytopenia. May have lymphatic vessel dysplasia. May have subcutaneous edema, particularly of the hands and feet.

MISCELLANEOUS: In 1980, Cole (14) pointed out that the blacksmith who posed for Ivan Le Lorraine Albright's painting, *Among Those Left*, appears to have had Noonan syndrome. His short stature, facial features, low-set ears, and probable pectus deformity are highly suggestive. Interestingly, the blacksmith's great-grandson also had the characteristic features of Noonan syndrome, including pulmonic stenosis. Ivan Le Lorraine Albright, best known for *The Picture of Dorian Gray*, was also a medical illustrator. In this instance, he was unaware of his contribution to the medical literature.

ANESTHETIC CONSIDERATIONS

Short or webbed neck, micrognathia, and dental malocclusion may make tracheal intubation very difficult. These problems usually become less marked with age.

Peripheral intravenous access may be difficult if there is significant subcutaneous edema. Chest deformities may lead to decreased functional residual capacity or restrictive lung disease. The presence of a bleeding diathesis may increase the amount of perioperative bleeding. Renal impairment may affect the metabolism of renally excreted drugs.

Regional and general anesthesia have been used for cesarean section in parturients with Noonan syndrome (7, 12), although keep in mind that there may be clotting abnormalities. Kyphoscoliosis and a relatively narrow spinal canal with a normal-sized spinal cord make identifying the epidural and subarachnoid spaces difficult. Because of the spinal deformities, insertion of an epidural catheter may be difficult, and spread of subarachnoid anesthetic may be unpredictable.

A decrease in peripheral vascular resistance, hypovolemia, or increased contractility should be avoided if HOCM is present. Intravenous hydration, halothane and beta-adrenergic blockade are useful in patients with HOCM. Patients with cardiac lesions require perioperative antibiotic prophylaxis as indicated.

There is a recent report of a patient with Noonan syndrome who developed malignant hyperthermia on induction of anesthesia (4). Previous reports in the literature have linked Noonan syndrome with malignant hyperthermia (13), but the patients described also had myopathies and are probably more legitimately classified as having had King syndrome (see earlier), which is clearly associated with malignant hyperthermia susceptibility. The relationship between Noonan syndrome and malignant hyperthermia, if any, remains unclear.

Bibliography:

1. Jongmans M, Sistermans EA, Rikken A, et al. Genotypic and phenotypic characterization of Noonan syndrome: new data and review of the literature. *Am J Med Genet A* 2005;134:165–170.
2. Yellon RF. Prevention and management of complications of airway surgery in children. *Paediatr Anaesth* 2004;14:107–111.
3. Holder-Espinasse M, Winter RM. Type 1 Arnold-Chiari malformation and Noonan syndrome: a new diagnostic feature? *Clin Dysmorphol* 2003;12:275.
4. Lee CK, Chang BS, Hong YM, et al. Spinal deformities in Noonan syndrome: a clinical review of sixty cases. *J Bone Joint Surg Am* 2001;83-A:1495–1502.
5. Shah N, Rodriguez M, St. Louis D, et al. Feeding difficulties and foregut dysmotility in Noonan's syndrome. *Arch Dis Child* 1999;81:28–31.
6. Grange CS, Heid R, Lucas SB, et al. Anaesthesia in a parturient with Noonan syndrome. *Can J Anaesth* 1998;45:332–336.
7. McLure HA, Yantis SM. General anaesthesia for Caesarean section in a parturient with Noonan's syndrome. *Br J Anaesth* 1996;77:665–668.
8. Burch M, Sharland M, Shinebourne E, et al. Cardiologic abnormalities in Noonan syndrome: phenotypic diagnosis and echocardiographic assessment of 118 patients. *Am J Coll Cardiol* 1993;22:1189–1192.
9. Campbell AM, Bousfield JD. Anaesthesia in a patient with Noonan syndrome and cardiomyopathy. *Anaesthesia* 1992;47:131–133.
10. Schwartz N, Eisenkraft JB. Anesthetic management of a child with Noonan syndrome and idiopathic subaortic stenosis. *Anesth Analg* 1992;74:464–466.
11. Sharland M, Patton MA, Talbot S, et al. Coagulation-factor deficiencies and abnormal bleeding in Noonan syndrome. *Lancet* 1992;339:19–21.
12. Dadabhoy ZP, Winnie AP. Regional anesthesia for cesarean section in a parturient with Noonan syndrome. *Anesthesiology* 1988;68:636–638.
13. Mendez HM, Opitz JM. Noonan syndrome: a review. *Am J Med Genet* 1985;21:493–506.
14. Cole RB. Noonan's syndrome: a historical perspective. *Pediatrics* 1980;66:468–469.

O

OAT Deficiency

See Ornithine delta-aminotransferase deficiency

Ochronosis

See Alcaptonuria

Oculoauriculovertebral Syndrome

See Goldenhar syndrome

Oculocerebral Hypopigmentation Syndrome

See Cross syndrome

Oculocerebrocutaneous Syndrome

See Delleman syndrome

Oculocerebrorenal Syndrome

See Lowe syndrome

Oculodentodigital Syndrome

SYNONYM: Oculodentoosseous dysplasia; ODOD

MIM #: 164200, 257850

This dysmorphic syndrome involves the eyes, nose, teeth, and bones. The most frequent manifestations are microphthalmia, small nose, enamel dysplasia, and camptodactyly. This syndrome is usually inherited in an autosomal dominant fashion, but there appears to be a more rare and more severe autosomal recessive form. A gene responsible for the autosomal dominant form has been mapped to the long arm of chromosome 6. The gene product, connexin 43, is a gap junction protein.

HEENT/AIRWAY: Microphthalmia, microcornea, short palpebral fissures, epicanthal folds. May have glaucoma, iris dysplasia. May have conductive hearing loss. Long, thin nose with hypoplastic alae nasi and small anteverted nostrils. May have high-arched palate, cleft lip or palate. Dental enamel hypoplasia or dysplasia. May have premature tooth loss. May have either mandibular overgrowth or micrognathia.

NEUROMUSCULAR: Intelligence is usually normal. May have abnormal white matter, calcification of the basal ganglia, dilated ventricles. May have dysarthria, ataxia, hyperactive reflexes, spastic paraparesis or quadriparesis, seizures. May have neurogenic bladder. Spinal cord compression from an enlarged C1 vertebra has been reported.

ORTHOPEDIC: Camptodactyly of fifth fingers. Syndactyly of fourth and fifth fingers, third and fourth toes. Hypoplastic or missing phalanges. There is a generalized problem with bone modeling. Broad clavicles, ribs, long bones. May have polydactyly. May have cubitus valgus, hip dislocation.

OTHER: Sparse, fine hair. Low serum calcium in some patients.

ANESTHETIC CONSIDERATIONS

Direct laryngoscopy and tracheal intubation may be difficult secondary to either mandibular overgrowth or micrognathia. The small nose with small nares may make nasotracheal intubation difficult. Dental abnormalities should be documented preoperatively. Dysplastic teeth are at risk for damage or loss during laryngoscopy. Clavicular abnormalities may alter the anatomic landmarks for the insertion of a subclavian venous catheter. Patients with paraparesis or quadriparesis may be at risk for hyperkalemia after the administration of succinylcholine.

Bibliography:

1. Frasson M, Calixto N, Cronemberger S, et al. Oculodentodigital dysplasia: study of ophthalmological and clinical manifestations in three boys with probably autosomal recessive inheritance. *Ophthalmic Genet* 2004;25:227–236.
2. Loddenkemper T, Grote K, Evers S, et al. Neurological manifestations of the oculodentodigital dysplasia syndrome. *J Neurol* 2002;249:584–595.
3. Thomsen M, Schneider U, Weber M, et al. The different appearance of the oculodentodigital dysplasia syndrome. *J Pediatr Orthop B* 1998;7:23–26.
4. Colreavy F, Colbert S, Dunphy J. Oculodento-osseous dysplasia: a review of anaesthetic problems. *Paediatr Anaesth* 1994;4:179–182.

Oculodentoosseous Dysplasia

See Oculodentodigital syndrome

Oculomandibulofacial Dyscephaly

See Hallermann-Streiff syndrome

ODOD

See Oculodentodigital syndrome

OEIS Complex

See Exstrophy of the cloaca sequence

Oligohydramnios Sequence

See Potter syndrome

Ollier Disease

SYNONYM: Osteochondromatosis syndrome. (Includes Maffucci syndrome)

MIM #: 166000

This sporadically occurring syndrome involves asymmetric enchondromas with associated asymmetric growth deficiency. When hemangiomas are also present, the condition is known as **Maffucci syndrome.**

HEENT/AIRWAY: Hemangiomas can involve the head and neck, the pharynx, and the airway.

NEUROMUSCULAR: May have intracranial lesions.

ORTHOPEDIC: Asymmetric long bone enchondromas (benign cartilaginous tumors). Limited growth of the affected bones results in asymmetric extremities. Long bones can become bowed and the spine scoliotic. Enchondromas can also develop in the bones of the hands, feet, and pelvis. Fractures related to enchondromas are common. Potential for malignant transformation of enchondromas (chondrosarcoma). Hemangiomas can involve the spine.

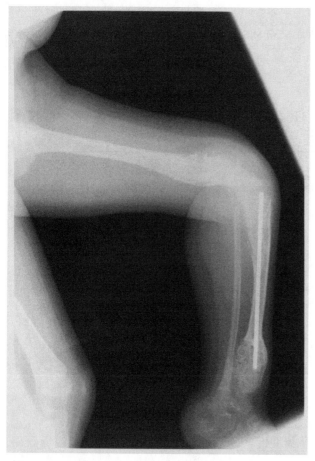

Ollier disease. FIG. 1. Note enchondroma of distal femur and distal tibia.

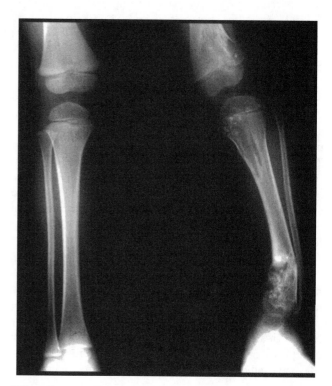

Ollier disease. FIG. 2. Note asymmetric involvement.

GI/GU: Maffucci syndrome may have associated splenomenagly and may develop low-grade splenic angiosarcoma. Rare granulosa cell tumor of the ovary.

OTHER: The Maffucci syndrome involves hemangiomas located in the subcutaneous fat and dermis adjacent to the enchondromas. Hemangiomas are usually cavernous, but can also be capillary or phlebectasia. Thrombosis of the dilated blood vessels with phlebolith formation frequently occurs. Consumptive coagulopathy can occur, but the etiology (splenic vs. hemangiomas) is not clear.

MISCELLANEOUS: On the day that the president of France, Marie François Sadi Carnot, made Ollier commander of the Légion d'Honneur (June 24,1894), Carnot was stabbed to death by an Italian anarchist. Although Ollier was summoned to aid the president, there was nothing he could do to save him.

ANESTHETIC CONSIDERATIONS
Hemangiomas can be located in many sites, including the oropharynx and trachea (3). Patients must be carefully positioned intraoperatively because of the risk of pathologic fractures related to enchondromas. The use of sequential venous compression devices over affected extremities during prolonged surgery might be considered to avoid stasis.

Bibliography:
1. Auyeung J, Mohanty K, Tayton K. Maffucci lymphangioma syndrome: an unusual variant of Ollier disease, a case report and a review of the literature. *J Pediatr Orthop B* 2003;12:147–150.
2. Lee NH, Choi EH, Choi WK, et al. Maffucci syndrome with oral and intestinal haemangioma [Letter]. *Br J Dermatol* 1999;140:968–969.
3. Chan SKC, Ng SK, Cho AM, et al. Anaesthetic implications of Maffucci syndrome. *Anaesth Intensive Care* 1998;26:586–589.
4. Kaplan RP, Wang JT, Amron DM, et al. Maffucci syndrome: case reports with a literature review. *J Am Acad Dermatol* 1994;29:894–899.

Omodysplasia

MIM #: 164745, 258315

There appear to be two forms of this disease, an autosomal dominant form and an autosomal recessive form. Common to the two forms are characteristic facies, growth defects of the distal humeri, and deformities of the elbows. In the autosomal dominant form, findings are restricted to the upper extremities. Findings are more generalized in the autosomal recessive form, with severe dwarfism.

HEENT/AIRWAY: Midline hemangiomas, short nose, depressed nasal bridge, long philtrum. May have short neck with short thyromental distance, large tongue, or hypoplastic mandible.

NEUROMUSCULAR: May have mental retardation.

ORTHOPEDIC: Micromelic dwarfism. Short humerus with characteristic hypoplastic distal humerus. Radioulnar diastasis. Hypoplastic, everted humeral condyle. Clubbed proximal femurs. Limited extension of elbows and knees. Anterolateral radial head dislocation.

GI/GU: Cryptorchidism.

MISCELLANEOUS: "Omo" comes from the Greek word for "shoulder," and is used to indicate a connection with the shoulder or scapula.

ANESTHETIC CONSIDERATIONS
Mandibular and neck findings may make laryngoscopy and intubation difficult.

Bibliography:
1. Elcioglu NH, Gustavson KH, Wilkie AO, et al. Recessive omodysplasia: five new cases and review of the literature. *Pediatr Radiol* 2004;34: 75–82.
2. Venditti CP, Farmer J, Russell KL, et al. Omodysplasia: an affected mother and son. *Am J Med Genet* 2002;111:169–177.
3. Di Luca BJ, Mitchell A. Anaesthesia in a child with autosomal recessive omodysplasia. *Anaesth Intensive Care* 2001;29:71–73.

Ondine's Curse

SYNONYM: Central hypoventilation syndrome

MIM #: 209880

This syndrome involves the failure of autonomic control of ventilation, particularly during sleep, which leads to complications of hypoventilation and chronic carbon dioxide retention. The syndrome may be genetic (congenital) or secondary to central nervous system injury. In congenital cases, the abnormal respiratory drive usually becomes apparent in the neonatal period. Inheritance is autosomal recessive or autosomal dominant with reduced penetrance. There is also a strong association with Hirschsprung disease (see earlier). In congenital cases, there is rarely an intracranial anatomic defect to account for the disorder. It is thought that the disorder could be secondary to a problem with migration of neural crest cells. The high incidence of Hirschsprung disease in association with the central hypoventilation syndrome has led to the suggestion of Ondine-Hirschsprung disease as a synonym for this disease. A mutation in the *PHOX2B* gene has been most frequently associated with congenital central hypoventilation syndrome, but mutations in several other genes have been implicated as well, including *RET, GDNF, EDN3, BDNF,* and *ASCL1.*

HEENT/AIRWAY: May have distinctive facial features such as downward-slanting palpebral fissures, low-set, posteriorly rotated ears, small nose, and triangular mouth. May have abnormalities of the eye. Loss of upper airway patency with onset of central apnea.

CHEST: The ventilatory response to carbon dioxide is blunted. Oxygen supplementation may exacerbate hypoventilation if the ventilatory drive depends on hypoxia. There has been some success with diaphragmatic pacing.

CARDIOVASCULAR: Pulmonary arterial hypertension, cor pulmonale. Pulmonary arterial hypertension may be improved with supplemental oxygen. Autonomic control of the heart rate can also be defective.

NEUROMUSCULAR: Central autonomic ventilatory failure, particularly during sleep, resulting in apnea and hypoventilation. Hypoventilation may improve during REM sleep. The patients are somnolent and lethargic. Arcuate nucleus may be absent. Many have mild to moderate developmental delay. May have seizures. May have hypotonia.

GI/GU: Up to 50% of the patients with Ondine's curse will also have Hirschsprung disease (see earlier). Esophageal motility is reduced.

OTHER: Polycythemia, in response to ventilatory failure. Inappropriate secretion of antidiuretic hormone with hyponatremic seizures has been reported. May be associated with neuroblastoma and ganglioneuroma.

MISCELLANEOUS: The legend of Ondine dates from 15th century Germany. Undine, the spirit of water, would acquire a soul on marrying a mortal. Her husband was cursed by the King of the Ondines for being unfaithful, and from thence forward had to actively command every bodily function: "One moment of inattention and I shall forget to hear, to breathe" (10). Although the disease entity had been described earlier, the sobriquet of "Ondine's curse" is from Severinghaus and Mitchell.

ANESTHETIC CONSIDERATIONS
Patients have frequently had a tracheostomy placed for nighttime positive-pressure ventilation. Hypoventilation is exacerbated by anesthesia. The ventilatory response to carbon dioxide is blunted, and perioperative supplemental oxygen may cause apnea. Patients usually require positive-pressure controlled ventilation during general anesthesia. They should not have narcotic or other premedication unless they can be carefully monitored. The use of short acting anesthetics of all classes would seem appropriate. Extubation should be delayed until patients are completely awake, and they should be observed closely for adequate ventilation after general anesthesia. Regional anesthesia would seem advantageous, if appropriate.

These patients have decreased esophageal motility, and are therefore at risk of perioperative aspiration. Anticonvulsant medications need to be continued (or a parenteral form substituted), and may alter the metabolism of some anesthetic drugs, requiring more frequent dosing. Inappropriate secretion of antidiuretic hormone with hyponatremic seizures has been reported at least twice.

In patients with significant pulmonary arterial hypertension, cor pulmonale and cardiac failure may have developed. Recall that autonomic control of heart rate may also be impaired (3). Complete heart block after induction with propofol has been reported (4).

Bibliography:

1. Ishibashi H, Umezawa K, Hayashi S, et al. Anesthetic management of a child with congenital central hypoventilation syndrome (CCHS, Ondine's curse) for dental treatment. *Anesth Prog* 2004;51:102–104.
2. Chen ML, Keens TG. Congenital central hypoventilation syndrome: not just another rare disorder. *Paediatr Respir Rev* 2004;5:182–189.
3. Silvestri JM, Hanna BD, Volgman AS, et al. Cardiac rhythm disturbances among children with idiopathic congenital central hypoventilation syndrome. *Pediatr Pulmonol* 2000;29:351–358.
4. Sochala C, Deenen D, Ville A, et al. Heart block following propofol in a child. *Paediatr Anaesth* 1999;9:349–351.
5. Strauser LM, Helikson MA, Tobias JD. Anesthetic care for the child with congenital central alveolar hypoventilation syndrome (Ondine's curse). *J Clin Anesth* 1999;11:431–437.
6. Urushihara N, Nakagawa Y, Tanaka N, et al. Ondine's curse and Hirschsprung disease: neurocristopathic syndrome. *Eur J Pediatr Surg* 1999;9:430–432.
7. Wiesel S, Fox GS. Anaesthesia for a patient with central alveolar hypoventilation syndrome (Ondine's curse). *Can J Anaesth* 1990;37:122–126.
8. Minutillo C, Pemberton PJ, Goldblatt J. Hirschsprung disease and Ondine's curse: further evidence for a distinct syndrome. *Clin Genet* 1989;36:200–203.
9. Mather SJ. Ondine's curse and the anaesthetist. *Anaesthesia* 1987;42:394–403.
10. Sugar OS. In search of Ondine's curse. *JAMA* 1978;240:236–237.

Ophthalmoplegia-Plus

See Kearns-Sayre syndrome

Opitz Syndrome

See Hypertelorism-hypospadias syndrome

Opitz-Frias Syndrome

See Hypertelorism-hypospadias syndrome

Opitz-Kaveggia Syndrome

See FG syndrome

Oral-Facial-Digital Syndrome, Type I

(Includes Oral-facial-digital syndromes, types III to X)

MIM #: 311200

This X-linked dominant syndrome is characterized by oral frenula, oral clefts, hypoplastic alae nasi, and asymmetric shortening of the digits. Neurologic manifestations occur in up to 40% of patients. Most patients are female, suggesting

X-linked dominant inheritance with lethality in boys. It is caused by a mutation in the *CXORF5* gene.

There are a total of ten different oral-facial-digital syndromes. Oral-facial-digital syndrome type II is also known as Mohr syndrome (see earlier). The other eight types have only subtle clinical distinctions. They are listed here for completeness:

Type III (Sugarman syndrome)
MIM # 258850
Autosomal recessive inheritance
Mental retardation, "metronome" eye movements
Type IV (Baraitser-Burn syndrome)
MIM # 258860
Autosomal recessive inheritance
Tibial dysplasia
Type V (Thurston syndrome)
MIM # 174300
Autosomal recessive inheritance
Median cleft lip
Type VI (Varadi-Papp syndrome)
MIM # 277170
Autosomal recessive inheritance

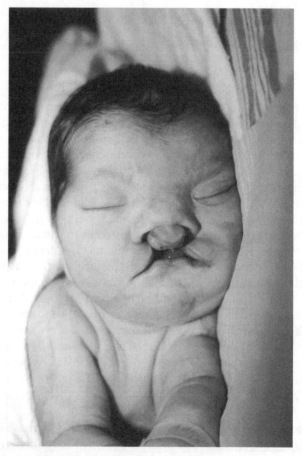

Oral-facial-digital syndrome, type I. FIG. 1. An infant with oral-facial-digital syndrome, type I showing cleft and widely spaced eyes.

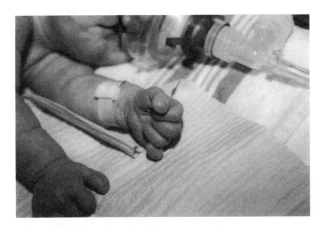

Oral-facial-digital syndrome, type I. FIG. 2. Short fingers with broad, hypoplastic nails.

Metacarpal abnormalities, central polydactyly, cerebellar abnormalities

Type VII (Whelan syndrome)
MIM # 608518
X-linked dominant or autosomal dominant inheritance
Facial asymmetry, hydronephrosis

Type VIII
MIM # 300484
X-linked recessive inheritance
Hypoplastic epiglottis and arytenoids

Type IX
MIM # 258865
Autosomal or X-linked recessive inheritance
Retinal abnormalities

Type X
MIM # 165590
Inheritance pattern unknown
Fibular aplasia, radial shortening, tarsal coalescence

HEENT/AIRWAY: Inner canthi are displaced laterally. Hypoplastic alae nasi. Midline cleft lip. Midline cleft tongue. Cleft alveolar ridge. Cleft palate. Papilliform protuberances on tongue. Hyperplastic frenulum, may have multiple oral frenula. Abnormal dentition, including missing lateral incisors, dental caries, enamel hypoplasia, supernumerary teeth. May have choanal atresia. May have mandibular hypoplasia.

CARDIOVASCULAR: Congenital heart disease is rare.

NEUROMUSCULAR: May have mental retardation. May have agenesis of the corpus callosum, seizures, hydrocephalus.

ORTHOPEDIC: Asymmetric shortening of the digits. Syndactyly, clinodactyly, or brachydactyly of the hands. Unilateral postaxial polydactyly of the feet. Irregular mineralization of the bones of the hands and feet.

GI/GU: Polycystic kidney disease can develop (in type I only).

OTHER: Facial milia (a common benign rash) in infancy. Sparse hair. May have spotty alopecia.

ANESTHETIC CONSIDERATIONS
Dental abnormalities should be documented preoperatively. Carious teeth may be more easily dislodged during laryngoscopy. Choanal atresia may cause respiratory distress in neonates, and precludes the use of nasotracheal and nasogastric tubes. Patients with polycystic kidney disease may have renal insufficiency or failure, which affects fluid management and the choice of anesthetic agents.

Bibliography:
1. Holub M, Potocki L, Bodamer OA. Central nervous system malformations in oral-facial-digital syndrome, type 1. *Am J Med Genet A* 2005;136: 218.
2. Ferrante MI, Giorgio G, Feather SA, et al. Identification of the gene for oral-facial-digital type I syndrome. *Am J Hum Genet* 2001;68:569–576.
3. Toriello HV. Oral-facial-digital syndromes, 1992. *Clin Dysmorphol* 1993;2:95–105.

Oral-Facial-Digital Syndrome, Type II

See Mohr syndrome

Oral-Facial-Digital Syndromes, Types III to X

Included in Oral-facial-digital syndrome, type I

Ornithine Carbamyltransferase Deficiency

See Ornithine transcarbamylase deficiency

Ornithine Delta-Aminotransferase Deficiency

SYNONYM: OAT deficiency; Hyperornithinemia with gyrate atrophy of the choroid and retina

MIM #: 258870
This autosomal recessive disease is due to diminished activity of ornithine delta-aminotransferase, a mitochondrial enzyme involved in ornithine synthesis and degradation. The hallmark is characteristic gyrate atrophy of the choroid and retina. This enzyme is pyridoxine dependent, and pyridoxine may be therapeutic in some patients. There are multiple alleles that can cause this disease.

HEENT/AIRWAY: Progressive retinal atrophy with myopia. The retinal lesions begin as small circular areas and gradually enlarge, coalesce, and extend to the posterior pole of the fundus. Decreased peripheral vision progressing to decreased night vision, and complete blindness by adulthood.

NEUROMUSCULAR: Normal intelligence. Tubular aggregates may be found in type 2 (fast-twitch) muscle fibers of skeletal muscle, but there is no documentable myopathy, although a few have mild proximal weakness. There is eventual atrophy of type 2 muscle fibers, but this occurs later than the eye changes. Electroencephalographic abnormalities without increased incidence of seizures.

OTHER: There may be a dibasic aminoaciduria. There is no associated hyperammonemia, either at rest, after fasting, or with stress.

ANESTHETIC CONSIDERATIONS
There are no specific anesthetic considerations other than an awareness of the visual loss.

Bibliography:

1. Kaiser-Kupfer MI, Caruso RC, Valle D. Gyrate atrophy of the choroid and retina: further experience with long-term reduction of ornithine levels in children. *Arch Ophthalmol* 2002;120:146–153.
2. Valtonen M, Nanto-Salonen K, Jaaskelainen S, et al. Central nervous system involvement in gyrate atrophy of the choroid and retina with hyperornithinaemia. *J Inherit Metab Dis* 1999;22:855–866.
3. Potter MJ, Berson EL. Diagnosis and treatment of gyrate atrophy. *Int Ophthalmol Clin* 1993;33:229–236.

Ornithine Transcarbamylase Deficiency

SYNONYM: Ornithine carbamyltransferase deficiency

MIM #: 311250

This urea cycle defect is a partially dominant X-linked disorder, the only urea cycle defect that is not autosomal recessive. It is a potential cause of hyperammonemia. The urea cycle degrades amino acids to urea. Symptoms can be triggered by stress such as surgery or infection, and episodes of protein catabolism such as involution of the postpartum uterus. Heterozygous, asymptomatic women are at risk for hyperammonemic coma, particularly during the puerperium. The clinical picture of deterioration is reminiscent of Reye syndrome. Patients may be relatively asymptomatic, and may spontaneously avoid protein-rich foods. Chronic treatment includes a low-protein diet and supplemental dietary arginine. Liver transplantation is curative. A single patient has been treated successfully with transplantation of isolated hepatocytes.

The clinical presentations of the urea cycle defects—carbamyl phosphate synthetase, ornithine transcarbamylase, argininosuccinic acid synthetase, and argininosuccinic acid lyase defects—are essentially identical.

NEUROMUSCULAR: Chronic findings include episodic lethargy, irritability, ataxia. Developmental delay. Seizures. Hyperammonemic encephalopathy is clinically similar to hepatic encephalopathy and proceeds through stages of lethargy and agitation to coma with cerebral edema. Sodium valproate can precipitate acute hyperammonemia.

GI/GU: Episodic vomiting. Hepatic synthetic function is normal, although there may be elevations in serum transaminases, both during and between episodes of hyperammonemia.

OTHER: Failure to thrive. Acrodermatitis. Episodes of hyperammonemia begin with anorexia and lethargy, and may progress through agitation, irritability, and confusion. Vomiting and headaches may be prominent. Untreated, central nervous system deterioration ensues, with worsening encephalopathy, coma, and eventually death with cerebral edema. Diminished nitric oxide synthesis (derived from arginine, produced only in the urea cycle).

MISCELLANEOUS: One boy was described who was very difficult and had a "volcanic temper." He became unconscious at age 14 years after a high-protein meal. After the diagnosis was made, he was treated with dietary modifications, and improved so much that he was accepted to medical school (albeit a few years later).

ANESTHETIC CONSIDERATIONS
Patients should not fast preoperatively for more than a few hours. They should maintain a high carbohydrate intake (and low protein intake) perioperatively. Dehydration and catabolism are particularly detrimental. Intravenous glucose alone does not prevent the accumulation of amino acids. In patients with intercurrent hyperammonemia, the perioperative maintenance intravenous solution should ideally contain sodium benzoate (0.25 g/kg/day), sodium phenylacetate (0.25 g/kg/day), and 10% arginine hydrochloride (0.21 g/kg/day). These chemicals optimize alternate pathways (nonurea cycle) for waste nitrogen removal. This intravenous solution may result in potassium wasting, so serum potassium levels should be followed and potassium chloride added to the maintenance intravenous fluids as needed. An orogastric tube or throat packs should be placed if the surgery has the potential to cause oral or intestinal bleeding because blood aspirated into the gastrointestinal tract after oral or nasal surgery might present an excessive protein load and trigger an acute exacerbation. Acute metabolic encephalopathy can present after anesthesia and surgery. Serum pH and ammonia levels should be followed throughout the perioperative period, and consideration should be given to postoperative observation in a pediatric intensive care unit (1).

FIGURE: See **Appendix C**

Bibliography:

1. Schmidt J, Kroeber S, Irouschek A, et al. Anesthetic management of patients with ornithine transcarbamylase deficiency. *Paediatr Anaesth* 2006;16:333–337.

2. Gordon N. Ornithine transcarbamylase deficiency: a urea cycle defect. *Eur J Paediatr Neurol* 2003;7:115–121.
3. Urea Cycle Disorders Conference group. Consensus statement from a conference for the management of patients with urea cycle disorders. *J Pediatr* 2001;138:S1-5.
4. Tazuke M, Murakawa M, Nakao S, et al. Living related liver transplantation for patients with ornithine transcarbamylase deficiency [Japanese]. *Masui* 1997;46:783–787.
5. Iida R, Nagai H, Iwasaki K, et al. Anesthetic management of a patient with ornithine transcarbamylase deficiency [Japanese]. *Masui* 1996;45:642–645.

Oromandibular-Limb Hypogenesis

SYNONYM: Aglossia-adactyly syndrome; Hypoglossia-hypodactyly syndrome; Hanhart syndrome

MIM #: 103300

This sporadically occurring syndrome is characterized by hypoglossia/aglossia, distal limb defects, and micrognathia. It has been hypothesized that the oromandibular-limb hypogenesis sequence is a consequence of fetal vascular disruption. The distal regions are most often affected, giving rise to tongue, distal limb, and mandibular abnormalities. In support of this hypothesis is the finding that fetal disturbance by chorionic villus sampling is associated with an increased risk for the development of this syndrome.

HEENT/AIRWAY: Small mouth with hypoglossia or aglossia. May have epicanthal folds, hypodontia, cleft palate, aberrant attachment of the tongue. Micrognathia.

NEUROMUSCULAR: Intelligence is usually normal. May have Moebius sequence (see earlier) or isolated cranial nerve palsies, thought also to be secondary to *in utero* vascular disruption.

ORTHOPEDIC: Variable distal limb defects, particularly hypoplastic phalanges, adactyly. Syndactyly.

GI/GU: May have "apple peel" bowel, thought to be due to disruption of the superior mesenteric artery *in utero*. One report of gastroschisis. May have splenogonadal fusion.

MISCELLANEOUS: This syndrome was probably represented in a series of illustrations from 16th century England. This is the earliest known report of oromandibular-limb hypogenesis.

ANESTHETIC CONSIDERATIONS
Microstomia and micrognathia may make tracheal intubation difficult, although the small or absent tongue may facilitate direct laryngoscopy and tracheal intubation (2). Dental abnormalities should be documented preoperatively. In the absence of a tongue, patients may have difficulty swallowing, and excess oral secretions may result. An antisialogogue may be indicated. Patients with facial (seventh cranial) nerve

palsy may be unable to close their eyelids. The eyes must be protected perioperatively to avoid corneal abrasions.

Bibliography:
1. Girshin M, Parikh SR, Leyvi G, et al. Intraoperative oxygen desaturation and electrocardiographic changes in a patient with Hanhart syndrome. *J Cardiothorac Vasc Anesth* 2005;19:546–547.
2. Karakaya D, Bariş S, Belet N, et al. Anaesthetic and airway management in a child with Hanhart syndrome. *Paediatr Anaesth* 2003;13:263–266.
3. De Smet L, Schollen W. Hypoglossia-hypodactyly syndrome: report of 2 patients. *Genet Couns* 2001;12:347–352.
4. Gruber B, Burton BK. Oromandibular-limb hypogenesis syndrome following chorionic villus sampling. *Int J Pediatr Otorhinolaryngol* 1994; 29:59–63.

Orotic Aciduria

MIM #: 258900, 258920

The classic disease (orotic aciduria I) involves diminished activity of two enzymes, orotidine-5'-pyrophosphorylase and orotidine-5'-phosphate-decarboxylase. These enzymes catalyze the two final steps in pyrimidine synthesis, the conversion of orotic acid to uridine monophosphate. It seems that both enzyme activities reside on the same gene, that encoding UMP synthase (uridine monophosphate synthetase). Orotic aciduria II is due to inadequate orotodine-5'-phosphate-decarboxylase activity only. Orotic aciduria can also result from urea cycle defects, essential amino acid deficiency, Reye syndrome, and parenteral nutrition. The major clinical findings are anemia and complications from orotic acid crystal formation in the urine. Symptoms resolve after treatment with uridine.

CARDIOVASCULAR: There may be an increased incidence of congenital heart disease.

NEUROMUSCULAR: Psychomotor retardation, sluggishness.

GI/GU: Urinary obstruction from orotic acid crystals in the urine has been reported. This has occurred at the renal, ureteral, and urethral levels.

OTHER: Failure to thrive. Megaloblastic anemia unresponsive to vitamin B_{12} or folate, hypochromic microcytic anemia unresponsive to iron or pyridoxine. There may be a predisposition to severe infections with abnormal cellular immunity, but the *in vitro* effects are variable, and most patients do not have excessive problems with infectious diseases. Sparse, short hair.

MISCELLANEOUS: When left standing, fine needle-shaped crystals form in urine.

ANESTHETIC CONSIDERATIONS
Perioperative fluid administration should be sufficient to maintain a reasonable diuresis to avoid increasing the concentration of urinary crystals, which may lead to urinary obstruction.

Bibliography:

1. Sumi S, Suchi M, Kidouchi K, et al. Pyrimidine metabolism in hereditary orotic aciduria. *J Inherit Metab Dis* 1997;20:104–105.
2. Suchi M, Mizuno H, Kawai Y, et al. Molecular cloning of the human UMP synthase gene and characterization of point mutations in two hereditary orotic aciduria families. *Am J Hum Genet* 1997;60:525–539.

Osgood-Schlatter Disease

MIM #: 165800

This is a fairly common, benign disorder involving pain and tenderness of the tibial tubercle in the preteen and early teenage years. Inflammation of the tibial tubercle at the point of insertion of the patellar tendon may be due to tiny stress fractures of the apophysis. Symptoms are exacerbated by vigorous running and jumping. Patients may need to limit vigorous exercise to control symptoms. The disease is self-limiting and resolves with maturation.

ORTHOPEDIC: Swelling and point tenderness over the tibial tubercle. Radiographs of the knee are usually normal. May have increased external tibial torsion. On rare occasions there is permanent prominence of the tibial tubercle as a sequela.

ANESTHETIC CONSIDERATIONS
There are no specific anesthetic implications.

Bibliography:

1. Demirag B, Ozturk C, Yazici Z, et al. The pathophysiology of Osgood-Schlatter disease: a magnetic resonance investigation. *J Pediatr Orthop B* 2004;13:379–382.
2. Bloom OJ, Mackler L, Barbee J. Clinical inquiries. What is the best treatment for Osgood-Schlatter disease? *J Fam Pract* 2004;53:153–156.
3. Rosenberg ZS, Kawelblum M, Cheung YY, et al. Osgood-Schlatter lesion: fracture or tendonitis? Scintigraphic, CT, and MR imaging features. *Radiology* 1992;185:853–858.

Osler-Weber-Rendu Syndrome

SYNONYM: Hereditary hemorrhagic telangiectasia

MIM #: 187300

This autosomal dominant, highly penetrant vasculopathy is marked by multiple telangiectases of the skin, mucosa, and viscera. These telangiectases are prone to recurrent bleeding. Recurrent epistaxis is the most common type of bleeding, and hemorrhage may be significant. There may also be gastrointestinal, pulmonary, or intracerebral bleeding. Thirty percent of patients require hospitalization for control of bleeding. Blood vessels in the telangiectatic areas have dilated, histologically abnormal vessel walls, and are likely to form aneurysms or arteriovenous fistulae. Osler-Weber-Rendu syndrome is likely genetically heterogeneous. Implicated genes include the gene encoding endoglin (a transforming growth factor-beta binding protein) and the gene activin receptor-like kinase (*ALK1*). Mutations in the gene *ALK1* can also be responsible for familial primary

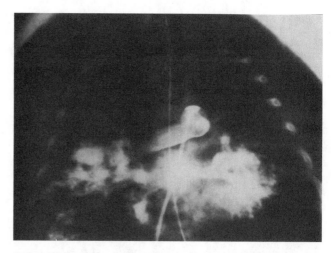

Osler-Weber-Rendu syndrome. Pulmonary arteriogram of a 4-day-old cyanotic infant showing massive left-sided and large right-sided pulmonary arteriovenous fistulae. Early drainage to the pulmonary veins and left atrium can be appreciated. This infant's systemic oxygen saturation was 56% while breathing 100% oxygen. His mother required a partial lung resection during pregnancy for worsening cyanosis, and his maternal grandfather died of a nosebleed.

pulmonary arterial hypertension. Arteriovenous malformations often can be successfully treated with transcatheter embolization.

HEENT/AIRWAY: Telangiectases of the face, lips, tongue, nasopharynx, and conjunctiva. Recurrent epistaxis.

CHEST: Pulmonary telangiectases. May have pulmonary bleeding. Pulmonary arteriovenous fistulae can cause significant systemic arterial desaturation from intrapulmonary right-to-left shunting. Hypoxemia may worsen during pregnancy. Pulmonary arterial hypertension.

CARDIOVASCULAR: Pulmonary arteriovenous fistulae increase the risk of paradoxical emboli. Some fistulae can be closed by catheter embolization techniques. Large shunts through hepatic or pulmonary arteriovenous fistulae have resulted in high-output congestive heart failure.

NEUROMUSCULAR: Neurologic complications most frequently result from pulmonary arteriovenous fistulae with paradoxical emboli or brain abscess formation. Other causes of neurologic complications include vascular malformations (arteriovenous fistulae or aneurysms) of the brain or spinal cord, bleeding from intracerebral telangiectases, or hypoxemic injury secondary to pulmonary arteriovenous fistulae.

ORTHOPEDIC: Fingertip and nailbed telangiectases.

GI/GU: Gastrointestinal, hepatic, and bladder telangiectases. Gastrointestinal bleeding. Hepatic arteriovenous fistulae. May have hepatic cirrhosis.

OTHER: Patients may be anemic from repeated hemorrhage. They may be taking oral iron or oral estrogen, which has been found to improve the integrity of the telangiectatic vessel walls. Patients with severe recurrent epistaxis may be receiving intranasal tranexamic acid. Pregnant patients are more likely to bleed.

MISCELLANEOUS: This disorder was differentiated from hemophilia by Rendu in 1896, and further described by Osler in 1901, who emphasized its familial nature. Weber expanded the clinical description in 1907. The term "hereditary hemorrhagic telangiectasia" was introduced in 1909, but the triple eponym is still more commonly used when referring to this syndrome.

Osler was a leading international medical figure of his time. He was a Canadian who was appointed to the chair of medicine at the University of Pennsylvania. He then became one of the founding figures at the Johns Hopkins University School of Medicine, serving there as the first professor of medicine. He became Regius Professor at Oxford 16 years later and was made a baronet in 1911. Osler married Grace Gross, a great-granddaughter of Paul Revere of American Revolution fame, and they named their son Revere in honor of his great-great-grandfather.

F. Parkes Weber was a British physician who had an interest in rare disorders and uncommon syndromes. Weber's father came from Germany to Britain (where he became physician to Queen Victoria), and Weber continued to pronounce his last name with the 'W' pronounced as the Germanic 'V.' He had an encyclopedic knowledge of rare disorders. It is said that when at a meeting of the Royal Society of Medicine he first announced that he had not heard of a certain syndrome, such cheers and applause broke out from the audience that the meeting had to be abandoned. He wrote a total of 1,200 medical papers.

Henri Rendu was a prominent French physician who also held a doctorate in geology. He served as a surgeon in the army in the Franco-Prussian war. He published over 100 medical articles.

ANESTHETIC CONSIDERATIONS

Nasal intubation, nasal trumpets, and nasogastric tubes are contraindicated because of the likelihood of nasopharyngeal telangiectases and the consequent risk of bleeding. Care must be taken to avoid trauma to oral telangiectases during laryngoscopy.

Although associated epidural bleeding has not been reported, this is a concern when considering epidural anesthesia.

Intravenous catheters need to be kept free of air bubbles because of the risk of right-to-left shunting through pulmonary arteriovenous fistulae.

Bibliography:

1. Sharma D, Pandia MP, Bithal PK. Anaesthetic management of Osler-Weber-Rendu syndrome with coexisting congenital methaemoglobinaemia. *Acta Anaesthesiol Scand* 2005;49:1391–1394.
2. Fuchizaki U, Miyamori H, Kitagawa S, et al. Hereditary haemorrhagic telangiectasia (Rendu-Osler-Weber disease). *Lancet* 2003;362:1490–1494.
3. Begbie ME, Wallace GM, Shovlin CL. Hereditary haemorrhagic telangiectasia (Osler-Weber-Rendu syndrome): a view from the 21st century. *Postgrad Med J* 2003;79:18–24.
4. Berg J, Porteous M, Reinhardt D, et al. Hereditary haemorrhagic telangiectasia: a questionnaire based study to delineate the different phenotypes caused by endoglin and ALK1 mutations. *J Med Genet* 2003;40:585–590.
5. Morgan T, McDonald J, Anderson C, et al. Intracranial hemorrhage in infants and children with hereditary hemorrhagic telangiectasia (Osler-Weber-Rendu syndrome). *Pediatrics* 2002;109:E12.
6. Le Corre F, Golkar B, Tessier C, et al. Liver transplantation for hepatic arteriovenous malformation with high-output cardiac failure in hereditary hemorrhagic telangiectasia: hemodynamic study. *J Clin Anesth* 2000;12:339–342.
7. Garcia-Tsao G, Korzenik JR, Young L, et al. Liver disease in patients with hereditary hemorrhagic telangiectasia. *N Engl J Med* 2000;343:931–936.
8. Shovlin CL, Guttmacher AE, Buscarini E, et al. Diagnostic criteria for hereditary hemorrhagic telangiectasia (Rendu-Osler-Weber syndrome). *Am J Med Genet* 2000;91:66–67.
9. Radu C, Reich DL, Tamman R. Anesthetic considerations in a cardiac surgical patient with Osler-Weber-Rendu disease. *J Cardiothorac Vasc Anesth* 1992;6:461–464.
10. Waring PH, Shaw DB, Brumfield CG. Anesthetic management of a parturient with Osler-Weber-Rendu syndrome and rheumatic heart disease. *Anesth Analg* 1990;71:96–99.

Osteitis Fibrosa Cystica

See McCune-Albright syndrome

Osteochondromatosis Syndrome

See Ollier disease

Osteogenesis Imperfecta

MIM #: 166200, 166210, 259420, 166220

Osteogenesis imperfecta (OI) is a disorder in which the bones are extremely fragile and can be fractured easily, even with only minor trauma. Four types of OI have been delineated. The genetic abnormality in OI is a mutation in one or both of the genes for type 1 collagen, *COL1A1 or COL1A2*. Pamidronate has been used in preliminary studies in children with severe disease, and mutant gene inactivation using mesenchymal stem cells has been proposed.

Type I OI is inherited in an autosomal dominant fashion, and is characterized by blue sclerae, fragile bones, hyperextensible joints, progressive conductive hearing loss, and dentinogenesis imperfecta. It is the most common form of OI. There is variability in expression, but most patients have fractures during childhood. Fractures are less common in adulthood.

Type II OI is lethal either *in utero* or in the perinatal period. It is characterized by blue sclerae, growth retardation, short, bent limbs with multiple fractures, and severe thoracic cage abnormalities. If not stillborn, most patients die in the

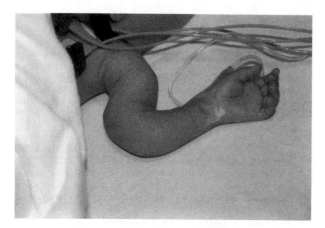

Osteogenesis imperfecta. FIG. 1. The arm of a young child with osteogenesis imperfecta type III. It has already been deformed by multiple fractures.

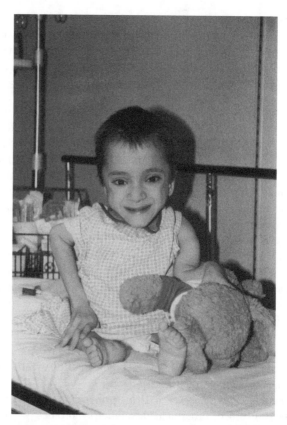

Osteogenesis imperfecta. FIG. 2. This 28-inch-tall (71 cm), 8-year-old boy weighs 8 kg. He has osteogenesis imperfecta type III.

perinatal period of respiratory insufficiency. Inheritance may be autosomal recessive or autosomal dominant lethal.

Type III OI is inherited in an autosomal dominant fashion, and is characterized by blue sclerae at birth that thereafter normalize, multiple fractures, and progressive bony deformities. The patients usually die in childhood or adolescence as a consequence of cardiorespiratory complications. A rare autosomal recessive form of type III OI has been described.

Type IV OI is inherited in an autosomal dominant fashion, and is characterized by bony fragility and multiple fractures without the scleral, audiologic, and dental abnormalities of type I OI. As in type I OI, there is improvement after puberty, and fractures are uncommon in adults.

HEENT/AIRWAY

Type I OI: Blue sclerae. Progressive conductive hearing loss—40% of the adults need a hearing aid. Dentinogenesis imperfecta—hypoplasia of dentin resulting in translucent yellow teeth, which are prone to development of caries. May have vertigo secondary to inner ear pathology.

Type II OI: Poorly mineralized, soft skull with large fontanelles and wormian bones. Blue sclerae. Apparent hypotelorism, shallow orbits. Low nasal bridge, small, beaked nose.

Type III OI: Macrocephaly with triangular facies. Poorly mineralized skull with wormian bones. Blue sclerae in infancy become progressively less blue with age. Hearing loss is rare. May have dentinogenesis imperfecta.

Type IV OI: Normal sclerae (may be bluish during infancy). Normal hearing. Rare dentinogenesis imperfecta.

CHEST

Type I OI: Severe kyphoscoliosis can lead to restrictive lung disease and respiratory compromise.

Type II OI: Severe thoracic cage abnormalities cause fatal respiratory insufficiency.

Type III OI: Severe kyphoscoliosis can lead to restrictive lung disease and respiratory compromise.

CARDIOVASCULAR

Type I OI: May have aortic root dilation, aortic insufficiency, mitral valve prolapse. Rare cor pulmonale from severe kyphoscoliosis.

Type III OI: Rare cor pulmonale from severe kyphoscoliosis.

NEUROMUSCULAR

Type II OI: Hypotonia, variable hydrocephalus.

ORTHOPEDIC

Type I OI: Short stature. Osteopenia. Fractures heal rapidly, with evidence of good callus formation. However, deformities of the limbs secondary to fractures occur, particularly bowing of the femurs and tibias. Metatarsus varus, flat feet. Hyperextensible joints. Progressive kyphoscoliosis.

Type II OI: Short, thick, long bones with multiple fractures and callus formation. The limbs, particularly the lower extremities, are bent. Flattened vertebrae.

Type III OI: Short stature. Osteopenia. Multiple fractures and progressive deformities of the limbs and the spine.

Type IV OI: May have short stature. Multiple fractures, bony deformities. Bowing of the lower limbs. Vertebral abnormalities.

GI/GU

Type I OI: May have inguinal hernias.

Type II OI: May have inguinal hernias.

OTHER

Type I OI: Thin, easily bruised skin. May have functional platelet abnormality, which is usually not clinically significant, but which has been shown to cause increased bleeding after cardiac and other surgeries. This can occur in the face of normal tests of coagulation, and is thought to be because of the effects of the abnormal collagen on platelet-endothelial interaction and capillary strength. May have hyperthyroidism.

Type II OI: Very thin skin.

ANESTHETIC CONSIDERATIONS

Significant perioperative morbidity results from the extreme bony fragility. Hyperextension of the neck may result in a fracture. The mandible may be fractured during laryngoscopy. Succinylcholine-induced fasciculations may cause fractures. In particular, positioning the patient for surgery may result in a fracture. Even inflation of the blood pressure cuff has resulted in fractures, and in severe cases of OI the anesthesiologist may decide not to use a blood pressure cuff. An arterial line may alternatively be used.

The larynx can be difficult to visualize secondary to distortion caused by thoracic kyphoscoliosis or decreased neck mobility. The laryngeal mask airway (LMA) and the intubating LMA have both been used successfully (1, 7, 8). Patients with dentinogenesis imperfecta are at increased risk of perioperative tooth loss. These patients should have their dental abnormalities documented preoperatively. Consideration should be given to using a mouth guard to protect the teeth. Some patients with type I OI may have excessive bleeding secondary to platelet dysfunction, and desmopressin (DDAVP) was utilized successfully in one patient (2). Cesarean section is often required because of cephalopelvic disproportion or a fetus with OI. Regional anesthesia has been reported for cesarean section (6, 16). Spinal anesthesia has been used in an adult with type IV OI (3), and caudal anesthesia has also been used successfully (11). However, bear in mind that the full implications of the coagulopathy associated with this disease have not been delineated. Given the short stature associated with severe disease, epidural dosing should be incremental. Patients with cardiac anomalies require perioperative prophylactic antibiotics as indicated.

Several patients have reportedly experienced a perioperative hypermetabolic state with fever (1, 15, 17). It is generally thought that this does not represent malignant hyperthermia. An association with malignant hyperthermia is very unlikely (10, 12). One patient has developed lactic acidosis during total intravenous anesthesia using propofol (5).

Bibliography:
1. Karabiyik L, Capan Z. Osteogenesis imperfecta: different anaesthetic approaches to two paediatric cases [Letter]. *Paediatr Anaesth* 2004;14:524–525.
2. Keegan MT, Whatcott BD, Harrison BA, et al. Osteogenesis imperfecta, perioperative bleeding, and desmopressin. *Anesthesiology* 2004;97:1011–1013.
3. Aly EE, Harris P. Spinal anesthesia in an obese patient with osteogenesis imperfecta [Letter]. *Can J Anaesth* 2004;51:420–421.
4. Rauch F, Glorieux FH. Osteogenesis imperfecta. *Lancet* 2004;363: 1377–1385.
5. Kill C, Leonhardt A, Wulf H. Lacticacidosis after short-term infusion of propofol for anaesthesia in a child with osteogenesis imperfecta. *Paediatr Anaesth* 2003;13:823–826.
6. Vogel TM, Ratner EF, Thomas RC, et al. Pregnancy complicated by severe osteogenesis imperfecta: a report of two cases. *Anesth Analg* 2002;94:1315–1317.
7. Karabiyik L, Parpucu M, Kurtipek O. Total intravenous anaesthesia and the use of an intubating laryngeal mask in a patient with osteogenesis imperfecta. *Acta Anaesthesiol Scand* 2002;46:618–619.
8. Kostopanagiotou G, Coussi T, Tsaroucha N, et al. Anaesthesia using a laryngeal mask airway in a patient with osteogenesis imperfecta. *Anaesthesia* 2000;55:506.
9. Edge G, Okafor B, Fennelly ME, et al. An unusual manifestation of bleeding diathesis in a patient with osteogenesis imperfecta. *Eur J Anaesthesiol* 1997;14:215–219.
10. Porsborg P, Astrup G, Bendixen D, et al. Osteogenesis imperfecta and malignant hyperthermia: is there a relationship? *Anaesthesia* 1996;51: 863–865.
11. Barros E. Caudal block in a child with osteogenesis imperfecta, type II [Letter]. *Paediatr Anaesth* 1995;5:202–203.
12. Peluso A, Cerullo M. Malignant hyperthermia susceptibility in patients with osteogenesis imperfecta [Letter]. *Paediatr Anaesth* 1995; 5:398–399.
13. Szmuk P, Ezri T, Soroker D. Total intravenous anaesthesia for patients with osteogenesis imperfecta [Letter]. *Paediatr Anaesth* 1994;4:344.
14. Cho E, Dayan SS, Marx GF. Anaesthesia in a parturient with osteogenesis imperfecta. *Br J Anaesth* 1992;68:422–423.
15. Ryan CA, Al-Ghamdi AS, Gayle M, et al. Osteogenesis imperfecta and hyperthermia. *Anesth Analg* 1989;68:811–814.
16. Cunningham AJ, Donnelly M, Comerford J. Osteogenesis imperfecta: anesthetic management of a patient for cesarean section: a case report. *Anesthesiology* 1984;61:91–93.
17. Rampton AJ, Kelly DA, Shanahan EC. Occurrence of malignant hyperpyrexia in a patient with osteogenesis imperfecta. *Br J Anaesth* 1984;56:1443–1446.

Osteopetrosis

SYNONYM: Albers-Schönberg disease

MIM #: 166600, 259700

This disease of the bone occurs in autosomal dominant and autosomal recessive forms, and results from defective

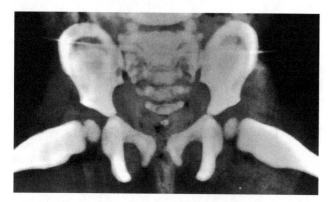

Osteopetrosis. FIG. 1. Pelvic radiograph showing markedly increased bone density. (Courtesy of the Division of Pediatric Radiology, University of Virginia Health System.)

osteoclastic resorption of immature bone. The autosomal dominant form is much more common and benign. Cardinal features are bony fragility and overgrowth, dental abscesses, and osteomyelitis, particularly of the mandible. The autosomal dominant form is usually nondebilitating, and life span is normal. The autosomal recessive form, although less common, is much more debilitating and uniformly lethal before adolescence. In addition to bony fragility and overgrowth, it involves secondary pancytopenia, cranial nerve compression, and visual impairment. The prognosis is poorest in patients with early onset of hematologic and ocular defects. Death is usually the result of anemia, bleeding, or overwhelming infection. Steroids, high-dose calcitriol, or interferon-gamma therapy may be beneficial, and bone marrow transplantation has been offered. Bone marrow transplantation is being investigated as a potentially curative therapy for this disorder, because it leads to restoration of osteoclast function. The autosomal recessive form is described here in detail.

HEENT/AIRWAY: Macrocephaly. Frontal bossing. Bone growth leading to proptosis may cause extraocular muscle paralysis or dysfunction of the optic nerve, leading to blindness. Obtuse mandibular angle may develop. Mandibular osteomyelitis. Teeth are distorted, and prone to early decay and loss. Dental abscesses. High-arched palate.

NEUROMUSCULAR: Bone growth causing compression of the cranial nerves may lead to deafness, vestibular nerve palsy, or other cranial nerve dysfunction. Increased intracranial pressure from bone growth into the cranial space. Mental retardation is common.

ORTHOPEDIC: Bone is thick, dense, and fragile. Pathologic fractures are common, including cervical vertebrae. Upper and lower end-plate sclerosis of vertebral bodies has been referred to as "sandwich vertebrae" on radiographs. Osteomyelitis.

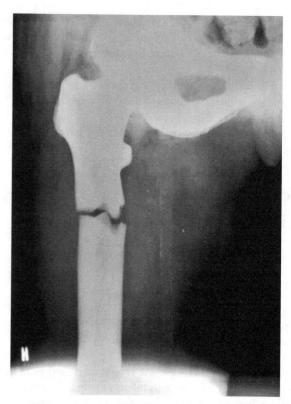

Osteopetrosis. FIG. 2. Pathologic fracture through dense bone. (Courtesy of the Division of Pediatric Radiology, University of Virginia Health System.)

OTHER: Bone growth causes bone marrow obliteration and leads to pancytopenia. Serum calcium levels may be low, and serum phosphorus and alkaline phosphatase may be elevated. Hepatosplenomegaly secondary to compensatory extramedullary hematopoiesis.

MISCELLANEOUS: Despite the hyphenated eponym, Heinrich Albers-Schönberg was one person. He was a German radiologist at the turn of the last century. In 1904 Albers-Schönberg received the Grand Prize at the World Fair in St. Louis because of the quality of his diagnostic x-rays. In a not uncommon scenario for early radiologists, he contracted radiation-induced tumors. He eventually required amputations, and lost the use of both arms. He requested that the results of his autopsy (at the age of 56) be published for the use of others.

ANESTHETIC CONSIDERATIONS
The hematocrit and platelet count should be evaluated preoperatively. Care must be taken in positioning the patient, because bones are fragile and prone to fracture. Limited mandibular joint movement may make oral intubation difficult, and the bony encroachment on the nasal turbinates may preclude nasal intubation (2). Periodontal attachment is poor, leading to risk of tooth loss. Hypocalcemic seizures or tetany may occur. Patients may be taking steroids, and should

receive stress doses of steroids perioperatively. Postoperative mortality is increased in these children (4).

Bibliography:
1. Tolar J, Teitelbaum SL, Orchard PJ. Osteopetrosis. *N Engl J Med* 2004;351:2839–2849.
2. Basaranoglu G, Erden V. Difficult tracheal intubation of a patient with cervical fracture due to osteopetrosis [Letter]. *Paediatr Anaesth* 2001;11:745–750.
3. Benichou OD, Laredo JD, De Vernejoul MC. Type II autosomal dominant osteopetrosis (Albers-Schonberg disease): clinical and radiological manifestations in 42 patients. *Bone* 2000;26:87–93.
4. Burt N, Haynes GR, Bailey MK, et al. Patients with malignant osteopetrosis are at high risk of anesthetic morbidity and mortality. *Anesth Analg* 1999;88:1292–1297.
5. Gerritsen EJA, Vossen JM, van Loo IHG, et al. Autosomal recessive osteopetrosis: variability of findings at diagnosis and during the natural course. *Pediatrics* 1994;93:247–253.

Otopalatodigital Syndrome, Type I

Synonym: Taybi syndrome

MIM #: 311300

This X-linked disorder is characterized by hearing loss, cleft palate, and broad thumbs and great toes with short nails. Female carriers have mild clinical expression. Like otopalatodigital syndrome, type II (see later), it is caused by a mutation in the gene encoding filamin A (*FLNA*).

The two types of otopalatodigital syndrome are probably allelic. Note that this syndrome is distinct from the more widely known Rubinstein-Taybi syndrome.

HEENT/AIRWAY: Thickened base of skull and frontal bone with frontal bossing, delayed closure of anterior fontanelle. Occipital prominence. Absent frontal and sphenoid sinuses. Facial bone hypoplasia. Hypertelorism. Conductive hearing loss. Broad nasal root, small nose. Small mouth, missing teeth, impacted teeth, small tonsils. Cleft palate.

CHEST: Pectus excavatum.

NEUROMUSCULAR: Mild mental retardation. Delayed speech.

ORTHOPEDIC: Small stature. Broad thumbs and great toes. Other digits may also be broad. Short nails. Clinodactyly. Limited elbow extension, dislocation of the radial head ("nursemaid's elbow"). Bowed tibia. Small iliac crests. May have dislocated hips, limited knee flexion. May have scoliosis.

ANESTHETIC CONSIDERATIONS
Recall that most patients have significant hearing loss. Dental abnormalities should be documented preoperatively. Postoperative respiratory arrest (occurring 5 hours after surgery) was reported in a child, and was thought to be secondary to brainstem compression from the thickened skull base (3).

Bibliography:
1. Robertson SP, Twigg SR, Sutherland-Smith AJ, et al. Localized mutations in the gene encoding the cytoskeletal protein filamin A cause diverse malformations in humans. *Nat Genet* 2003;33:487–491.
2. Robertson SP, Walsh S, Oldridge M, et al. Linkage of otopalatodigital syndrome type 2 (OPD2) to distal Xq28: evidence for allelism with OPD1. *Am J Hum Genet* 2001;69:223–227.
3. Clark JR, Smith LJ, Kendall BE, et al. Unexpected brainstem compression following routine surgery in a child with oto-palato-digital syndrome. *Anaesthesia* 1995;50:641–643.

Otopalatodigital Syndrome, Type II

Synonym: Cranioorofacial digital syndrome

MIM #: 304120

This X-linked syndrome is characterized by hearing loss, cranial and facial abnormalities, cleft palate, digital abnormalities, and bowing of the long bones. The manifestations in male patients are much more severe than in otopalatodigital syndrome, type I. Most patients are stillborn, or die in infancy secondary to respiratory failure. Female carriers have only mild manifestations of the syndrome. Like otopalatodigital syndrome, type I (see earlier), it is caused by a mutation in the gene encoding filamin A (*FLNA*). The two types of otopalatodigital syndrome are probably allelic.

HEENT/AIRWAY: Microcephaly. Prominent forehead, wide sutures, late closure of anterior fontanelle. Flat midface. Hypertelorism, downward-slanting palpebral fissures. Abnormal, low-set ears. Conductive hearing loss. Flat nasal bridge. Very small mouth. May have dental abnormalities. Cleft palate. Severe micrognathia.

CHEST: Pectus excavatum. Small thorax with irregular clavicles and ribs. Respiratory insufficiency commonly develops.

NEUROMUSCULAR: Mental retardation. May have cerebellar hypoplasia, hydrocephalus.

ORTHOPEDIC: Growth deficiency. Short, broad thumbs and great toes. Flexed, overlapping fingers. Hypoplastic phalanges. Abnormal proximal phalangeal epiphyses. Polydactyly, syndactyly, clinodactyly, brachydactyly. Short first metacarpal, extra bone in the capitate-hamate complex. Bowed radius, ulna, femur, tibia. Hypoplastic fibula. Subluxation at elbows, wrists, and knees. Small iliac crests. Hip dislocation. Rocker-bottom feet. May have abnormalities of the cervical spine.

GI/GU: May have omphalocele. May have cryptorchidism, hypospadias, hydronephrosis, hydroureter.

ANESTHETIC CONSIDERATIONS
Most patients have severe restrictive lung disease, and are at risk for perioperative respiratory failure. Clavicular anomalies may make placement of a subclavian venous catheter

more difficult. Direct laryngoscopy and tracheal intubation are difficult secondary to the very small mouth and very severe micrognathia. Recall that most patients have significant hearing loss. Dental abnormalities should be documented preoperatively. Consider preoperative evaluation of renal function in patients with a history of renal abnormalities which predispose to renal insufficiency.

Bibliography:
1. Robertson SP, Twigg SR, Sutherland-Smith AJ, et al. Localized mutations in the gene encoding the cytoskeletal protein filamin A cause diverse malformations in humans. *Nat Genet* 2003;33:487–491.
2. Robertson SP, Walsh S, Oldridge M, et al. Linkage of otopalatodigital syndrome type 2 (OPD2) to distal Xq28: evidence for allelism with OPD1. *Am J Hum Genet* 2001;69:223–227.
3. Savarirayan R, Cormier-Daire V, Unger S, et al. Oto-palato-digital syndrome, type II: report of three cases with further delineation of the chondro-osseous morphology. *Am J Med Genet* 2000;95:193–200.

Oxalosis

Synonym: Hyperoxaluria

MIM #: 259900, 260000

There are two separate autosomal recessive disorders that can present with excessive production and excretion of oxalic acid. Type I disease, by far the more common, is due to an abnormality in the enzyme alanine:glyoxylate aminotransferase (AGXT), which should be present in liver peroxisomes. There may be three abnormalities: no AGXT protein in hepatocytes, inactive AGXT protein in peroxisomes, or AGXT protein misdirected to mitochondria instead of to peroxisomes. In the absence of adequate peroxisomal AGXT, glyoxylate is not metabolized to less toxic metabolites, but is instead converted to oxalate and glycolate. Oxalate is renally excreted, and excessive amounts of oxalate lead to the formation of calcium oxalate crystals in the urine. Type II disease is due to a defect in hydroxypyruvate metabolism, which results in its conversion to L-glyceric acid with eventual formation of oxalate. Other causes of hyperoxaluria include ingestion of ethylene glycol or ascorbic acid, pyridoxine deficiency (a cofactor for the enzyme AGXT), resection or disease of the terminal ileum, or other fat malabsorption. It is thought that excessive fatty acids compete with oxalate for intestinal calcium, leaving the oxalate to form salts more soluble than calcium oxalate, with increased absorption.

Treatment of oxalosis includes chronic diuresis with a diuretic, administration of magnesium and phosphates (limiting calcium oxalate stone formation), ascorbic acid, and avoidance of oxalate-rich foods. Oxalate is found in high concentrations in leafy plants such as spinach and rhubarb, in cocoa, and in tea. Its high concentration in some ornamental plants has led them to be classified as toxic. Pyridoxine has helped a few patients with type I disease. Dialysis does not remove oxalate adequately, and patients on dialysis have extrarenal oxalate deposits. Combined hepatic and renal transplantation might be curative.

HEENT/AIRWAY: There may be deposits of calcium oxalate crystals in the retina.

CARDIOVASCULAR: Arrhythmias, particularly complete atrioventricular block (oxalate crystals have been seen near the conduction system) and peripheral vascular insufficiency from oxalate deposits.

ORTHOPEDIC: Short stature (possibly secondary to renal tubular acidosis). There may be oxalate crystal deposition in the joints and in bone.

GI/GU: Recurrent abdominal pain. Hematuria, urolithiasis, nephrocalcinosis, renal insufficiency, renal tubular acidosis. May rarely present as renal failure (without lithiasis) in infancy. Calcium oxalate stones are radiopaque. The natural history of the disease is progression to renal failure and death. The disease rapidly recurs in transplanted kidneys.

OTHER: There may be oxalate deposits in the skin.

MISCELLANEOUS: Although the presence of oxalate stones in the urine has been recognized for over 200 years, the disease was formally described only in 1925.

ANESTHETIC CONSIDERATIONS
Prolonged preoperative fasting should be avoided and a brisk diuresis should be maintained. Patients with renal tubular acidosis should have alkali therapy maintained perioperatively. Renal failure has implications for the titration of perioperative fluids and the choice of perioperative medications. Careful positioning may be needed in patients with disabling bone involvement. A single patient who developed hepatitis two days after a sevoflurane anesthetic has been reported, but no link to oxalosis could be identified or theorized (2).

Hyperoxaluria and nephrocalcinosis have been reported after the administration of methoxyflurane, without subsequent renal failure (4–8). This is presumably due to secondary hyperoxalosis from metabolism of methoxyflurane to oxalate, rather than a genetic disease.

Bibliography:
1. Milliner DS. The primary hyperoxalurias: an algorithm for diagnosis. *Am J Nephrol* 2005;25:154–160.
2. Reich A, Everding AS, Bulla M, et al. Hepatitis after sevoflurane exposure in an infant suffering from primary hyperoxaluria type 1. *Anesth Analg* 2004;99:370–372.
3. Cochat P, Nogueira PC, Mahmoud MA, et al. Primary hyperoxaluria in infants: medical, ethical, and economic issues. *J Pediatr* 1999;135:746–750.
4. Bergstrand A, Collste LG, Franksson C, et al. Oxalosis in renal transplants following methoxyflurane anesthesia. *Br J Anaesth* 1972;44:569–574.
5. Frascino JA. Tetracycline, methoxyflurane anaesthesia, and renal dysfunction. *Lancet* 1972;1:1127.
6. Aufderheide AC. Renal tubular calcium oxalate crystal deposition: its possible relation to methoxyflurane anesthesia. *Arch Pathol* 1971;92:162–166.
7. Mazze RI, Cousins MJ. Methoxyflurane anesthesia. *Arch Pathol* 1971;92:484.
8. Frascino JA, Vanamee P, Rosen PP. Renal oxalosis and azotemia after methoxyflurane anesthesia. *N Engl J Med* 1970;283:676–679.

P

Pachydermoperiostosis Syndrome

MIM #: 167100

This autosomal dominant disorder is distinguished by thick, coarse skin (pachyderma), clubbing of the fingers and thickening of the periosteum. There is wide variability in expression, but the disease is consistently more severe in male patients. The disorder can be diagnosed in childhood, but is usually diagnosed in adolescence, when it becomes clinically more apparent. The responsible gene and gene product are unknown.

HEENT/AIRWAY: Acromegalic facial features. Ptosis may develop. May have periodontal abnormalities.

ORTHOPEDIC: Clubbing of the fingers. Thickening of the periosteum, especially of the distal extremities. Joint and muscle pain.

GI/GU: May have gastrointestinal tract polyps.

OTHER: Progressive coarsening and thickening of the skin, particularly over the face (pachyderma). Hyperhidrosis. Peripheral vascular stasis.

ANESTHETIC CONSIDERATIONS

Note that clubbing of the fingers is secondary to periostosis, and is not in this case reflective of any cardiopulmonary disease. Skin changes might make vascular access more difficult. Patients with acromegaly may have excessive pharyngeal soft tissue, thickened vocal cords, and an enlarged tongue and epiglottis, all of which may make laryngoscopy and tracheal intubation difficult. Mandibular enlargement increases the lip-to-vocal cord distance. Hypertrophy of the turbinates may make passage of a nasogastric or nasotracheal tube difficult or impossible. A good mask fit may be difficult in patients with pronounced acromegalic features. There is significant clinical variability, and it is unclear if the acromegalic features in this syndrome can be severe enough routinely to affect airway management.

Bibliography:

1. Thappa DM, Sethuraman G, Kumar GR, et al. Primary pachydermoperiostosis: a case report. *J Dermatol* 2000;27:106–109.
2. Shimizu C, Kubo M, Kijima H, et al. A rare case of acromegaly associated with pachydermoperiostosis. *J Endocrinol Invest* 1999;22:386–389.
3. Sinha GP, Curtis P, Haigh D, et al. Pachydermoperiostosis in childhood. *Br J Rheumatol* 1997;36:1224–1227.
4. Singh GR, Menon PS. Pachydermoperiostosis in a 13-year-old boy presenting as an acromegaly-like syndrome. *J Pediatr Endocrinol Metab* 1995;8:51–54.

Pachyonychia Congenita Syndrome

MIM #: 167200, 167210

This autosomal dominant syndrome of ectodermal dysplasia is characterized by hypertrophic nails, hyperkeratosis, hyperhidrosis, and palmar and plantar bullae. There are two forms of this syndrome, a more common form that includes oral leukokeratosis, and a rarer form that includes epidermal cysts. The two forms of this syndrome are caused by mutations in the keratin 16 or 6A genes (type 1), or the keratin 17 or 6B genes (type 2).

HEENT/AIRWAY: Leukokeratosis of the oral membranes occurs in the more common form of pachyonychia congenita syndrome. Dental abnormalities, including neonatal teeth, malformed teeth, early eruption of primary teeth, caries. May have cataracts. May have hoarseness secondary to laryngeal leukokeratosis. May have recurrent oral candidiasis.

CHEST: Laryngeal leukokeratosis may result in recurrent upper respiratory tract irritation and infection. Severe laryngeal involvement has required tracheostomy.

NEUROMUSCULAR: May have mental deficiency.

ORTHOPEDIC: Arthritis may develop in large joints.

GI/GU: May have intestinal diverticula.

OTHER: Hyperkeratosis of palms, soles, knees, elbows. Hyperhidrosis. Palmar and plantar bullae. Hypertrophic nails become thick, discolored, and misshapen. Recurrent cutaneous candidiasis may exacerbate the nail dystropy. Nails often eventually need to be surgically removed. Keratosis pilaris. Epidermal cysts on the face, neck, and upper chest in the rarer form of pachyonychia congenita syndrome. Verrucous lesions on elbows, knees, and lower legs. May have sparse, dry hair.

ANESTHETIC CONSIDERATIONS

Patients may have significant oral, laryngeal, or tracheal leukokeratosis, which may interfere with visualization of

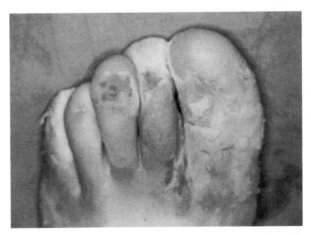

Pachyonychia congenita syndrome. Typical changes of the toes. (Courtesy of Dr. Kenneth E. Greer, Department of Dermatology, University of Virginia Health System.)

the larynx or cause respiratory compromise. Dental abnormalities should be documented preoperatively. Abnormal or carious teeth are susceptible to damage during laryngoscopy.

Bibliography:

1. Leachman SA, Kaspar RL, Fleckman P, et al. Clinical and pathological features of pachyonychia congenita. *J Invest Dermatol Symp Proc* 2005;10:3–17.
2. Kaspar RL. Challenges in developing therapies for rare diseases including pachyonychia congenita. *J Invest Dermatol Symp Proc* 2005;10:62–66.
3. Vijaikumar M, Thappa DM, Laxmisha C. Pachyonychia congenita: a case report. *Pediatr Dermatol* 2001;18:541–543.

Palizaeus-Merzbacher Disease

See Pelizaeus-Merzbacher disease

Pallister-Hall Syndrome

MIM #: 146510

This autosomal dominant disorder consists of hypothalamic hamartoblastoma, panhypopituitarism, anal defects, and postaxial polydactyly. Most patients die in infancy or early childhood. If treated adequately with replacement therapy, some patients may reach adulthood. Replacement therapy consists of L-thyroxine, growth hormone, and corticosteroids. This disorder is due to frameshift mutations in the gene *GLI3*, an oncogene that maps to the short arm of chromosome 7.

HEENT/AIRWAY: Bathrocephaly. Midline capillary hemangioma. Flattened midface. May have downward-slanting palpebral fissures, ptosis, microphthalmia. Abnormal external ear. Flat nasal bridge, short nose, anteverted nares. May have choanal atresia. Microglossia, multiple oral frenula. May have cleft lip, palate, or uvula. Micrognathia. Bifid, hypoplastic, or absent epiglottis in more than 50%. Laryngeal cleft. May have posterior subglottic web. Dysplastic tracheal cartilage, may have cricoid stenosis.

CHEST: Hypoplastic or absent lung. May have abnormal lung lobation. May have rib anomalies.

CARDIOVASCULAR: Congenital cardiac defects include patent ductus arteriosus, ventricular septal defects, endocardial cushion defects, mitral and aortic valve defects, and coarctation of the aorta.

NEUROMUSCULAR: Intelligence is usually normal. Hypothalamic hamartoblastoma, which replaces the normal hypothalamus. Pituitary aplasia/dysplasia leading to panhypopituitarism. May have occipital encephalocele, holoprosencephaly, polymicrogyria, Dandy-Walker malformation. May have seizures.

ORTHOPEDIC: Postaxial polydactyly. Oligodactyly, syndactyly, brachydactyly, camptodactyly. Nail dysplasia. Short limbs. May have vertebral abnormalities. May have congenital hip dislocation.

GI/GU: Anal defects, including imperforate anus, rectal atresia. May have Hirschprung disease. Hypoplasia of the adrenal glands. May have hypoplasia of the pancreas. May have hypospadias, micropenis. Renal agenesis or dysplasia.

OTHER: Hypoplasia of the thyroid gland. May have hypoparathyroidism. May have precocious puberty.

ANESTHETIC CONSIDERATIONS

Micrognathia may make direct laryngoscopy and tracheal intubation more difficult. Patients with abnormal tracheal cartilage or a posterior subglottic web may require a smaller-than-expected endotracheal tube. Choanal atresia, if present, precludes the use of a nasal airway or a nasogastric tube. Patients with lung hypoplasia or abnormal lung lobation are at increased risk for postoperative respiratory complications.

Patients will likely be on steroid replacement therapy, and require perioperative stress doses of steroids as well as postoperative continuation of steroids. The presence of renal disease has implications for fluid therapy and the choice of anesthetic drugs. Patients with congenital cardiac defects require perioperative antibiotic prophylaxis as indicated.

Bibliography:

1. Kalff-Suske M, Paparidis Z, Bornholdt D, et al. Gene symbol: GLI3. Disease: Pallister-Hall syndrome. *Hum Genet* 2004;114:403.
2. Stoll C, De Saint Martin A, Donato L, et al. Pallister-Hall syndrome with stenosis of the cricoid cartilage and microphallus without hypopituitarism. *Genet Couns* 2001;12:231–235.
3. Ondrey F, Griffith A, Van Waes C, et al. Asymptomatic laryngeal malformations are common in patients with Pallister-Hall syndrome. *Am J Med Genet* 2000;94:64–67.
4. Biesecker LG, Abbott M, Allen J, et al. Report from the workshop on Pallister-Hall syndrome and related phenotypes. *Am J Med Genet* 1996;65:76–81.

Pallister-Killian Syndrome

MIM #: 601803

This syndrome is due to mosaicism for tetrasomy of chromosome 12p. The phenotype can be somewhat variable.

HEENT/AIRWAY: Prominent forehead. Coarse facial features develop. Sparse anterior scalp hair. Sparse eyebrows and eyelashes. Hypertelorism, ptosis, strabismus, epicanthal folds, cataracts, exophthalmos. Deafness. Large ears. Stenotic external auditory canals. Short anteverted nose. Micrognathia. Cupid-bow lip, macroglossia, protruding lower lip, cleft palate, bifid uvula. Delayed dental eruption. Short webbed neck.

CHEST: Pulmonary hypoplasia. Diaphragmatic hernia. Accessory nipples.

CARDIOVASCULAR: Congenital cardiac defects, pericardial agenesis, hypertrophic cardiomyopathy.

NEUROMUSCULAR: Profound mental retardation, seizures. Hypotonic when newborn, hypertonic with aging.

ORTHOPEDIC: Kyphoscoliosis. Sacral appendage. Congenital hip dislocation. Hypermobile joints. Contractures with age. Mesomelic/rhizomelic limb shortening. Broad hands, clinodactyly of the fifth finger. Short fingers and toes, hypoplasia of distal digits. Postaxial polydactyly. Transverse (simian) palmar crease.

GI/GU: Umbilical hernia, omphalocele. Malrotation of the gut. Anal atresia, imperforate anus, anal stenosis. Cystic or dysplastic kidneys. Urogenital cloaca. Inguinal hernia. Cryptorchidism, hypospadias, small scrotum. Hypoplastic labia majora, absent upper vagina or uterus.

OTHER: Obesity. Hypo- and hyperpigmented hair streaks.

ANESTHETIC CONSIDERATIONS
Macroglossia and micrognathia are potential problems for intubation, but were not problematic in the only case report in the anesthesia literature.

Bibliography:
1. Sanchez-Carpintero R, McLellan A, Parmeggiani L, et al. Pallister-Killian syndrome: an unusual cause of epileptic spasms. *Dev Med Child Neurol* 2005;47:776–779.
2. Iacobucci T, Galeone M, De Francisci G. Anaesthetic management of a child with Pallister-Killian syndrome. *Paediatr Anaesth* 2003;13:457–459.
3. Genevieve D, Cormier-Daire V, Sanlaville D, et al. Mild phenotype in a 15-year-old boy with Pallister-Killian syndrome. *Am J Med Genet A* 2003;116:90–93.

Papillon-Lefevre Syndrome

MIM #: 245000

This autosomal recessive disorder, which maps to the long arm of chromosome 11, is characterized by hyperkeratosis of the palms and soles and periodontal disease. It is caused by a mutation in the gene for cathepsin C (*CTSC*), which is a lysosomal protease. The disease is treated with retinoids, which appear successfully to preserve adult teeth.

HEENT/AIRWAY: Eyelid cysts. Periodontal disease with premature loss of primary and adult teeth. Early eruption of adult teeth.

NEUROMUSCULAR: Calcification of the dura mater.

ORTHOPEDIC: Fragile nails.

GI/GU: May develop pyogenic liver abscess.

OTHER: Hyperkeratosis of the palms and soles. Hypotrichosis. Depressed neutrophil chemotaxis.

ANESTHETIC CONSIDERATIONS
Dental abnormalities should be documented preoperatively. Patients may have loose teeth at an age when it is not expected. Care must be taken to avoid dental damage during laryngoscopy.

Bibliography:
1. Janjua SA, Khachemoune A. Papillon-Lefevre syndrome: case report and review of the literature. *Dermatol Online J* 2004;10:13.
2. Ullbro C, Crossner CG, Nederfors T, et al. Dermatologic and oral findings in a cohort of 47 patients with Papillon-Lefevre syndrome. *J Am Acad Dermatol* 2003;48:345–351.
3. Wiebe CB, Hakkinen L, Putnins EE, et al. Successful periodontal maintenance of a case with Papillon-Lefevre syndrome: 12-year follow-up and review of the literature. *J Periodontol* 2001;72:824–830.

Papillorenal Syndrome

(Includes Morning glory syndrome)

MIM #: 120330

Morning glory syndrome refers specifically to a retinal finding which resembles a 'morning glory' flower. It was originally thought to be a retinal coloboma, but may represent abnormal regression of embryonic mesoderm of the optic disc. When associated with renal failure, it is the papillorenal syndrome. It is thought to be due to a mutation in the *PAX2* gene, even though several patients with this phenotype have not demonstrated a *PAX2* mutation.

HEENT/AIRWAY: Funnel-shaped, excavated optic disc with surrounding pigmentary changes. May have myopia, exotropia, retinal vascular abnormalities, and retinal detachment. May have high frequency hearing loss. May have midline defects including cleft lip and palate and hypertelorism.

NEUROMUSCULAR: May have basal myelomeningocele. May have agenesis of the corpus callosum. May have Arnold-Chiari malformation.

GI/GU: Vesicoureteral reflux. Congenital renal hypoplasia. Congenital and progressive renal insufficiency. Renal cysts.

OTHER: Morning glory syndrome has been found with the CHARGE association (see earlier).

ANESTHETIC CONSIDERATIONS
There is a single report of difficult intubation and difficulty in fitting a laryngeal mask (2).

Bibliography:
1. Parsa CF, Silva ED, Sundin OH, et al. Redefining papillorenal syndrome: an underdiagnosed cause of ocular and renal morbidity. *Ophthalmology* 2001;108:738–749.

2. Shevchenko Y, Rehman M, Dorsey AT. Unexpected difficult intubation in the patient with Morning Glory syndrome. *Paediatr Anaesth* 1999; 9:359–361.
3. Eccles MR, Schimmenti LA. Renal-coloboma syndrome: a multi-system developmental disorder caused by PAX2 mutations. *Clin Genet* 1999;56:1–9.

Paramyotonia Congenita

SYNONYM: Eulenburg disease

MIM #: 168300

This syndrome is due to a mutation in the alpha subunit of the type IV sodium channel (*SCN4A*) on the long arm of chromosome 17. As such, it is allelic with hyperkalemic periodic paralysis (see earlier) and the phenotypes of the two disorders overlap. Abnormal inactivation of the mutant channels allows additional sodium to enter the cells. Cells remain excitable during the delayed inactivation. The hallmarks of this autosomal dominant disease are myotonia (failure of timely muscle relaxation) which is exaggerated by cold, intermittent flaccidity, lability of serum potassium, and lack of histologic muscle changes. The disease is manifest in infancy or early childhood, is nonprogressive, and does not affect life expectancy. The phenotype is variable.

CARDIOVASCULAR: There are no myopathic or arrhythmogenic implications.

NEUROMUSCULAR: Cold-sensitive myotonia, predominantly of the face, neck, and hands. Grip myotonia, may have percussion myotonia. Myotonia increases with exercise ("paradoxical myotonia"), unlike other myotonic disorders. Myotonia is also precipitated by rest after exercise. Often will develop weakness on muscle warming, or after cooling. May have episodic weakness unrelated to myotonia. May have paresis.

OTHER: Hypokalemia and hyperkalemia have been reported. Cold-induced abortion has been reported.

MISCELLANEOUS: Exacerbation by cold means that eating ice cream (even the low-fat kind) can be dangerous to these patients. Unlike myotonia congenita, stiffness and weakness are exacerbated by activity, thus the term para(doxical) myotonia.

ANESTHETIC CONSIDERATIONS

Patients need to be kept warm, utilizing warm operating rooms, warmed surgical prep solutions, warmed intravenous fluids, and external warming devices as appropriate. Propofol may be the anesthetic agent of choice (3). Succinylcholine should be avoided as it can induce myotonia (see figure, Myotonic dystrophy). Nondepolarizing muscle relaxants have been used without complication. Anticholinesterases may aggravate the myotonia (1). There appears to be no intrinsic reason for preoperative potassium manipulation. Postoperative hypokalemia has been observed (7). A case of cardiac surgery utilizing moderate hypothermia (and adequate rewarming) resulted in no sequelae. Respiratory status must be monitored carefully perioperatively, as there is potential for respiratory insufficiency during an episode of flaccid paresis.

In the event of a myotonic crisis, serum potassium should be measured emergently. Drugs which have been used include type I antiarrhythmics (e.g., quinidine, procainamide, mexiletine, and tocainide). Other drugs which have been tried include epinephrine, acetazolamide, albuterol, and calcium gluconate.

Bibliography:
1. Ay B, Gerçek A, Dodan V, et al. Pyloromyotomy in a patient with paramyotonia congenital. *Anesth Analg* 2004;98:68–69.
2. Rosenbaum HK, Miller JD. Malignant hyperthermia and myotonic disorders. *Anesthesiol Clin North America* 2002;20:623–664.
3. Haeseler G, Stormer M, Mohammadi B, et al. The anesthetic propofol modulates gating in paramyotonia congenita mutant muscle sodium channels. *Muscle Nerve* 2001;24:736–743.
4. Davies NP, Eunson LH, Gregory RP, et al. Clinical, electrophysiological, and molecular genetic studies in a new family with paramyotonia congenita. *J Neurol Neurosurg Psychiatry* 2000;68:504–507.
5. Grace RF, Roach VJ. Caesarean section in a patient with paramyotonia congenita. *Anaesth Intensive Care* 1999;27:534–537.
6. Howell PR, Douglas MJ. Lupus anticoagulant, paramyotonia congenita and pregnancy. *Can J Anaesth* 1992;39:992–996.
7. Streib EW. Hypokalemic paralysis in two patients with paramyotonia congenita (PC) and known hyperkalemic/exercise-induced weakness. *Muscle Nerve* 1989;12:936–937.

Parenti-Fraccaro Achondrogenesis

Included in Achondrogenesis

Parry-Romberg Disease

See Romberg disease

Patau Syndrome

See Trisomy 13

Pearson Syndrome

MIM #: 557000

This is a syndrome of sideroblastic anemia, vacuolization of marrow precursors, and exocrine pancreatic dysfunction. The disorder is due to deletions and duplications in mitochondrial DNA. The clinical variations in the manifestations of the syndrome are thought to reflect the tissue distribution and relative proportion of the abnormal DNA. The clinically similar Shwachman syndrome (see later) also involves anemia and exocrine pancreatic dysfunction. The Shwachman syndrome additionally involves pancytopenia (particularly neutropenia), immunologic abnormalities, and metaphyseal chondrodysplasia. Pancreatic dysfunction is associated with pancreatic fatty infiltration in Shwachman syndrome and with pancreatic fibrosis in Pearson syndrome. Patients have been reported with Pearson syndrome who later acquired Kearns-Sayre syndrome, another disease of mitochondria (see earlier).

CARDIOVASCULAR: May develop heart block. May develop left ventricular failure.

GI/GU: Pancreatic exocrine dysfunction with pancreatic fibrosis. Splenic atrophy. Fanconi syndrome (see earlier). May have renal cysts.

OTHER: Low birth weight, failure to thrive. Sideroblastic anemia. Normal marrow cellularity with vacuolization of marrow precursors. Insulin-dependent diabetes, metabolic acidosis, which may be chronic. A case has been reported with fibrosis of the thyroid.

ANESTHETIC CONSIDERATIONS

The hematocrit should be evaluated preoperatively. Patients may have Fanconi syndrome, so consideration should be given to evaluating renal function and electrolyte status preoperatively. In the presence of Fanconi syndrome, urine output may not adequately reflect intravascular volume. Patients may acquire Kearns-Sayre syndrome (see earlier for anesthetic considerations with the Kearns-Sayre syndrome).

Bibliography:
1. Knerr I, Metzler M, Niemeyer CM, et al. Hematologic features and clinical course of an infant with Pearson syndrome caused by a novel deletion of mitochondrial DNA. *J Pediatr Hematol Oncol* 2003;25:948–951.
2. Krauch G, Wilichowski E, Schmidt KG, et al. Pearson marrow-pancreas syndrome with worsening cardiac function caused by pleiotropic rearrangement of mitochondrial DNA. *Am J Med Genet* 2002;110: 57–61.
3. Lacbawan F, Tifft CJ, Luban NL, et al. Clinical heterogeneity in mitochondrial DNA deletion disorders: a diagnostic challenge of Pearson syndrome. *Am J Med Genet* 2000;95:266–268.
4. Kerr DS. Protean manifestations of mitochondrial diseases: a minireview. *J Pediatr Hematol Oncol* 1997;19:279–286.

Pelizaeus-Merzbacher Disease

SYNONYM: Palizaeus-Merzbacher disease

MIM #: 312080

This is an X-linked recessive leukodystrophy with onset in infancy. There is significant genetic and clinical heterogeneity. The disease is due to an abnormality in the gene for proteolipid protein, or lipophilin, a major constituent of myelin.

HEENT/AIRWAY: Microcephaly. Head shaking and rotatory nystagmus. Copious oral secretions, poor airway tone, tracheomalacia and neonatal stridor.

NEUROMUSCULAR: Slowly progressive psychomotor retardation with eventual dementia. Neonatal hypotonia. Seizures. Choreoathetosis, spasticity, pyramidal signs, Parkinsonian symptoms. The neuropathologic findings include diffuse demyelination with interspersed areas of normal myelin, the "tigroid appearance." Magnetic resonance imaging scans show multiple areas of hyperintensity in the periventricular and subcortical white matter areas. Myelination of peripheral nerves and electrophysiologic studies of peripheral nerves are normal.

ORTHOPEDIC: Poor growth.

GI/GU: Increased incidence of gastroesophageal reflux.

MISCELLANEOUS: One of the leukodystrophies, the others being adrenoleukodystrophy, metachromatic leukodystrophy, Krabbe disease, Canavan disease, and Alexander disease. Leukodystrophies involve defective formation of myelin. The analogous defect of Pelizaeus-Merzbacher disease in mice is the "jimpy" defect, and Pelizaeus-Merzbacher disease seems similar or identical to "paralytic tremor" in chinchillas.

ANESTHETIC CONSIDERATIONS

Copious secretions and airway hypotonia make close perioperative observation of respiratory adequacy important. Consideration should be given to anticholinergic premedication to dry oral secretions. Patients are at increased risk for perioperative aspiration because of poor airway tone, copious oral secretions, and an increased incidence of gastroesophageal reflux. Patients should be carefully positioned and padded perioperatively secondary to their poor nutritional status. The risk of excessive potassium release with succinylcholine is unknown, but is theoretically possible in bedridden patients with atrophic muscles. Anticonvulsant medications need to be continued (or a parenteral form substituted), which may alter the metabolism of some anesthetic drugs, requiring more frequent dosing.

Phenothiazines, butyrophenones, and other dopaminergic blockers may exacerbate movement disorders. Metoclopramide may cause extrapyramidal effects and should be avoided if possible. Ondansetron should be safe as an antiemetic because it does not have antidopaminergic effects.

Bibliography:
1. Inoue K. PLP1-related inherited dysmyelinating disorders: Pelizaeus-Merzbacher disease and spastic paraplegia type 2. *Neurogenetics* 2005;6:1–16.
2. Koeppen AH, Robitaille Y. Pelizaeus-Merzbacher disease. *J Neuropathol Exp Neurol* 2002;61:747–759.
3. Tobias JD. Anaesthetic considerations for the child with leukodystrophy. *Can J Anaesth* 1992;39:394–397.

Pena-Shokeir Syndrome, Type I

See Fetal akinesia/hypokinesia sequence

Pena-Shokeir Syndrome, Type II

See Cerebrooculofacioskeletal syndrome

Pendred Syndrome

MIM #: 274600

This autosomal recessive syndrome is characterized by congenital deafness and abnormal organification of thyroid hormone. It is caused by a mutation in the *SLC26A4* gene, located on the long arm of chromosome 7. The function of the gene product, termed "pendrin," is not certain, but it may act as an iodide-specific transporter which is responsible for iodide efflux in the thyroid gland. Of interest, this gene maps to a similar location on the long arm of chromosome 7 as another recessive gene for deafness, *DFNB4*.

HEENT/AIRWAY: Congenital neurosensory deafness, sometimes associated with cochlear malformation and vestibular dysfunction. Widened vestibular aqueduct. Goiter.

NEUROMUSCULAR: Mental retardation.

OTHER: Defect in thyroid hormone organification with compensated (euthyroid) hypothyroidism. Exaggerated response to thyroid-releasing hormone. Because of the very abnormal appearance of the thyroid on histologic study, an incorrect diagnosis of thyroid cancer may be made. However, thyroid carcinoma may develop.

MISCELLANEOUS: Described by Pendred in 1896, it took exactly 100 years to map the gene to the long arm of chromosome 7.

ANESTHETIC CONSIDERATIONS

Preoperative thyroid studies should be obtained, and patients should be euthyroid before elective surgery is undertaken. Be sensitive to the fact that patients may have hearing loss and vestibular dysfunction.

Bibliography:
1. Taylor JP, Metcalfe RA, Watson PF, et al. Mutations of the PDS gene, encoding pendrin, are associated with protein mislocalization and loss of iodide efflux: implications for thyroid dysfunction in Pendred syndrome. *J Clin Endocrinol Metab* 2002;87:1778–1784.
2. Wilcox ER, Everett LA, Li XC, et al. The PDS gene, Pendred syndrome and non-syndromic deafness DFNB4. *Adv Otorhinolaryngol* 2000;56:145–151.
3. Reardon W, Coffey R, Chowdhury T, et al. Prevalence, age of onset, and natural history of thyroid disease in Pendred syndrome. *J Med Genet* 1999;36:595–598.

Penta X Syndrome

SYNONYM: XXXXX syndrome

MIM #: None

This chromosomal syndrome consists primarily of mental retardation, growth retardation, small hands, and patent ductus arteriosus. This syndrome is due to five copies of the X chromosome. Of interest, the X chromosomes appear to be of maternal origin.

HEENT/AIRWAY: Microcephaly, low posterior hairline. Upward-slanting palpebral fissures, hypertelorism, epicanthal folds, iris colobomas. Low nasal bridge. Malocclusion. Premature loss of deciduous teeth. May have cleft palate, macroglossia, micrognathia.

CARDIOVASCULAR: Patent ductus arteriosus or ventricular septal defect.

NEUROMUSCULAR: Moderate to severe mental retardation. Hypotonia. May have hydrocephalus.

ORTHOPEDIC: Short stature. Small hands with clinodactyly of fifth fingers. Excessively lax joints with risk of dislocations of multiple joints, including shoulder, elbow, hips, knees, wrists, and fingers.

GI/GU: Occasional renal dysplasia, horseshoe kidney. May have ovarian agenesis.

OTHER: Small for gestational age, failure to thrive.

ANESTHETIC CONSIDERATIONS

Difficult intubation has not been reported, but may be a concern, given the incidence of macroglossia and micrognathia. Deciduous teeth may be prematurely loose, particularly the anterior teeth. Baseline renal function should be established. Patients must be carefully positioned secondary to joint laxity. Patients with patent ductus arteriosus or ventricular septal defect require perioperative antibiotic prophylaxis as indicated.

Bibliography:
1. Cho YG, Kim DS, Lee HS, et al. A case of 49,XXXXX in which the extra X chromosomes were maternal in origin. *J Clin Pathol* 2004;57:1004–1006.
2. Biroli E, Ghimenti C, Ricci I, et al. Sex chromosome abnormality: report of three clinical cases of X pentasomy. *Pathologica* 2003;95:444–446.
3. Linden MG, Bender BG, Robinson A. Sex chromosome tetrasomy and pentasomy. *Pediatrics* 1995;96:672–682.

Pentalogy of Cantrell

SYNONYM: Thoracoabdominal syndrome; Cantrell pentalogy

MIM #: 313850

This disease is a defect in midline fusion that is probably inherited in an X-linked fashion and involves defects in the (a) abdominal wall, (b) sternum, (c) diaphragm, (d) pericardium, and (e) heart. Infants often require a multistaged surgical repair.

HEENT/AIRWAY: Hydrocephalus or anencephaly. Cystic hygroma. Cleft lip or palate.

CHEST: Failure of sternal fusion. Diaphragmatic hernia, hypoplastic lungs.

CARDIOVASCULAR: Ectopia cordis (heart protrudes through an open sternum) with a variety of congenital cardiac defects, including ventricular septal defect, atrial septal defect, tetralogy of Fallot, and left ventricular diverticulum. Absent pericardium.

GI/GU: Omphalocele. Hypospadias. Renal agenesis.

ANESTHETIC CONSIDERATIONS

Infants may be quite ill with multiorgan involvement. Anesthetic management depends on the specific anatomic anomalies and their severity. Displacement of intraabdominal organs can interfere with fetal ultrasound, and associated intracardiac defects could be missed (1). Surgeons must be particularly careful not to place undue pressure on the abdomen or chest by resting on a draped patient. Closure of an omphalocele has resulted in dislocation of abdominal contents through an anterior diaphragmatic hernia, with acute cardiopulmonary deterioration. Patients with congenital heart disease require perioperative antibiotic prophylaxis as indicated.

Bibliography:

1. Saito T, Suzuki A, Takahara O, et al. Anesthetic management of a patient with Cantrell pentalogy diagnosed prenatally [Letter]. *Can J Anaesth* 2004;51:946–947.
2. Correa-Rivas MS, Matos-Llovet I, Garcia-Fragoso L. Pentalogy of Cantrell: a case report with pathologic findings. *Pediatr Dev Pathol* 2004;7:649–652.
3. Agrawal N, Sehgal R, Kumar R, et al. Cantrell pentalogy [Letter]. *Anaesth Intensive Care* 2003;31:120–121.
4. Laloyaux P, Veyckemans F, van Dyck M. Anaesthetic management of a prematurely born infant with Cantrell Pentalogy. *Paediatr Anaesth* 1998;8:163–166.
5. Martin RA, Cunniff C, Erickson L, et al. Pentalogy of Cantrell and ectopia cordis, a familial developmental field complex. *Am J Med Genet* 1992;42:839–841.

Perheentupa Syndrome

See Mulibrey nanism syndrome

Periodic Paralysis

See Familial periodic paralysis

Peters-Plus Syndrome

MIM #: 261540

Peters anomaly (corneal clouding and adhesions between the iris and lens) is a defect in the embryonic development of the anterior chamber of the eye. It can occur in isolation or with many genetic and nongenetic syndromes. Peters-Plus syndrome is an autosomal recessive disorder of Peters anomaly, short limb dwarfism, and mental retardation.

HEENT/AIRWAY: Round face, hypertelorism, corneal clouding, anterior lens adhesions, lens opacity, glaucoma, decreased vision. Narrowed external auditory canals with hearing loss. "Cupid-bow" thin upper lip, smooth philtrum, short frenulum. Mild micrognathia. Cleft lip and/or palate. Broad neck.

CHEST: Occasional pectus excavatum.

CARDIOVASCULAR: A variety of acyanotic cardiac defects.

NEUROMUSCULAR: Mental retardation ranging from mild to severe. Occasional dilated lateral ventricles, seizures, spastic diplegia. Agenesis of the corpus callosum has been reported.

ORTHOPEDIC: Short limb dwarfism, primarily rhizomelic. Limited range of motion of the elbows, with hypermobility of other joints. Broad, short hands and feet, fifth-finger clinodactyly.

GI/GU: Hydronephrosis, duplication of kidneys, cryptorchidism. Occasional hypospadias.

OTHER: Prenatal onset of growth deficiency. May have growth hormone deficiency.

ANESTHETIC CONSIDERATIONS

Although there may be mild micrognathia, difficult laryngoscopy and tracheal intubation have not been reported. Recall that patients are likely to have visual impairment. Patients should be carefully positioned secondary to joint hypermobility. Consider preoperative evaluation of renal function in patients with a history of renal abnormalities which predispose to renal insufficiency. Chronic use of anticonvulsant medications may affect the metabolism of some anesthetic drugs.

Bibliography:

1. Maillette de Buy Wenniger-Prick LJ, Hennekam RCM. The Peters' plus syndrome: a review. *Ann Genet* 2002;45:97–103.
2. Hennekam RCM, van Schooneveld MJ, Ardinger HH, et al. The Peters'-Plus syndrome: description of 16 patients and review of the literature. *Clin Dysmorphol* 1993;2:283–300.

Peutz-Jeghers Syndrome

MIM #: 175200

This autosomal dominant disease is characterized by intestinal polyposis and melanin spots on the oral mucosa, lips, and digits. Cutaneous spots fade with age, but the oral spots persist. Malignant degeneration of the intestinal polyps can occur. There also appears to be an increased incidence of various other neoplasms. This syndrome is due to a mutation in the gene for serine/threonine kinase (*STK11/LKB1*), located on the short arm of chromosome 19. This gene may act as a tumor suppressor gene.

HEENT/AIRWAY: Melanin spots on the oral mucosa and lips. Nasal polyps.

CHEST: Bronchial polyps.

ORTHOPEDIC: Melanin spots on the digits. These are actually classified as lentigines. Lentigines are macules similar to freckles but, unlike freckles, are not restricted to sun-exposed areas. They are dark brown to black, and round to oval.

GI/GU: Multiple intestinal polyps (hamartomas), particularly jejunal. Rare malignant degeneration of intestinal polyps. Intussusception, gastrointestinal bleeding, rectal prolapse (all secondary to polyps). May have esophageal polyps, as well as polyps of the kidney, ureter, and bladder. Increased incidence of gonadal tumors (ovarian and testicular), and increased incidence of pancreatic cancer.

OTHER: Pigmented macules can develop in preexisting psoriatic lesions that are in otherwise atypical locations. Increased incidence of breast cancer.

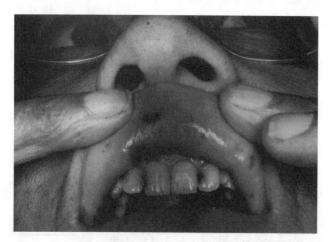

Peutz-Jeghers syndrome. Typical melanin spots of the lips. (Courtesy of Dr. Kenneth E. Greer, Department of Dermatology, University of Virginia Health System.)

MISCELLANEOUS: In 1895 Connor described twins with darkly pigmented spots on their lips and oral mucosa, likely the first description in the literature of the Peutz-Jeghers syndrome. The paper by Peutz (1921, in Dutch) came 28 years before that of Jeghers. Bruwer introduced the eponym Peutz-Jeghers syndrome in 1954. During his career, Jeghers kept an extensive collection of medical articles, systematically filed and annotated, which is currently accessible as the Jeghers Medical Index (www.jeghers.com).

ANESTHETIC CONSIDERATIONS
The possibility of nasal polyps should be appreciated before passing nasal tubes or catheters. Similarly, caution should be taken in endotracheal suctioning because of the possibility of bronchial polyps.

Bibliography:
1. Amos CI, Keitheri-Cheteri MB, Sabripour M, et al. Genotype-phenotype correlations in Peutz-Jeghers syndrome. *J Med Genet* 2004;41: 327–333.
2. Keller JJ, Westerman AM, de Rooij FW, et al. Molecular genetic evidence of an association between nasal polyposis and the Peutz-Jeghers syndrome. *Ann Intern Med* 2002;136:855–856.
3. Westerman AM, Wilson JHP. Peutz-Jeghers syndrome: risks of a hereditary condition. A clinical review. *Scand J Gastroenterol* 1999;34: S64–S70.
4. Fernandez Seara MJ, Martinez Soto MI, Fernandez Lorenzo JR, et al. Peutz-Jeghers syndrome in a neonate. *J Pediatr* 1995;126: 965–967.

Pfeiffer Syndrome

SYNONYM: Acrocephalosyndactyly type V

MIM #: 101600

This autosomal dominant syndrome is marked by craniosynostosis, mild syndactyly, and broad thumbs and great toes. Although most cases are due to mutations in the genes encoding fibroblast growth factor receptors 1 or 2 (*FGFR1* or *FGFR2*), some cases cannot be ascribed to either. Different mutations in *FGFR2* are also responsible for Antley-Bixler, Apert, Beare-Stevenson, and Crouzon syndromes (see earlier).

Three clinical subtypes have been described. Type 1 is an autosomal dominant disorder, whereas types 2 and 3 have occurred sporadically. The classic syndrome is type 1. Types 2 and 3 have more severe involvement. Type 2 involves the typical hand and foot anomalies as well as Kleeblattschaedel (cloverleaf skull, see earlier), severe proptosis and ankylosis of the elbows. Patients with type 2 have had diminished life expectancy. Type 3 is similar to type 2 but without cloverleaf skull. Ocular proptosis in type 3 is also severe. Various visceral malformations have been found in association with type 3.

HEENT/AIRWAY: Brachycephaly with coronal and possibly also sagittal craniosynostosis. Maxillary hypoplasia. Kleeblattschaedel anomaly (cloverleaf skull). Hypertelorism, shallow orbits with proptosis. Can have atresia of external auditory canal. Conductive hearing loss. Small nose with flat bridge. Rare choanal atresia. There has been a report of a cartilaginous trachea and a calcified trachea, also laryngomalacia, tracheomalacia, and bronchomalacia.

CHEST: Obstructive sleep apnea.

CARDIOVASCULAR: A variety of congenital cardiac malformations have been reported.

NEUROMUSCULAR: Intelligence is usually normal, occasional mental retardation. May have seizures, hydrocephalus, Arnold-Chiari malformation. May have increased intracranial pressure if craniosynostosis is severe.

ORTHOPEDIC: Broad thumbs and great toes. Polysyndactyly. Occasional fifth finger clinodactyly, radiohumeral synostosis of elbow, fused vertebrae. Vertebral fusion, usually upper cervical spine.

GI/GU: A variety of intestinal defects have been reported, including Prune-belly syndrome (see later), malrotation, and duplication.

ANESTHETIC CONSIDERATIONS

It has not been reported, but it has been suggested that these children may have a difficult airway (3). Certainly upper cervical vertebral fusion would limit mobility and make laryngoscopy and tracheal intubation more difficult. The placement of a maxillary distraction device may increase the difficulty of tracheal intubation (2). Tracheal abnormalities may lead to tracheal stenosis. Choanal atresia, if present, precludes the use of a nasal airway or placement of a nasogastric tube. Because of the incidence of obstructive apnea, patients should be observed carefully postoperatively. The eyes must be carefully protected perioperatively secondary to proptosis. Patients may have elevated intracranial pressure, in which case precautions should be taken to avoid further elevation in pressure. Chronic use of anticonvulsant medications may affect the metabolism of some anesthetic drugs. Patients with congenital heart disease need perioperative antibiotic prophylaxis as indicated.

Bibliography:

1. Harb E, Kran B. Pfeiffer syndrome: systemic and ocular implications. *Optometry* 2005;76:352–362.
2. Roche J, Frawley G, Heggie A. Difficult tracheal intubation induced by maxillary distraction devices in craniosynostosis syndromes. *Paediatr Anaesth* 2002;12:227–234.
3. Tobias JD, Jones B, Jimenez DF, et al. Anesthetic implications of Pfeiffer syndrome. *Am J Anesthesiol* 1998;25:79–83.
4. Plomp AS, Hamel BCJ, Cobben JM, et al. Pfeiffer syndrome type 2: further delineation and review of the literature. *Am J Med Genet* 1998;75:245–251.
5. Perkins JA, Sie KC, Milczuk H, et al. Airway management in children with craniofacial anomalies. *Cleft Palate Craniofac J* 1997;34:135–140.

PHACE Association

MIM #: 606519

Because it occurs almost exclusively in females, this neurocutaneous disorder may be X-linked dominant, with lethality in males. PHACE stands for **P**osterior fossa brain malformations, **H**emangiomas of the face, **A**rterial anomalies, **C**ardiac anomalies, and **E**ye abnormalities. The association has been referred to as PHACES when ventral defects, such as **S**ternal clefting or **S**upraumbilical raphe, are also present.

HEENT/AIRWAY: Facial hemangiomas—usually large and/or complex. Ocular anomalies include congenital cataracts, choroidal hemangiomas, cryptophthalmos, exophthalmos, microphthalmos, colobomas, optic atrophy, esotropia, optic nerve hypoplasia and congenital glaucoma. May have micrognathia. May have a subglottic hemangioma.

CHEST: May have sternal clefting.

CARDIOVASCULAR: Coarctation of the aorta or other cardiac anomalies. Arterial anomalies, such as aberrant arterial origins, stenosis, atresia and aneurysms, including one report of aortic aneurysm.

NEUROMUSCULAR: Cerebral vascular malformations, particularly aneurysm formation and the presence of anomalous branches of the internal carotid artery. May have ischemic strokes. Structural malformations of the brain, most commonly a Dandy-Walker malformation. May have agenesis of the corpus callosum. Neurologic sequelae include seizures, developmental delay, and contralateral hemiparesis.

GI/GU: May have supraumbilical raphe.

OTHER: Hemangiomas occur in locations other than the face in 30% of cases. May have congenital hypothyroidism.

ANESTHETIC CONSIDERATIONS

Be sensitive is to the fact that patients may have some loss of vision. Subglottic hemangiomas might bleed with instrumentation or intubation of the airway. Patients with aortic or cerebral aneurysms warrant tight control of blood pressure. Patients with congenital heart disease require perioperative antibiotic prophylaxis as indicated.

Bibliography:

1. Smith DS, Lee KK, Milczuk HA. Otolaryngologic manifestations of PHACE syndrome. *Int J Pediatr Otorhinolaryngol* 2004;68:1445–1450.
2. Bronzetti G, Giardini A, Patrizi A, et al. Ipsilateral hemangioma and aortic arch anomalies in posterior fossa malformations, hemangiomas, arterial anomalies, coarctation of the aorta, and cardiac defects and eye abnormalities (PHACE) anomaly: report and review. *Pediatrics* 2004;113:412–415.
3. Metry DW, Dowd CF, Barkovich AJ, et al. The many faces of PHACE syndrome. *J Pediatr* 2001;139:117–123.

Phenylketonuria

SYNONYM: PKU [includes Tetrahydrobiopterin (BH4) deficiency]

MIM #: 261600, 261630

This autosomal recessive disease is due to a defect in phenylalanine hydroxylase. This enzyme converts phenylalanine to tyrosine. There are multiple alleles, and some patients have defects that allow partial enzyme activity. These patients may have only moderately elevated levels of phenylalanine, not high enough to warrant treatment. Approximately 1% to 2% of patients with phenylketonuria do not have a defect in phenylalanine hydroxylase, but instead have a defect in the gene coding for the cofactor **tetrahydrobiopterin (BH4)** or for the cofactor's regeneration (dihydropteridine reductase deficiency). This cofactor is also needed for hydroxylation of tryptophan and tyrosine in the central nervous system, and limited BH4 causes decreased synthesis of the neurotransmitters serotonin and the catecholamines.

Treatment is by dietary restriction of phenylalanine, an essential amino acid. Commercial infant formulas are available. The artificial sweetener aspartame is hydrolyzed in the intestinal lumen to phenylalanine and aspartic acid. It needs to be studiously avoided by patients with phenylketonuria. Unfortunately, dietary restriction of phenylalanine does not affect the biopterin-deficient types. Phenylalanine hydroxylase is resident in the liver. Interestingly, liver transplantation in a boy with coincident end-stage liver disease also cured his phenylketonuria.

It is recommended that the restricted diet be continued until at least adolescence for boys and longer for girls. Elevated phenylalanine levels have been shown to be toxic to the fetus (see Maternal PKU syndrome, earlier). Fetal effects are proportional to maternal phenylalanine levels, and toxicity to the fetus is preventable with strict maternal dietary control at the time of conception and for the duration of pregnancy. Reasons not to stop the special diet in women of childbearing age include (a) pregnancy may be unexpected, and (b) the diet is so unpleasant that once people are off it, it is hard to get them back on.

HEENT/AIRWAY: Blue eyes.

NEUROMUSCULAR: If untreated, will have severe psychomotor retardation, poor head growth, seizures, increased deep tendon reflexes, abnormal gait and sitting posture. Slightly lower than average IQ in treated patients. Patients with the biopterin-deficient variant have a Parkinson-like progressive deterioration, and they often die young, even with good dietary phenylalanine control. There is evidence of abnormal brain myelin on magnetic resonance imaging, even without neurologic symptoms.

ORTHOPEDIC: Osteopenia.

GI/GU: If untreated, will have episodes of vomiting. (Some have been misdiagnosed as having pyloric stenosis during the neonatal period.)

OTHER: Treated patients compliant with a protein-restricted diet may have vitamin B$_{12}$ deficiency and megaloblastic anemia if they fail to take adequate vitamin supplementation.

If untreated, patients will have a mousy, pungent odor. Patients usually have less pigmentation than the rest of the family, including lighter hair ("dilute" pigmentation), although it will have been normal at birth. Indolent, often perirectal, eczema-like or scleroderma-like skin rash.

MISCELLANEOUS: Old names for this disease included "imbecilitas phenylpyrouvica" and "phenylpyruvic oligophrenia." This disease is an important historical paradigm for inborn errors of metabolism, and the first for which widespread testing of newborns was offered (the Guthrie test). The two children in whom it was first described were brought for medical attention because the pungent, musty odor they exuded induced asthma in their father. The odor is caused by an oxidation product of phenylalanine, phenylacetic acid.

It has been suggested that the heterozygous state may offer selective protection against the mycotoxin ochratoxin A. This toxin can be found in moldy stored grains and foods. Interestingly, the Celtic and Scandinavian regions, which have had repeated famines during which moldy foods were frequently eaten, also have a particularly high incidence of phenylketonuria.

ANESTHETIC CONSIDERATIONS

The special phenylalanine-restricted diet must be maintained perioperatively. Proconvulsant anesthetic agents should be avoided. Chronic use of anticonvulsant medications may alter the metabolism of some anesthetic drugs. Protracted fasting could result in a catabolic state with increased tissue catabolism and elevated phenylalanine levels. There is a single case report of a patient who developed paraparesis after an anesthetic which included nitrous oxide (5). By inactivating the B$_{12}$-dependent enzyme methionine synthetase, nitrous oxide is a known cause of myeloneuropathy. The authors postulated that their patient was vitamin B$_{12}$ deficient, and that the further effect of nitrous oxide led to his neurologic symptoms. Avoidance of nitrous oxide in patients with phenylketonuria, particularly if they are known or suspected to be vitamin B$_{12}$ deficient, seems reasonable.

Bibliography:

1. Blau N, Scriver CR. New approaches to treat PKU: how far are we? *Mol Genet Metab* 2004;81:1–2.
2. Kulkarni PR. Anesthetic management of a strabismus patient with phenylketonuria [Letter]. *Paediatr Anaesth* 2004;14:701.
3. Dal D, Çeliker V. Anaesthetic management of a strabismus patient with phenylketonuria [Letter]. *Paediatr Anaesth* 2003;13:740–741.
4. Cederbaum S. Phenylketonuria: an update. *Curr Opin Pediatr* 2002;14:702–706.

5. Lee P, Smith I, Piesowicz A, et al. Spastic paraparesis after anaesthesia. *Lancet* 1999;353:554.

Phosphoenolpyruvate Carboxykinase Deficiency

MIM #: 261680, 261650

This disease is a cause of lactic acidemia in childhood. Phosphoenolpyruvate carboxykinase is important in the conversion of pyruvate to glucose. Pyruvate is converted to oxaloacetate, and then by this enzyme to phosphoenolpyruvate, which is then converted to glucose. There are two genes implicated in the pathogenesis of this syndrome: one coding for enzyme which resides in the cytosol (*PCK1*) and the other coding for enzyme which resides in mitochondria (*PCK2*). Symptoms in patients with the mitochondrial enzyme defect tend to be more persistent, whereas activity of the cytosolic enzyme is influenced by insulin, glucocorticoids, diet, cyclic adenosine monophosphate, and thyroid hormone to maintain appropriate glucose production.

NEUROMUSCULAR: Hypotonia.

GI/GU: Hepatomegaly, fatty liver, rarely hepatic failure. Fatty kidney.

OTHER: Lactic acidemia. Impaired gluconeogenesis, hypoglycemia. Failure to thrive.

ANESTHETIC CONSIDERATIONS
Serum glucose levels should be monitored perioperatively. Prolonged perioperative fasting should be avoided. Adequate perioperative glucose intake must be ensured.

Bibliography:
1. Beale EG, Hammer RE, Antoine B, et al. Glyceroneogenesis comes of age. *FASEB J* 2002;16:1695–1696.
2. Leonard JV, Hyland K, Furukawa N, et al. Mitochondrial phosphoenolpyruvate carboxykinase deficiency. *Eur J Pediatr* 1991;150:198–199.
3. Clayton PT, Hyland K, Brand M, et al. Mitochondrial phosphoenolpyruvate carboxykinase deficiency. *Eur J Pediatr* 1986;145:46–50.

Phosphofructokinase Deficiency

See Glycogen storage disease VII

Phosphoglycerate Kinase Deficiency

MIM #: 311800

This X-linked abnormality (PGK 1) is characterized by hemolytic anemia and neurologic manifestations in boys, and occasional hemolytic anemia in girls. This important enzyme in glycolysis catalyzes the interconversion of 3-phosphoglycerate and 1,3-diphosphoglycerate, with the production of adenosine triphosphate. There are several variants of this disorder, with differing levels of enzyme activity. In addition, it is thought that the variable involvement of red blood cells, muscles, and nervous system may in part be due to organ-specific isozymes that are secondary to organ-specific posttranslational modifications. Bypass of the phosphoglycerate kinase enzyme in the Embden-Meyerhof pathway by triose results in its diversion to form 2,3-diphosphoglycerate (2,3-DPG) in red blood cells. Phosphoglycerate kinase may also be secreted by tumor cells, and participate in tumor-associated angiogenesis, which is necessary for tumor expansion and metastasis.

A second, autosomal recessive, form of this enzyme defect (PGK 2) is localized to spermatozoa.

NEUROMUSCULAR: Behavioral problems, emotional lability, impaired speech, variable mental retardation, seizures, extrapyramidal tract disease, weakness after exercise. Hemiplegia or coma during exacerbations of hemolysis. Recovery from exacerbations is rapid. Some variants are associated with myopathic symptoms and rhabdomyolysis without hemolysis.

GI/GU: Postexercise nausea and anorexia. Occasional hemoglobinuria. May develop renal failure.

OTHER: Chronic hemolytic anemia with spherocytosis, and occasional hemolytic crises. 2,3-DPG levels are elevated.

ANESTHETIC CONSIDERATIONS
The hematocrit should be evaluated preoperatively. Ensuring adequate perioperative glucose would seem reasonable. Brisk diuresis should be maintained perioperatively if there is hemoglobinuria. Fluids and medications should be titrated carefully in patients with renal failure. Elevated 2,3-DPG levels might be expected to have mild effects on the correlation of oxygen saturation and partial pressure of oxygen (pO_2), with lower saturation for the same pO_2 because of a rightward shift in the oxyhemoglobin dissociation curve. Chronic use of anticonvulsant medications may affect the metabolism of some anesthetic drugs. Given the possible myopathic symptoms and rhabdomyolysis, succinylcholine should be used with care. Phenothiazines, butyrophenones, and other dopaminergic blockers may exacerbate movement disorders. Ondansetron should be safe as an antiemetic because it does not have antidopaminergic effects.

Bibliography:
1. Spanu C, Oltean S. Familial phosphoglycerate kinase deficiency associated with rhabdomyolysis and acute renal failure: abnormality in mRNA splicing? *Nephrol Dial Transplant* 2003;18:445–446.
2. Lay AJ, Jiang XM, Kisker O, et al. Phosphoglycerate kinase acts in tumour angiogenesis as a disulphide reductase. *Nature* 2000;408:869–873.
3. DiMauro S, Dalakas M, Miranda AS. Phosphoglycerate kinase deficiency: another cause of recurrent myoglobinuria. *Ann Neurol* 1983;13:11–19.

Phosphohexose Isomerase Deficiency

See Glucose phosphate isomerase deficiency

Phosphorylase b Kinase Deficiency

See Hers disease

Phosphorylase Kinase Deficiency

See Glycogen storage disease VIII

Pierre Robin Syndrome

SYNONYM: Robin sequence

MIM #: 261800

This syndrome of micrognathia, glossoptosis, and a cleft soft palate is a well-known cause of difficult intubations in children. The mandible may demonstrate significant catch-up growth with aging. The etiologic defect is probably early mandibular hypoplasia *in utero*, placing the tongue posteriorly, which keeps the palatal shelves (which normally must grow over the tongue) from closing in the midline, causing a cleft. The rounded contour of the cleft differs from the usual inverted "V" shape of most palatal clefts. Neonates may require prone positioning, a nasopharyngeal airway, suturing of the tongue to the lip, or even urgent tracheostomy to preserve an airway. As an isolated finding in an otherwise healthy infant, the prognosis is good if the neonatal airway problems can be managed. Pierre Robin syndrome can occur, however, as a component of many multiple-malformation syndromes.

HEENT/AIRWAY: Severe micrognathia. Glossoptosis. Cleft soft palate. Obstructive apnea. Airway obstruction usually improves with age.

CHEST: Hypoxia from airway obstruction.

CARDIOVASCULAR: Cor pulmonale can develop with severe chronic airway obstruction. May have vagal hyperactivity.

NEUROMUSCULAR: Patients may have brainstem dysfunction, with periods of central apnea.

GI/GU: Feeding difficulties are common secondary to anatomic abnormalities, and also possibly to swallowing problems due to brainstem dysfunction.

MISCELLANEOUS: Pierre Robin (one person) was the leading French dental surgeon of his day.

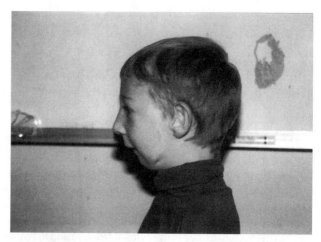

Pierre Robin syndrome. FIG. 1. A 4-year-old boy with Pierre Robin syndrome. He has already had mandibular augmentation surgery, but still has a very small mandible. Orotracheal intubation by a senior pediatric anesthesiologist had been impossible during a prior surgery, and he required fiberoptic intubation, which was reportedly very difficult. For his current surgery (tympanostomy tubes, resection of frenulum and dental surgery), a laryngeal mask airway was easily placed. The dentist worked around the airway and the anesthesia was uncomplicated and uneventful.

ANESTHETIC CONSIDERATIONS

Direct laryngoscopy and tracheal intubation can be extremely difficult. A variety of alternative intubation techniques have been suggested, including the laryngeal mask airway (LMA) (13–15, 17, 19, 20, 22), the Shikani Optical Stylet (S.O.S.) (1), intubation through a laryngeal mask airway (9), fiberoptic intubation through a laryngeal mask airway (8, 10), digitally assisted intubation (18), fiberoptic nasal intubation (4, 21, 23), retrograde tracheal intubation (26), laryngoscopy with the Bullard laryngoscope (16), and blind nasal intubation in the prone position with hyperextension

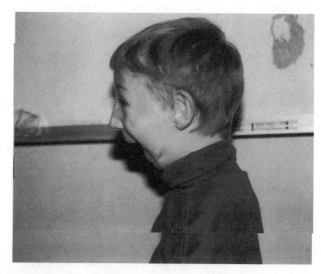

Pierre Robin syndrome. FIG. 2. Patient from figure 1, laughing.

of the neck (25). Intervening procedures, such as cleft palate repair, may make a once-uncomplicated laryngoscopy difficult in the future by altering visualization of the larynx.

Neonates may require prone positioning, a nasopharyngeal airway, suturing of the tongue to the lip, or even urgent tracheostomy to preserve an airway. Spontaneous ventilation may be improved by placing the patient prone so the tongue does not fall posteriorly into the pharynx. Patients should be closely observed postoperatively for evidence of airway obstruction (2).

Bibliography:

1. Shukry M, Hanson RD, Koveleskie JR, et al. Management of the difficult pediatric airway with Shikani optical stylet. *Paediatr Anaesth* 2005;15:342–345.
2. Dell'Oste C, Savron F, Pelizzo G, et al. Acute airway obstruction in an infant with Pierre Robin syndrome after palatoplasty. *Acta Anaesthesiol Scand* 2004;48:787–789.
3. Nargozian C. The airway in patients with craniofacial abnormalities. *Paediatr Anaesth* 2004;14:53–59.
4. Blanco G, Melman E, Cuairan V, et al. Fibreoptic nasal intubation in children with anticipated and unanticipated difficult intubation. *Paediatr Anaesth* 2001;11:49–53.
5. Schwarz U, Weiss M. Endotracheal intubation of patients with Pierre-Robin sequence. Successful use of video intubation laryngoscope. *Anaesthesist* 2001;50:118–121.
6. Taylor MR. Consultation with the specialist: The Pierre Robin sequence: a concise review for the practicing pediatrician. *Pediatr Rev* 2001;22:125–130.
7. Barker I. Anaesthesia for Pierre-Robin syndrome [Letter]. *Hosp Med* 2000;61:72.
8. Selim M, Mowafi H, Al-Ghamdi A, et al. Intubation via LMA in pediatric patients with difficult airways. *Can J Anaesth* 1999;46:891–893.
9. Osses H, Poblete M, Asenjo F. Laryngeal mask for difficult intubation in children. *Paediatr Anaesth* 1999;9:399–401.
10. Otuwa S, Mayhew JF, Woodson L, et al. Fiberoptic intubation through a laryngeal mask airway in a child with Pierre-Robin syndrome. *Am J Anesthesiol* 1999;26:221–222.
11. Jones SE, Derrick GM. Difficult intubation in an infant with Pierre Robin syndrome and concomitant tongue tie. *Paediatr Anaesth* 1998;8:510–511.
12. Perkins JA, Sie KC, Milczuk H, et al. Airway management in children with craniofacial anomalies. *Cleft Palate Craniofac J* 1997;34:135–140.
13. Ofer R, Dworzak H. The laryngeal mask–a valuable instrument for cases of difficult intubation in children. Anesthesiologic management in the presence of Pierre-Robin syndrome. *Anaesthesist* 1996;45:268–270.
14. Baraka A. Laryngeal mask airway for resuscitation of a newborn with Pierre-Robin syndrome. *Anesthesiology* 1996;83:645–646.
15. Hansen TG, Joensen H, Henneberg SW, et al. Laryngeal mask airway guided tracheal intubation in a neonate with the Pierre Robin syndrome. *Acta Anaesthesiol Scand* 1995;39:129–131.
16. Baraka A, Muallem M. Bullard laryngoscopy for tracheal intubation in a neonate with Pierre-Robin syndrome. *Paediatr Anaesth* 1994;4:111–113.
17. Wheatley RS, Stainthorp SE. Intubation of a one-day-old baby with the Pierre-Robin syndrome via a laryngeal mask [Letter]. *Anaesthesia* 1994;49:733.
18. Sutera PT, Gordon GJ. Digitally assisted tracheal intubation in a neonate with Pierre Robin syndrome. *Anesthesiology* 1993;78:983–985.
19. Chadd GD, Crane DL, Phillips RM, et al. Extubation and reintubation guided by the laryngeal mask airway in a child with the Pierre Robin syndrome. *Anesthesiology* 1992;76:640–641.
20. Markakis DA, Sayson SC, Schreiner MS. Insertion of the laryngeal mask airway in awake infants with the Robin sequence. *Anesth Analg* 1992;75:822–824.
21. Schelle JG, Schulman SR. Fiberoptic bronchoscopic guidance for intubation of a neonate with Pierre-Robin syndrome. *J Clin Anesth* 1991;3:45–47.
22. Beveridge ME. Laryngeal mask anaesthesia for repair of cleft palate. *Anaesthesia* 1989;44:656–657.
23. Howardy-Hansen P, Berthelsen P. Fibreoptic bronchoscopic nasotracheal intubation of a neonate with Pierre Robin syndrome. *Anaesthesia* 1988;43:121–122.
24. Rasch DK, Browder F, Barr M, et al. Anaesthesia for Treacher Collins and Pierre Robin syndromes: a report of three cases. *Can Anaesth Soc J* 1986;33:364–370.
25. Populaire C, Lundi JN, Pinaud M, et al. Elective tracheal intubation in the prone position for a neonate with Pierre Robin syndrome [Letter]. *Anesthesiology* 1985;62:214–215.
26. Yonfa AE, Klein E, Mackall LL. Retrograde approach to nasotracheal intubation in a child with severe Pierre Robin syndrome: a case report. *Anesthesiol Rev* 1983;10:28–29.

PKU

See Phenylketonuria

Plott Syndrome

MIM #: 308850

This autosomal dominant or X-linked recessive disorder is one of congenital bilateral laryngeal abductor paralysis and mental retardation. There is also sixth nerve palsy and possible visual or auditory impairment. The laryngeal motor defect is thought to be because of abnormal formation of the medullary nucleus ambiguous. Nonfunctioning of the posterior cricoarytenoid, the only cord abductor, results in a midline, adducted position of the vocal cords at rest, with complete adduction with crying. The other clinical manifestations are thought to be due to developmental abnormalities of other cranial nerve nuclei. It is unclear if mental retardation is a primary event, or is a sequela of episodes of perinatal asphyxia. A gene for the autosomal dominant disorder has been localized to the long arm of chromosome 6.

HEENT/AIRWAY: Possible abnormal vision and hearing. Sixth nerve palsy. High-arched palate. Micrognathia. Bilateral congenital laryngeal abductor paralysis with neonatal stridor at rest that may be severe enough to cause asphyxia.

NEUROMUSCULAR: Psychomotor retardation.

ANESTHETIC CONSIDERATIONS

Psychomotor retardation may make a gentle induction of anesthesia more difficult. Difficult laryngoscopy and tracheal intubation have not been reported. Patients are at risk for development of postanesthesia stridor. One child has had severe bouts of postanesthesia coughing (2).

Bibliography:

1. Manaligod JM, Skaggs J, Smith RJ. Localization of the gene for familial laryngeal abductor paralysis to chromosome 6q16. *Arch Otolaryngol Head Neck Surg* 2001;127:913–917.
2. McDonald D. Anaesthetic management of a patient with Plott syndrome. *Paediatr Anaesth* 1998;8:155–157.
3. Manaligod JM, Smith RJ. Familial laryngeal paralysis. *Am J Med Genet* 1998;77:277–280.

Poikiloderma Congenitale Syndrome

See Rothmund-Thomson syndrome

Poland Sequence

MIM #: 173800

This disorder involves unilateral hypoplasia or aplasia of the chest wall muscles, hypoplasia of chest wall structures, and ipsilateral syndactyly. It has been suggested that the Klippel-Feil sequence, the Moebius sequence, and the Poland sequence, all of which can occur in various combinations in the same patient, be grouped together; and that they represent anomalies from fetal disruption of the subclavian artery, the vertebral artery, or one of their branches around the sixth week of development. Therefore, some advocates call these the "subclavian artery supply disruption syndromes." The Poland sequence is sporadic, although rare familial instances have occurred. It is three times as common in boys as in girls.

CHEST: Unilateral hypoplasia or aplasia of the pectoralis major muscle, nipple, and areola. Rib defects. Breast aplasia in girls.

CARDIOVASCULAR: Occasional dextrocardia in left-sided Poland sequence.

NEUROMUSCULAR: Unilateral hypoplasia or aplasia of pectoralis minor, the sternal head of the pectoralis major, latissimus dorsi, and serratus anterior.

ORTHOPEDIC: Ipsilateral hypoplasia of distal limbs with varying degrees of syndactyly, brachydactyly, oligodactyly, and, rarely, a more severe limb reduction defect. Occasional hemivertebrae or winged scapulae.

GI/GU: Occasional renal anomaly.

OTHER: Patchy absence of axillary hair.

MISCELLANEOUS: Poland's account (1841) was based on George Elt, a deceased convict he dissected.

ANESTHETIC CONSIDERATIONS

Patients with significant chest wall muscle abnormalities may be at increased risk for perioperative respiratory complications, including paradoxical respirations while under general anesthesia. Peripheral vascular access may be limited in patients with significant limb abnormalities.

Bibliography:

1. Marui Y, Nitahara K, Iwakiri S, et al. Anesthetic management of patients with Poland syndrome: report of two cases [Japanese]. *Masui* 2003;52:274–276.

2. Fokin AA, Robicsek F. Poland syndrome revisited. *Ann Thorac Surg* 2002;74:2218–2225.
3. Kuklik M. Poland-Mobius syndrome and disruption spectrum affecting the face and extremities: a review paper and presentation of five cases. *Acta Chir Plast* 2000;42:95–103.
4. Kupper HJ. Anesthesia in Poland syndrome [Letter]. *Can J Anaesth* 1999;46:513–514.
5. Sethuraman R, Kannan S, Bala I, et al. Anaesthesia in Poland-syndrome. *Can J Anaesth* 1998;45:277–279.

Polyostotic Fibrous Dysplasia

See McCune-Albright syndrome

Polysplenia

SYNONYM: Ivemark syndrome; Heterotaxy syndrome

MIM #: 208530

Polysplenia, and the related syndrome of asplenia, are often thought of as disorders of laterality. Patients with asplenia are bilaterally right sided (i.e., they have two copies of right-sided structures and they lack normal left-sided structures, the spleen being one), and patients who are polysplenic are bilaterally left-sided (left isomerism). Thus, they have neither situs solitus nor situs inversus, but are said to have situs ambiguous. Patients with asplenia often have primitive hearts and cardiac right-sided obstructive lesions. The responsible gene or genes have not yet been identified.

CHEST: There are two left lungs [bilobed with the bronchial–arterial relationship of the left lung (a hyparterial bronchus below the pulmonary artery)].

CARDIOVASCULAR: Patients with polysplenia have a wider variety of cardiac defects than patients with asplenia, and they have a lower incidence of pulmonary stenosis. Patients with polysplenia have two left atria. Thus, there is no true sinoatrial node. There is absence of the inferior vena caval connection to the right atrium, with azygos continuation to the superior vena cava. Because there are two left atria, there may be abnormal pulmonary venous return.

NEUROMUSCULAR: May have agenesis of the corpus callosum.

GI/GU: There may be multiple small spleens, all located to the left of the spine. There is laterality to the "tacking down" of the fetal GI tract in normal fetuses (which is why the appendix fairly reliably ends up in the right lower quadrant). In this disease of abnormal laterality, there may be malrotation of the gut, which can present with volvulus. There are two left lobes to the liver and often no gallbladder, also a right-sided structure. May have horseshoe adrenal gland.

MISCELLANEOUS: From a semantic point of view, it is unfortunate that the genes *LEFTY A* and *LEFTY B* have been cleared of having a role in the causation of this syndrome.

ANESTHETIC CONSIDERATIONS

Specific anesthetic management varies with the individual cardiac lesion. Patients with cardiac anomalies require perioperative antibiotic prophylaxis as indicated. Although not reported, presumably there would be no relative advantage to using a left-sided, double-lumen endobronchial tube, because both lungs have the anatomy of a left lung.

Bibliography:

1. Noack F, Sayk F, Ressel A, et al. Ivemark syndrome with agenesis of the corpus callosum: a case report with a review of the literature. *Prenat Diagn* 2002;22:1011–1015.
2. Strouse PJ, Haller JO, Berdon WE, et al. Horseshoe adrenal gland in association with asplenia: presentation of six new cases and review of the literature. *Pediatr Radiol* 2002;32:778–782.
3. Winer-Muram HT. Adult presentation of heterotaxic syndromes and related complexes. *J Thorac Imaging* 1995;10:43–57.
4. Gagner M, Munson JL, Scholz FJ. Hepatobiliary anomalies associated with polysplenia syndrome. *Gastrointest Radiol* 1991;16:67–71.
5. Winer-Muram HT, Tonkin IL. The spectrum of heterotaxic syndromes. *Radiol Clin North Am* 1989;27:1147–1170.

Pompe Disease

SYNONYM: Glycogen storage disease type II; Acid maltase deficiency; Alpha-1,4-glucosidase deficiency

MIM #: 232300

This autosomal recessive glycogen storage disease due to the absence of lysosomal acid maltase (alpha-1,4-glucosidase), results in glycogen deposition in a wide variety of organs, including the heart, skeletal muscle, smooth muscle, brain, spinal cord, kidney, liver, spleen, and tongue. In the other glycogen storage diseases, glycogen is stored diffusely in the cytoplasm. In Pompe disease, it is stored in the lysosomes. There are multiple alleles. A high-protein, low-carbohydrate diet has been found to be beneficial in several adults with the disease.

The juvenile form, classic Pompe disease, is marked by hypotonia and cardiomegaly. In both the juvenile and adult forms, skeletal muscle involvement is predominant. The adult form is genetically distinct, and is thought to be due to absence of lysosomal alpha-glucosidase.

HEENT/AIRWAY: The large tongue and muscle weakness can cause significant airway obstruction.

CHEST: Decreased cough and uncoordinated swallowing increase the risk of aspiration. Massive cardiomegaly can compress the bronchi, causing atelectasis. Respiratory insufficiency from muscle weakness can be severe even in the milder adult-onset type.

CARDIOVASCULAR: Cardiomegaly is prominent. Ventricular hypertrophy. Cardiomyopathy with congestive heart failure usually develops by 2 to 3 months of age. The electrocardiogram typically shows left ventricular hypertrophy, a wide QRS complex, a short PR interval and T-wave inversion. There can be hypertrophy of the ventricular septum sufficient to cause outflow obstruction.

There does not appear to be cardiac involvement in the adult form.

NEUROMUSCULAR: Normal intellectual development. Hypotonia, progressive muscle weakness.

GI/GU: There can be hepatomegaly, but not to the massive degree seen with von Gierke disease. Hepatic function is normal. There is no hepatic enlargement in the adult form.

OTHER: There is no hypoglycemia.

MISCELLANEOUS: Johannes Pompe, a Dutch pathologist, was killed by the Nazis shortly before the liberation of the Netherlands. He had maintained a clandestine radio in his laboratory and was executed for blowing up a strategic rail line.

ANESTHETIC CONSIDERATIONS

Macroglossia may compromise the airway during induction of anesthesia and may also complicate laryngoscopy. Succinylcholine should be used with caution in this muscle disease because of the risk of exaggerated hyperkalemia. A regional technique with ketamine sedation has been used successfully in infants who have required a muscle biopsy (2, 7). Patients with muscle weakness are at risk for perioperative respiratory compromise (5).

Anesthetics with myocardial depressant effects should be avoided in most cases, and a cardiac arrest with a sevoflurane induction (and propofol infusion) has been reported (2) as has arrest with halothane (8). The specific cardiac lesion must be delineated because the optimal anesthetic technique for cardiomyopathy with poor ventricular function is at odds with the optimal anesthetic technique for obstructive cardiomyopathy. Ejection fraction can be overestimated in the presence of profound myocardial hypertrophy leading to unwarranted reassurance. Higher ventricular filling pressures are required by hypertrophied hearts and are required in the face of dynamic left ventricular outflow obstruction; and systemic vascular resistance needs to be maintained to assure adequate coronary perfusion. Anesthetic agents which decrease systemic vascular resistance should be used sparingly if at all.

FIGURE: See **Appendix E**

Bibliography:

1. Hagemans MLC, Winkel LPF, Hop WCJ, et al. Disease severity in children and adults with Pompe disease related to age and disease duration. *Neurology* 2005;64:2139–2141.

2. Ing RJ, Cook DR, Bengur RA, et al. Anaesthetic management of infants with glycogen storage disease type II: a physiological approach. *Paediatr Anaesth* 2004;14:514–519.
3. Krishnani PS, Howell RR. Pompe disease in infants and children. *J Pediatr* 2004;144:S35–S48.
4. van den Hout HM, Hop W, van Diggelen OP, et al. The natural course of infantile Pompe disease: 20 original cases compared with 133 cases from the literature. *Pediatrics* 2003;112:332–340.
5. Kotani N, Hashimoto H, Hirota K, et al. Prolonged respiratory depression after anesthesia for parathyroidectomy in a patient with juvenile type of acid maltase deficiency. *J Clin Anesth* 1996;8:620.
6. Gitlin MC, Jahr JS, Garth KL. Ureteroscopic removal of left ureteral lithiasis in a patient with acid maltase deficiency disease. *Anesth Analg* 1993;76:662–664.
7. Rosen KR, Broadman LM. Anaesthesia for diagnostic muscle biopsy in an infant with Pompe disease. *Can Anaesth Soc J* 1986;33:790–794.
8. McFarlane HJ, Soni N. Pompe disease and anaesthesia. *Anaesthesia* 1986;41:1219–1224.
9. Kaplan R. Pompe disease presenting for anesthesia: two case reports. *Anesthesiol Rev* 1980;7:21–28.

Popliteal Pterygium Syndrome

SYNONYM: Faciogenitopopliteal syndrome

MIM #: 119500

This autosomal dominant disorder is characterized by lower lip mucous cysts, cleft lip or palate, genital anomalies, and popliteal pterygia (webs). There is marked variability in expression. The disorder is allelic with van der Woude syndrome (see later), and both are due to defects in the gene encoding interferon regulatory factor 6. In mildly affected patients, this syndrome is easily confused with van der Woude syndrome.

HEENT/AIRWAY: Ankyloblepharon filiforme adnatum (webbing between the eyelids). Occasional conductive hearing loss. Lower lip mucous cysts. Cleft lip or palate. May have intraoral webbing (syngnathia). Syngnathia can vary from a few thin connections to bony fusion.

CHEST: Short sternum. May have bifid ribs.

NEUROMUSCULAR: Normal intelligence.

ORTHOPEDIC: Popliteal webs, which can extend from the ischial tuberosity to the heel. Can also have muscle or other lower extremity anomaly, such that repair of webs does not completely restore lower extremity function. Syndactyly of toes and fingers. Dysplastic nails.

GI/GU: Genital anomalies, including hypoplastic labia majora, bifid scrotum, cryptorchidism. Genital anomalies may be secondary to intercrural pterygia. May have inguinal hernias.

MISCELLANEOUS: Single-nucleotide polymorphisms in interferon regulatory factor 6 are thought to be a major contributor to the development of cleft lip with or without cleft palate.

ANESTHETIC CONSIDERATIONS

Mouth opening and access to the larynx may be severely limited by intraoral webbing which connects the mandibular and maxillary alveolar ridges. Division of oral bands can be done with no anesthesia if the bands are small enough. Awake intubation of neonates has been suggested for the potentially difficult airway (3). The lower extremities must be carefully positioned because the sciatic nerve and the popliteal artery are often contained within the popliteal web.

Bibliography:

1. Ghassibe M, Revencu N, Bayet B, et al. Six families with van der Woude and/or popliteal pterygium syndrome: all with a mutation in the IRF6 gene. *J Med Genet* 2004;41:e15.
2. Parikh SN, Crawford AH, Do TT, et al. Popliteal pterygium syndrome: implications for orthopaedic management. *J Pediatr Orthop B* 2004;13:197–201.
3. Patel V, Theroux MC, Reilly J. Popliteal pterygium syndrome with syngnathia. *Paediatr Anaesth* 2003;13:80–82.
4. Soekarman D, Cobben JM, Vogels A, et al. Variable expression of the popliteal pterygium syndrome in two 3-generation families. *Clin Genet* 1995;47:169–174.

Porphyria

MIM #: 176000, 176090, 176100, 176200, 121300, 125270, 263700

The several porphyrias are associated with defects in heme synthesis and the overproduction of heme precursors (see **Appendix F**). There is great clinical heterogeneity. The porphyrias can be separated into the erythropoietic or hepatic porphyrias, depending on the major site of heme precursor overproduction. In all forms, environmental factors can alter the clinical expression. Decreased heme concentration stimulates the regulatory enzyme delta-aminolevulinic acid synthetase (ALA synthetase) which stimulates porphyrins produced proximal to the enzymatic block. Acute attacks are manifest by abdominal pain, autonomic instability, electrolyte disturbances, and neuropsychiatric changes. Most attacks occur between puberty and menopause. Attacks range from mild to fatal. Factors that have triggered attacks include starvation, infection, pregnancy, estrogens, exposure to sunlight, and drugs, including barbiturates, sulfonamides, oral contraceptives, anticonvulsants, and alcohol (Table 4). Barbiturates trigger a crisis by stimulating the cytochrome P450 system, incorporating more heme into new cytochromes, decreasing heme levels, and thereby decreasing negative feedback on ALA synthetase activity. Latent carriers, such as prepubertal children of porphyric families, can have acute attacks on exposure to porphyrinogenic drugs. The mortality rate with an acute attack is approximately 10%, usually secondary to infection, respiratory failure, or arrhythmia. More than 50% of pregnant women with porphyria experience an attack during pregnancy, with the mortality rate reported to be as high as 42%.

The erythropoietic porphyrias include congenital erythropoietic porphyria (CEP), erythropoietic protoporphyria

TABLE 4. *Anesthetic drugs and porphyria*

Drug class	Likely safe	Likely unsafe	Unclear
Intravenous anesthetics	Midazolam	Barbiturates	Diazepam
	Lorazepam	Etomidate	Ketamine
	Propofol	Chlordiazepoxide	
		Flunitrazepam	
		Nitrazepam	
Inhalational anesthetics	Nitrous oxide	Enflurane (based on animal data)	Desflurane
	Halothane		Sevoflurane
	Isoflurane		
Muscle relaxants	Succinylcholine		Pancuronium
	Vecuronium		cis-Atracurium
	d-Tubocurarine		Rocuronium
	Atracurium		
Premedications	Scopolamine		
	Benzodiazepines		
	Atropine		
	Droperidol		
	Promethazine		
	Chloral hydrate		
	Diphenhydramine		
	Cimetidine		
Opioids	Morphine	Pentazocine	Sufentanil
	Fentanyl		
Anticholinesterases	Neostigmine		
Local anesthetics	Bupivacaine	Mepivacaine	Prilocaine
	Lidocaine		
	Procaine		
Cardiovascular	Epinephrine		
	Beta-blockers	Alpha-methyldopa	
	Labetolol	Hydralazine	
	Guanethidine	Phenoxybenzamine	
	Reserpine	Nifedipine	
	Alpha-blockers		
Others			
	Glucose loading	Oral contraceptives	
	Anticonvulsants	Griseofulvin	
	Metoclopramide	Cimetidine	Ranitidine

(Modified from Jensen NF, Fiddler DS, Striepe V. Anesthetic considerations in porphyries. *Anesth Analg* 1995;80:591–599; Harrison GG, Meissner PN, Hift RJ. Anaesthesia for the porphyric patient. *Anaesthesia* 1993;48:417–421; and James MFM, Hift RJ. Porphyrias. *Br J Anaesth* 2000;85:143–153.)

(EPP) and hepatoerythropoietic porphyria (HEP). CEP is an uncommon autosomal recessive disorder of uroporphyrinogen III cosynthetase. EPP is an autosomal dominant disorder due to deficient activity of ferrochelatase, and the clinical findings are similar to CEP, with the exception of milder skin findings. EPP is the most common of the erythropoietic porphyrias. HEP is a rare autosomal recessive disorder due to decreased activity of uroporphyrinogen decarboxylase. Clinical findings are similar to CEP.

The hepatic porphyrias include the more widely known variants, acute intermittent porphyria (AIP), porphyria cutanea tarda (PCT), hereditary coproporphyria (HC) and variegate porphyria (VP). AIP is an autosomal dominant disorder due to the diminished activity of uroporphyrinogen I synthase (PBG deaminase). It is one of the more common porphyrias and has variable clinical manifestations, depending on environmental factors, such as drug exposure. Patients are usually asymptomatic between episodes

of clinical attacks. PCT is also relatively common. It is autosomal dominant, and may occur sporadically. PCT is due to decreased activity of uroporphyrinogen decarboxylase. There is incomplete penetrance, and not all carriers of the gene have symptoms. Acute attacks, as with AIP, do not occur. HC is an autosomal dominant disorder due to diminished activity of coproporphyrinogen oxidase. There is variable expression of the disease, which is similar to, but milder than, AIP. VP is an autosomal dominant disorder due to a defect in the gene for protoporphyrinogen oxidase. This enzyme, located on the inner membrane of mitochondria, catalyzes the conversion of protoporphyrinogen IX to protoporphyrin IX.

Acute attacks are found with AIP, HC, VP and also with aminolevulinic acid dehydratase deficiency (the very uncommon plumboporphyria). PCT and the erythropoietic porphyrias CEP and EPP are not associated with drug-induced crises.

HEENT/AIRWAY

CEP: Deformation of the nose, ears, eyelids and corneas from secondary skin infections. Reddish-brown teeth.

HEP: Discoloration of teeth.

CHEST

AIP: Chest or back pain with attacks. Respiratory failure from neuropathy, which may be fatal.

CARDIOVASCULAR

AIP: Tachycardia or hypertension with an attack.

VP: Hypertension during attacks.

NEUROMUSCULAR

AIP: Muscle weakness, sensory disturbances, or psychiatric disturbances (disorientation, hallucinations, paranoia, anxiety, depression) with attacks. There may also be a neuropathy (motor > sensory) that can include cranial nerve and bulbar dysfunction during an acute attack, and which may predict impending respiratory failure from paralysis. The neuropathy can also involve the hypothalamus and splanchnics. There may be neuronal damage and axonal degeneration followed by demyelination. There may be residual weakness after a severe attack, which may take several months for full recovery. Twenty percent of patients in crisis have seizures during the crisis.

HC: Similar to, but milder than, AIP.

VP: Similar to AIP.

ORTHOPEDIC

CEP and HEP: Deformation of the digits from secondary skin infections, pathologic fractures.

AIP: Bone pain with attacks.

GI/GU

CEP and HEP: Hemolytic anemia with hypersplenism, cirrhosis. Reddish-brown urinary staining of diaper in infants.

EPP: Protoporphyrin-containing biliary stones, cirrhosis, hepatic failure.

AIP: Abdominal pain, vomiting, ileus, and constipation during episodic attacks. Urinary dysfunction (retention or incontinence) with attacks. The urine turns reddish-brown ("port wine") on standing. Some women have attacks related to the menstrual cycle.

PCT: Hepatic involvement common by adulthood. Cirrhosis, focal necrosis, hepatoma.

VP: Minimal hepatic involvement.

OTHER

CEP and HEP: Severe cutaneous photosensitivity with formation of bullae and subsequent scarring and hyperpigmentation. Friable skin and hypertrichosis.

EPP: Similar, but less severe. Scarring and hyperkeratosis, if present, are mild.

AIP: Syndrome of inappropriate secretion of antidiuretic hormone (SIADH).

PCT: Cutaneous photosensitivity with bullae, scarring, hyperpigmentation, friable skin, hypertrichosis, lichenification.

HC: Similar to PCT.

VP: Similar to PCT. Attacks of VP result in hyperpigmentation and hypertrichosis.

MISCELLANEOUS: Hematin (used to treat acute attacks of porphyria) was the first drug approved under the Orphan Drug Act.

Plumboporphyria derives its name from the increased levels of ALA analogs in the urine, similar to that found in lead poisoning. Lead levels in plumboporphyria are, however, normal.

Variegate porphyria is particularly common in South Africans of Afrikaans descent, where its arrival can be traced back to a single Dutch settler (or his wife, who was one of the orphan girls sent to South Africa to provide wives for the early Dutch settlers).

The malady of George III of England has been suggested (and hotly debated) to be porphyria. Although the symptoms of George suggest AIP, the skin and other manifestations of his family suggest the variegate type. In addition, it has recently been suggested that his condition was exacerbated by high levels of arsenic, delivered in arsenic containing medications (1).

ANESTHETIC CONSIDERATIONS

Abdominal findings may lead to the misdiagnosis of a surgical abdomen during an acute attack of AIP. Dehydration, fever, infection, stress (including surgery), and endogenous steroids can all induce ALA synthetase (the initial and rate-limiting step in heme synthesis). Psychological stress has been reported to precipitate crises, so good premedication is indicated in patients with porphyria. Care needs to be taken perioperatively to avoid causing inadvertent skin infections from skin trauma. Lighting should be as dim as practical, or an appropriate light filter used for patients with photosensitivity. Maintenance of adequate hemoglobin levels will minimize heme synthesis and minimize protoporphyrin levels.

Ketamine has been implicated in porphyrinogenesis (13), although it has also been used uneventfully (28, 31, 32). There are many reports of the successful use of propofol in patients with porphyria (10, 12, 19, 23–25). However, an asymptomatic increase in porphyrinogenesis has been described in one patient who was given propofol (17). Also, a prolonged alteration in consciousness with transient neurologic symptoms and elevated porphyrins was described in a patient who received propofol who did not have a prior diagnosis of porphyria (11). However, in this patient the diagnosis of porphyria remains unproven (9). Despite its contraindication in patients with porphyrias, barbiturates have been given during latent phases without causing clinical manifestations (30, 33), making interpretation of claims for the safety of other agents difficult if they were administered during latent phases of the disease. In fact, it is rare for any anesthetic drug to cause symptoms in latent disease. Morphine or other narcotics can be used for pain, but may worsen constipation or urinary retention during an acute attack.

Because cold can induce stress and increased steroid synthesis, minimal hypothermia (32°C) has been suggested for cardiac surgery (14), although others have performed surgeries with patient temperatures of less than 30°C (21, 27, 29). One of these patients had postoperative biochemical evidence of an acute crisis (29).

Treatment of an acute episode includes hematin 1 to 4 mg/kg/day (possible side effects include renal failure, thrombophlebitis, and coagulopathy) or hemoperfusion to remove porphyrin precursors. Oral or intravenous carbohydrate or glucose loading may be helpful during an acute attack. Electrolytes, including magnesium, should be measured and repleted appropriately. Hypovolemia and autonomic neuropathy during an acute attack may be an indication for invasive blood pressure monitoring. A crisis may occur up to 5 days postoperatively.

Not surprisingly, regional anesthesia has been used successfully (20, 22). However, regional techniques during an acute attack may cloud neuropathic changes, and mental status changes and cooperation may also be a problem. Hypovolemia and autonomic instability during an acute attack increase the risk of hemodynamic instability associated with the sympathectomy of major regional techniques. Although theoretical differences exist, there does not appear to be any advantage or disadvantage with any specific local anesthetic.

It is likely that single, acute exposures to potent inducers, such as short term exposure to anesthetic drugs, are tolerated in the stable patient, but can be problematic in the patient in whom a crisis has already developed. Exposure to multiple inducers is likely significantly worse than exposure to a single inducing drug.

Bibliography:

1. Cox TM, Jack N, Lofthouse S, et al. King George III and porphyria: an elemental hypothesis and investigation. *Lancet* 2005;366: 332–335.

2. Sheppard L, Dorman T. Anesthesia in a child with homozygous porphobilinogen deaminase deficiency: a severe form of acute intermittent porphyria. *Paediatr Anaesth* 2005;15:426–428.

3. Durmus M, Turkoz A, Togal T, et al. Remifentanil and acute intermittent porphyria. *Eur J Anaesthesiol* 2002;19:839–840.

4. Rigal JC, Blanloeil Y. Anaesthesia and porphyria. *Minerva Anestesiol* 2002;68:326–331.

5. James MFM, Hift RJ. Porphyrias. *Br J Anaesth* 2000;85:143–153.

6. Torrance JM. Anaesthetic management of erythropoietic protoporphyria [Letter]. *Paediatr Anaesth* 2000;10:571.

7. Sarantopoulos CD, Bratanow NC, Stowe DF, et al. Uneventful propofol anesthesia in a patient with coexisting hereditary coproporphyria and hereditary angioneurotic edema. *Anesthesiology* 2000;92:607–609.

8. Asokumar B, Kierney K, James TW, et al. Anaesthetic management of a patient with erythropoietic protoporphyria for ventricular septal defect closure. *Paediatr Anaesth* 1999;9:356–358.

9. Mamet R, Schoenfeld N. A reliable diagnosis of porphyria should precede any conclusion concerning the safety of a drug in porphyria. *Anesthesiology* 1999;91:583–584.

10. Pazvanska EE, Hinkov OD, Stojnovska LV. Uneventful propofol anaesthesia in a patient with acute intermittent porphyria. *Eur J Anaesthesiol* 1999;16:485–492.

11. Asirvatham SJ, Johnson TW, Oberoi MP, et al. Prolonged loss of consciousness and elevated porphyrins following propofol administration. *Anesthesiology* 1998;89:1029–1031.

12. Shaw HI, Mckeith IG. Propofol and electroconvulsive therapy in a patient at risk from acute intermittent porphyria. *Br J Anaesth* 1998;80:260–262.

13. Kanbak M. Ketamine in porphyria [Letter]. *Anesth Analg* 1997;84:1395.

14. Stevens JWM, Kneeshaw JD. Mitral valve replacement in a patient with acute intermittent porphyria. *Anesth Analg* 1996;82:416–418.

15. Ashley EM. Anaesthesia for porphyria. *Br J Hosp Med* 1996;56:37–42.

16. Jensen NF, Fiddler DS, Striepe V. Anesthetic considerations in porphyrias. *Anesth Analg* 1995;80:591–599.

17. Elcock D, Norris A. Elevated porphyrins following propofol anaesthesia in acute intermittent porphyria. *Anaesthesia* 1994;49:957–958.

18. Harrison GG, Meissner PN, Hift RJ. Anaesthesia for the porphyric patient. *Anaesthesia* 1993;48:417–421.

19. Kantor G, Rolbin SH. Acute intermittent porphyria and Caesarean delivery. *Can J Anaesth* 1992;39:282–285.

20. Bohrer H, Schmidt H. Regional anesthesia as anesthetic technique of choice in acute hepatic porphyria [Letter]. *J Clin Anesth* 1992;4:259.

21. Campos GH, Stein DK, Michel NK, et al. Anesthesia for aortic valve replacement in a patient with acute intermittent porphyria. *J Cardiothorac Vasc Anesth* 1991;5:258–261.

22. McNeill MJ, Bennet A. Use of regional anaesthesia in a patient with acute porphyria. *Br J Anaesth* 1990;64:371–373.

23. Hughes PJ. Propofol in acute porphyrias. *Anaesthesia* 1990;45:415.

24. Mitterschiffthaler G, Theiner A, Hetzel H, et al. Safe use of propofol in a patient with acute intermittent porphyria. *Br J Anaesth* 1988;60:109–111.

25. Weir PM, Hodkinson BP. Is propofol a safe agent in porphyria? *Anaesthesia* 1988;43:1022–1023.

26. Mostert JW. Porphyria variegata: a problem for the anesthesiologist. *Perspect Biol Med* 1988;31:567–571.

27. Shipton EA, Roelofse JA. Anaesthesia in a patient with variegated porphyria undergoing coronary bypass surgery. *S Afr Med J* 1984;65:53–54.

28. Bancroft GH, Lauria JI. Ketamine induction for cesarean section in a patient with acute intermittent porphyria and achondroplastic dwarfism. *Anesthesiology* 1983;59:143–144.

29. Ruby HP, Harison GA. Anaesthesia for coronary artery bypass in a patient with Porphyria variegata. *Anaesth Intensive Care* 1982;10:276–278.

30. Mustajoki P, Heinonen J. General anesthesia and "inducible" porphyrias. *Anesthesiology* 1980;53:15–20.

31. Rizk SF, Jacobson JH, Silvay G. Ketamine as an induction agent for acute intermittent porphyria. *Anesthesiology* 1977;46:305–306.

32. Downing JW, Mahomedy MC, Deal DE, et al. Anaesthesia for caesarean section with ketamine. *Anaesthesia* 1976;31:883–892.

33. Slavin SA, Christoforides C. Thiopental administration in acute intermittent porphyria without adverse effect. *Anesthesiology* 1976;44: 77–79.

Postaxial Acrofacial Dysostosis Syndrome

See Miller syndrome

Potter Syndrome

SYNONYM: Oligohydramnios sequence

MIM #: None

When Potter described this dysmorphic syndrome, she described it in association with bilateral renal agenesis. However, it has become clear that it is due to the *in utero* fetal effects of oligohydramnios. The etiology of the oligohydramnios is unimportant. For example, decreased amniotic fluid production, as with renal agenesis or obstruction, or amniotic fluid loss from chronic amniotic fluid leak, both result in similar features.

HEENT/AIRWAY: Hypertelorism, epicanthal folds, low-set ears, flattened, beaked nose, micrognathia.

CHEST: Pulmonary hypoplasia. Respiratory failure is a common cause of immediate postnatal death.

ORTHOPEDIC: Spade-like hands.

GI/GU: May have renal agenesis.

OTHER: Maternal oligohydramnios.

MISCELLANEOUS: Edith Potter was a prominent pediatric pathologist at the Chicago Lying-in Hospital. The condition now bearing her name has been described sporadically since the 1600s. Dr. Potter delineated the characteristics of this syndrome after performing a series of 5,000 fetal and neonatal autopsies.

ANESTHETIC CONSIDERATIONS
Pulmonary hypoplasia may require urgent intubation after delivery and sophisticated mechanical ventilatory strategies. Direct laryngoscopy may be difficult secondary to micrognathia. Renal dysfunction in infants requires precise titration of perioperative fluids, and has implications for the choice of anesthetic drugs.

Bibliography:

1. Abe Y, Mizuno K, Horie H, et al. Potter sequence complicated by congenital cystic lesion of the bladder. *Am J Perinatol* 2002;19:267–272.
2. Christianson C, Huff D, McPherson E. Limb deformations in oligohydramnios sequence: effects of gestational age and duration of oligohydramnios. *Am J Med Genet* 1999;86:430–433.
3. Scott RJ, Goodburn SF. Potter's syndrome in the second trimester-prenatal screening and pathological findings in 60 cases of oligohydramnios sequence. *Prenat Diagn* 1995;15:519–525.
4. Marras A, Mereu G, Dessi C, et al. Oligohydramnios and extrarenal abnormalities in Potter syndrome. *J Pediatr* 1983;102:597–598.

Prader-Willi Syndrome

MIM #: 176270

This autosomal dominant disorder is classically characterized by hypotonia, hypomentia, and hypogonadism that is associated with obesity. There is phenotypic variability, and many patients do not display the classic body habitus. This disorder is due to a partial deletion of the long arm of chromosome 15 between 15q11 and 15q13. Similar deletions are present in Angelman syndrome (see earlier), although the origin of the chromosomal deletion is maternal in Angelman syndrome and paternal in Prader-Willi syndrome. Contiguous genes involved in the deletion are the paternal copies of the imprinted *SNRPN* (small nuclear ribonucleotide polypeptide N) gene, the *necdin* gene, and possibly other genes. The main clinical features of the syndrome include decreased fetal activity, obesity, hypotonia, mental retardation, short stature, hypogonadotropic hypogonadism, and small hands and feet.

HEENT/AIRWAY: Narrow bifrontal diameter. Strabismus, myopia. Dental enamel hypoplasia. Viscous saliva.

CHEST: Neonatal asphyxia secondary to hypotonia and hypoventilation. Poor cough and restrictive lung disease from hypotonia may result in recurrent pulmonary infections. May be pickwickian (chronic pulmonary hypoventilation secondary to obesity). May have sleep apnea. Hypoventilation and sleep apnea may be related, at least in part, to an abnormality of peripheral chemoreceptor pathways (9).

CARDIOVASCULAR: May have pulmonary hypertension secondary to chronic hypoventilation. Arrhythmias may develop, primarily premature ventricular contractions. May have hypertension.

NEUROMUSCULAR: Hypotonia beginning at birth, which may require gavage feedings for several months. Improvement in cough, crying, and feeding over the first year. Psychomotor retardation with average IQ 50 to 60. There are food-related behavior problems. Labile temperament and temper tantrums are common. May have psychotic episodes. Tend to be relatively insensitive to pain. Tend to pick excessively at sores.

ORTHOPEDIC: Short stature. Small hands and feet with tapered fingers. Hypermobile joints. Scoliosis and kyphosis.

GI/GU: Prolonged feeding problems as infants. Ischemic gastroenteritis has been reported. There is an increased incidence of rumination. Cryptorchidism and hypoplastic penis and scrotum in boys, hypoplastic labia in girls, and hypogonadotropic hypogonadism in both sexes. Precocious puberty has been reported.

OTHER: Decreased fetal activity, mild prenatal growth retardation. Morbid obesity with insatiable hunger and hypoglycemia beginning at approximately 1 year of age.

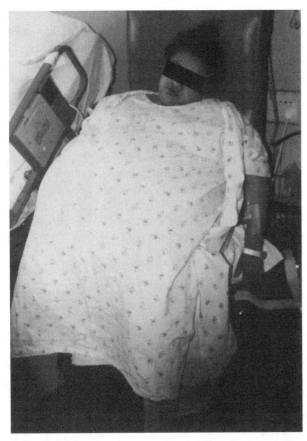

Prader-Willi syndrome. This 125 kg 19-year-old young lady with Prader-Willi syndrome has massive central obesity. She has severe mental and motor retardation. She does not talk, is not ambulatory, and has a history of seizures.

Plethoric obesity and striae are common. Non–insulin-dependent diabetes mellitus in the adolescent/adult. Survival is probably normal if weight and diabetes can be controlled, but is shortened otherwise. May have increased risk of myeloid leukemia. May have abnormal temperature control, most likely on a central basis. Erythrocytosis may develop secondary to chronic hypoventilation. Hypopigmented, photosensitive skin with light hair and blue eyes. Growth hormone treatment has been used to increase height velocity and decrease body mass index (BMI).

MISCELLANEOUS: Charles Dickens in *The Pickwick Papers* described "a fat and red-faced boy in a state of somnolency," which may have been the first written description of Prader-Willi syndrome. *The Pickwick Papers* is also the origin of the term "pickwickian," a term used to describe someone who has chronic pulmonary hypoventilation secondary to obesity.

ANESTHETIC CONSIDERATIONS
Laryngoscopy and tracheal intubation may be difficult secondary to morbid obesity. Patients may steal food and may not be truly NPO as expected. This, plus obesity and the increased incidence of rumination, suggests that all of these patients should be considered at high risk of gastric aspiration (10). Secretions may be viscous. Obesity may result in desaturation with induction of anesthesia because of increased airway closure and decreased functional residual capacity. Bronchospasm has been reported after induction (8). Venous access and identification of landmarks for regional anesthesia may be difficult secondary to morbid obesity. Obese patients require lower-than-expected drug doses on a per-kilogram basis.

Perioperative blood glucose should be monitored, and younger patients may require glucose-containing intravenous fluids, whereas older patients with type II diabetes may require insulin to maintain normoglycemia. Patients may have cor pulmonale, or exhibit intraoperative arrhythmias (primarily premature ventricular contractions). Most patients have decreased pulmonary reserve, and are at risk for postoperative respiratory complications (1). Postoperative pulmonary edema has been reported. Temperature regulation may be impaired, and patients may exhibit perioperative hypothermia or hyperthermia. Succinylcholine has been used without problems. Growth hormone treatment has been implicated in an increased risk of obstructive apnea, respiratory infection, and sudden death (2).

Bibliography:
1. Lirk P, Keller C, Colvin J, et al. Anaesthetic management of the Prader-Willi syndrome. *Eur J Anaesthesiol* 2004;21:831–833.
2. Van Vliet G, Deal CL, Crock PA, et al. Sudden death in growth hormone-treated children with Prader-Willi syndrome. *J Pediatr* 2004;144:129–131.
3. Zipf WB. Prader-Willi syndrome: the care and treatment of infants, children, and adults. *Adv Pediatr* 2004;51:409–434.
4. Rinaldi S, Rizzo L, Di Filippo A, et al. Monopharmacologic general anaesthesia with sevoflurane in paediatric patient with Prader-Willi syndrome. *Minerva Anestesiol* 2002;68:783–790.
5. Sharma AD, Erb T, Schulman SR, et al. Anaesthetic considerations for a child with combined Prader-Willi syndrome and mitochondrial myopathy. *Paediatr Anaesth* 2001;11:488–490.
6. Gunay-Aygun M, Schwartz S, Heeger S, et al. The changing purpose of Prader-Willi syndrome clinical diagnostic criteria and proposed revised criteria. *Pediatrics* 2001;108:e92.
7. Dearlove OR, Dobson A, Super M. Anaesthesia and Prader-Willi-syndrome. *Paediatr Anaesth* 1998;8:267–271.
8. Kawahito S, Kitahata H, Kimura H, et al. Bronchospasm during anesthesia in a patient with Prader-Willi syndrome [Japanese]. *Masui* 1995;44:1675–1679.
9. Gozal D, Arens R, Omlin KJ, et al. Absent peripheral chemosensitivity in Prader-Willi syndrome. *J Appl Physiol* 1994;77:2231–2236.
10. Sloan TB, Kaye CI. Rumination risk of aspiration of gastric contents in the Prader-Willi syndrome. *Anesth Analg* 1991;73:492–495.
11. Yamashita M, Koishi K, Yamaya R, et al. Anaesthetic considerations in the Prader-Willi syndrome: report of four cases. *Can Anaesth Soc J* 1983;30:179–184.
12. Palmer SK, Atlee JL. Anesthetic management of the Prader-Willi syndrome. *Anesthesiology* 1976;44:161–163.
13. Milliken RA, Weintraub DM. Cardiac abnormalities during anesthesia in a child with Prader-Willi syndrome. *Anesthesiology* 1975;43:590–592.

Progeria

SYNONYM: Hutchinson-Gilford syndrome

MIM #: 176670

This rare disorder is characterized by accelerated aging. There is progressive alopecia, decreased subcutaneous fat, and skeletal degeneration. There is early and progressive coronary artery disease, with death usually occurring in the mid-teens secondary to ischemic heart disease. Although the inheritance pattern is not certain, there is evidence to support both autosomal dominant and autosomal recessive inheritance. The syndrome is caused by a mutation in the lamin A gene (*LMNA*).

HEENT/AIRWAY: Thin calvarium, facial hypoplasia. May have microphthalmia, cataracts. May have conductive hearing loss. Beak-like nose. Dental anomalies include missing, hypoplastic, and discolored teeth with dental caries. May have decreased temporomandibular joint mobility. Micrognathia. High-pitched voice.

CHEST: Thin ribs and small thoracic cage.

CARDIOVASCULAR: Progressive coronary artery disease in childhood. Progressive aortic atherosclerosis. Early onset of hypertension. Death is usually secondary to myocardial infarction or congestive heart failure. Patients may benefit from percutaneous transluminal coronary angioplasty or coronary artery bypass grafting. May develop premature calcific degeneration of aortic and mitral valves.

NEUROMUSCULAR: Intelligence is normal. Cerebrovascular disease may develop in childhood.

ORTHOPEDIC: Short stature. Arthritic, stiff joints. "Horse-riding" stance. Thin, fragile long bones. Early osteoporosis, pathologic fractures. Skeletal hypoplasia, dysplasia, and degeneration. Nail hypoplasia. Coxa valga.

OTHER: Thin skin, with progressive pigmentary changes. Alopecia. Decreased subcutaneous fat. Prominent scalp veins. No sexual maturation. May have diabetes.

MISCELLANEOUS: The first reference to this syndrome may have been in the *St. James Gazette* in 1754: "March 19, 1754 died in Glamorganshire of mere old age and a gradual decay of nature at seventeen years and two months, Hopkins Hopkins, the little Welshman, lately shown in London. He never weighed more than 17 pounds." The first description of this syndrome in the medical literature was by Hutchinson in 1886. It was later called "progeria" by Gilford in 1904. The word *progeria* means "premature aging." Hutchinson wrote his own epitaph: "A Man of Hope and Forward-Looking Mind."

ANESTHETIC CONSIDERATIONS

Although patients appear old, they are emotionally and developmentally appropriate for their chronological age, and need to be related to as such. Lack of subcutaneous fat may make a good mask fit difficult. Limited mouth opening and fragile skin has resulted in lip and buccal tears from placement of an oral bite block (3). Micrognathia and decreased temporomandibular joint mobility may make direct laryngoscopy and endotracheal intubation very difficult (4). Patients may require a smaller-than-expected endotracheal tube. Patients are likely to have abnormal dentition (2), and their teeth are susceptible to loss.

Patients are assumed to have coronary artery disease, with myocardium at risk for ischemia. Patients may be on chronic beta-blockers, which should be continued. Patients may also have significant cerebrovascular disease.

Patients must be carefully positioned because of osteoporosis and the potential for pathologic fractures. The thin, fragile skin must be properly padded. Lack of subcutaneous fat may lead to perioperative hypothermia.

Bibliography:

1. Pollex RL, Hegele RA. Hutchinson-Gilford progeria syndrome. *Clin Genet* 2004;66:375–381.
2. Arai T, Yamashita M. An abnormal dentition in progeria. *Paediatr Anaesth* 2002;12:287.
3. Liessmann CD. Anaesthesia in a child with Hutchinson-Gildford [sic] progeria. *Paediatr Anaesth* 2001;11:611–614.
4. Nguyen NH, Mayhew JF. Anaesthesia for a child with progeria. *Paediatr Anaesth* 2001;11:370–371.
5. Ha JW, Shim WH, Chung NS. Cardiovascular findings of Hutchinson-Gilford syndrome: a Doppler and two-dimensional echocardiographic study. *Yonsei Med J* 1993;34:352–355.
6. Chapin JW, Kahre J. Progeria and anesthesia. *Anesth Analg* 1979;58:424–425.

Progressive Diaphyseal Dysplasia

See Camurati-Engelmann syndrome

Progressive Hereditary Nephritis

See Alport syndrome

Progressive Myoclonus Epilepsies Syndrome

See Ramsay Hunt syndrome

Prolidase Deficiency

MIM #: 170100

This autosomal recessive disease results in mental retardation, chronic dermatitis and recurrent infections. Prolidase (peptidase D) is one of the peptidases. It is involved in the metabolism of certain dietary oligopeptides (imidopeptides, as found in gelatin) in the intestinal epithelium, and in the metabolism of collagen. It is found in a wide variety of organs, including the brain. There is wide variability in the clinical expression of this disorder, and there are also codominantly expressed alleles that can affect prolidase structure without affecting function.

HEENT/AIRWAY: Severely affected patients may have prominent skull sutures, ptosis, and proptosis. Chronic ear and sinus infections are common.

NEUROMUSCULAR: Variable mental retardation. Abnormal gait and posture.

ORTHOPEDIC: Foot amputation has been required because of severe lower leg ulcerations.

GI/GU: Hepatosplenomegaly, abnormal spleen histology.

OTHER: The skin rash consists of diffuse telangiectasis, purpura, ecchymosis, or ulceration, particularly of the lower leg. Increased incidence of infection.

ANESTHETIC CONSIDERATIONS
Patients must be carefully positioned perioperatively, particularly if they have lower leg ulcerations.

Bibliography:
1. Cabrera HN, Giovanna PD, Bozzini NF, et al. Prolidase deficiency: case reports of two Argentinian brothers. *Int J Dermatol* 2004;43:684–686.
2. Kokturk A, Kaya TI, Ikizoglu G, et al. Prolidase deficiency. *Int J Dermatol* 2002;41:45–48.
3. Milligan A, Graham-Brown RA, Burns DA, et al. Prolidase deficiency: a case report and literature review. *Br J Dermatol* 1989;121:405–409.
4. Leoni A, Cetta G, Tenni R, et al. Prolidase deficiency in two siblings with chronic leg ulcerations: clinical, biochemical, and morphologic aspects. *Arch Dermatol* 1987;123:493–499.

Proline Oxidase (Dehydrogenase) Deficiency

See Hyperprolinemia type I

Prolonged QT Syndrome

See Long QT syndrome

Propionic Acidemia

SYNONYM: Ketotic hyperglycinemia

MIM #: 606054

This autosomal recessive disease is the result of a defect in the gene for the mitochondrial enzyme propionyl-CoA carboxylase. This enzyme occurs as a tetrameric protein whose two protein subunits are encoded by genes located on chromosome 13 and chromosome 3. Propionyl-CoA carboxylase is important near the end of the catabolic pathway for several essential amino acids, including isoleucine and valine, as well as three-carbon fatty acids. The result is accumulation of propionyl-CoA. Propionyl-CoA is an inhibitor of the synthesis of *N*-acetylglutamate, which is required for the conversion of ammonia to urea. Some of the highest ammonia levels ever recorded have been in patients with this disease. Propionyl-CoA is split into propionic acid and coenzyme A. The propionic acid is responsible for acidosis in this disease. The disease usually presents with life-threatening episodes of ketoacidosis. Clinical exacerbations are associated with increased dietary protein or intercurrent infection. Symptoms are usually exacerbated when weaning from breast milk because breast milk is relatively low in protein. Propionyl-CoA carboxylase is also affected by abnormalities of biotinidase and holocarboxylase synthetase, both of which affect the availability of biotin.

HEENT/AIRWAY: Puffy cheeks, exaggerated "Cupid's bow" upper lip. May have optic nerve atrophy.

CHEST: Respiratory insufficiency secondary to neuromuscular involvement.

CARDIOVASCULAR:: May develop cardiomyopathy.

NEUROMUSCULAR: Mental retardation, which can be minimized or completely avoided with dietary protein restriction. Hypotonia. If untreated, anorexia progresses to lethargy, obtundation, seizures, coma, and death. There are spongiform changes in the white matter similar to those seen with other aminoacidemias. Magnetic resonance imaging scans show occasional basal ganglia changes.

GI/GU: Severe vomiting during episodes of acidosis.

OTHER: Hyperammonemia. Ketoacidosis during acute exacerbations. Anorexia, failure to thrive. Neutropenia. Anemia and thrombocytopenia in infancy. Hypogammaglobulinemia.

MISCELLANEOUS: Propionic acid is one of the things that gives Swiss cheese its taste (made by the bacterium *Propionibacterium*). Since the enyme defect is found throughout the body, liver transplantation is not curative, but will ameliorate symptoms.

ANESTHETIC CONSIDERATIONS
Glucose level, ammonia level, and pH should be obtained preoperatively. The hematocrit and platelet count should be ascertained preoperatively in infants. Anesthetic management is directed towards avoiding the events that precipitate metabolic acidosis in these patients. Protein-restricted diets should be continued perioperatively. One child became comatose when tube feedings were instituted for failure to thrive. If the patient is receiving bicarbonate and/or carnitine, these should be continued in the perioperative period. Hypoxia, hypotension, and dehydration must be avoided. Patients should receive adequate perioperative glucose (intravenously if necessary) to minimize protein catabolism. It is advisable to avoid lactic acid-containing

fluids such as lactated Ringer's solution. An orogastric tube or throat packs should be placed if the surgery has the potential to cause oral or intestinal bleeding because blood aspirated into the gastrointestinal tract after oral or nasal surgery might present an excessive protein load, and trigger an acute decompensation. Medications which decrease gut motility should be curtailed (2). Propofol may be contraindicated because its emulsion is high in polyunsaturated fats (5). Drugs derived from propionic acid, including ibuprofen, naproxen, ketoprofen, and oxaprozin, should be avoided (5).

Patients may have increased aspiration risk due to hypotonia or abnormal gag reflex from acid metabolites. Peripheral venous access may be difficult. Chronic use of anticonvulsant medications may alter the metabolism of some anesthetic drugs. Postoperatively, patients are at risk for respiratory embarrassment secondary to fatigue, hypotonia and/or upper airway obstruction.

FIGURE: See **Appendix D**

Bibliography:
1. Mardach R, Verity MA, Cederbaum SD. Clinical, pathological, and biochemical studies in a patient with propionic acidemia and fatal cardiomyopathy. *Mol Genet Metab* 2005;85:286–290.
2. Prasad C, Nurko S, Borovoy J, et al. The importance of gut motility in the metabolic control of propionic acidemia. *J Pediatr* 2004;144:532–535.
3. Sass JO, Hofmann M, Skladal D, et al. Propionic acidemia revisited: a workshop report. *Clin Pediatr* 2004;43:837–843.
4. Yorifuji T, Muroi J, Uematsu A, et al. Living-related liver transplantation for neonatal-onset propionic acidemia. *J Pediatr* 2000;137:572–574.
5. Harker HE, Emhardt JD, Hainline BE. Propionic acidemia in a four-month-old male: a case study and anesthetic implications. *Anesth Analg* 2000;91:309–311.

Protein C Deficiency

MIM #: 176860

Protein C deficiency is one of the causes of hereditary thrombophilia, a familial propensity to develop venous thromboembolism. Protein C deficiency is usually inherited in an autosomal dominant fashion, with marked phenotypic variability. There is a more severe form of protein C deficiency which is inherited in an autosomal recessive fashion. Protein C is a vitamin K-dependent plasma protein which is activated by thrombin. Once activated, it functions as an important anticoagulant by inactivating factors VIIIa and Va, thereby permitting fibrinolysis. Two major subtypes of heterozygous protein C deficiency have been described. Type I deficiency (most common) is characterized by diminished synthesis of protein C, with plasma protein C levels approximately 50% of normal. In type II deficiency, plasma protein C levels are in the normal range but the protein is dysfunctional. Protein C deficiency is present in approximately 10% of families with inherited thrombophilia, and in approximately 5% of individuals with deep vein thromboses. Heterozygous protein C deficiency is associated with an almost sevenfold increase in the incidence of deep vein thrombosis over that in a normal person.

CARDIOVASCULAR: Recurrent thrombosis of the deep veins of the legs, the iliofemoral veins, and the mesenteric veins. Approximately 40% will develop pulmonary emboli. May develop superficial thrombophlebitis. May develop cerebral venous thrombosis. Thromboses may be spontaneous or associated with other risk factors (contraceptive pill use, pregnancy, surgery, or trauma). Onset of thrombotic events is usually in the third decade of life.

OTHER: Patients with protein C deficiency may develop skin necrosis when placed on warfarin therapy. Infants with protein C deficiency may rarely develop *purpura fulminans*, with plasma protein C levels less than 1% of normal, and frank disseminated intravascular coagulation.

MISCELLANEOUS: First described in 1981 when Griffin et al. were investigating the cause of recurrent thrombophlebitis and pulmonary emboli in a 22-year-old whose family history included a father with recurrent thrombophlebitis and pulmonary emboli who had a stroke at the age of 43 and a myocardial infarction at the age of 45, a paternal uncle with recurrent thrombophlebitis and pulmonary emboli, a paternal grandfather who died suddenly at the age of 45 after a period of immobility (presumptive pulmonary embolism), and a paternal great-grandfather who died unexpectedly of a stroke at the age of 61.

ANESTHETIC CONSIDERATIONS
Prophylactic perioperative anticoagulation is recommended for all patients where warranted, and identification of a hypercoagulable state would not alter this recommendation. Neuraxial anesthesia should be avoided in patients who are anticoagulated. Hypovolemia, hypotension, and hypothermia should be avoided as they may increase the risk of thrombosis.

Bibliography:
1. Johnson CM, Mureebe L, Silver D. Hypercoagulable states: a review. *Vasc Endovascular Surg* 2005;39:123–133.
2. Sievert A, McCall M, Blackwell M, et al. Use of aprotinin during cardiopulmonary bypass in a patient with protein C deficiency. *J Extra Corpor Technol* 2003;35:39–43.
3. Morrissey PE, Ramirez PJ, Gohh RY, et al. Management of thrombophilia in renal transplant patients. *Am J Transplant* 2002;2: 872–876.
4. Kumagai K, Nishiwaki K, Sato K, et al. Perioperative management of a patient with purpura fulminans syndrome due to protein C deficiency. *Can J Anaesth* 2001;48:1070–1074.
5. Kogure S, Makita K, Saitoh Y, et al. Anesthetic management of a patient with protein C deficiency associated with pulmonary thromboembolism [Japanese]. *Masui* 1998;47:831–834.
6. Grocott HP, Clements F, Landolfo K. Coronary artery bypass graft surgery in a patient with hereditary protein S deficiency. *J Cardiothorac Vasc Anesth* 1996;10:915–917.
7. Lawson DS, Darling EM, Ware RE, et al. Management considerations for a heterozygous protein C deficient patient undergoing open heart surgery with cardiopulmonary bypass. *J Extra Corpor Technol* 1995; 27:172–176.
8. Ridley PD, Ledingham SJ, Lennox SC, et al. Protein C deficiency associated with massive cerebral thrombosis following open heart surgery. *J Cardiovasc Surg* 1990;31:249–251.

Protein S Deficiency

MIM #: 176880

Protein S deficiency is one of the causes of hereditary thrombophilia, a familial propensity to develop venous thromboembolism. Protein S deficiency is usually inherited in an autosomal dominant fashion, with significant phenotypic variability. There is a more severe form of protein S deficiency which is inherited in an autosomal recessive fashion. Protein S is a vitamin K-dependent plasma protein. Protein S is a cofactor for protein C, and its presence accelerates the inactivation of factors VIIIa and Va by protein C. In plasma, approximately 60% of the total protein S exists in a complex with complement, and 40% is free. Only the free fraction is active in modulating the anticoagulant effects of protein C. Three subtypes of heterozygous protein S deficiency have been identified. Type I deficiency (classic) is characterized by a decrease in total protein S, a decrease in free protein S and a decrease in the functional activity of the free fraction. Type II deficiency is characterized by a decrease in the functional activity of free protein S with normal levels of total and free protein S. Type III deficiency is characterized by normal levels of total protein S, with a decrease in the amount and functionality of the free fraction. Protein S deficiency is present in approximately 10% of families with inherited thrombophilia, and in approximately 5% of individuals with deep vein thrombosis. Protein S deficiency is associated with a risk of thrombosis similar to that in protein C deficiency, approximately a sevenfold increase in the incidence of deep vein thrombosis over that in normal persons. Because of its pronounced phenotypic variability, protein S deficiency is the most difficult of the hereditary thrombophilias to diagnose.

CARDIOVASCULAR: Deep vein thromboses, superficial thrombophlebitis, pulmonary emboli. May also have thrombosis of the mesenteric, renal, axillary, or cerebral veins. Thromboses may be spontaneous or associated with other risk factors (contraceptive pill use, pregnancy, surgery, or trauma). Onset of thrombotic events is usually in the third decade of life.

OTHER: Purpura fulminans has been described in association with homozygous protein S deficiency.

MISCELLANEOUS: First described in 1984 by Comp et al. 3 years after the elucidation of protein C deficiency.

ANESTHETIC CONSIDERATIONS

Prophylactic perioperative anticoagulation is recommended for all patients where warranted, and identification of a hypercoagulable state would not alter this recommendation. Neuraxial anesthesia should be avoided in patients who are anticoagulated. Hypovolemia, hypotension, and hypothermia should be avoided as they may increase the risk of thrombosis.

Bibliography:

1. Johnson CM, Mureebe L, Silver D. Hypercoagulable states: a review. *Vasc Endovascular Surg* 2005;39: 123–133.
2. Gupta B, Prakash S, Gujral K. Anaesthetic management of the parturient with protein S deficiency and lumboperitoneal shunt. *Anaesth Intensive Care* 2003;31:573–575.
3. Crean SJ, Sivarajasingam V, Muhammed J, et al. Thrombophilia and dental surgery: a report of dental extraction in a patient with protein S deficiency. *Dent Update* 2000;27:302–305.
4. Abramovitz SE, Beilin Y. Anesthetic management of the parturient with protein S deficiency and ischemic heart disease. *Anesth Analg* 1999;89:709–710.
5. Grocott HP, Clements F, Landolfo K. Coronary artery bypass graft surgery in a patient with hereditary protein S deficiency. *J Cardiothorac Vasc Anesth* 1996;10:915–917.
6. Fan SZ, Yeh M, Tsay W. Caesarean section in a patient with protein S deficiency. *Anaesthesia* 1995;50:251–253.
7. Cecil ML, Fenton PJ, Jackson WT. The perioperative management of protein S deficiency in total hip arthroplasty. *Clin Orthop* 1994;303:170–172.

Proteus Syndrome

MIM #: 176920

Occurring sporadically, this disease becomes apparent soon after birth, with hemihypertrophy or partial gigantism. Gross deformities develop by late childhood. The syndrome has manifestations in a variety of organs. The main characteristics are hemihypertrophy, subcutaneous tumors (hamartomas), and macrodactyly. Patients often require plastic surgery or amputations. The clinical manifestations are highly variable.

HEENT/AIRWAY: Macrocephaly with cranial hyperostosis (calvarium, facial bones or mandible). May have retinal and/or optic nerve abnormalities. Epibulbar dermoids. A thickened epiglottis has been reported. Fixed torticollis has been reported.

CHEST: Cystic lung disease, may become symptomatic. Occasional pectus excavatum.

CARDIOVASCULAR: Occasional hypertrophic cardiomyopathy and cardiac conduction defects. Pulmonary embolism has been reported with or without deep venous thrombosis.

NEUROMUSCULAR: Intelligence is usually normal, but some may have moderate mental retardation. Seizures. Vertebral anomalies or tumor infiltration have caused spinal stenosis with neurologic sequelae. Meningiomas.

ORTHOPEDIC: Tall. Hemihypertrophy—somatic overgrowth can be generalized or focal. Macrodactyly (partial gigantism of the hands and feet), syndactyly. Soft tissue hypertrophy of the hands or feet. The neck may be elongated from vertebral enlargement. Hemivertebrae, dysplastic vertebrae, dystrophic discs, and spondylomegaly are common. Scoliosis, kyphosis.

GI/GU: Occasional renal abnormalities. Ovarian cystadenoma, testicular tumors.

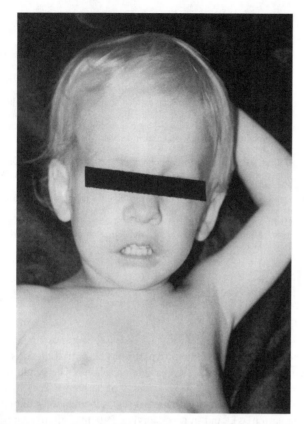

Proteus syndrome. FIG. 1. This young boy has obvious body asymmetry. (Courtesy of Dr. K. Lin and the Craniofacial Anomalies Clinic, University of Virginia Health System.)

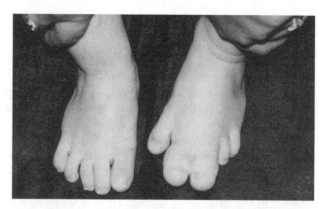

Proteus syndrome. FIG. 2. Asymmetric macrodactyly of the toes of the boy in figure 1. (Courtesy of Dr. K. Lin and the Craniofacial Anomalies Clinic, University of Virginia Health System.)

OTHER: Subcutaneous hamartomatous tumors. Hyperpigmented areas that look like pigmented nevi. Thickened skin on the palms and soles. Lipomas, lymphangiomas. May have hypogammaglobulinemia.

MISCELLANEOUS: This syndrome was first described by Cohen and Hayden. The name "Proteus syndrome" was used by Wiedemann. It alludes to Proteus, a figure in Greek mythology who took on many forms to avoid capture. This syndrome also has variable ("protean") presentations. Joseph Merrick, the "Elephant Man," probably had Proteus syndrome, and not neurofibromatosis, as was suggested in the past.

ANESTHETIC CONSIDERATIONS

The high incidence of cervical spine abnormalities makes difficult laryngoscopy and endotracheal intubation likely. Patients may also exhibit a thickened epiglottis. A 4-month-old baby has been anesthetized without difficulty (6), a 7-year-old boy has required the use of a McCoy levering laryngoscope because of an enlarged epiglottis (3), and a 14-year-old boy has been intubated using awake fiberoptic bronchoscopy because of fixed torticollis (7). The presence of cystic lung disease is a relative contraindication to the use of nitrous oxide and high peak airway pressures

with positive-pressure ventilation. There is emerging evidence that these patients are at increased risk of death from pulmonary embolism (4).

Bibliography:

1. Turner JT, Cohen MM, Biesecker LG. Reassessment of the Proteus syndrome literature: application of diagnostic criteria to published cases. *Am J Med Genet A* 2004;130:111–122.
2. Cekmen N, Zengin A, Tuncer B, et al. Anesthesia for Proteus syndrome. *Paediatr Anaesth* 2004;14:689–692.
3. Pradhan A, Sen I,Batra YK, et al. Proteus syndrome: a concern for the anesthesiologist [Letter]. *Anesth Analg* 2003;96:915–916.
4. Cohen MM. Causes of premature death in Proteus syndrome. *Am J Med Genet* 2001;101:1–3.
5. Biesecker LG. The multifaceted challenges of Proteus syndrome. *JAMA* 2001;285:2240–2243.
6. Ceyhan A, Gulhan Y, Cakan T. Anesthesia for Proteus syndrome. *Eur J Anaesthesiol* 2000;17:645–647.
7. Pennant JH, Harris ME. Anaesthesia for Proteus syndrome. *Anaesthesia* 1991;46:126–128.
8. Cohen MM. Understanding Proteus syndrome, unmasking the elephant man, and stemming elephant fever. *Neurofibromatosis* 1988;1:260.

Prune-Belly Syndrome

SYNONYM: Eagle-Barrett syndrome

MIM #: 100100

This disease is characterized by absent abdominal wall musculature with wrinkled overlying skin, urinary tract dilatation, and cryptorchidism. It occurs much more commonly in boys, with a male:female ratio of 20:1. Most cases have been sporadic, and the etiology of this syndrome is unknown. The pathogenesis of this syndrome is also frequently debated. There may be a primary defect in mesenchymal development that is responsible for both the muscle deficiency and the genitourinary abnormalities. Alternatively, this syndrome may be secondary to distal urinary tract obstruction that occurs *in utero,* leading to the characteristic abdominal and genitourinary findings. Less likely, there may be a vascular etiology for this syndrome,

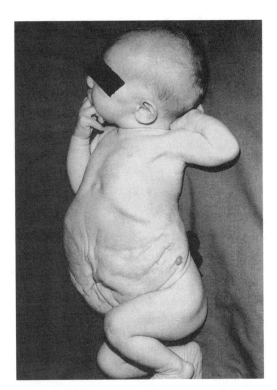

Prune-belly syndrome. Typical infant with relatively severe deficiency of abdominal wall musculature. (Courtesy of Dr. Kenneth E. Greer, Department of Dermatology, University of Virginia Health System.)

which has been proposed to account for the high incidence of associated lower extremity anomalies. However, the lower extremity anomalies are just as likely to be due to the compression of the iliac vessels by the dilated urinary tract *in utero* as they are to any primary vascular insufficiency.

HEENT/AIRWAY: Oligohydramnios can result in Potter facies (hypertelorism, epicanthal folds, low-set ears, flattened, beaked nose, micrognathia) from *in utero* compression (see Potter syndrome, earlier).

CHEST: Pulmonary hypoplasia can occur as a consequence of distal urinary tract obstruction and oligohydramnios. Severely affected patients may die in the neonatal period from pulmonary hypoplasia. Deficient abdominal musculature weakens the ability to cough effectively and increases the risk of respiratory infections. Chronic bronchitis is common. The diaphragm is relatively flat and the accessory muscles are relatively more important. Pneumothorax and pneumomediastinum occur in infants even without significant pulmonary hypoplasia. May have pectus excavatum.

CARDIOVASCULAR: Associated cardiac defects occur in 10%, and include patent ductus arteriosus, atrial septal defect, ventricular septal defect, and tetralogy of Fallot.

ORTHOPEDIC: Congenital dislocation of the hips and clubfoot deformity are common. May have polydactyly,

syndactyly. May have scoliosis, torticollis. Compression of the iliac vessels by the dilated urinary tract *in utero* may lead to lower limb deficits.

GI/GU: Absent or deficient anterior abdominal wall musculature. Overlying skin lies in redundant folds, hence the name "prune-belly." Chronic constipation secondary to abdominal muscle deficiency. May have imperforate anus, malrotation of the gut. Bilateral cryptorchidism. Severe bladder and ureteral dilatation, usually with no apparent obstruction. Hydronephrosis with small dysplastic kidneys is common. Recurrent urinary tract infections are a common complication. Renal failure may develop.

ANESTHETIC CONSIDERATIONS
Renal function should be evaluated preoperatively. Renal insufficiency has implications for perioperative fluid management and the choice of anesthetic drugs. An infant has been reported whose micrognathia resulted in unsuccessful intubation attempts, but easy and successful placement of a laryngeal mask airway (LMA) (1). The response to neuromuscular blockers is normal, although neuromuscular blockade is unnecessary for abdominal surgery because of the paucity of abdominal wall musculature. If respiratory dysfunction is suspected, intubation and controlled ventilation should be employed intraoperatively. Postoperative respiratory complications are common secondary to pulmonary hypoplasia (if present) and a weak cough. An abdominal binder may improve the efficacy of coughing. Medications that produce respiratory depression should be used sparingly. A thoracic epidural has been shown to improve postoperative respiratory function (3). Patients with congenital heart disease require perioperative antibiotic prophylaxis as indicated.

Bibliography:
1. Bariş S, Karakaya D, Üstün E, et al. Complicated airway management in a child with prune-belly syndrome. *Paediatr Anaesth* 2001;11:501–504.
2. Jennings RW. Prune belly syndrome. *Semin Pediatr Surg* 2000;9: 115–120.
3. Heisler DB, Lebowitz P, Barst SM. Pectus excavatum repair in a patient with prune belly syndrome. *Paediatr Anaesth* 1994;4:267–269.
4. Crompton CH, MacLusky IB, Geary DF. Respiratory function in the prune-belly syndrome. *Arch Dis Child* 1993;68:505–506.
5. Henderson AM, Vallis CJ, Sumner E. Anaesthesia in the prune-belly syndrome. *Anaesthesia* 1987;42:54–60.

Pseudoachondroplasia

SYNONYM: Pseudoachondroplastic spondyloepiphyseal dysplasia

MIM #: 177170

This autosomal dominant disorder is due to a mutation in the gene encoding cartilage oligomeric matrix protein (COMP). Mutations in the same gene are responsible for at least some cases of Fairbank type multiple epiphyseal dysplasia (see earlier). Children with pseudoachondroplasia appear normal at birth, but have progressive and disproportionate short stature by 2 years of age, and eventually resemble patients with achondroplasia. Unlike achondroplasia, the head and face remain normal in pseudoachondroplasia.

HEENT/AIRWAY: Normal head and face.

CHEST: Spatulate ribs.

NEUROMUSCULAR: Normal intelligence. Compression of the cervical cord from chronic atlantoaxial dislocation has been reported.

ORTHOPEDIC: Acquired short-limb dwarfism. Odontoid hypoplasia. Short, hyperlax fingers (allowing "telescoping" of the fingers). Ulnar deviation of the wrists and limited extension of the elbows. Ligamentous laxity of the legs. Genu valgum or varum. All long bones are short with widened metaphyses and irregularities of developing epiphyses. Platyspondyly in childhood, normalizing somewhat in adulthood. Kyphosis, scoliosis, lumbar lordosis. Premature osteoarthritis.

MISCELLANEOUS: This syndrome was first described by Maroteaux and Lamy, but their names are given to a different syndrome.

ANESTHETIC CONSIDERATIONS
Careful and stable positioning of the head, particularly during laryngoscopy, is necessary because of the possibility of odontoid hypoplasia and joint laxity. Patients must be carefully positioned perioperatively secondary to limited extension of the elbows and generalized joint laxity.

Bibliography:
1. Briggs MD, Chapman KL. Pseudoachondroplasia and multiple epiphyseal dysplasia: mutation review, molecular interactions, and genotype to phenotype correlations. *Hum Mutat* 2002;19:465–478.
2. McKeand J, Rotta J, Hecht IT. Natural history study of pseudoachondroplasia. *Am J Med Genet* 1996;63:406–410.
3. Berkowitz ID, Raja SN, Bender KS, et al. Dwarfs: pathophysiology and anesthetic implications. *Anesthesiology* 1990;73:739–759.

Pseudoachondroplastic Spondyloepiphyseal Dysplasia

See Pseudoachondroplasia

Pseudohermaphroditism, Male

See 17-ketosteroid reductase deficiency; 5α-reductase deficiency; 17,20-desmolase deficiency

Pseudohyperaldosteronism

See Liddle syndrome

Pseudo-Hurler Syndrome

SYNONYM: Mucolipidosis III; Pseudo-Hurler polydystrophy

MIM #: 252600

This autosomal recessive disorder is due to a deficiency in *N*-acetylglucosamine-1-phosphotransferase. This disease has many of the features of Hurler syndrome, but develops more slowly and lacks mucopolysacchariduria. In this disease, newly synthesized enzyme is released into the extracellular stroma rather than being stored in the lysosomes. The defect is the same as that found in mucolipidosis II (I-cell disease, see earlier), and the reason for the more benign progression of pseudo-Hurler syndrome is unknown.

Before the biochemistry of the mucolipidoses was understood, it was recognized that these patients had features of both the mucopolysaccharidoses and the sphingolipidoses, hence the name "mucolipidosis."

HEENT/AIRWAY: Thickened skull with prominent occiput. Coarse facies with prominent forehead and broad nose. Corneal opacities on slit-lamp examination, mild retinopathy, hyperopic astigmatism. Mucolipid storage with enlarged tongue, particularly the base. May also have mucolipid storage in the epiglottis, tonsils, larynx, and trachea. May have temporomandibular joint destruction. Short neck.

CARDIOVASCULAR: Thickened valves, aortic insufficiency. Symptomatic involvement is rare.

NEUROMUSCULAR: Intelligence is usually normal. May have mild mental retardation.

ORTHOPEDIC: Short stature. Odontoid hypoplasia. Dysostosis of multiple bones, generally more severe in boys than in girls. Multiple stiff joints, including the spine. Flexion contracture of the fingers and toes causing "claw hand/claw foot." Carpal tunnel syndrome. Progressive destruction of the hip. Avascular necrosis of the talus. Lumbar lordosis.

GI/GU: Umbilical hernia. Hepatosplenomegaly.

OTHER: Thickened skin. Patients may be taking pamidronate for bone pain.

MISCELLANEOUS: Although first described by Maroteaux and Lamy, that eponym goes to a completely different disease.

ANESTHETIC CONSIDERATIONS
Anesthetic management of patients with pseudo-Hurler syndrome has not been reported, and the following refers to the

related, but usually more severe, I-cell disease (see earlier). Direct laryngoscopy and tracheal intubation may be very difficult, and may become more difficult as the patient ages. It may be difficult to maintain a patent airway with a mask, even with an oral airway. In one case, a laryngeal mask airway helped, and in another it did not (1). Odontoid hypoplasia has been reported in pseudo-Hurler syndrome, and the possibility of an unstable neck should be considered. If the patient's tracheal wall is thickened, an endotracheal tube that is smaller than predicted may be required. Patients with chronic airway obstruction must be observed closely postoperatively. Patients should be carefully positioned secondary to joint stiffness. Patients with valvular heart disease require perioperative antibiotic prophylaxis as indicated.

Bibliography:

1. Tylki-Szymanska A, Czartoryska B, Groener JE, et al. Clinical variability in mucolipidosis III (pseudo-Hurler polydystrophy). *Am J Med Genet* 2002;108:214–218.
2. Baines DB, Street N, Overton JH. Anaesthetic implications of mucolipidosis. *Paediatr Anaesth* 1993;3:303–306.
3. King DH, Jones RM, Barrett MB. Anaesthetic considerations in the mucopolysaccharidoses. *Anaesthesia* 1984;39:126–131.
4. Baines D, Kenneally J. Anaesthetic management of the mucopolysaccharidoses: a fifteen-year experience in a children's hospital. *Anaesth Intensive Care* 1983;11:198–202.
5. Kempthorne PM, Brown TCK. Anaesthesia and the mucopolysaccharidoses: a survey of techniques and problems. *Anaesth Intensive Care* 1983;11:203–207.

Pseudo-Hurler Polydystrophy

See Pseudo-Hurler syndrome

Pseudohypohyperparathyroidism

Included in Pseudohypoparathyroidism

Pseudohypoparathyroidism

SYNONYM: Albright hereditary osteodystrophy. (Includes pseudopseudohypoparathyroidism and pseudohypohyperparathyroidism)

MIM #: 103580, 603233

Pseudohypoparathyroidism is a group of diseases characterized by target cell (renal tubular or osseous) insensitivity to parathyroid hormone. Hypocalcemia and hyperphosphatemia are prominent features. There are two types of pseudohypoparathyroidism.

Type I is caused by the inability of parathyroid hormone to activate renal cell adenylyl cyclase, with subsequent deficient production of cyclic adenosine monophosphate (cAMP). Type Ia, the most common form of pseudohypoparathyroidism, is due to a defect in the alpha subunit of the gene encoding stimulatory G protein ($G_{s\alpha}$), with loss of the protein, and resistance of target tissues to the effects of parathyroid hormone. The affected gene is called *GNAS1*. It is inherited in an autosomal dominant fashion, and the defect is due to inactivation of one allele; all patients are heterozygous. The situation is more complex as exons and promoter regions are methylated on one parental side, and transcripts are derived from only the nonmethylated allele. There are also a variety of splice variants. In several tissues (including the proximal renal tubule) only the maternally derived allele is expressed. Because this G protein is required for responsiveness to multiple hormones, there are usually other associated endocrinopathies, including hypothyroidism and gonadal dysfunction. The distinctive skeletal and developmental features of type Ia represent classic Albright hereditary osteodystrophy. Type Ib is probably due to abnormalities in signal transduction at the parathyroid hormone receptor limited to the kidney. $G_{s\alpha}$ is normal, and clinical manifestations are limited to those associated with parathyroid hormone activity. The physical appearance in type Ib is normal. Most cases of type Ib have occurred sporadically, but inheritance may be autosomal dominant. Type I disease is treated with vitamin D (1,25-dihydroxyvitamin D_3 or dihydrotachysterol) and oral phosphate binders.

In some families with type Ia pseudohypoparathyroidism, some members exhibit the abnormal habitus but are not resistant to parathyroid hormone. They have normal serum calcium and phosphate levels. These individuals have **pseudopseudohypoparathyroidism**. This may be determined by whether the abnormal gene is maternally (pseudohypoparathyroidism) or paternally (pseudopseudohypoparathyroidism) derived.

Type II disease is due to the inability of cAMP to initiate parathormone-directed metabolic events. Patients have a normal physical appearance. Treatment is the same as for type I.

Pseudohypohyperparathyroidism describes a group of patients with parathyroid hormone resistance that is limited to the renal tubules. There is normal bone response to the elevated parathyroid hormone levels, and these patients have the osseous manifestations of hyperparathyroidism, namely subperiosteal resorption and osteitis fibrosa cystica.

HEENT/AIRWAY: Thickened skull, round face. Subcapsular cataracts. Enamel hypoplasia and failure of teeth to erupt. Short neck. May have laryngeal spasm from hypocalcemia.

CARDIOVASCULAR: The QT interval is prolonged in the presence of hypocalcemia.

NEUROMUSCULAR: May have mental retardation. Hypocalcemia may lead to muscle hyperexcitability, with tetany, seizures, or muscle cramps. Perivascular calcifications in the region of the basal ganglia.

ORTHOPEDIC: Short stature. Short metacarpals, metatarsals and phalanges (brachydactyly). The hallmark finding is short fourth (or fifth) metacarpals. Increased bone density.

Patients with type II may have subperiosteal bone resorption and osteitis fibrosa cystica.

GI/GU: Renal function is normal.

OTHER: Hypocalcemia, hyperphosphatemia. Obese or stocky habitus. Cutaneous or subcutaneous calcifications. Serum calcium levels fluctuate, and may be in the normal range.

MISCELLANEOUS: Albright, the Boston physician who is a founder of the subspecialty of endocrinology, postulated in his original report that the defect was one of end-organ hormone resistance. This is the same Albright of McCune-Albright syndrome. He also described vitamin D-resistant rickets (once known as Albright-Butler-Bloomberg syndrome).

ANESTHETIC CONSIDERATIONS

Serum calcium level should be evaluated and corrected pre-operatively. Hypocalcemia may lead to laryngeal spasm, a prolonged QT interval, and/or tetany. Patients should be assessed preoperatively for the presence of other endocrinopathies. Direct laryngoscopy and tracheal intubation may be difficult secondary to obesity and a short neck.

Bibliography:
1. Weinstein LS, Liu J, Sakamoto A, et al. Minireview: GNAS: normal and abnormal functions. *Endocrinology* 2004;145:5459–5464.
2. Jüppner H. The genetic basis of progressive osseous heteroplasia. *N Engl J Med* 2002;366:128–130.
3. Wilson LC, Hall CM. Albright's hereditary osteodystrophy and pseudo-hypoparathyroidism. *Semin Musculoskelet Radiol* 2002;6:273–283.
4. Farfel Z, Bourne HR, Iiri T. The expanding spectrum of G protein diseases. *N Engl J Med* 1999;340:1012–1020.
5. Axelrod L. Bones, stones and hormones: the contributions of Fuller Albright. *N Engl J Med* 1970;283:964–970.

Pseudometatrophic Dysplasia

See Kniest syndrome

Pseudopseudohypoparathyroidism

Included in Pseudohypoparathyroidism

Pseudothalidomide Syndrome

SYNONYM: SC phocomelia syndrome; Roberts syndrome

MIM #: 269000, 268300

This autosomal recessive disorder is characterized by symmetric limb reduction deformities that resemble phocomelia, flexion contractures, craniofacial anomalies, and a variety of other minor abnormalities. Patients with this disorder appear to have abnormal centromere separation, caused by mutations in the *ESCO2* gene. Mutations in the same gene cause SC phocomelia syndrome and Roberts syndrome, and it is likely that the two syndromes are the same entity, often referred to as the "pseudothalidomide syndrome." There is wide clinical variability, even within families.

HEENT/AIRWAY: Microcephaly. Occasional frontal encephalocele or craniosynostosis. Capillary hemangiomas of face, forehead, and ears. Hypertelorism. Corneal clouding. Hypoplastic ear cartilage. Thin nares with hypoplastic nasal cartilage. May have cleft lip or palate. Micrognathia. Short neck, nuchal cystic hygroma.

CARDIOVASCULAR: Atrial septal defect, valvar aortic stenosis, and premature myocardial infarction have all been reported.

NEUROMUSCULAR: Mild to severe mental retardation.

ORTHOPEDIC: Short stature. Symmetrical limb reduction defects (phocomelia), more severe in the upper limbs. The long bones of the extremities can be hypoplastic to absent. Flexion contractures of multiple joints. Radiohumeral synostosis. Malformed hands. Syndactyly.

GI/GU: Accessory spleen. Cryptorchidism, hypospadias. Occasional renal anomaly, including polycystic kidneys, horseshoe kidney.

OTHER: Prenatal growth failure. Children may have sparse, silvery blond hair. Occasional thrombocytopenia.

MISCELLANEOUS: John Roberts was a plastic surgeon from Philadelphia. Clearly, the name "pseudothalidomide" came later, because Roberts practiced at the turn of the last century, long before there were cases of phocomelia caused by maternal use of thalidomide. The "SC" comes from the initials of the surnames of the two families described by Herrmann in 1969. The earliest description of pseudothalidomide syndrome may have been by Bouchard in 1672, who reported the autopsy of a deceased infant who had been put on public display.

ANESTHETIC CONSIDERATIONS

Thrombocytopenia may occur, and consideration should be given to obtaining a preoperative platelet count. Direct laryngoscopy and tracheal intubation may be difficult secondary to micrognathia and a short neck. Limb reduction deformities may severely limit sites for peripheral vascular access, and radial anomalies may affect ease of access to the radial artery. Phocomelia may make fixation of an appropriately sized blood pressure cuff difficult, and falsely high pressures may be displayed by noninvasive monitors. An appropriate blood pressure cuff should cover two-thirds of the upper arm length. Contractures may make proper positioning difficult.

Bibliography:

1. Mandal AK, Singh AP, Rao L, et al. Roberts pseudothalidomide syndrome. *Arch Ophthalmol* 2000;118:1462–1463.
2. Camlibel T, Mocan H, Kutlu N, et al. Roberts SC phocomelia with isolated cleft palate, thrombocytopenia, and eosinophilia. *Genet Couns* 1999;10:157–161.
3. Van Den Berg DJ, Francke U. Roberts syndrome: a review of 100 cases and a new rating system for severity. *Am J Med Genet* 1993;47: 1104–1123.

Pseudovaginal Perineoscrotal Hypospadias

See 5α-reductase deficiency

Pseudoxanthoma Elasticum

MIM #: 177850, 264800

This usually autosomal recessive, but occasionally autosomal dominant, disorder is marked by abnormal elastic fibers that degenerate and calcify over time. Most of the clinical manifestations are due to disease of medium-sized arteries. Multiple organ systems can be affected, most prominently the skin, the eyes, and the cardiovascular system. It is caused by mutations in the *ABCC6* gene, which encodes an ATP-dependent transmembrane transporter.

HEENT/AIRWAY: Angioid streaks on the retina (secondary to degeneration of elastic tissue) are often diagnostic. Visual acuity is decreased, particularly when vascular changes result in vitreous or subretinal hemorrhage. The oral mucosa may be involved. Involvement of the larynx has been reported in a single patient (5).

CHEST: Benign breast calcifications.

CARDIOVASCULAR: Endocardial thickening and calcification. Calcified endocardial bands have been reported. Involvement of the conduction tissues may result in arrhythmias and sudden death. There can also be valve involvement, including mitral valve prolapse. Early calcification (1 year) of a heterograft mitral valve has been reported. Premature coronary arterial disease. Hypertension. There can be calcification of the peripheral arteries, and patients may have symptomatic peripheral vascular disease (claudication).

NEUROMUSCULAR: Cerebrovascular involvement includes aneurysms, premature occlusive disease, hemorrhage, or infarction. Calcified falx cerebri. Increased incidence of psychiatric problems.

GI/GU: High incidence of gastrointestinal hemorrhage, even after minor mucosal trauma. There are intestinal submucosal lesions similar to the xanthoma-like skin lesions. May have hematuria secondary to renal artery involvement. The vaginal mucosa may be involved. Uterine bleeding on occasion requires hysterectomy.

OTHER: Skin changes are often the earliest manifestation. Yellowish xanthoma-like skin patches ("pseudoxanthoma") are found primarily on the neck, axillary and inguinal folds, cubital area, and periumbilical area. They have a "Moroccan leather" quality, which has more prosaically been likened to plucked chicken skin. The disease may be accelerated during pregnancy. Placental involvement may result in intrauterine growth retardation.

ANESTHETIC CONSIDERATIONS

Laryngeal involvement precluding routine laryngoscopy and intubation has been reported in one patient (5). Vascular access, both venous and arterial, may be difficult because of vascular involvement and involvement of overlying skin (6). The effect of invasive arterial catheters on the progression of local vascular disease is not known. The high incidence of gastric bleeding is a relative contraindication to nasogastric tubes and transesophageal echocardiography. Regional anesthesia has been successfully used in parturients (3). The possibility of cerebrovascular disease and intracranial aneurysms should be considered. Involvement of the endocardium or the cardiac valves, and the possibility of premature cardiovascular disease should also be considered. Patients with valvular disease should receive perioperative prophylactic antibiotics as indicated.

Bibliography:

1. Laube S, Moss C. Pseudoxanthoma elasticum. *Arch Dis Child* 2005;90: 754–756.
2. Chassaing N, Martin L, Calvas P, et al. Pseudoxanthoma elasticum: a clinical, pathophysiological and genetic update including 11 novel ABCC6 mutations. *J Med Genet* 2005;42:881–892.
3. Douglas MJ, Gunka VB, von Dadelszen P. Anesthesia for the parturient with pseudoxanthoma elasticum. *Int J Obstet Anesth* 2003;12:45–47.
4. Solgonick RM, Trubiano PB. Elective coronary revascularization in a patient with pseudoxanthoma elasticum. *Am J Anesthesiol* 1998;25: 77–78.
5. Levitt MW, Collison JM. Difficult endotracheal intubation in a patient with pseudoxanthoma elasticum. *Anaesth Intensive Care* 1992;10:62–64.
6. Krechel SLW, Ramirez-Inawat RC, Fabian LW. Anesthetic considerations in pseudoxanthoma elasticum. *Anesth Analg* 1981;60:344–347.

Pterygium Syndrome

See Multiple pterygium syndrome

Purine Nucleoside Phosphorylase Deficiency

MIM #: 164050

This disease is inherited in an autosomal recessive fashion. Purine nucleoside phosphorylase catalyzes the lysis of the purine nucleosides (deoxy)inosine and (deoxy)guanosine to their purine bases and the corresponding ribose-1-phosphate. Deficiency of this enzyme results in accumulation of deoxyguanosine and deoxyinosine, which are particularly toxic to T cells. Accumulation of deoxyguanosine triphosphate, which inhibits ribonucleotide reductase, blocks DNA synthesis and prevents the cellular proliferation required for an immune response. Purine nucleoside phosphorylase deficiency therefore leads to defective T-cell immunity. With time, there can also be B-cell dysfunction because of abnormal interaction with T cells. Patients are particularly susceptible to viral infections, which can be fatal, and patients have succumbed to disseminated vaccinia or varicella infections, lymphosarcoma, or graft-versus-host disease from nonirradiated transfused blood.

CHEST: Recurrent upper respiratory tract infections.

NEUROMUSCULAR: Mental retardation, developmental delay, behavioral disorders. Spastic diplegia or tetraparesis, dysequilibrium syndrome, pyramidal tract signs, Babinski sign, exaggerated reflexes.

OTHER: Failure to thrive. Repeated infections, particularly viral, which may be fatal. T-cell function is more severely affected than B-cell function. Autoimmune disease (autoimmune hemolytic anemia, idiopathic thrombocytopenic purpura, systemic lupus erythematosus). B-immunoblastic type malignant lymphoma. Hypouricemia.

MISCELLANEOUS: Adenosine deaminase is the next enzyme in this metabolic pathway, and its absence results in severe combined immune deficiency. Intermittent transfusions with (irradiated) red blood cells supply adequate exogenous enzyme. Bone marrow transplantation is curative.

ANESTHETIC CONSIDERATIONS
Good aseptic technique is imperative. Blood products must be irradiated to avoid graft-versus-host disease. Patients with autoimmune disease may be taking steroids, and may require perioperative stress doses of steroids.

Bibliography:
1. Nyhan WL. Disorders of purine and pyrimidine metabolism. *Mol Genet Metab* 2005;86:25–33.
2. Myers LA, Hershfield MS, Neale WT, et al. Purine nucleoside phosphorylase deficiency (PNP-def) presenting with lymphopenia and developmental delay: successful correction with umbilical cord blood transplantation. *J Pediatr* 2004;145:710–712.
3. Markert ML. Purine nucleoside phosphorylase deficiency. *Immunodefic Rev* 1991;3:45–81.

Pyknodysostosis

MIM #: 265800

This autosomal recessive disease is due to a mutation of the cathepsin K gene. The cathepsins are in the papain family of cysteine proteases. These proteases are involved with multiple functions. In this disorder, osteoclasts demineralize bone appropriately, but are unable to adequately degrade the organic material. Cathepsin K is highly expressed in osteoclasts. The primary clinical manifestations are osteosclerosis and short stature. Patients often require

medical attention for fractures, which can be sustained even after relatively mild trauma.

HEENT/AIRWAY: Frontal and occipital prominence, wormian bones, wide sutures with delayed closure. Persistence of anterior fontanelle, absent frontal sinus and mastoid air cells. Midface hypoplasia. Prominent nose and narrow, grooved palate. Dental abnormalities including delayed eruption, hypodontia, irregular permanent teeth, dental caries. Hypoplastic mandible and mandibular rami, with obtuse angle of the mandible. May have mandibular fractures. Pharyngeal narrowing, associated with an increased risk of obstructive sleep apnea.

CHEST: Hypoplastic clavicles, with loss of lateral end. Clavicular fractures.

NEUROMUSCULAR: Mental retardation has been reported in some.

ORTHOPEDIC: Short stature (adult height less than 5 ft). Osteosclerosis with bone fragility and fractures even after mild trauma, particularly in the lower extremities. Osteolysis of the distal phalanges, especially of the index finger. Wrinkled skin over the dorsum of distal fingers. Flattened, grooved nails. Spondylolysis of L4 and L5.

MISCELLANEOUS: First described by Maroteaux and Lamy. The artist Toulouse-Lautrec (whose parents were first cousins) is thought to have had pyknodysostosis, but this assertion has also been contested (4, 5). The spelling "pykno . . . " tends to be used by American authors and "pycno . . . " by British authors (and by Maroteaux and Lamy originally).

ANESTHETIC CONSIDERATIONS
Recall that despite the child-size stature, the patient's intelligence is usually normal for his or her chronologic age. Dental abnormalities should be documented preoperatively. Spondylolysis of L4-5 may have an impact on the decision to perform a regional anesthetic in this location. Clavicular anomalies may make placement of a subclavian venous catheter more difficult. Patients must be carefully positioned secondary to bone fragility. Patients with a history of obstructive sleep apnea may have postoperative airway obstruction.

Bibliography:
1. Muto T, Yamazaki A, Takeda S, et al. Pharyngeal narrowing as a common feature in pycnodysostosis—a cephalometric study. *Int J Oral Maxillofac Surg* 2005;34:680–685.
2. Motyckova G, Fisher DE. Pycnodysostosis: role and regulation of cathepsin K in osteoclast function and human disease. *Curr Mol Med* 2002;2:407–421.
3. Soliman AT, Ramadan MA, Sherif A, et al. Pycnodysostosis: clinical, radiologic, and endocrine evaluation and linear growth after growth hormone therapy. *Metabolism* 2001;50:905–911.
4. Frey JB. What dwarfed Toulouse-Lautrec? *Nat Genet* 1995;10:128–130.
5. Maroteaux P. Toulouse-Lautrec diagnosis [Letter]. *Nat Genet* 1995;11: 363–364.

Pyle Disease

See Pyle metaphyseal dysplasia

Pyle Metaphyseal Dysplasia

SYNONYM: Pyle disease; Metaphyseal dysplasia, Pyle type

MIM #: 265900

There are many types of metaphyseal chondrodysplasia—see also Jansen type, McKusick type (cartilage-hair hypoplasia syndrome), Schmid type, Shwachman syndrome, and Spahr type [not included in this text (*MIM #* 250400)]. This autosomal recessive type of metaphyseal chondrodysplasia is distinguished by characteristic radiographic findings. Despite the impressive radiographic findings, patients usually are asymptomatic. The most common clinical finding is genu valgum. Minimal involvement of the cranial bones distinguishes this syndrome from the craniometaphyseal dysplasias. The responsible gene and gene product are unknown.

HEENT/AIRWAY: Mild thickening of the calvarium. May have supraorbital hyperplasia. Dental caries and misplaced teeth. May have prognathism.

ORTHOPEDIC: "Erlenmeyer flask-like" flaring of long bones, most prominently of the distal femur and proximal tibia. Broad proximal humerus, distal radius, and ulna. Cortical thinning and osteoporosis in the long bones. Limited elbow extension. May have scoliosis. Genu valgum. Fractures.

MISCELLANEOUS: Edwin Pyle was an orthopedic surgeon in Waterbury, Connecticut.

ANESTHETIC CONSIDERATIONS
Carious teeth may be dislodged during laryngoscopy. Distal radial and ulnar abnormalities may affect ease of access to the radial artery. Patients must be carefully positioned secondary to osteoporosis and the risk of fracture.

Bibliography:
1. Percin EF, Percin S, Koptagel E, et al. A case with Pyle type metaphyseal dysplasia: clinical, radiological and histological evaluation. *Genet Couns* 2003;14:387–393.
2. Beighton P. Pyle disease (metaphyseal dysplasia). *J Med Genet* 1987;24: 321–324.

Pyruvate Dehydrogenase Deficiency

MIM #: 312170

Pyruvate dehydrogenase deficiency is a relatively common X-linked defect of mitochondrial energy metabolism. Deficiency of pyruvate dehydrogenase prevents entry of pyruvate into the citric acid cycle by preventing the conversion of pyruvate to acetyl CoA, with the subsequent accumulation of lactate and pyruvate. Pyruvate dehydrogenase is actually a complex of three catalytic enzymes: pyruvate decarboxylase (El), dihydrolipoyl transacetylase (E2), and dihydrolipoyl dehydrogenase (E3). Also involved are two cofactors: thiamine pyrophosphate and lipoate. Regulation of the enzyme system is further modified by stimulation from a specific phosphatase, and inhibition from a specific kinase.

The clinical manifestation of this disorder ranges from benign intermittent ataxia without acidosis (chronic form) to severe acidosis with death in early infancy (early fatal form). Patients with the chronic form often have acute exacerbations that are precipitated by infection, prolonged fasting, or other stimuli of gluconeogenesis. Acute exacerbations are characterized by lactic acidosis, hypotonia, ataxia, confusion, lethargy, and coma. The clinical phenotype may resemble Leigh disease (see earlier). Girls usually have the chronic form, whereas boys usually have the early fatal form. Affected girls are carriers of the X-linked trait, and this is one of the few X-linked conditions in which female heterozygotes manifest significant clinical symptoms.

HEENT/AIRWAY: Dysmorphic facial features in some, similar to those seen with fetal alcohol syndrome, including microcephaly, short palpebral fissures, ptosis, microphthalmia, maxillary hypoplasia, posteriorly rotated, prominent ears, eustachian tube dysfunction, short nose, thin upper lip with smooth philtrum, cleft lip or palate, malocclusion, micrognathia, short neck. E3 deficiency is associated with optic atrophy and laryngeal stridor.

CHEST: May have episodes of hyperventilation secondary to acidosis.

NEUROMUSCULAR: El and E2 deficiencies are associated with progressive and severe neurologic dysfunction. E3 deficiency is associated with lethargy and irritability.

Stress has been reported to exacerbate neurologic symptoms. May have seizures. May have central respiratory depression. May have agenesis of the corpus callosum.

OTHER: E2 and E3 deficiencies are associated with lactic acidosis. Acidosis may be precipitated by a high-carbohydrate diet with E2 (but not with E3) deficiency.

MISCELLANEOUS: Elevated fetal acid aldehyde has been suggested as the common link with fetal alcohol syndrome, explaining the similar facial features. Interestingly, this gene is autosomal in marsupials, and is known to be located on a fragment of marsupial chromosome that was later translocated to the short arm of the X chromosome after the divergence of marsupials and primordial mammals.

ANESTHETIC CONSIDERATIONS
Avoid hypothermia, decreases in cardiac output, and other physiologic conditions which may lead to lactic acidosis (1, 3). It has been suggested that the inhibition

of gluconeogenesis by halothane may exacerbate the lactic acidosis in these patients (5). Lactate-containing intravenous fluids such as Ringer's lactate should be avoided because they increase the lactate load. Patients who are acidotic may need treatment with bicarbonate. Patients should receive ample perioperative glucose to maintain serum glucose in the high–normal range. Although barbiturates and volatile anesthetics can inhibit mitochondrial respiration, induction of anesthesia with thiopental has been used without any complications in the phenotypically similar Leigh disease (see earlier). Patients are predisposed to central respiratory depression, and should be closely monitored for respiratory depression perioperatively.

Bibliography:

1. Mayhew JF. Anesthesia in a child with pyruvate dehydrogenase deficiency [Letter]. *Paediatr Anaesth* 2006;16:93.
2. De Meirleir L. Defects of pyruvate metabolism and the Krebs cycle. *J Child Neurol* 2002;17:3S26–3S33.
3. Acharya D, Dearlove OR. Anaesthesia in pyruvate dehydrogenase deficiency. *Anaesthesia* 2001;56:808–809.
4. Keyes MA, Van de Wiele BV, Stead SW. Mitochondrial myopathies: an unusual cause of hypotonia in infants and children. *Paediatr Anaesth* 1996;6:329–335.
5. Dierdorf SF, McNiece WL. Anaesthesia and pyruvate dehydrogenase deficiency. *Can Anaesth Soc J* 1983;30:413–416.

Pyruvate Kinase Deficiency

MIM #: 266200

Pyruvate kinase (PK) deficiency is an autosomal recessive disease. There are four PK isozymes: L in liver, R in red blood cells, M_1 in muscle, and M_2 in white blood cells and platelets. M_1 and M_2 are derived from the same gene, by alternative RNA splicing. PK converts phosphoenolpyruvate to pyruvate in red blood cells, one of the last steps in the anaerobic glycolytic pathway. Thus, PK-deficient red blood cells are depleted of adenosine triphosphate and have an abbreviated life span. The clinical presentation varies from chronic, compensated hemolytic anemia to severe hemolytic anemia. PK deficiency is the most common cause of hereditary nonspherocytic hemolytic anemia. Pregnancy and intercurrent viral infections may exacerbate hemolysis. There are many genetic variants, and most patients are in fact compound heterozygotes (two different mutations) rather than homozygotes (two copies of the same mutation).

HEENT/AIRWAY: Severely affected children have frontal bossing secondary to excessive erythropoiesis in the cranial marrow cavity.

CARDIOVASCULAR: Rare phlebitis and arterial thrombosis, including carotid artery thrombosis.

NEUROMUSCULAR: Rare spinal cord compression from extramedullary hematopoietic tissue.

GI/GU: Splenomegaly. Chronic hemolysis may require a splenectomy, which usually results in improvement, but not cure. Increased incidence of bilirubinate gallstones and cholecystitis.

OTHER: Normocytic anemia, thrombocytosis, hyperbilirubinemia. Levels of glycolytic intermediaries such as 2,3-diphosphoglycerate are increased, which causes a shift in the oxygen–hemoglobin desaturation curve to the right, reducing the symptoms of anemia. Patients who have received multiple transfusions may have iron overload.

MISCELLANEOUS: PK deficiency is the most common enzyme abnormality of the glycolytic pathway in humans. It is common in basenji dogs, and also occurs naturally in beagles. PK deficiency in mice protects against malaria.

ANESTHETIC CONSIDERATIONS

The patient's hematocrit should be evaluated preoperatively.

Bibliography:

1. Zanella A, Fermo E, Bianchi P, et al. Red cell pyruvate kinase deficiency: molecular and clinical aspects. *Br J Haematol* 2005;130:11–25.
2. Marshall SR, Saunders PW, Hamilton PJ, et al. The dangers of iron overload in pyruvate kinase deficiency. *Br J Haematol* 2003;120:1090–1091.
3. Chou R, DeLoughery TG. Recurrent thromboembolic disease following splenectomy for pyruvate kinase deficiency. *Am J Hematol* 2001;67:197–199.

R

Ramsay Hunt Syndrome

SYNONYM: Progressive myoclonus epilepsies syndrome
Note: "Ramsay Hunt syndrome" is also used to describe postherpetic (varicella-zoster) otitis.

MIM #: 159700

This Ramsay Hunt syndrome represents a heterogeneous collection of disorders that are distinguished by cerebellar ataxia, seizure disorder and myoclonus. "Ragged-red" fibers are seen on muscle biopsy. Ragged-red fibers represent mitochondria, and this entity is probably a pathophysiologic process of mitochondria.

NEUROMUSCULAR: Cerebellar ataxia, myoclonus, intention tremor. Grand mal seizures. There are lesions of the dentate nucleus, as was postulated by Hunt, and degeneration of the globus pallidus.

OTHER: May have psychiatric disease, including psychosis.

MISCELLANEOUS: Given the heterogeneity of this syndrome, some have argued that Ramsay Hunt syndrome does not represent a useful clinical rubric and should be discarded.

ANESTHETIC CONSIDERATIONS

Although there is a paucity of clinical evidence, succinylcholine should be used with caution in these myopathic patients because of the risk of an exaggerated hyperkalemic response. Myoclonus is common, and is difficult to differentiate from true motor seizures.

Bibliography:
1. Shahwan A, Farrell M, Delanty N. Progressive myoclonic epilepsies: a review of genetic and therapeutic aspects. *Lancet Neurol* 2005;4:239–248.
2. Hsiao MC, Liu CY, Yang YY, et al. Progressive myoclonic epilepsies syndrome (Ramsay Hunt syndrome) with mental disorder: report of two cases. *Psychiatry Clin Neurosci* 1999;53:575–578.

Rapp-Hodgkin Ectodermal Dysplasia

SYNONYM: Hypohidrotic ectodermal dysplasia, autosomal dominant type

MIM #: 129400

This autosomal dominant type of hypohidrotic ectodermal dysplasia is marked by hypohidrosis or anhydrosis (decreased or absent sweating), cleft lip or palate, and ectodermal dysplasia. There are actually many syndromes of ectodermal dysplasia, all having different degrees of hypohidrosis, different degrees of ectodermal dysplasia, and different inheritance patterns. (See also AEC syndrome, Clouston syndrome, EEC syndrome, Pachyonychia congenita syndrome.)

HEENT/AIRWAY: High forehead. Ptosis. Lacrimal duct anomalies. May have hearing loss, usually secondary to chronic otitis media, which is more likely in patients with palatal incompetence. Flat nasal bridge, narrow nose, hypoplastic alae nasi. Maxillary hypoplasia. Small mouth. Hypoplastic teeth. Cleft lip or palate, cleft uvula, velopharyngeal incompetence.

NEUROMUSCULAR: Speech development may be delayed secondary to velopharyngeal incompetence or hearing loss.

ORTHOPEDIC: Nail dysplasia. May have syndactyly, ectrodactyly.

GI/GU: Hypospadias. May have labial anomalies.

OTHER: Hypohidrosis or anhydrosis, secondary to hypoplastic sweat glands. Thin skin. Thin, wiry hair. Alopecia.

ANESTHETIC CONSIDERATIONS

Patients may become hyperthermic perioperatively secondary to hypohidrosis or anhydrosis. Dental anomalies should be documented preoperatively. Patients must be carefully padded perioperatively to protect thin skin.

Bibliography:
1. Chan I, McGrath JA, Kivirikko S. Rapp-Hodgkin syndrome and the tail of p63. *Clin Exp Dermatol* 2005;30:183–186.

2. Neilson DE, Brunger JW, Heeger S, et al. Mixed clefting type in Rapp-Hodgkin syndrome. *Am J Med Genet* 2002;108:281–284.
3. O'Donnell BP, James WD. Rapp-Hodgkin ectodermal dysplasia. *J Am Acad Dermatol* 1992;27:323–326.

Refsum Disease

(Includes Infantile Refsum disease)

MIM #: 266500, 266510

This autosomal recessive disease is a disorder of lipid metabolism caused by a defect in the gene coding the enzyme phytanoyl-CoA hydroxylase or the gene encoding peroxin-7. Affected patients are unable to metabolize phytanic acid, which comes from dietary sources. Phytanic acid then accumulates in the body. The hallmark findings are retinitis pigmentosa, chronic polyneuropathy and cerebellar abnormalities. Most patients also have nonspecific electrocardiographic changes. The general course is one of progressive deterioration, although exacerbations may accompany infections, surgery, or pregnancy. There may be some recovery after an acute exacerbation. The disease may be controlled and neural function improved by a diet lacking chlorophyll, phytol, and phytanic acid. Phytol, a component of chlorophyll, is converted to phytanic acid.

Infantile Refsum disease is a genetically and biochemically distinct disorder, and is therefore probably inappropriately named (1). It is an autosomal recessive peroxisomal biogenesis disorder due to an abnormality in the genes peroxin-1 (*PEX1*), peroxin-2 (*PEX2*) or peroxin-26 (*PEX26*). Patients are unable to transport proteins into peroxisomes appropriately. Peroxisomal function is deficient, and peroxisomes may be absent. This leads to an accumulation of phytanic acid as in Refsum disease, but also to an accumulation of very long chain fatty acids, dihydroxycholestanoic and trihydroxycholestanoic acids, and pipecolic acid. In addition to the clinical features of Refsum disease, patients with the infantile form may have flattened facies, mental retardation, hepatomegaly, skeletal changes with osteoporosis, protracted diarrhea, and episodic bleeding. There are genetic and biochemical similarities among infantile Refsum disease, neonatal adrenoleukodystrophy (see earlier, Adrenoleukodystrophy) and Zellweger syndrome (see later). These three disorders may represent a continuum, with Zellweger syndrome being the most severe, neonatal adrenoleukodystrophy intermediate, and infantile Refsum disease being the least severe.

The clinical features described in the following sections pertain to Refsum disease.

HEENT/AIRWAY: Retinitis pigmentosa, poor vision in low light, diminished peripheral vision, lens opacities, miosis, nystagmus, ptosis. Nerve deafness. Anosmia.

CARDIOVASCULAR: Nonspecific electrocardiographic (EKG) changes, including atrioventricular conduction block and bundle branch block. Congestive cardiomyopathy.

NEUROMUSCULAR: Chronic polyneuropathy (motor and sensory). Cerebellar ataxia, diminished or absent deep tendon reflexes, intention tremor. Elevated cerebrospinal fluid protein without pleocytosis.

ORTHOPEDIC: Multiple epiphyseal dysplasia. Syndactyly, bilaterally short fourth metacarpals. Pes cavus, hammer toe.

OTHER: Ichthyosis, ranging from mild hyperkeratosis of the palms and soles to full truncal ichthyosis.

MISCELLANEOUS: A leading Norwegian neurologist in his day, Refsum described this disorder as his medical thesis. Phytol is found in many dietary fats and dairy products. The phytol in chlorophyll, the major dietary source, is not well absorbed.

ANESTHETIC CONSIDERATIONS

Exacerbations of this disease can accompany surgery, infection, or pregnancy. A baseline EKG with rhythm strip should be evaluated preoperatively. Because of the risk of hyperkalemia, succinylcholine should be avoided in patients with significant motor neuropathy.

Bibliography:

1. Jansen GA, Waterham HR, Wanders RJ. Molecular basis of Refsum disease: sequence variations in phytanoyl-CoA hydroxylase (PHYH) and the PTS2 receptor (PEX7). *Hum Mutat* 2004;23:209–218.
2. Wierzbicki AS, Lloyd MD, Schofield CJ, et al. Refsum disease: a peroxisomal disorder affecting phytanic acid alpha-oxidation. *J Neurochem* 2002;80:727–735.
3. Wanders RJ, Jansen GA, Skjeldal OH. Refsum disease, peroxisomes and phytanic acid oxidation: a review. *J Neuropathol Exp Neurol* 2001;60: 1021–1031.
4. Bader PI, Dougherty S, Cangany N, et al. Infantile Refsum disease in four Amish sibs. *Am J Med Genet* 2000;90:110–114.
5. Nyberg-Hansen R. Obituary: Sigvald Refsum (1907–1991). *J Neurol Sci* 1992;107:125–126.

Respiratory Chain Disorders

See Complex I-V deficiencies

Retinoic Acid Embryopathy

MIM #: 243440

This syndrome is due to the teratogenic effects of retinoic acid [isotretinoin, 1,3-*cis*-retinoic acid (Accutane, Roche Laboratories, Nutley, NJ)]. Abnormalities occur primarily in the face, heart and central nervous system. The DiGeorge syndrome (see earlier) may be seen in association with *in utero* exposure to retinoic acid.

HEENT/AIRWAY: Microcephaly, facial asymmetry. Hypertelorism. Small ears or absent external ears with stenosis of the external auditory canal. Facial nerve paralysis ipsilateral to the ear abnormality. Mottled teeth. Cleft palate. Micrognathia.

CARDIOVASCULAR: A variety of congenital cardiac malformations, particularly conotruncal malformations and aortic arch abnormalities.

NEUROMUSCULAR: Mental retardation. Hydrocephalus. Structural brain defects, particularly in the posterior fossa. Facial nerve paralysis ipsilateral to the ear anomalies.

OTHER: Abnormalities of the thymus and parathyroid. May have DiGeorge syndrome.

MISCELLANEOUS: The risk to the fetus appears to occur only when maternal ingestion occurs after the 15th day of pregnancy. Maternal use before conception is not thought to be teratogenic. Exposure to topical tretinoin (Retin-A, Ortho McNeil Pharmaceutical, Inc., Titusville, NJ) does not appear to be associated with fetal malformations (1).

ANESTHETIC CONSIDERATIONS

Direct laryngoscopy and tracheal intubation may be difficult secondary to micrognathia. Patients with parathyroid dysfunction may have abnormal levels of serum calcium. Patients with congenital heart disease require perioperative antibiotic prophylaxis as indicated.

Bibliography:

1. Loureiro KD, Kao KK, Jones KL, et al. Minor malformations characteristic of the retinoic acid embryopathy and other birth outcomes in children of women exposed to topical tretinoin during early pregnancy. *Am J Med Genet A* 2005;136:117–121.
2. Centers for Disease Control and Prevention (CDC). Accutane-exposed pregnancies—California, 1999. *MMWR Morb Mortal Wkly Rep* 2000;49:28–31.
3. Coberly S, Lammer E, Alashari M. Retinoic acid embryopathy: case report and review of literature. *Pediatr Pathol Lab Med* 1996;16: 823–836.

Rett Syndrome

MIM #: 312750

This syndrome of progressive encephalopathy occurs almost exclusively in girls. It is thought to be X-linked dominant, usually lethal in male hemizygotes, or it may be due to a particular X-inactivation pattern. It is caused by mutations in the X-linked gene *MECP2*, encoding methyl-CpG-binding protein-2, resulting in arrested development of neuronal cells. Patients are normal at birth, and develop normally until 6 to 18 months of age, when developmental regression begins. After a period of neurologic decline, there can be a prolonged phase of stability or improvement. Survival into adulthood is possible. Some patients maintain a degree of hand and speech use, and have been classified as having the preserved speech variant (PSV) of Rett syndrome.

An early onset, and a more severe, form of Rett syndrome can be caused by mutations in the gene *CDKL5*. This early onset form is characterized by neonatal hypotonia and seizures.

HEENT/AIRWAY: Acquired microcephaly (head circumference is normal at birth). There may be an increased incidence of upper airway obstruction.

CHEST: Wakefulness is associated with periods of abnormal respiration, characterized by intermittent hyperventilation and occasional apnea. This normalizes with sleep. Kyphoscoliosis may result in restrictive lung disease.

CARDIOVASCULAR: Prolonged QT interval. May have reduced heart rate variability. May be at increased risk for sudden cardiac death. Vasomotor change in the lower extremities.

NEUROMUSCULAR: Normal development until 6 to 18 months of age, then rapid regression to severe dementia and autism. Behavioral problems. Axial hypotonia and limb spasticity are common. Also have choreoathetosis, dystonia, ataxia, and myoclonic jerks. Stereotypic hand movements (hand wringing). Decreased sensitivity to pain. Seizures (both absence and tonic-clonic).

ORTHOPEDIC: Acquired short stature. Kyphoscoliosis, hip dislocation, osteopenia, pathologic fractures. Hands and feet are small, with short fourth or fifth metacarpals and metatarsals.

OTHER: Poor growth. Rett described increased ammonia concentrations, but this is not a consistent finding. Increased serum and cerebrospinal fluid lactate have also been reported.

Children classically exhibit stereotypical hand movements, described as "hand washing" or "hand wringing." Music is said to have a calming effect and to stop such stereotypical behavior. May awaken at night with uncontrollable screaming. Depo-Provera is said to worsen behavioral problems.

MISCELLANEOUS: Rett was a Viennese pediatrician who described this syndrome after observing two unrelated girls exhibiting similar hand movements while sitting next to each other in his waiting room.

ANESTHETIC CONSIDERATIONS

Medical procedures may induce behavioral problems. May be more sensitive to sedative drugs, with faster onset of anesthesia and prolonged period of emergence (4, 9). Patients may have a prolonged QT interval, and may be at risk for sudden cardiac death. Patients with advanced disease are at increased risk for perioperative aspiration. Chronic use of anticonvulsant medications affects the metabolism of some anesthetic drugs. Muscle wasting makes careful intraoperative positioning necessary. The thin body habitus may predispose patients to intraoperative cooling. Abnormalities in the control of respiration and kyphoscoliosis predispose these patients to postoperative respiratory complications. When titrating analgesics, recall that these patients often exhibit decreased sensitivity to pain.

Bibliography:

1. Nomura Y, Segawa M. Natural history of Rett syndrome. *J Child Neurol* 2005;20:764–768.
2. Weaving LS, Christodoulou J, Williamson SL, et al. Mutations of CDKL5 cause a severe neurodevelopmental disorder with infantile spasms and mental retardation. *Am J Hum Genet* 2004;75:1079–1093.
3. Coleman P. Rett syndrome: anaesthesia management [Letter]. *Paediatr Anaesth* 2003;13:180.
4. Khalil SN, Hanna E, Armendartz G. Rett syndrome: anaesthesia management [Letter]. *Paediatr Anaesth* 2002;12:374–379.
5. Konen AA, Joshi GP, Kelly CK. Epidural analgesia for pain relief after scoliosis surgery in a patient with Rett syndrome. *Anesth Analg* 1999;89:451–452.
6. Ellaway CJ, Sholler G, Leonard H, et al. Prolonged QT interval in Rett syndrome. *Arch Dis Child* 1999;80:470–472.
7. Guideri F, Acampa M, Hayek G, et al. Reduced heart rate variability in patients affected with Rett syndrome: a possible explanation for sudden death. *Neuropediatrics* 1999;30:146–148.
8. Dearlove OR, Walker RWM. Anaesthesia for Rett syndrome. *Paediatr Anaesth* 1996;6:155–158.
9. Konarzewski WH, Misso S. Rett syndrome and delayed recovery from anaesthesia. *Anaesthesia* 1994;49:357.
10. Maguire D, Bachman C. Anaesthesia and Rett syndrome: a case report. *Can J Anaesth* 1989;36:478–481.

Rhizomelic Chondrodysplasia Punctata

See Chondrodysplasia punctata—autosomal recessive type

Ribbing Type Multiple Epiphyseal Dysplasia

Included in Multiple epiphyseal dysplasia

Richner-Hanhart Syndrome

See Tyrosinemia II

Rieger Syndrome

See also Axenfeld syndrome

MIM #: 180500

This autosomal dominant syndrome is an association of the originally described Rieger anomaly of the anterior segment of the eye with later-described dental abnormalities. The Rieger anomaly (findings limited to the peripheral anterior segment of the eye plus abnormalities of the iris) can also occur with several other dysmorphic syndromes. This disorder is most often due to a mutation in the homeobox transcription factor gene, *PITX2*, which maps to the long arm of chromosome 4. A second type of Rieger syndrome (type 2) maps to the long arm of chromosome 13.

HEENT/AIRWAY: Maxillary hypoplasia. Microcornea with corneal opacity, hypoplasia of the iris, anterior synechiae. Glaucoma is common. Hypertelorism, telecanthus. Broad nasal bridge, thin upper lip, short philtrum, protruding lower lip. Underdeveloped maxilla. Microdontia and hypodontia, usually of upper incisors.

NEUROMUSCULAR: A single kindred has been described that also had myotonic dystrophy.

GI/GU: Failure of involution of the periumbilical skin. Anal stenosis or imperforate anus. Hypospadias.

OTHER: May have growth hormone deficiency.

MISCELLANEOUS: In the mouse embryo, *PITX2* gene mRNA localizes to the periocular mesenchyme, the maxillary and mandibular epithelium, and the umbilicus, all areas affected in the human syndrome. Herwigh Rieger was an Austrian ophthalmologist with an interest in genetic diseases of the eye.

ANESTHETIC CONSIDERATIONS

Dental abnormalities should be documented preoperatively. Care should be taken to prevent dental damage during laryngoscopy. Patients may have glaucoma. A case of difficult intubation and post extubation airway obstruction in a neonate has been reported (3).

Bibliography:

1. Jena AK, Kharbanda OP. Axenfeld-Rieger syndrome: report on dental and craniofacial findings. *J Clin Pediatr Dent* 2005;30:83–88.
2. Amendt BA, Semina EV, Alward WL. Rieger syndrome: a clinical, molecular, and biochemical analysis. *Cell Mol Life Sci* 2000;57: 1652–1666.
3. Asai T, Matsumoto H, Shingu K. Difficult airway management in a baby with Axenfeld-Rieger syndrome [Letter]. *Paediatr Anaesth* 1998;8:444.

Rigid Spine Syndrome

MIM #: 602771

This autosomal recessive disorder is characterized by skeletal muscle myopathy and fibrous shortening of the spine extensor muscles, leading to limited flexion of the thoracolumbar and, in particular, the cervical spine. Movement of other joints may also be limited, particularly the elbow joint. The disorder is caused by a mutation in the *SEPN1* gene. It bears similarities to Emery-Dreifuss muscular dystrophy (see earlier), but is distinguished from Emery-Dreifuss muscular dystrophy by lack of consistent cardiac involvement and by its autosomal recessive inheritance.

HEENT/AIRWAY: The neck is extremely hyperlordotic. The trachea is significantly narrowed.

CHEST: Most patients have clinically significant respiratory muscle weakness. May also have restrictive lung disease secondary to restricted chest wall mobility and the development of kyphoscoliosis. Respiratory failure develops in some patients.

CARDIOVASCULAR: May have a cardiomyopathy. May have right ventricular failure due to respiratory insufficiency.

NEUROMUSCULAR: Skeletal muscle myopathy.

ORTHOPEDIC: Markedly restricted cervical spine flexion. Restricted movement of the thoracolumbar spine. Kyphoscoliosis. Contractures of multiple joints, particularly the elbow joint.

ANESTHETIC CONSIDERATIONS

Direct laryngoscopy and tracheal intubation may be very difficult secondary to the extremely hyperlordotic cervical spine and restrictions in cervical spine movement. Note that the normal kyphotic bend of endotracheal tubes opposes the curve of the trachea in these patients. The trachea may be significantly narrowed. An endotracheal tube that is smaller than predicted may be appropriate. Tracheal rupture has been reported, possibly due to multiple attempts at laryngoscopy and tracheal intubation (5).

Most patients have clinically significant respiratory muscle weakness, and some have a restrictive lung disease secondary to restricted chest wall mobility and kyphoscoliosis. Patients may have a cardiomyopathy or right ventricular failure secondary to respiratory insufficiency. Succinylcholine should be avoided in patients with skeletal muscle myopathy because of the risk of exaggerated hyperkalemia. Patients must be carefully positioned perioperatively secondary to multiple joint contractures. Patients are at risk for postoperative respiratory complications and may experience postoperative respiratory failure.

Bibliography:

1. Flanigan KM, Kerr L, Bromberg MB, et al. Congenital muscular dystrophy with rigid spine syndrome: a clinical, pathological, radiological, and genetic study. *Ann Neurol* 2000;47:152–161.
2. Jørgensen BG, Laub M, Knudsen RH. Anaesthetic implications of rigid spine syndrome. *Paediatr Anaesth* 1999;9:352–355.
3. Kitayama M, Ohtomo N, Sakai T, et al. Airway management and rigid spine syndrome. *Anesth Analg* 1997;84:690–691.
4. Ras GJ, van Staden M, Schultz C, et al. Respiratory manifestations of rigid spine syndrome. *Am J Respir Crit Care Med* 1994;150:540–546.
5. Bein T, Lenhart FP, Berger H, et al. Rupture of the trachea during difficult intubation. *Anaesthetist* 1991;40:456–457.

Riley-Day Syndrome

See Familial dysautonomia

Riley-Smith Syndrome

Synonym: Bannayan-Riley-Ruvalcaba syndrome; Bannayan-Zonana syndrome; Ruvalcaba-Myhre syndrome

MIM #: 153480

This autosomal dominant syndrome is characterized by macrocephaly, intestinal hamartomatous polyps, multiple benign neoplasms, abnormal pigmentation of the penis, and frequently a lipid storage myopathy. It results from a mutation of the gene *PTEN* (for "phosphatase and tensin homologue deleted on chromosome ten"), which is probably a tumor suppressor gene. It has been suggested that the defect is allelic with Cowden disease, with which it has overlapping clinical features (see earlier). Intestinal polyps are often diagnosed in childhood when patients present with intussusception or rectal bleeding. In patients exhibiting myopathy, a deficiency in muscle carnitine has been documented, and carnitine replacement therapy has been beneficial. Malignant transformation has not been found in Riley-Smith syndrome, unlike Cowden syndrome.

HEENT/AIRWAY: Macrocephaly, scaphocephaly. Hypertelorism, down-slanting palpebral fissures, strabismus. High-arched palate. Occasional tongue polyps.

CHEST: May have pectus excavatum.

NEUROMUSCULAR: Mild mental retardation, gross motor delay, and speech delay are common. May have pseudopapilledema. Most patients have a lipid storage myopathy, primarily involving the proximal muscles. Hypotonia. Intracranial hemangiomas may bleed. Seizures, particularly in those with intracranial bleeds.

ORTHOPEDIC: Scoliosis. May exhibit joint hypermobility.

GI/GU: Ileal and colonic hamartomatous polyps. Nonelevated pigmentary penile lesions.

OTHER: Subcutaneous, cranial, or osseous neoplasms—usually lipomas, occasionally hemangiomas. Diabetes mellitus and Hashimoto thyroiditis have been reported. May have supernumerary nipples.

ANESTHETIC CONSIDERATIONS

Patients with a significant myopathy probably should not receive succinylcholine secondary to the risk of hyperkalemia. Chronic use of anticonvulsant medications may affect the metabolism of some anesthetic drugs. Care should be taken with the perioperative positioning of patients with hyperextensible joints.

Bibliography:
1. Shimpuku G, Fujimoto K, Okazaki K. A case of Bannayan-Zonana syndrome [Japanese]. *Masui* 2005;54:535–537.
2. Schreibman IR, Baker M, Amos C, et al. The hamartomatous polyposis syndromes: a clinical and molecular review. *Am J Gastroenterol* 2005;100:476–490.
3. Merg A, Howe JR. Genetic conditions associated with intestinal juvenile polyps. *Am J Med Genet C Semin Med Genet* 2004;129:44–55.
4. Corredor J, Wambach J, Barnard J. Gastrointestinal polyps in children: advances in molecular genetics, diagnosis and management. *J Pediatr* 2001;138:621–628.

Roberts Syndrome

See Pseudothalidomide syndrome

Robin Sequence

See Pierre Robin syndrome

Robinow Syndrome

Synonym: Fetal face syndrome

MIM #: 180700, 268310

A type of mesomelic dysplasia, this usually autosomal dominant disorder has as its main features short stature, flat facies ("fetal face"), short forearms, and hypoplastic genitalia. This syndrome is etiologically heterogeneous. An autosomal recessive form has been shown to be caused by mutations in the gene *ROR2*, a receptor tyrosine kinase. The autosomal recessive form tends to be more severe than the autosomal dominant form.

HEENT/AIRWAY: Macrocephaly, frontal bossing, large anterior fontanelle. Flat facies, depressed nasal bridge. Hypertelorism, prominent eyes, down-slanting palpebral fissures. Posteriorly rotated ears. Small, upturned nose, long philtrum. Triangular shaped mouth, malaligned teeth. May have cleft lip or palate. Ankyloglossia (adhesion of the tongue to the palate). Micrognathia.

CHEST: Rib anomalies. May have pectus excavatum.

CARDIOVASCULAR: Congenital cardiac defect, particularly right ventricular outlet obstruction.

NEUROMUSCULAR: Normal intelligence in most. Occasional mental retardation or developmental delay. May have seizures.

ORTHOPEDIC: Mild short stature. Short forearms. Clinodactyly. Nail dysplasia. May have congenital hip dislocation. Hemivertebrae, especially thoracic. Scoliosis.

GI/GU: Hypoplastic genitalia—cryptorchidism, small penis, hypoplastic labia majora, small clitoris. May have vaginal atresia. Primary hypogonadism, although women may have normal fertility. May have renal anomalies. May have inguinal hernias.

OTHER: May have growth hormone deficiency. Low testosterone levels in boys. Impaired hypothalamic-pituitary axis or hormonal response of ovaries in girls.

ANESTHETIC CONSIDERATIONS

Micrognathia may make laryngoscopy and tracheal intubation more difficult, although this has not been encountered in the small number of patients whose anesthetic course has been reported. Patients with cardiac defects require perioperative antibiotic prophylaxis as indicated. Impairment of pulmonary function by scoliosis has not yet been reported in this syndrome.

Bibliography:

1. Tufan F, Cefle K, Turkmen S, et al. Clinical and molecular characterization of two adults with autosomal recessive Robinow syndrome. *Am J Med Genet A* 2005;136:185–189.
2. Lirk P, Rieder J, Schuerholz A, et al. Anaesthetic implications of Robinow syndrome. *Paediatr Anaesth* 2003;13:725–727.
3. Sleesman JB, Tobias JD. Anaesthetic implications of the child with Robinow syndrome. *Paediatr Anaesth* 2003;13:629–632.
4. Patton MA, Afzal AR. Robinow syndrome. *J Med Genet* 2002;39: 305–310.
5. MacDonald I, Dearlove OR. Anaesthesia and Robinow syndrome [Letter]. *Anaesthesia* 1995;50:1097.
6. Berkowitz I, Raja S, Bender K, et al. Dwarfs: pathophysiology and anesthetic implications. *Anesthesiology* 1990;73:739–759.

Rokitansky Malformation Sequence

See Rokitansky-Kuster-Hauser syndrome

Rokitansky-Kuster-Hauser Syndrome

SYNONYM: Mayer-Rokitansky-Kuster syndrome; Rokitansky malformation sequence

MIM #: 277000

This disorder involves hypoplasia or absence of the vagina and a rudimentary, usually bicornuate, uterus. The lower vagina, derived from the urogenital sinus, is normal, but ends blindly. The fallopian tubes and ovaries are normal. Endocrinologic function is normal. Secondary sexual characteristics are normal. There is primary amenorrhea. It is caused by a mutation in the gene *WNT4*. Most cases are sporadic, but there are some instances of familial occurrence. The Rokitansky-Kuster-Hauser syndrome may be a part of another malformation sequence, such as the MURCS association (see earlier).

CARDIOVASCULAR: One report of associated pulmonary stenosis.

ORTHOPEDIC: One report of associated scoliosis.

ANESTHETIC CONSIDERATIONS

There are no specific anesthetic concerns other than exhibiting sensitivity towards young girls having gynecologic procedures.

Bibliography:

1. Pittock ST, Babovic-Vuksanovic D, Lteif A. Mayer-Rokitansky-Kuster-Hauser anomaly and its associated malformations. *Am J Med Genet A* 2005;135:314–316.
2. Kula S, Saygili A, Tunaoglu FS, et al. Mayer-Rokitansky-Kuster-Hauser syndrome associated with pulmonary stenosis. *Acta Paediatr* 2004;93:570–572.
3. Fisher K, Esham RH, Thorneycroft I. Scoliosis associated with typical Mayer-Rokitansky-Kuster-Hauser syndrome. *South Med J* 2000;93: 243–246.

Romano-Ward Syndrome

Included in Long QT syndrome

Romberg Disease

SYNONYM: Parry-Romberg disease

MIM #: 141300

This syndrome of uncertain etiology is characterized by progressive atrophy of the soft tissue and bone on one side of the face, trigeminal neuralgia, changes of the hair and skin, and Jacksonian seizures that occur contralateral to the facial changes. It has been suggested that this syndrome may represent focal scleroderma. Immunosuppressive agents may be beneficial.

HEENT/AIRWAY: Slowly progressive atrophy of the soft tissue on one side of the face. There may be atrophy of the underlying facial bones. Heterochromia. Enophthalmos. Hemiatrophy of the tongue. Delayed eruption of the teeth, malocclusion.

NEUROMUSCULAR: Trigeminal neuralgia. Jacksonian seizures, which occur contralateral to the facial changes. Migraine-like headaches.

OTHER: Hyperpigmentation, vitiligo. Alopecia, hair color changes.

MISCELLANEOUS: Romberg was the world's first clinical neurologist, having been appointed lecturer in neurology at the University of Berlin in 1834. He is also the Romberg of Romberg's sign, an indicator of posterior column dysfunction.

ANESTHETIC CONSIDERATIONS

Although there is facial asymmetry, the ease of laryngoscopy and tracheal intubation should not be affected. Chronic use

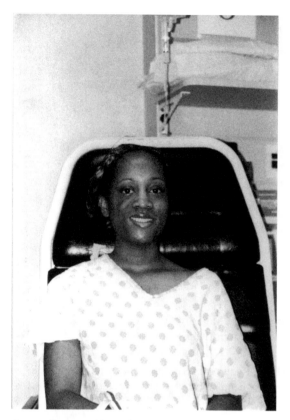

Romberg disease. Note the asymmetric facial hypoplasia in this 17-year-old girl admitted for plastic surgery.

of anticonvulsant medications may affect the metabolism of some anesthetic drugs.

Bibliography:

1. Anderson PJ, Molony D, Haan E, et al. Familial Parry-Romberg disease. *Int J Pediatr Otorhinolaryngol* 2005;69:705–708.
2. Korkmaz C, Adapinar B, Uysal S. Beneficial effect of immunosuppressive drugs on Parry-Romberg syndrome: a case report and review of the literature. *South Med J* 2005;98:940–942.
3. Blaszczyk M, Krolicki L, Krasu M, et al. Progressive facial hemiatrophy: central nervous system involvement and relationship with scleroderma en coup de sabre. *J Rheumatol* 2003;30:1997–2004.
4. Stone J. Parry-Romberg syndrome: a global survey of 205 patients using the Internet. *Neurology* 2003;61:674–676.

Rothmund-Thomson Syndrome

SYNONYM: Poikiloderma congenitale syndrome

MIM #: 268400

This autosomal recessive disorder is characterized by poikiloderma, cataracts, and possibly other ectodermal dysplasias. There is wide variability in the clinical expression. At least some cases are caused by mutations in the DNA helicase gene *RECQL4*, leading to defective repair of DNA.

HEENT/AIRWAY: Microcephaly. Juvenile cataracts, corneal dystrophy. Saddle nose. Dental abnormalities include microdontia, hypodontia, ectopic eruption, dental caries. Prognathism.

NEUROMUSCULAR: May have mental retardation.

ORTHOPEDIC: Proportionate short stature. May have small hands and feet, hypoplastic to absent thumbs, syndactyly, forearm reduction defects. May have absent patella, clubfoot deformity. Osteoporosis. Development of osteosarcomas has been described in a number of patients.

GI/GU: Hypogonadism, cryptorchidism. May have anteriorly placed anus, annular pancreas.

OTHER: There are many skin changes including irregular erythema progressing to poikiloderma (telangiectasis, scarring, irregular pigmentation and depigmentation, atrophic dermatitis), most marked in sun-exposed areas. Anhydrosis. Hyperkeratotic lesions may be verrucous. Photosensitivity, sparse hair or progressive alopecia, prematurely gray. Dysplastic nails. Anemia.

MISCELLANEOUS: August von Rothmund was a 19th-century, Bulgarian-born German ophthalmologist. Matthew Thomson, a British dermatologist, reported a similar disorder 55 years later.

ANESTHETIC CONSIDERATIONS
When meeting patients preoperatively, recall that they may have loss of vision. If anemia is suspected, a preoperative hematocrit should be obtained. Dental abnormalities should be documented preoperatively. Patients may become hyperthermic perioperatively secondary to hypohidrosis or anhydrosis. Vascular access may be challenging secondary to skin changes and small hands and feet. These patients must be carefully positioned and padded secondary to atrophic changes in the skin.

Bibliography:

1. Wang LL, Levy ML, Lewis RA, et al. Clinical manifestations in a cohort of 41 Rothmund-Thomson syndrome patients. *Am J Med Genet* 2001;102:11–17.
2. Pujol LA, Erickson RP, Heidenreich RA, et al. Variable presentation of Rothmund-Thomson syndrome. *Am J Med Genet* 2000;95:204–207.

Rotor Syndrome

MIM #: 237450

This autosomal recessive disease leads to conjugated hyperbilirubinemia. Clinically it is very similar to the Dubin-Johnson syndrome (see earlier). The gene and gene product responsible for the disorder are unknown. The disease is benign, with an unaltered life expectancy. Other diseases of hepatic bilirubin metabolism include Crigler-Najjar and Gilbert syndromes (see earlier).

GI/GU: Intermittent jaundice. Routine liver function tests are negative. The absence of abnormal hepatic pigmentation is one way to differentiate this disorder from Dubin-Johnson syndrome.

MISCELLANEOUS: Rotor was an orchid breeder. In addition to having a syndrome named after him he also has an orchid named after him (Vanda merrillii var. rotorii).

ANESTHETIC CONSIDERATIONS
These patients are asymptomatic and there are no specific anesthetic considerations. Some drugs, the most common being rifampin, cause enzyme inhibition with increased serum bilirubin levels and jaundice. Although sulfonamides, some cephalosporins, and intravenous contrast agents can increase free bilirubin levels by displacing bilirubin from albumin, no currently used anesthetic agents are known to displace bilirubin to a degree that would contraindicate their use. The stress of surgery or a perioperative infection may exacerbate the hyperbilirubinemia.

Bibliography:
1. Cichoz-Lach H, Celinski K, Slomka M. Congenital nonhemolytic hyper-bilirubinemias. *Ann Univ Mariae Curie Sklodowska* 2004;59:449–452.
2. Teh CP, Nevard CH, Lawson N. Clinical quiz. Dubin-Johnson syndrome or Rotor syndrome. *Pediatr Nephrol* 1999;13:627–628.

Rubella

See Fetal rubella syndrome

Rubinstein-Taybi Syndrome

MIM #: 180849

This autosomal dominant disorder is characterized by mental retardation, broad thumbs and first toes, and craniofacial abnormalities. There is significant variation in the clinical presentation. Rubinstein-Taybi syndrome can be caused by a defect in the gene encoding the CREB binding protein, a transcriptional coactivator that is involved in the cyclic adenosine monophosphate mediated induction of intracellular protein synthesis. Production of this coactivator is stimulated by protein kinase A. There is genetic heterogeneity, however, as the disease can also be caused by a mutation in the gene *EP300*.

HEENT/AIRWAY: Microcephaly. Prominent forehead. May have large anterior fontanelle with delayed closure of the fontanelle. Apparent hypertelorism. Thick, arched eyebrows. Nasolacrimal duct stenosis, downward-slanting palpebral fissures, ptosis, glaucoma, strabismus, iris coloboma. Low-set or malformed external ears. Hypoplastic maxilla, broad nasal bridge. Beaked nose, deviated nasal septum. May have choanal atresia. Short upper lip and pouting lower lip. Microstomia. High-arched palate. Dental crowding.

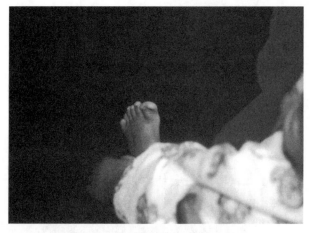

Rubinstein-Taybi syndrome. **FIG. 1.** Typical broad first toe and polydactyly of a 12-month-old child with Rubinstein-Taybi syndrome. His thumbs were equally broad.

Micrognathia. May have easily collapsible larynx. One report of congenital tracheal stenosis (1).

CHEST: Recurrent respiratory infections. Obstructive sleep apnea has been reported. May have sternal anomalies, pectus excavatum.

CARDIOVASCULAR: Approximately one-third have congenital cardiac defects of a variety of acyanotic types. One patient has been reported with Wolff-Parkinson-White syndrome (see later).

NEUROMUSCULAR: Moderate to severe mental and motor retardation. Speech delay. Hypotonia. Stiff, unsteady gait. May have seizures, hyperreflexia. Large foramen magnum, agenesis of the corpus callosum.

ORTHOPEDIC: Short stature. Broad thumbs and first toes. Clinodactyly of the fifth finger. Flaring of the ilia, slipped capital femoral epiphyses, flat feet. Scoliosis, cervical kyphosis. Stiff gait. Spina bifida occulta. Retarded osseous maturation.

GI/GU: Constipation. Cryptorchidism, shawl scrotum, hypospadias. Occasional renal anomaly.

OTHER: Feeding difficulties. Postnatal growth deficiency. Hirsutism. Premature telarche. Asthma and other allergic manifestations are common.

MISCELLANEOUS: Dr. Rubinstein and Dr. Taybi did not know each other while independently preparing to publish a report of this syndrome. A third physician known to both of them realized that the descriptive features in their case reports were the same. Rubinstein and Taybi then jointly published the first paper on this syndrome.

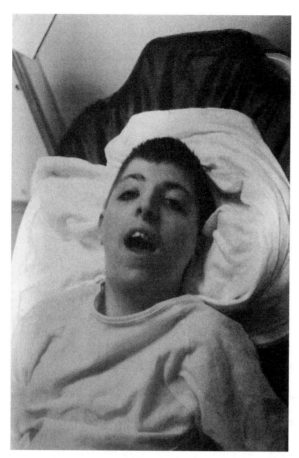

Rubinstein-Taybi syndrome. FIG. 2. This 16-year-old with Rubinstein-Taybi syndrome has had obstructive sleep apnea and delayed emergence from several anesthetics, including desflurane.

ANESTHETIC CONSIDERATIONS

Craniofacial abnormalities may make direct laryngoscopy and tracheal intubation difficult (6, 7). Hyperkyphosis may affect patient positioning, particularly at induction. Choanal atresia, if present, precludes the use of a nasal airway or placement of a nasogastric tube. The high incidence of feeding difficulties in these patients suggests that they routinely be considered an aspiration risk (2, 10, 14). Use of a ProSeal laryngeal mask airway in an adult patient has been reported with passage of a gastric tube to decompress the stomach (6). The collapsible larynx may be problematic perioperatively, particularly in the postanesthesia care unit (12). A single patient with Rubinstein-Taybi syndrome has been described in whom arrhythmias developed after succinylcholine and atropine/neostigmine (13, 14). This is likely to have been an isolated case, and has not been reported since (11). Succinylcholine has subsequently been used without incident in a patient with Rubinstein-Taybi syndrome (10). One patient was reported to have had delayed awakening after anesthesia, with both isoflurane and propofol given on separate occasions (9). Postoperatively, there is a risk of apnea, respiratory obstruction, and respiratory failure (5). Patients with congenital heart disease require perioperative antibiotic prophylaxis as indicated.

Bibliography:

1. Magillo P, Della Rocca M, Campus R, et al. Images in anesthesia: congenital tracheal stenosis in a boy with Rubinstein-Taybi syndrome. *Can J Anaesth* 2005;52:990–991.
2. Altintas F, Cakmakkaya S. Anesthetic management of a child with Rubinstein-Taybi syndrome. *Paediatr Anaesth* 2004;14:610–611.
3. Dearlove OR, Perkins R. Anaesthesia in an adult with Rubinstein-Taybi syndrome [Letter]. *Br J Anaesth* 2003;90:399–400.
4. Wiley S, Swayne S, Rubinstein JH, et al. Rubinstein-Taybi syndrome medical guidelines. *Am J Med Genet A* 2003;119:101–110.
5. Tokarz A, Gaszynski T, Gaszynski W, et al. General anaesthesia for a child with Rubinstein-Taybi syndrome. *Eur J Anaesthesiol* 2002;19:896–897.
6. Twigg SJ, Cook TM. Anaesthesia in an adult with Rubinstein-Taybi syndrome using the ProSeal laryngeal mask airway. *Br J Anaesth* 2002;89:786–787.
7. Bozkirli F, Gunaydin B, Celebi H, et al. Anesthetic management of a child with Rubinstein-Taybi syndrome for cervical dermoid cyst excision. *J Anesth* 2000;14:214–215.
8. Isayama S, Nakayama R, Sakamoto M, et al. General anesthesia for an infant with Rubinstein-Taybi syndrome [Japanese]. *Masui* 1997;46:1094–1096.
9. Dunkley CJA, Dearlove OR. Delayed recovery from anaesthesia in Rubinstein-Taybi syndrome [Letter]. *Paediatr Anaesth* 1996;6:245–246.
10. Critchley LAH, Gin T, Stuart JC. Anaesthesia in an infant with Rubinstein-Taybi syndrome. *Anaesthesia* 1995;50:37–38.
11. Baer GA, Lempinen J, Oikkonen M. No complications during anesthesia in patients with Rubinstein-Taybi syndrome [Letter]. *Paediatr Anaesth* 1994;4:272–273.
12. Hennekam RCM, Van Doorne JM. Oral aspects of Rubinstein-Taybi syndrome. *Am J Med Genet Suppl* 1990;6:42–47.
13. Stirt JA. Succinylcholine in Rubinstein-Taybi syndrome [Letter]. *Anesthesiology* 1982;57:429.
14. Stirt JA. Anesthetic problems in Rubinstein-Taybi syndrome. *Anesth Analg* 1981;60:534–536.

Russell-Silver Dwarf

See Russell-Silver syndrome

Russell-Silver Syndrome

SYNONYM: Russell-Silver dwarf

MIM #: 180860

This syndrome is characterized by short stature of prenatal onset, triangular facies, skeletal asymmetry, and clinodactyly of the fifth finger. Most cases have been sporadic, and inheritance pattern is uncertain. The specific gene and gene product are unknown, but a gene for this syndrome may reside on the short arm of chromosome 7. There is likely more than one genetic defect that can cause this syndrome (genetic heterogeneity).

HEENT/AIRWAY: Late closure of the anterior fontanelle. The head appears large in relation to the face, which is small and triangular, and to the body, which is also small ("pseudohydrocephalus"). Head circumference is actually in

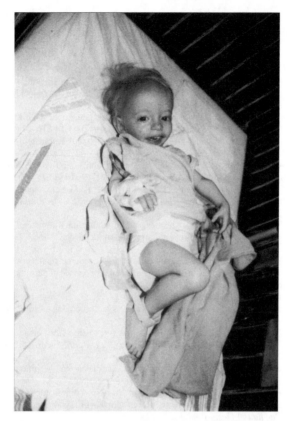

Russell-Silver syndrome. FIG. 1. A 7 kg, 2-year-old boy with Russell-Silver syndrome. Note the wide forehead and narrow mandible. He had chronic problems with hypoglycemia and received 10% dextrose perioperatively. His trachea was difficult to intubate. At another hospital, after a prior surgery, he crawled out of bed and fell to the floor in the postanesthesia care unit. The staff had been misled by his small size and had assumed he was too young to crawl.

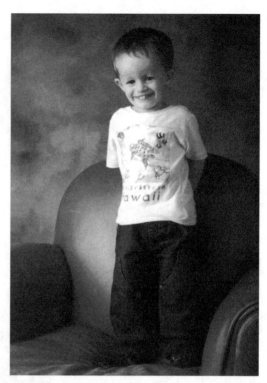

Russell-Silver syndrome. FIG. 2. An older boy with Russell-Silver syndrome. Note that the head is disproportionately large in comparison to the face.

the normal range. The sclerae may be bluish in early infancy. Micrognathia.

NEUROMUSCULAR: Intelligence is usually normal. Occasional developmental delay. Infants tend to be weak.

ORTHOPEDIC: Short stature; children improve in weight and height throughout childhood and adolescence. May have scoliosis. Skeletal asymmetry, particularly of the limbs. Hemihypertrophy. May have congenital hip dysplasia. Camptodactyly. Clinodactyly of the fifth finger.

GI/GU: Gastroesophageal reflux, esophagitis. Cryptorchidism. Precocious sexual development. May have hypospadias, posterior urethral valves, renal anomalies. May have inguinal hernia.

OTHER: Small for gestational age. Feeding problems. Occasional growth hormone deficiency. Café au lait spots. Excessive sweating during infancy. Elevated urinary gonadotrophins. Risk of fasting hypoglycemia from

approximately 10 months until 2 to 3 years of age. May be associated with a variety of cancers, including testicular seminoma, hepatocellular carcinoma, Wilms tumor, and craniopharyngioma.

MISCELLANEOUS: Henry Silver was a leading figure in American pediatrics. He was the Chair of Pediatrics at the University of Colorado and was one of the first to describe the battered child syndrome. He was also a leading early proponent of nurse practitioners.

ANESTHETIC CONSIDERATIONS
Recall that despite the child-size stature, these patients have intelligence that is normal for their chronologic age. Direct laryngoscopy and tracheal intubation may be difficult secondary to facial deformities and micrognathia. Obtaining a good mask seal may be difficult secondary to facial asymmetry. Because of their extremely small size, patients may require an endotracheal tube that is smaller than predicted by age. There is a high incidence of gastroesophageal reflux, and patients may be at risk for perioperative aspiration (2). These patients often exhibit fasting hypoglycemia, particularly during the toddler years (1). Extended perioperative fasting must be avoided. Intravenous glucose-containing fluids should be used and serum glucose levels monitored perioperatively in all patients, not just those with a history of hypoglycemia (3). If drug doses are calculated on a per-kilogram basis, the increased surface area-to-weight ratio in these patients may

result in underdosing. The absence of significant fat stores may allow for more rapid awakening after the use of volatile anesthetics. Poor insulation from inadequate subcutaneous fat, high surface-to-mass ratio, and a relatively large head all contribute to the development of intraoperative hypothermia.

Bibliography:
1. Azcona C, Stanhope R. Hypoglycaemia and Russell-Silver syndrome. *J Pediatr Endocrinol* 2005;18:663–670.
2. Anderson J, Viskochil D, O'Gorman M, et al. Gastrointestinal complications of Russell-Silver syndrome: a pilot study. *Am J Med Genet* 2002;113:15–19.
3. Tomiyama H, Ibuki T, Nakajima Y, et al. Late intraoperative hypoglycemia in a patient with Russell-Silver syndrome. *J Clin Anesth* 1999;11:80–82.
4. Price SM, Stanhope R, Garrett C, et al. The spectrum of Silver-Russell syndrome: a clinical and molecular genetic study and new diagnostic criteria. *J Med Genet* 1999;36:837–842.
5. Dinner M, Goldin EZ, Ward R, et al. Russell-Silver syndrome: anesthetic implications. *Anesth Analg* 1994;78:1197–1199.

Ruvalcaba Syndrome

Note: This disorder is distinct from Ruvalcaba-Myhre syndrome/Bannayan-Riley-Ruvalcaba syndrome (see earlier, Riley-Smith syndrome).

MIM #: 180870

Ruvalcaba syndrome is an autosomal dominant disorder with neurologic and facial manifestations. The responsible gene and gene product are not known.

HEENT/AIRWAY: Microcephaly. Oval face, high forehead. Upward-slanting palpebral fissures. Hooked nose. Small mouth.

CHEST: Narrow thoracic cage. Pectus carinatum.

NEUROMUSCULAR: Mental retardation. Congenital hydrocephalus. Dandy-Walker malformation.

ORTHOPEDIC: Short stature. Short metatarsals and metacarpals, proximally displaced thumbs, clinodactyly. Small feet.

GI/GU: Hiatal hernia with gastroesophageal reflux has been reported. Renal abnormalities.

OTHER: Hypoplastic skin lesions.

ANESTHETIC CONSIDERATIONS
Laryngoscopy may be difficult in patients with a small mouth. Patients with a hiatal hernia or gastroesophageal reflux are at increased risk for perioperative aspiration, and consideration should be given to a rapid-sequence anesthetic induction and intubation.

Bibliography:
1. Bialer MG, Wilson WG, Kelly TE. Apparent Ruvalcaba syndrome with genitourinary abnormalities. *Am J Med Genet* 1989;33:314–317.

2. Bianchi E, Livieri C, Arico M, et al. Ruvalcaba syndrome: a case report. *Eur J Pediatr* 1984;142:301–303.

Ruvalcaba-Myhre Syndrome

See Riley-Smith syndrome

S

Sacral Agenesis

See Caudal regression syndrome

Saethre-Chotzen Syndrome

SYNONYM: Acrocephalosyndactyly type III

MIM #: 101400

This autosomal dominant disorder, one of the acrocephalosyndactyly syndromes, is characterized by brachycephaly, maxillary hypoplasia, and syndactyly. There is wide variability in clinical expression. There is some evidence for genetic heterogeneity. Most cases are due to a defect in the *TWIST* gene. The product of the *TWIST* gene is a transcription factor.

HEENT/AIRWAY: Craniosynostosis of one or more sutures, brachycephaly, plagiocephaly. Maxillary hypoplasia. Late closure of fontanelles, ossification defects and hyperostosis of the skull. Facial asymmetry, low frontal hairline. Shallow orbits with orbital asymmetry, ptosis, strabismus. Prominent crus across external ear. May have sensorineural hearing loss. Long, thin, pointed nose, deviated nasal septum. Narrow palate, cleft palate. Facial appearance tends to improve with age through childhood.

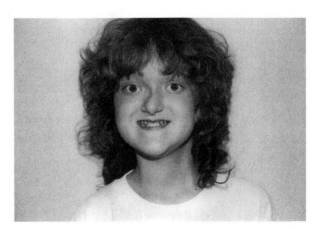

Saethre-Chotzen syndrome. **FIG. 1.** This young girl with Saethre-Chotzen syndrome was scheduled for Laforte III midface advancement surgery.

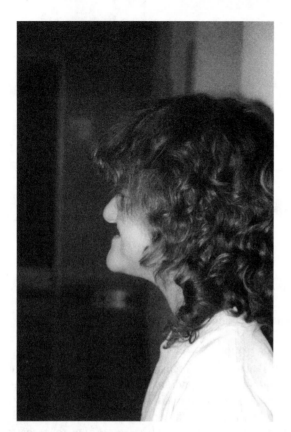

Saethre-Chotzen syndrome. FIG. 2. Lateral view of the girl in figure 1.

CHEST: Short clavicles.

NEUROMUSCULAR: Intelligence is usually normal, may have some developmental delay. Rarely, craniosynostosis causes increased intracranial pressure, leading to mental deterioration. May have seizures.

ORTHOPEDIC: Occasional small stature. Cutaneous syndactyly. Small distal phalanges, clinodactyly of fifth finger, digitalization of thumbs, limited elbow extension. Broad great toes with valgus deformity. Contractures of elbows and knees. May have cervical vertebral fusion, which may be progressive throughout childhood.

GI/GU: May have cryptorchidism. Occasional renal anomalies. Occasional anorectal malformation.

MISCELLANEOUS: Mice with mutations in the *TWIST* gene have skull and limb abnormalities similar to those of Saethre-Chotzen syndrome. Saethre was a Norwegian psychiatrist. The first patient he saw with this syndrome was referred to him for schizophrenia.

ANESTHETIC CONSIDERATIONS
Unlike the other acrocephalosyndactyly syndromes, Saethre-Chotzen syndrome does not involve craniofacial features that are likely to increase the difficulty of direct laryngoscopy and

tracheal intubation, although significant cervical vertebral fusion might make laryngoscopy and tracheal intubation more difficult. Patients may have elevated intracranial pressure, in which case precautions should be taken to avoid further elevations in pressure. Excessive premedication and intraoperative hypoventilation may exacerbate preexisting increases in intracranial pressure. Clavicular anomalies may make placement of a subclavian venous catheter more difficult. Patients must be carefully positioned secondary to contractures.

Bibliography:
1. Dollfus H, Biswas P, Kumaramanickavel G, et al. Saethre-Chotzen syndrome: notable intrafamilial phenotypic variability in a large family with Q28X TWIST mutation. *Am J Med Genet* 2002;109:218–225.
2. Clauser L, Galie M, Hassanipour A, et al. Saethre-Chotzen syndrome: review of the literature and report of a case. *J Craniofac Surg* 2000;11:480–486.
3. Perkins JA, Sie KC, Milczuk H, et al. Airway management in children with craniofacial anomalies. *Cleft Palate Craniofac J* 1997;34:135–140.
4. Anderson PJ, Hall CM, Evans RD, et al. The cervical spine in Saethre-Chotzen syndrome. *Cleft Palate Craniofac J* 1997;34:79–82.

Saldino-Noonan Type Short Rib-Polydactyly Syndrome

See Short rib-polydactyly syndrome

Sandhoff Disease

SYNONYM: GM$_2$ gangliosidosis, type II

MIM #: 268800

This autosomal recessive disease with multiple alleles is due to abnormal accumulation of GM$_2$ ganglioside in neural tissue. Tay-Sachs disease (see later) is also due to accumulation of GM$_2$ ganglioside. Gangliosides are components of the outer cell membrane. They have a hydrophobic ceramide moiety anchoring them in the cell membrane, and a hydrophilic oligosaccharide chain extending into the extracellular space. Although their function is unknown, they have been implicated as binding sites for a variety of viruses, bacterial toxins, growth factors, and interferons. Defects may occur in the alpha subunit of hexosaminidase (Tay-Sachs disease, deficient hexosaminidase A isoenzyme, see later) or the beta subunit of hexosaminidase (Sandhoff disease, deficient hexosaminidase A and B), or there may be a defect in the GM$_2$ activator protein (both isoenzymes are present, but hexosaminidase A is nonfunctional). The clinical presentation of Sandhoff disease is generally similar to that of the biochemically related Tay-Sachs disease. The presence of hepatosplenomegaly in Sandhoff disease differentiates the two. Autonomic dysfunction is a prominent clinical manifestation.

HEENT/AIRWAY: Macrocephaly. Coarse facies. Cherry-red spot in the macular area, blindness. Macroglossia. Dysarthria.

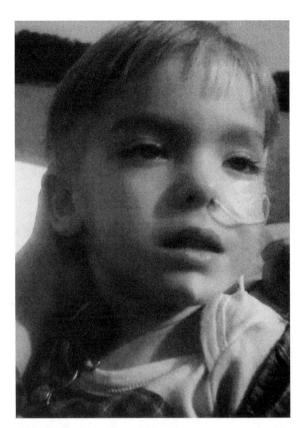

Sandhoff disease. A young boy with Sandhoff disease. Note the need for head support.

CARDIOVASCULAR: Cardiomegaly. Orthostatic hypotension.

NEUROMUSCULAR: Progressive mental and motor deterioration. Autonomic dysfunction. Cerebellar ataxia, pyramidal tract signs, hyperreflexia with exaggerated startle reflex. Muscle weakness and muscle wasting with fasciculations.

ORTHOPEDIC: High lumbar gibbus deformity.

GI/GU: Hepatosplenomegaly, recurrent abdominal pain, chronic diarrhea. Impotence, mild urinary incontinence.

OTHER: Impaired sweating.

ANESTHETIC CONSIDERATIONS
Direct laryngoscopy and tracheal intubation may be more difficult secondary to macroglossia. Perioperative intravascular volume should be optimally maintained secondary to autonomic dysfunction and the possibility of orthostatic hypotension. Similarly, patients should ambulate carefully postoperatively because of the risk of postural hypotension. Widespread autonomic dysfunction may affect perioperative cardiovascular stability and temperature regulation. Succinylcholine is contraindicated in patients with significant muscle wasting because of the risk of hyperkalemia.

Bibliography:
1. Hendriksz CJ, Corry PC, Wraith JE, et al. Juvenile Sandhoff disease—nine new cases and a review of the literature. *J Inherit Metab Dis* 2004;27:241–249.
2. Tay SK, Low PS, Ong HT, et al. Sandhoff disease—a case report of 3 siblings and a review of potential therapies. *Ann Acad Med Singapore* 2000;29:514–517.
3. Modigliani R, Lemann M, Melancon SB, et al. Diarrhea and autonomic dysfunction in a patient with hexosaminidase B deficiency (Sandhoff disease). *Gastroenterology* 1994;106:775–781.

Sandifer Syndrome

MIM #: None

This disorder describes the paroxysmal dystonic posturing in children that is caused by gastroesophageal reflux. The posturing resolves completely after resolution of the reflux.

HEENT/AIRWAY: Episodic extension and lateral deviation of the head.

GI/GU: Gastroesophageal reflux. Hiatal hernia should be strongly suspected. May have delayed gastric emptying.

ANESTHETIC CONSIDERATIONS
By definition, these patients have gastroesophageal reflux. They also often have delayed gastric emptying. A rapid-sequence induction with tracheal intubtion is indicated. These episodes can look superficially like seizures, and must be differentiated from true seizures.

Bibliography:
1. Somjit S, Lee Y, Berkovic SF, et al. Sandifer syndrome misdiagnosed as refractory partial seizures in an adult. *Epileptic Disord* 2004;6:49–50.
2. Kotagal P, Costa M, Wyllie E, et al. Paroxysmal nonepileptic events in children and adolescents. *Pediatrics* 2002;110:e46.
3. Cardi E, Corrado G, Cavaliere M, et al. Delayed gastric emptying in an infant with Sandifer syndrome. *Ital J Gastroenterol* 1996;28:518–519.
4. Gorrotxategi P, Reguilon MJ, Arana J, et al. Gastroesophageal reflux in association with the Sandifer syndrome. *Eur J Pediatr Surg* 1995;5:203–205.

Sanfilippo Syndrome

SYNONYM: Mucopolysaccharidosis III

MIM #: 252900, 252920, 252930, 252940

There are four biochemically distinct forms of Sanfilippo syndrome, all autosomal recessive, which are essentially indistinguishable clinically. They are all associated with the accumulation of heparan sulfate. Type A involves a defect in *N*-sulfoglucosamine sulfohydrolase, type B involves a defect in alpha-*N*-acetylglucosaminidase, type C involves a defect in alpha-glucosaminide *N*-acetyltransferase, and type D involves a defect in *N*-acetylglucosamine-6-sulfatase. Compared with the other mucopolysaccharidoses, Sanfilippo syndrome has relatively severe central nervous system involvement and relatively mild systemic organ involvement. Typically, progressive neurodegeneration occurs over the

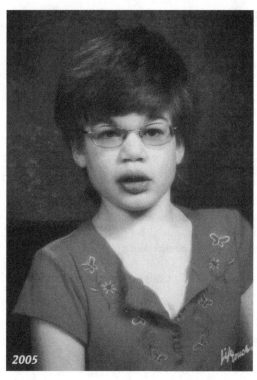

2005

Sanfilippo syndrome. Fourth grade school photo of a 10-year-old girl with Sanfilippo syndrome.

first decade of life, with death following shortly thereafter, although some patients experience a more benign clinical course.

HEENT/AIRWAY: Thickened skull. Mild coarsening of facies. Corneas are clear. Hearing loss. Poor speech.

CHEST: Patients with mucopolysaccharidoses are susceptible to pulmonary hemorrhage after bone marrow transplantation.

CARDIOVASCULAR: Cardiac involvement is rare, but mitral insufficiency requiring surgical valvuloplasty has been reported.

NEUROMUSCULAR: Severe mental retardation. Behavioral problems including hyperactivity. Patients may be aggressive and destructive. May have ventricular enlargement. May have seizures.

ORTHOPEDIC: Usually have normal stature, occasional short stature. Claw-hand deformity. Stiff joints. May have osteoporosis.

GI/GU: Mild hepatosplenomegaly in children, but not in adolescents or adults. Recurrent diarrhea in childhood. Umbilical and inguinal hernias.

OTHER: Sleep disturbances. Hypertrichosis.

ANESTHETIC CONSIDERATIONS

Preoperative management can be challenging in patients with severe behavioral problems, particularly because they have normal strength. Difficult intubations may develop with increasing age (13), although the incidence and severity are much less than with other mucopolysaccharidoses (4). The laryngeal mask airway has been used successfully in patients with mucopolysaccharidoses (3). Patients must be carefully positioned intraoperatively secondary to stiff joints. Treatment with anticonvulsant medications may affect the metabolism of some anesthetic drugs.

Bibliography:

1. Ingrosso M, Picilli MM, Capasso A, et al. Anaesthetic problems in Sanfilippo syndrome. A rare case of adult patient. *Minerva Anestesiol* 2003;69:641–645.
2. Yogalingam G, Hopwood JJ. Molecular genetics of mucopolysaccharidosis type IIIA and IIIB: Diagnostic, clinical, and biological implications. *Hum Mutat* 2001;18:264–281.
3. Walker RWM, Allen DL, Rothera MR. A fibreoptic intubation technique for children with mucopolysaccharidoses using the laryngeal mask airway. *Paediatr Anaesth* 1997;7:421–426.
4. Moores C, Rogers JG, McKenzie IM, et al. Anaesthesia for children with mucopolysaccharidoses. *Anaesth Intensive Care* 1996;24:459–463.
5. Walker RWM, Darowski M, Morris P. Anaesthesia and mucopolysaccharidoses. A review of airway problems in children. *Anaesthesia* 1994;49:1078–1084.
6. Diaz JH, Belani K. Perioperative management of children with mucopolysaccharidoses. *Anesth Analg* 1993;77:1261–1270.
7. Mahoney A, Soni N, Vellodi A. Anaesthesia and the mucopolysaccharidoses: a review of patients treated by bone marrow transplantation. *Paediatr Anaesth* 1992;2:317–324.
8. Myles PS, Westhorpe RN. A patient with Sanfilippo syndrome and pseudocholinesterase deficiency, further complicated by post-tonsillectomy haemorrhage. *Anaesth Intensive Care* 1989;17:86–88.
9. Herrick IA, Rhine EJ. The mucopolysaccharidoses and anaesthesia: a report of clinical experience. *Can J Anaesth* 1988;35:67–73.
10. Sjögren P, Pedersen T, Steinmetz H. Mucopolysaccharidoses and anaesthetic risks. *Acta Anaesthesiol Scand* 1987;31:214–218.
11. King DH, Jones RM, Barrett MB. Anaesthetic considerations in the mucopolysaccharidoses. *Anaesthesia* 1984;39:126–131.
12. Baines D, Kenneally J. Anaesthetic management of the mucopolysaccharidoses: a fifteen-year experience in a children's hospital. *Anaesth Intensive Care* 1983;11:198–202.
13. Kempthorne PM, Brown TCK. Anaesthesia and the mucopolysaccharidoses: a survey of techniques and problems. *Anaesth Intensive Care* 1983;11:203–207.

SC Phocomelia Syndrome

See Pseudothalidomide syndrome

SCAD Deficiency

See Short-chain acyl-CoA dehydrogenase deficiency

Scheie Syndrome

SYNONYM: Mucopolysaccharidosis IS

MIM #: 607016

This autosomal recessive disorder is due to an absence of alpha-L-iduronidase, which is involved in the degradation of glycosaminoglycans (mucopolysaccharides). There is accumulation of dermatan sulfate. Different mutations in this same gene are responsible for Hurler syndrome, Scheie syndrome, and the intermediate Hurler-Scheie syndrome. These more correctly represent a spectrum of mucopolysaccharidosis I, with Scheie syndrome being the most benign. Treatment with recombinant human alpha-L-iduronidase can significantly improve some clinical manifestations of the disease, and bone marrow transplantation has provided very good long term results. However, bone marrow transplantation appears to have minimal effects on the progression of skeletal diseases.

HEENT/AIRWAY: Clouding of corneas, glaucoma, myopia. Hearing loss. Broad mouth with full lips. Macroglossia. Prognathism.

CHEST: Obstructive sleep apnea. Patients with mucopolysaccharidoses are susceptible to pulmonary hemorrhage after bone marrow transplantation.

CARDIOVASCULAR: Aortic valve involvement with stenosis or insufficiency. Severe airway obstruction may lead to pulmonary hypertension and cor pulmonale.

NEUROMUSCULAR: Intelligence is normal. Compression of the spinal cord from thickened meninges ("pachymeningitis cervicalis") can occur, but less frequently than in Hurler-Scheie syndrome. Mental deterioration and psychosis may develop.

ORTHOPEDIC: Normal stature. Joint limitation. Short, broad hands and feet. Claw hand, small carpal bones, carpal tunnel syndrome. Trigger thumb. Dysplasia of the femoral head.

GI/GU: Umbilical and inguinal hernias, hepatomegaly.

OTHER: Hirsutism.

MISCELLANEOUS: Harold Scheie was the chair of ophthalmology at the University of Pennsylvania. During WWII, Scheie treated Lord Louis Mountbatten who had injured his eye in a jeep accident. Scheie was able to save Mountbatten's eye, and they remained friends for the rest of their lives.

A deficiency of lysosomal alpha-L-iduronidase also occurs in Plott hound dogs. Treatment with recombinant human alpha-L-iduronidase can significantly improve some clinical manifestations of the disease.

ANESTHETIC CONSIDERATIONS

A case has been reported in the Japanese literature of a 35-year old with Scheie syndrome with normal mouth opening, in whom limited mouth opening developed after induction of anesthesia with fentanyl, thiopental, and vecuronium. The tracheas of patients with Hurler syndrome, which is more severe, may be extremely difficult to intubate successfully (see Hurler syndrome, earlier). The laryngeal mask airway has been used successfully in patients with mucopolysaccharidoses (2).

Patients must be carefully positioned perioperatively because of limitations in joint mobility. Patients with cardiac valve involvement need perioperative antibiotic prophylaxis, as clinically appropriate.

Bibliography:
1. Brooks DA. Alpha-L-iduronidase and enzyme replacement therapy for mucopolysaccharidosis I. *Expert Opin Biol Ther* 2002;2:967–976.
2. Walker RWM, Allen DL, Rothera MR. A fibreoptic intubation technique for children with mucopolysaccharidoses using the laryngeal mask airway. *Paediatr Anaesth* 1997;7:421–426.
3. Moores C, Rogers JG, McKenzie IM, et al. Anaesthesia for children with mucopolysaccharidoses. *Anaesth Intensive Care* 1996;24:459–463.
4. Walker RWM, Darowski M, Morris P. Anaesthesia and mucopolysaccharidoses: a review of airway problems in children. *Anaesthesia* 1994;49:1078–1084.
5. Diaz JH, Belani K. Perioperative management of children with mucopolysaccharidoses. *Anesth Analg* 1993;77:1261–1270.
6. Mahoney A, Soni N, Vellodi A. Anaesthesia and the mucopolysaccharidoses: a review of patients treated by bone marrow transplantation. *Paediatr Anaesth* 1992;2:317–324.
7. Steven IM. Domiciliary use of nasopharyngeal intubation for obstructive sleep apnoea in a child with mucopolysaccharidosis. *Anaesth Intensive Care* 1988;16:493–494.
8. Sjogren P, Pedersen T, Steinmetz H. Mucopolysaccharidoses and anaesthetic risks. *Acta Anaesthesiol Scand* 1987;31:214–218.
9. King DH, Jones RM, Barrett MB. Anaesthetic considerations in the mucopolysaccharidoses. *Anaesthesia* 1984;39:126–131.
10. Baines D, Kenneally J. Anaesthetic management of the mucopolysaccharidoses: a fifteen-year experience in a children's hospital. *Anaesth Intensive Care* 1983;11:198–202.
11. Kempthorne PM, Brown TCK. Anaesthesia and the mucopolysaccharidoses: a survey of techniques and problems. *Anaesth Intensive Care* 1983;11:203–207.

Scheuermann Disease

MIM #: 181440

This autosomal dominant form of juvenile kyphosis is the most frequent cause of kyphosis in adolescents. The responsible gene and gene product are not known.

CHEST: Severe kyphosis can cause restrictive lung disease.

ORTHOPEDIC: Kyphosis. Wedging of vertebral bodies and disk space narrowing seen radiographically. Rare spinal cord compression.

ANESTHETIC CONSIDERATIONS

Patients will need to be carefully positioned secondary to kyphosis. Patients with severe kyphosis may have restrictive lung disease. They are at increased risk for perioperative respiratory complications. Good perioperative chest physiotherapy may be beneficial.

Bibliography:
1. Soo CL, Noble PC, Esses SI. Scheuermann kyphosis: long-term follow-up. *Spine J* 2002;2:49–56.

2. Graat HC, van Rhijn LW, Schrander-Stumpel CT, et al. Classical Scheuermann disease in male monozygotic twins: further support for the genetic etiology hypothesis. *Spine* 2002;27:e485–e487.
3. Ali RM, Green DW, Patel TC. Scheuermann kyphosis. *Curr Opin Pediatr* 1999;11:70–75.
4. Lowe TG. Scheuermann disease. *Orthop Clin North Am* 1999;30: 475–487.

Schilder Disease

MIM #: 272100

This term is of historic interest only. It was used to refer to the entities that are now known as Krabbe disease, metachromatic leukodystrophy, and adrenoleukodystrophy. Now that these specific diagnoses can be made, it is no longer useful to use this term. For more information, see the discussions of each of these individual entities.

MISCELLANEOUS: Born in Vienna, and later practicing at New York University, Paul Schilder was an early pioneer of psychoanalysis, although his ideas differed from some of Freud's concepts. The archetypal absent-minded professor, Schilder was killed in 1940 at the age of 54 years when he was hit by an automobile in New York City while crossing the street against traffic with an armload of books.

ANESTHETIC CONSIDERATIONS
See the discussions of each of these individual entities.

Schindler Disease

SYNONYM: Alpha-*N*-acetylgalactosaminidase deficiency; Alpha-galactosidase B deficiency. (Includes Kanzaki disease)

MIM #: 609241, 609242

This autosomal recessive disease is due to a deficiency in the lysosomal enzyme alpha-*N*-acetylgalactosaminidase (alpha-NAGA) (also called alpha-galactosidase B), which leads to neuroaxonal dystrophy and severe neurologic impairment. This enzyme cleaves terminal alpha-galactosyl and alpha-*N*-acetylgalactosaminyl residues in glycoproteins and sphingolipids. The specific material that is stored has not been identified. Alpha-galactosidase A is the enzyme that is deficient in Fabry disease (see earlier).

There is a separate mutation of this gene that results in a significantly milder disease of adulthood, referred to as type II Schindler disease, or **Kanzaki disease.** This disease is marked by disseminated angiokeratomas of the skin, cytoplasmic vacuoles of the skin and kidney, dilated conjunctival vessels and tortuous retinal vessels, and gastric mucosal telangiectasis. In Kanzaki disease, there is no neuroaxonal dystrophy or neurodegeneration.

The following discussion refers to Schindler disease, and not to the more mild Kanzaki disease.

HEENT/AIRWAY: Strabismus, nystagmus, optic atrophy, cortical blindness.

NEUROMUSCULAR: Development is normal for the first 9 to 12 months, and is then followed by profound neurodevelopmental regression. Hypotonia. Muscle atrophy. Myoclonic seizures, spasticity. By 4 to 5 years of age, children are essentially unresponsive to external stimuli. Decorticate posturing. The myenteric plexus is also affected by the storage of abnormal material, possibly leading to gastroparesis.

MISCELLANEOUS: The parents of the propositi of this disease preferred not to have it named after their family or their village (in Germany), so it was named after the physician who labored to diagnose their children, Dr. Schindler.

ANESTHETIC CONSIDERATIONS
Succinylcholine is contraindicated in patients with significant muscle atrophy because of the risk of hyperkalemia. If there is diffuse enteric autonomic involvement with gastroparesis, a rapid-sequence induction of anesthesia is indicated.

Bibliography:
1. Sakuraba H, Matsuzawa F, Aikawa S, et al. Structural and immunocytochemical studies on alpha-N-acetylgalactosaminidase deficiency (Schindler/Kanzaki disease). *J Hum Genet* 2004;49:1–8.
2. Umehara F, Matsumuro K, Kurono Y, et al. Neurologic manifestations of Kanzaki disease. *Neurology* 2004;62:1604–1606.
3. Bakker HD, de Sonnaville ML, Vreken P, et al. Human alpha-N-acetylgalactosaminidase (alpha-NAGA) deficiency: no association with neuroaxonal dystrophy? *Eur J Hum Genet* 2001;9:91–96.

Schinzel-Giedion Syndrome

Note: This syndrome is distinct from both Schinzel syndrome (ulnar-mammary syndrome, not discussed in this text) and Langer-Giedion syndrome (see earlier).

MIM #: 269150

This disorder, most likely inherited in an autosomal recessive fashion, has as its primary manifestations severe postnatal growth deficiency and profound mental retardation. Death often occurs before the age of 2 years, usually secondary to profound central nervous system dysfunction. The responsible gene and gene product are not known.

HEENT/AIRWAY: Sclerotic skull base, multiple wormian bones, long patent metopic suture, large fontanelles. Prominent forehead, midface hypoplasia. Occasional facial hemangiomas. Apparent proptosis due to shallow orbits, hypertelorism. Alacrima, corneal hypoesthesia. Low-set ears. Short nose with anteverted nares. Choanal atresia or stenosis. Occasional macroglossia. Short neck with redundant skin.

CHEST: Broad ribs, hypoplastic first ribs. Long clavicles, short sternum. Hypoplastic nipples.

CARDIOVASCULAR: Approximately one-third have congenital heart disease.

NEUROMUSCULAR: Profound mental retardation. Seizures, spasticity, opisthotonos. Ventriculomegaly secondary to cerebral atrophy. Intraventricular bands, subependymal pseudocysts.

ORTHOPEDIC: Postnatal growth deficiency—short stature. Broad cortex and increased density of long bones. Shortened forearms and legs. Simian crease, hypoplasia of distal phalanges, hyperconvex nails, occasional postaxial polydactyly. Hypoplastic/aplastic pubic bones. Widening of distal femurs, tibial bowing, clubfoot deformity. Occasionally the fifth toe overlaps the fourth.

GI/GU: Hypospadias, cryptorchidism, short penis, hypoplastic scrotum in boys; hypoplasia of labia majora or minora, hymenal atresia, short perineum in girls. Renal and ureteral anomalies. Hydronephrosis.

OTHER: Hypertrichosis. Embryonal tumors have been reported.

ANESTHETIC CONSIDERATIONS
Choanal atresia precludes placement of a nasal airway, nasal intubation, or placement of a nasogastric tube. Care must be taken when passing one of these tubes in patients with choanal stenosis. Chronic use of anticonvulsant medications may affect the metabolism of some anesthetic drugs. Patients with congenital heart disease require perioperative antibiotic prophylaxis as indicated.

Bibliography:
1. Minn D, Christmann D, De Saint-Martin A, et al. Further clinical and sensorial delineation of Schinzel-Giedion syndrome: report of two cases. *Am J Med Genet* 2002;109:211–217.
2. Shah AM, Smith MF, Griffiths PD, et al. Schinzel-Giedion syndrome: evidence for a neurodegenerative process. *Am J Med Genet* 1999;82:344–347.
3. Elliott AM, Meagher-Villemure K, Oudjhane K, et al. Schinzel-Giedion syndrome: further delineation of the phenotype. *Clin Dysmorphol* 1996;5:135–142.

Schizencephaly

MIM #: 269160

Schizencephaly is a unilateral or bilateral brain defect in which there is infolding of gray matter along a hemispheric cleft. It can be caused by a mutation in the gene *EMX2*, leading to a defect in neuronal migration. Patients with small clefts not involving the motor strip have a good prognosis. Some cases of schizencephaly appear to be familial.

NEUROMUSCULAR: Mental retardation. Seizures. Hypotonia. Spasticity, hemiparesis.

ANESTHETIC CONSIDERATIONS
Succinylcholine is relatively contraindicated in patients with hemiparesis because of the risk of hyperkalemia in patients with denervation of muscle.

Bibliography:
1. Granata T, Freri E, Caccia C, et al. Schizencephaly: clinical spectrum, epilepsy, and pathogenesis. *J Child Neurol* 2005;20:313–318.
2. Guerrini R, Filippi T. Neuronal migration disorders, genetics, and epileptogenesis. *J Child Neurol* 2005;20:287–299.

Schmid Type Metaphyseal Dysplasia

See Metaphyseal chondrodysplasia, Schmid type

Schönlein-Henoch Purpura

See Henoch-Schönlein purpura

Schwartz-Jampel Syndrome

SYNONYM: Chondrodystrophica myotonia

MIM #: 255800

This autosomal recessive disorder is one of the myotonic syndromes. The most common myotonic syndrome is myotonic dystrophy (see earlier). Schwartz-Jampel syndrome is characterized by myotonia, blepharophimosis, and joint limitation. Schwartz-Jampel syndrome is due to a mutation in the gene which encodes perlecan, the major proteoglycan component of basement membranes. There are clinical similarities to the Whistling face syndrome (see later) and the Marden-Walker syndrome (see earlier).

HEENT/AIRWAY: Fixed facies. Narrow palpebral fissures, blepharophimosis, myopia. Very small mouth and micrognathia from tense puckering of the perioral muscles. Short neck with decreased range of motion. Small larynx with high-pitched voice. May have obstructive sleep apnea.

CHEST: Pectus carinatum. Severe kyphoscoliosis may cause restrictive lung disease. Severely affected neonates may have recurrent aspiration pneumonia and respiratory distress.

CARDIOVASCULAR: No cardiac involvement.

NEUROMUSCULAR: Generalized myotonia, which refers to delayed relaxation of contracted muscles. Examples include the inability to release a handshake ("action myotonia"), or the sustained contraction with direct tapping or stimulation of a tendon reflex ("percussion myotonia"—best elicited by tapping the thenar eminence or finger extensors). In some mildly affected patients, myotonia may be apparent only on electromyography. There may be muscle hypertrophy or muscle atrophy. May have some degree of mental retardation.

ORTHOPEDIC: Short stature. Progressive joint contractures, with joint limitation. Carpal tunnel syndrome. Bowing of the long bones, ankle valgus, pes planus. May have shortened long bones. Kyphoscoliosis, lumbar lordosis. The skeletal abnormalities cause a particular gait, called by Schwartz and Jampel "marionette-like," whereas others have likened it to a "winding-doll."

GI/GU: Umbilical and inguinal hernias. Small testes.

MISCELLANEOUS: This syndrome was actually first reported by Catel and by Pinto and de Sousa.

ANESTHETIC CONSIDERATIONS
Laryngoscopy and tracheal intubation may be very difficult in these patients because of a very small mouth, limited mouth opening, micrognathia, short neck with limited range of motion and a small larynx (1,3,8,10). The laryngeal mask airway (LMA) has been used successfully (1).The passage of an endotracheal tube through a laryngeal mask airway has been reported in an awake 2.5-kg neonate after unsuccessful direct laryngoscopy and fiberoptic intubation (8).

Anesthetic or surgical manipulations may induce myotonic contractions, as can cold or shivering. The patient's body temperature should be maintained as close to normal as possible for this reason. Even pain from the intravenous injection of propofol may cause myotonic contractions. Neither regional anesthesia nor muscle relaxants prevent or reverse the myotonic contractions. Drugs that have been used to attenuate the contractions are quinine, procainamide, phenytoin, volatile anesthetics, and steroids. When all else fails, infiltration of the muscle with a local anesthetic has been recommended.

These patients may have abnormal drug reactions. Succinylcholine is best avoided in patients with muscle disuse, secondary to the risk of an exaggerated hyperkalemic response. Resistance to rocuronium has been demonstrated (4). Anticholinesterase drugs used to reverse nondepolarizing muscle relaxants can precipitate myotonia, and the use of shorter-acting muscle relaxants that do not require reversal has been recommended.

Patients with lung disease secondary to recurrent aspiration or skeletal deformities are at increased risk for postoperative pulmonary complications. Patients with a history of obstructive sleep apnea must be monitored vigilantly postoperatively. Patients must be carefully positioned because of joint contractures and joint limitation. Malignant hyperthermia has been reported in association with this syndrome (11). It is thought that this incident represented abnormal thermoregulation rather than true malignant hyperthermia, though others have subsequently used nontriggering anesthetics (1,3).

Bibliography:
1. Oue T, Nishimoto M, Kitaura M, et al. Anesthetic management of a child with Schwartz-Jampel syndrome [Japanese]. *Masui* 2004;53:782–784.
2. Ho NC, Sandusky S, Madike V, et al. Clinico-pathogenetic findings and management of chondrodystrophic myotonia (Schwartz-Jampel syndrome): a case report. *BMC Neurol* 2003;3:3.
3. Stephen LX, Beighton PH. Oro-dental manifestations of the Schwartz-Jampel syndrome. *J Clin Pediatr Dent* 2002;27:67–70.
4. Eikermann M, Bredendiek M, Schaper J, et al. Resistance to rocuronium in a child with Schwartz-Jampel syndrome type 1 B. *Neuropediatrics* 2002;33:43–46.
5. Rosenbaum HK, Miller JD. Malignant hyperthermia and myotonic disorders. *Anesthesiol Clin North America* 2002;20:623–664.
6. Spranger J, Hall BD, Hane B, et al. Spectrum of Schwartz-Jampel syndrome includes micromelic chondrodysplasia, kyphomelic dysplasia, and Burton disease. *Am J Med Genet* 2000;94:287–295.
7. Cook SP, Borkowski WJ. Obstructive sleep apnea in Schwartz-Jampel syndrome. *Arch Otolaryngol Head Neck Surg* 1997;123:1348–1350.
8. Theroux MC, Kettrick RG, Khine HH. Laryngeal mask airway and fiberoptic endoscopy in an infant with Schwartz-Jampel syndrome [Letter]. *Anesthesiology* 1995;82:605.
9. Russell SH, Hirsch NP. Anaesthesia and myotonia. *Br J Anaesth* 1994;72:210–216.
10. Ray S, Rubin AP. Anaesthesia in a child with Schwartz-Jampel syndrome. *Anaesthesia* 1994;49:600–602.
11. Seay AR. Malignant hyperthermia in a patient with Schwartz-Jampel syndrome. *J Pediatr* 1978;93:82–87.

SCIDS

See Severe combined immunodeficiency syndrome

Scimitar Syndrome

MIM #: 106700

Scimitar syndrome is a type of partial anomalous pulmonary venous return that occurs in families, and is possibly inherited in an autosomal dominant fashion. Anomalous pulmonary venous return occurs when the venous return from one or more lobes of the lung returns to the right atrium rather than to the left atrium. In Scimitar syndrome, there is a hypoplastic right lower lobe that gets its arterial supply directly from the aorta and whose venous return is to the inferior vena cava, below the diaphragm. The angiographic picture of this anomalous venous return was dubbed "Scimitar syndrome" by Catherine Neill and coworkers because of its resemblance to the broad, curved scimitar, a Middle Eastern sword.

CHEST: Hypoplastic right lower lung lobe, recurrent pulmonary infections. Possible pulmonary hypertension.

CARDIOVASCULAR: Anomalous pulmonary venous return. Cor pulmonale may develop.

ANESTHETIC CONSIDERATIONS
Recurrent infections of the abnormal lobe are common, and must be differentiated from the persistent density due to the abnormal vasculature on the chest radiograph that may mimic pneumonia. Pulmonary hypertension and cor pulmonale may be late manifestations.

Bibliography:

1. Khan A, Ring NJ, Hughes PD. Scimitar syndrome (congenital pulmonary venolobar syndrome). *Postgrad Med* 2005;81:216.
2. Riedelp M, Hausleiter J, Martinoff S. Scimitar syndrome. *Lancet* 2004;363:356.
3. Vanderheyden M, Goethals M, Van Hoe L. Partial anomalous pulmonary venous connection or Scimitar syndrome. *Heart* 2003;89:761.

Sclerosteosis

MIM #: 269500

This autosomal recessive disorder is characterized by osseous hyperostosis and syndactyly. Thick, dense bones can produce distortion of the face and compression of neural structures. This disorder is caused by a mutation in the gene encoding sclerostin (*SOST*), which is important in modulating osteoblastic activity. The pathogenesis is thought to be related to hyperactivity of osteoblasts.

HEENT/AIRWAY: Facial distortion with relative midface hypoplasia. Proptosis, which may lead to blindness in adulthood. Strabismus. Deafness secondary to occlusion of foramina by cranial hyperostosis. Dental malocclusion. Prominent, sometimes asymmetric jaw.

NEUROMUSCULAR: Facial and other cranial nerve palsies secondary to impingement of foramina by cranial hyperostosis. Intracranial pressure may be elevated. Impaction of the medulla has resulted in sudden death. Most patients require prophylactic craniectomy.

ORTHOPEDIC: Cutaneous syndactyly of second and third fingers, which may be asymmetric. Tall stature. Metaphyseal dysplasia. Radial deviation of terminal phalanges. Atrophic nails. Genu valgum.

MISCELLANEOUS: Most reported cases have been in the Afrikaaner population of South Africa. Interestingly, this disorder has also been reported in a part of Brazil that had been occupied by the Dutch in the 16th century.

ANESTHETIC CONSIDERATIONS

Facial asymmetry and bony overgrowth may make mask ventilation and/or tracheal intubation difficult. The proptotic eyes must be carefully protected intraoperatively. May have elevated intracranial pressure. Possible medullary compression suggests close postoperative observation for respiratory depression.

Bibliography:

1. Hamersma H, Gardner J, Beighton P. The natural history of sclerosteosis. *Clin Genet* 2003;63:192–197.
2. Stephen LX, Hamersma H, Gardner J, et al. Dental and oral manifestations of sclerosteosis. *Int Dent J* 2001;51:287–290.

Sebaceous Nevus Syndrome

See Nevus sebaceus of Jadassohn

Sebastian Syndrome

Included in Fechtner syndrome

Seckel Syndrome

MIM #: 210600

This autosomal recessive dysmorphic syndrome is characterized by extreme short stature, microcephaly, and a beak-like nose. Many patients survive well into adulthood. There is evidence of genetic heterogeneity with causative loci mapping to chromosomes 3, 14 and 18.

HEENT/AIRWAY: Microcephaly. Premature synostosis, receding forehead. Large eyes, down-sloping palpebral fissures. Retinal degeneration. May have optic lens dislocation. Low-set, malformed ears. Beak-like nose. May have cleft lip/palate. Partial anodontia, enamel hypoplasia. Retrognathia. May have laryngeal stenosis.

CHEST: Eleven pairs of ribs.

CARDIOVASCULAR: One report of atrioventricular canal defect. May have systemic hypertension.

NEUROMUSCULAR: May have mental retardation, which can be severe. Brain is small, with simple folding pattern. Pleasant personality, may be easily distracted. May have Arnold-Chiari malformation. May have intracranial aneurysm. May have seizures.

ORTHOPEDIC: Extreme short stature. Simian crease, clinodactyly of the fifth finger, hypoplasia of the proximal radius with dislocation of the radial head. Gap between the first and second toes, clubfoot deformity, hypoplasia of proximal fibula, inability to fully extend knee, dislocation of the hip. May have pes planus, scoliosis.

GI/GU: Cryptorchidism. Occasional hypoplastic external genitalia. May have renal insufficiency.

OTHER: Prenatal onset of severe growth deficiency. Proportional dwarfism. Sparse hair. Friable veins. Occasional hypoplastic anemia. May have increased risk of hematologic malignancies.

MISCELLANEOUS: This syndrome was given the rather derogatory name "bird-headed dwarfism" by Virchow. Seckel wrote the defining paper in 1960.

Caroline Crachami, a Sicilian-born dwarf who gained notoriety as one of the most extreme cases of dwarfism ever recorded when she was exhibited in England in 1824, probably had Seckel syndrome.

ANESTHETIC CONSIDERATIONS

Patients have extremely short stature, and should be addressed in a manner that is appropriate for their chronologic and mental age rather than their height age. Dental abnormalities should be documented preoperatively. Retrognathia may make direct laryngoscopy and tracheal intubation difficult. Endotracheal tube calculations based on age will overestimate the appropriate tube size. May have friable veins. Postoperative apneic spells were reported in one patient (1).

Bibliography:

1. Rajamani A, Kamat V, Murthy J. Anesthesia for cleft lip surgery in a child with Seckel syndrome—a case report. *Paediatr Anaesth* 2005; 15:338–341.
2. Faivre L, Le Merrer M, Lyonnet S, et al. Clinical and genetic heterogeneity of Seckel syndrome. *Am J Med Genet* 2002;112:379–383.
3. Kjaer I, Hansen N, Becktor KB, et al. Craniofacial morphology, dentition, and skeletal maturity in four siblings with Seckel syndrome. *Cleft Palate Craniofac J* 2001;38:645–651.
4. Shanske A, Caride DG, Menasse-Palmer L. Central nervous system anomalies in Seckel syndrome: report of a new family and review of the literature. *Am J Med Genet* 1997;70:155–158.

Segawa Syndrome

MIM #: 128230

This usually autosomal dominant disorder is one of levodopa-responsive, progressive dystonia with diurnal variation. There is dystonic posturing and disordered movement, beginning in one limb in childhood, but involving all limbs by approximately 5 years after clinical onset. The symptoms are somewhat similar to Parkinson disease. There is evidence of genetic heterogeneity, but it is usually caused by a mutation in the gene encoding guanosine triphosphate (GTP) cyclohydrolase I. This enzyme is the rate-limiting step in the conversion of GTP to tetrahydrobiopterin (BH4), a cofactor for tyrosine hydroxylase, in turn the rate-limiting step for the synthesis of dopamine. Tetrahydrobiopterin has a relatively short half-life, and it may be that synthesis is inadequate, and levels fall during daytime activity, resulting in the clinical worsening at the end of the day. Mutations in the gene encoding tyrosine hydroxylase can also cause an autosomal recessive form of this disease.

HEENT/AIRWAY: May have hearing loss. Torticollis.

NEUROMUSCULAR: Dystonic posturing, slowed movement, rigidity. Truncal involvement is uncommon. Symptoms are improved after sleep, and worsen toward evening. Symptoms are markedly improved by levodopa. Exaggerated deep tendon responses, and apparent Babinski sign (pseudopyramidal signs).

OTHER: May have a variety of psychiatric manifestations-anxiety, depression, obsessive-compulsive and eating disorders—probably secondary to defects in central dopamine, serotonin and/or norepinephrine synthesis.

ANESTHETIC CONSIDERATIONS

Regional and general anesthesia have been used successfully. Torticollis may make airway management more challenging. Because this disease affects muscle, succinylcholine should probably be used with care, although both succinylcholine and a nondepolarizing neuromuscular blocker have been used without problems (3). Phenothiazines, butyrophenones, metoclopramide, and other dopaminergic blockers may exacerbate movement disorders in general, and should be specifically avoided in this disorder of dopamine synthesis. Ondansetron should be safe as an antiemetic because it does not have antidopaminergic effects.

There are potential complications associated with higher-dose levodopa therapy in general, including tachycardia and increased cardiac irritability, increased glomerular filtration rate with lower intravascular volume and orthostatic hypotension, and decreased production of norepinephrine with substitution of dopamine, which is a less potent pressor. Ketamine, which has several sympathomimetic effects, has been used successfully in patients taking levodopa. There were no untoward effects in a patient who was taking relatively low doses of levodopa and had both general and epidural anesthesia for cesarean sections (3).

Bibliography:

1. Segawa M, Nomura Y, Nishiyama N. Autosomal dominant guanosine triphosphate cyclohydrolase I deficiency (Segawa disease). *Ann Neurol* 2003;54:S32–S45.
2. Hahn H, Trant MR, Brownstein MJ, et al. Neurologic and psychiatric manifestations in a family with a mutation in exon 2 of the guanosine triphosphate-cyclohydrolase gene. *Arch Neurol* 2001;58:749–755.
3. Priscu V, Lurie S, Savir I, et al. The choice of anesthesia in Segawa's syndrome. *J Clin Anesth* 1998;10:153–155.

Seip Syndrome

See Lipodystrophy

Senter Syndrome

SYNONYM: Senter-KID syndrome; KID syndrome

MIM #: 148210, 242150

This congenital ectodermal disorder has been documented to occur in both autosomal dominant and autosomal recessive forms. The primary manifestations are an ichthyosiform rash with focal hyperkeratosis and sensorineural deafness. KID is an acronym for **K**eratitis, **I**chthyosis, and **D**eafness. A corneal dystrophy can also be disabling. Autosomal dominant cases are caused by a mutation in the connexin-26 gene (*GJB2*), a gap junction protein. Since most cases are sporadic, they likely represent fresh mutations. The recessive form involves hepatic disease, growth failure, and mental retardation in addition to the features of the dominant form. The responsible gene and gene product are not known.

HEENT/AIRWAY: Progressive corneal opacification with progressive vascularization and photophobia. Eventual destruction of the cornea and development of keratoderma, a scar-like deposition over the cornea with vision loss. Sensorineural deafness. Malformed teeth, lesions of the mouth, scrotal tongue.

NEUROMUSCULAR: Occasional mental deficiency.

ORTHOPEDIC: Tight heel cords, variable flexion contractures.

GI/GU: Cryptorchidism. Occasional Hirschsprung disease (see earlier).

OTHER: Ichthyosiform rash with hyperkeratosis of the palms, soles, elbows, and knees. Hypohydrosis (decreased sweating). Variable alopecia. Variable nail dystrophy. Squamous cell carcinoma of skin and tongue. Fungal and bacterial skin infections, which may lead to septicemia.

ANESTHETIC CONSIDERATIONS
When meeting the patient before surgery, recall that he or she may have significant vision and/or hearing loss. Patients with photophobia may be extremely sensitive to the bright lights in operating rooms. Hypohydrosis may lead to overheating. Proper intraoperative positioning may be difficult secondary to contractures.

Bibliography:
1. Messmer EM, Kenyon KR, Rittinger O, et al. Ocular manifestations of keratitis-ichthyosis-deafness (KID) syndrome. *Ophthalmology* 2005;112:e1–e6.
2. Miteva L. Keratitis, ichthyosis, and deafness (KID) syndrome. *Pediatr Dermatol* 2002;19:513–516.
3. Szymko-Bennett YM, Russell LJ, Bale SJ, et al. Auditory manifestations of Keratitis-Ichthyosis-Deafness (KID) syndrome. *Laryngoscope* 2002;112:272–280.

Senter-KID Syndrome

See Senter syndrome

Septo-Optic Dysplasia

MIM #: 182230

This syndrome is characterized by optic nerve hypoplasia with midline defects of the prosencephalon. Most patients have hypothalamic hypopituitarism with associated multiple hormone deficiencies. It can be caused by a mutation in the murine homeobox gene *HESX1*. In some patients there is evidence of a vascular pathogenetic etiology. Children are at risk of sudden death from an intercurrent viral infection, presumably secondary to adrenal insufficiency (4).

HEENT/AIRWAY: Diminished visual acuity from optic nerve hypoplasia, occasionally including visual field defects. Congenital nystagmus.

NEUROMUSCULAR: Agenesis of the corpus callosum. Absence or abnormality of the septum pellucidum and hypothalamic/pituitary dysfunction. Schizencephaly. Neurologic signs and symptoms are variable. Some patients may have almost no neurologic findings and are of normal intelligence, whereas others have mental retardation, learning disabilities, delayed motor development, spastic quadriparesis, corticospinal tract involvement, and hypotonia or clumsiness. Occasional athetosis, seizures, autism, cranial nerve palsy, attention deficit disorders.
   May have neonatal apnea.

ORTHOPEDIC: Small stature. May have digital anomalies.

OTHER: Hypothalamic hypopituitarism with low levels of growth hormone, prolactin, thyroid-stimulating hormone, adrenocorticotrophic hormone (ACTH), luteinizing hormone, follicle-stimulating hormone, and antidiuretic hormone. Hypopituitarism may result in recurrent hypoglycemia.

MISCELLANEOUS: First described by Reeves, named "septo-optic dysplasia" by De Morsier, and fully delineated by Selna Kaplan and coworkers.

ANESTHETIC CONSIDERATIONS
Patients with hypothalamic hypopituitarism require chronic hormone and steroid replacement. Glucocorticoid and antidiuretic hormone deficiency are the most problematic perioperatively. Most patients require perioperative stress doses of steroids. Urine output may be an inadequate measure of intravascular volume in the face of both treated and inadequately treated diabetes insipidus.

Bibliography:
1. Stevens CA, Dobyns WB. Septo-optic dysplasia and amniotic bands: further evidence for a vascular pathogenesis. *Am J Med Genet A* 2004;125: 12–16.
2. Campbell CL. Septo-optic dysplasia: a literature review. *Optometry* 2003;74:417–426.
3. Birkebaek NH, Patel L, Wright NB, et al. Endocrine status in patients with optic nerve hypoplasia: relationship to midline central nervous system abnormalities and appearance of the hypothalamic-pituitary axis on magnetic resonance imaging. *J Clin Endocrinol Metab* 2003;88:5281–5286.
4. Brodsky MC, Conte FA, Taylor D, et al. Sudden death in septo-optic dysplasia: report of 5 cases. *Arch Ophthalmol* 1997;115:66–70.
5. Sherlock DA, McNichol LR. Anaesthesia and septo-optic dysplasia: implications of missed diagnosis in the peri-operative period. *Anaesthesia* 1987;42:1302–1305.

Severe Combined Immunodeficiency Syndrome

SYNONYM: SCIDS. (Includes Bare lymphocyte syndrome and Swiss-type agammaglobulinemia)

MIM #: 102700, 300400, 209920, and others

This rubric covers at least eleven distinct entities, both autosomal recessive and X-linked, which in general result in deficiency of both T- and B-cell function. All are marked by severe, life threatening infections. One form also has agranulocytosis, and another has just a deficiency of T cells. X-linked SCIDS has been diagnosed by linkage studies to a region of the X chromosome that codes for the gamma chain of interleukin-2R. Autosomal recessive SCIDS may also be associated with deficiency of the enzyme adenosine deaminase (see earlier, Adenosine deaminase deficiency). SCIDS has been associated with cartilage-hair hypoplasia syndrome, a type of metaphyseal chondrodysplasia (see earlier), and acrodermatitis enteropathica secondary to dietary zinc deficiency. Treatment with zinc is curative in this group. Otherwise, the treatment of SCIDS most commonly involves bone marrow transplantation. *Ex vivo* gene therapy has been used successfully to restore the immune system in patients with X-linked SCIDS (5).

The **Bare lymphocyte syndrome** is an autosomal recessive disorder in which lymphocytes do not express the major histocompatibility antigens. It involves a defect in a gene regulating surface expression of these antigens, rather than a defect in the structural gene for them. T cells (but not B cells) recognize antigens only when they are presented by another cell in association with a class II major histocompatibility antigen. These antigens are also required for a variety of cytotoxic and immunoregulatory functions.

Swiss-type agammaglobulinemia is more of an historical term, describing autosomal recessive SCIDS that is associated with thymic aplasia and the absence of both T and B cells.

HEENT/AIRWAY: Persistent candidiasis of the mouth and face.

CHEST: Recurrent pneumonia.

GI/GU: Persistent esophageal candidiasis. Diarrhea.

OTHER: Failure to thrive. Persistent candidal diaper rash. May have graft-versus-host disease if transfused. Children are anergic to skin tests. Variable deficiency in immunoglobulins.

MISCELLANEOUS: When vaccination for smallpox was universal, disseminated vaccinia was a common cause of death for these infants. Live polio virus may cause paralytic

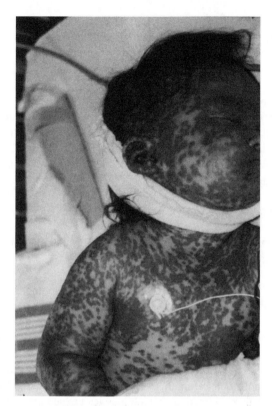

Severe combined immunodeficiency syndrome. A 17-month-old boy with severe combined immunodeficiency syndrome and disseminated varicella (chickenpox). The rash had become confluent on his face, and at the time this photograph was taken a second crop of vesicles had developed, some superimposed on the earlier, healing lesions. He required transfer to the intensive care unit.

polio. Other live vaccines, such as measles and bacille Calmette-Guerin (BCG), may cause serious disease.

ANESTHETIC CONSIDERATIONS

Transfused blood products must be irradiated to prevent graft-versus-host disease. Meticulous perioperative sterile technique is required. Electrolyte and fluid status should be evaluated preoperatively in the presence of diarrhea. Severe esophageal candidiasis may be a relative contraindication to the use of an esophageal stethoscope or nasogastric tube. Recurrent pulmonary infections may complicate intraoperative and/or postoperative ventilation.

Bibliography:

1. Cavazzana-Calvo M, Lagresle C, Hacein-Bey-Abina S, et al. Gene therapy for severe combined immunodeficiency. *Annu Rev Med* 2005;56: 585–602.
2. Buckley RH. Pulmonary complications of primary immunodeficiencies. *Paediatr Respir Rev* 2004;5:S225–S233.
3. Cooper MD, Lanier LL, Conley ME, et al. Immunodeficiency disorders. *Hematology (Am Soc Hematol Educ Program)* 2003;314–330.
4. Sikora AG, Lee KC. Otolaryngologic manifestations of immunodeficiency. *Otolaryngol Clin North Am* 2003;36:647–672.
5. Hacein-Bey-Abina S, Le Deist F, Carlier F, et al. Sustained correction of X-linked severe combined immunodeficiency by *ex vivo* gene therapy. *N Engl J Med* 2002;346:1185–1193.

Shah-Waardenburg Syndrome

Included in Waardenburg syndrome

Shone Complex

MIM #: None

Shone complex is a syndrome of multiple left-sided obstructive cardiac lesions. Findings are limited to the heart and aorta, and the etiology is unknown.

CARDIOVASCULAR: Levels of possible obstruction include supravalvar mitral (supravalvar mitral ring), mitral valvar (typically parachute mitral valve—all of the mitral chordae are attached to a single papillary muscle, invoking the image of the lines of a parachute from a billowing parachute collected together to a harness), subvalvar aortic stenosis, and coarctation of the aortic isthmus. Children may require multiple cardiac operations. Mitral valve surgery has particularly poor results in children.

ANESTHETIC CONSIDERATIONS
Anesthetic management depends on the specific lesions present, and their severity. Patients should receive perioperative antibiotic prophylaxis as indicated.

Bibliography:
1. Prunier F, Furber AP, Laporte J, et al. Discovery of a parachute mitral valve complex (Shone anomaly) in an adult. *Echocardiography* 2001;18(2):179–182.
2. Terry SM, Picone AL, Brandt B. Reconstruction of the mitral and aortic annuli for advanced management of the Shone complex. *J Heart Valve Dis* 1999;8:343–345.
3. Bolling SF, Iannettoni MD, Dick M II, et al. Shone anomaly: operative results and late outcome. *Ann Thorac Surg* 1990;49:887–893.

Short-Chain Acyl-CoA Dehydrogenase Deficiency

SYNONYM: SCAD deficiency

MIM #: 201470

This autosomal recessive disease is due to a defect in the gene for short-chain acyl-CoA dehydrogenase (SCAD), which is a mitochondrial enzyme required for the metabolism of short-chain fatty acids. SCAD is much less common than medium-chain acyl-CoA dehydrogenase deficiency (MCAD, see earlier). There are two distinct phenotypes of SCAD. One type presents in infants with acute acidosis and muscle weakness. The other type is a chronic myopathic disease of middle-aged adults. The infantile type is due to a generalized deficiency of SCAD, whereas the adult type is due to a deficiency of short-chain acyl-CoA (butyryl-CoA) that is limited to skeletal muscle mitochondria and a secondary deficiency of muscle carnitine.

Fatty acids are oxidized in mitochondria. After mobilization from the adipose tissue, they are taken up by the liver and other tissues, and converted to acyl-CoA esters in the cytoplasm. They enter mitochondria as carnitine esters, and become reesterified as acyl-CoA esters. Beta-oxidation results in the liberation of electrons. As beta-oxidation proceeds, the acyl chain is gradually shortened, and this first step in the oxidation process is catalyzed by acyl-CoA dehydrogenases with differing, but overlapping, chain-length specificities. These are very-long-chain, long-chain, medium-chain, and short-chain acyl-CoA dehydrogenases.

Treatment is with a fat-restricted diet and supplemental carnitine, but is only partially effective. Episodes of nonketotic hypoglycemia, common in medium- and long-chain acyl-CoA dehydrogenase deficiencies, are rare because most of the fatty acid chain can be metabolized in patients with SCAD deficiency.

NEUROMUSCULAR: Developmental delay, hypotonia, progressive muscle weakness (neonatal type). Lipid accumulation in type I fibers. Lipid storage myopathy of type I fibers (adult type).

GI/GU: Hepatosplenomegaly with fatty changes, cholestasis, and focal hepatic necrosis.

OTHER: Neonatal acidosis, poor feeding, failure to thrive, hyperammonemia. Occasional hypoglycemia. Secondary carnitine deficiency. May have cyclic vomiting.

ANESTHETIC CONSIDERATIONS
Although not as critical an issue as with the other disorders of beta-oxidation where hypoglycemia is more common (e.g., LCAD, MCAD and VLCAD deficiencies), prolonged perioperative fasting should be avoided. Serum glucose levels should be monitored, and patients may need perioperative glucose supplementation. Lactated Ringer's solution is not contraindicated in this disorder. The use of propofol is at least of theoretical concern in patients with disorders of fatty acid metabolism (1). Patients with a significant myopathy probably should not receive succinylcholine secondary to the risk of hyperkalemia.

Bibliography:
1. Turpin B, Tobias JD. Perioperative management of a child with short-chain acyl-CoA dehydrogenase deficiency. *Paediatr Anaesth* 2005;15:771–777.
2. Bok LA, Vreken P, Wijburg FA, et al. Short-chain Acyl-CoA dehydrogenase deficiency: studies in a large family adding to the complexity of the disorder. *Pediatrics* 2003;112:1152–1155.

Short Rib-Polydactyly Syndrome

[Includes Type I (Saldino-Noonan type), type II (Majewski type)]

MIM #: 263520, 263530

This lethal autosomal recessive disorder is characterized by short ribs, thoracic dysplasia, and polydactyly. There are four types of short rib-polydactyly syndrome, which may be four genetically distinct disorders or may be phenotypic variations of the same genetic disorder. **Type I (Saldino-Noonan type)** and **type II (Majewski type)** are described here.

HEENT/AIRWAY

Type I: Occasional neonatal teeth.

Type II: Low-set, small, malformed ears. Short, flat nose. Midline cleft lip, cleft palate. Hypoplasia of the epiglottis and/or larynx. Occasional microglossia, lobulated tongue.

CHEST

Type I: Short, horizontal ribs and narrow thorax.

Type II: Short, horizontal ribs. Very narrow thorax, pulmonary hypoplasia. High clavicles.

CARDIOVASCULAR

Type I: Cardiac defects include transposition of the great vessels, double-outlet left ventricle, double-outlet right ventricle, endocardial cushion defect, and hypoplastic right heart.

Type II: Occasional persistent left superior vena cava.

NEUROMUSCULAR

Type II: Occasional brain anomalies—pachygyria, a small vermis, and absence of olfactory bulbs.

ORTHOPEDIC

Type I: Short stature, short limbs. Postaxial polydactyly of hands or feet. Occasional preaxial polydactyly. Syndactyly, underossified phalanges. Metaphyseal irregularities of long bones, with spurs extended longitudinally from medial and lateral segments. Small iliac bones with horizontal acetabular roof.

Type II: Short stature with disproportionately short limbs. Both preaxial and postaxial polydactyly of hands or feet. Syndactyly, brachydactyly, underossified phalanges. Short, rounded metacarpals and metatarsals. Premature ossification of proximal epiphyses of humeri and femora. Short tibiae.

GI/GU

Type I: Imperforate anus. Defects of cloacal development. Occasional sex reversal (female phenotype with a 46XY karyotype). Polycystic kidneys.

Type II: May have absent gallbladder. Ambiguous genitalia. Multiple glomerular cysts and focal dilatation of distal tubules of kidney.

ANESTHETIC CONSIDERATIONS

Patients may have severe respiratory disease secondary to thoracic dysplasia or pulmonary hypoplasia. Clavicular anomalies may make placement of a subclavian venous catheter more difficult. Patients with renal insufficiency need careful titration of perioperative fluids. Renal insufficiency also affects the choice of perioperative drugs and drug dosages.

Bibliography:
1. Naki MM, Gur D, Zemheri E, et al. Short rib-polydactyly syndrome. *Arch Gynecol Obstet* 2005;272:173–175.
2. Chen CP, Shih JC, Tzen CY, et al. Recurrent short-rib polydactyly syndrome: prenatal three-dimensional ultrasound findings and associations with congenital high airway obstruction and pyelectasia. *Prenat Diagn* 2005;25:417–418.
3. Elcioglu NH, Hall CM. Diagnostic dilemmas in the short rib-polydactyly syndrome group. *Am J Med Genet* 2002;111:392–400.
4. Sarafoglou K, Funai EF, Fefferman N, et al. Short rib-polydactyly syndrome: more evidence of a continuous spectrum. *Clin Genet* 1999;56: 145–148.

Shprintzen Syndrome

See Velocardiofacial syndrome

Shprintzen-Goldberg Syndrome

MIM #: 182212

This autosomal dominant syndrome combines most of the features of Marfan syndrome with craniosynostosis. It is due, at least in some cases, to a mutation in the gene for fibrillin-1, which is also responsible for Marfan syndrome. Like Marfan syndrome, this is a generalized connective tissue dysplasia.

HEENT/AIRWAY: Craniosynostosis. Exophthalmos. Hypertelorism. Downslanting palpebral fissures. Myopia. Low-set, posteriorly rotated ears. Maxillary and mandibular hypoplasia. Soft tissue hypertrophy of the palate (causing "pseudocleft" palate). Unlike patients with the Marfan syndrome, these patients do not have ectopia lentis.

CHEST: Obstructive apnea. Pectus carinatum and excavatum, twisted ribs.

CARDIOVASCULAR: Aortic root dilatation, aortic dissection.

NEUROMUSCULAR: Infantile hypotonia. Mental retardation, developmental delay.

ORTHOPEDIC: Arachnodactyly and camptodactyly. Hammer toe. Bowing of the long bones, flared metaphyses. Scoliosis.

GI/GU: Multiple abdominal and inguinal hernias.

OTHER: Fragile skin. Lack of subcutaneous fat.

ANESTHETIC CONSIDERATIONS

The anesthetic management of Shprintzen-Goldberg syndrome has not been reported. However, mandibular hypoplasia may make direct laryngoscopy and tracheal intubation difficult. Patients must be carefully positioned and padded because of skin fragility and lack of subcutaneous fat. Hemodynamic stability is crucial in patients with aortic dilatation or dissection.

Bibliography:

1. Robinson PN, Neumann LM, Demuth S, et al. Shprintzen-Goldberg syndrome: 14 new patients and a clinical analysis. *Am J Med Genet A* 2005;135:251–262.
2. Stoll C. Shprintzen-Goldberg marfanoid syndrome: a case followed up for 24 years. *Clin Dysmorphol* 2002;11:1–7.
3. Greally MT, Carey JC, Milewicz DM, et al. Shprintzen-Goldberg syndrome: a clinical analysis. *Am J Med Genet* 1998;76:202–212.

Shwachman Syndrome

SYNONYM: Shwachman-Diamond syndrome

MIM #: 260400

There are many types of metaphyseal chondrodysplasia—see also Jansen type, McKusick type (cartilage-hair hypoplasia syndrome), Pyle type, Schmid type, and Spahr type [not included in this text (*MIM #250400*)]. Shwachman syndrome is a type of metaphyseal chondrodysplasia that is inherited in an autosomal recessive fashion. It is characterized by metaphyseal chondrodysplasia, exocrine pancreatic insufficiency, intermittent pancytopenia, and other hematologic and immunologic abnormalities. Both deficiencies in myeloid precursors and diminished neutrophil chemotaxis have been described. The hematologic and immunologic abnormalities that can be seen with this syndrome are similar to those that can be seen in the McKusick type of metaphyseal chondrodysplasia (cartilage-hair hypoplasia syndrome, see earlier). The disease is due to a mutation in the *SBDS* (Shwachman-Bodian-Diamond syndrome) gene which may play a role in RNA metabolism. It has been suggested that primary atrophy of the pancreas presenting in middle age may represent one end of the spectrum of this disease.

HEENT/AIRWAY: Otitis media.

CHEST: Short ribs with widely flared costochondral junctions. Recurrent pneumonia.

NEUROMUSCULAR: May have mild mental retardation, hypotonia, motor delay.

ORTHOPEDIC: Moderate short stature. Short extremities. Metaphyseal chondrodysplasia—irregular metaphyses, focal hypomineralization of epiphyses. Cubitus valgus, syndactyly, clinodactyly. Kyphoscoliosis. Osteomyelitis.

GI/GU: Malabsorption and diarrhea secondary to exocrine pancreas dysfunction, which improves with age. Inexplicably, steatorrhea is not a prominent feature. Type I renal tubular acidosis. Nephrocalcinosis.

OTHER: The exocrine pancreas is replaced by fat. The islets of Langerhans cells remain functional. Intermittent pancytopenia—normocytic/normochromic anemia, thrombocytopenia, leukopenia, neutropenia. Immunologic abnormalities, with frequent bacterial infections. Hematologic malignancy may develop.

MISCELLANEOUS: Scott Hamilton, the well-known figure skater and 1984 Olympic Gold Medal winner, has Shwachman syndrome.

The Diamond here is Dr. Louis Diamond, also of Diamond-Blackfan syndrome. Dr. Shwachman cared for many children with cystic fibrosis. He noted a subgroup of children with exocrine pancreatic insufficiency who had neutropenia, and mentioned it to his colleague Dr. Diamond, a hematologist.

ANESTHETIC CONSIDERATIONS

Baseline hematocrit and platelet count should be obtained. Patients may have immunologic abnormalities and are at increased risk for development of a perioperative infection. Good aseptic technique is imperative. Patients must be carefully positioned perioperatively because of their orthopedic abnormalities. Severe thoracic cage involvement causing asphyxiating thoracic dysplasia as in Jeune syndrome (see earlier) has been described. Poor nutrition, fatty acid deficiency and fat-soluble vitamin deficiency should not be a problem with appropriate pancreatic replacement therapy.

Bibliography:

1. Kuijpers TW, Alders M, Tool AT, et al. Hematologic abnormalities in Shwachman-Diamond syndrome: lack of genotype-phenotype relationship. *Blood* 2005;106:356–361.
2. Grinspan ZM, Pikora CA. Infections in patients with Shwachman-Diamond syndrome. *Pediatr Infect Dis J* 2005;24:179–181.
3. Tamhane P, Newton NI, White S. Anaesthetic management of quinsy in a patient with Shwachman-Diamond syndrome [Letter]. *Anaesthesia* 2003;58:821.
4. Ip WF, Dupuis A, Ellis L, et al. Serum pancreatic enzymes define the pancreatic phenotype in patients with Shwachman-Diamond syndrome. *J Pediatr* 2002;141:259–265.
5. Rothbaum R, Perrault J, Vlachos A, et al. Shwachman-Diamond syndrome: report from an international conference. *J Pediatr* 2002;141:266–270.
6. Dror Y, Freedman MH. Shwachman-Diamond syndrome. *Br J Haematol* 2002;118:701–713.

Shwachman-Diamond Syndrome

See Shwachman syndrome

Sialidosis

SYNONYM: Mucolipidosis I

MIM #: 256550

This autosomal recessive disease is due to a deficiency in neuraminidase (sialidase) which cleaves the sialyl linkages of several oligosaccharides and glycopeptides with the resultant accumulation or excretion of sialic acid bound to a variety of oligosaccharides and/or glycoproteins. Sialidosis type I is the milder form, and type II the more severe, with an earlier onset. It more resembles the phenotypes of the mucopolysaccharidoses. Type II has been subdivided into juvenile and infantile forms. Type I is marked by cherry-red macular spots and progressive myoclonus.

HEENT/AIRWAY

Type I: Cherry-red macular spots. Decreased visual acuity. Impaired color vision. Night blindness.

Type II: Hurler-like facies. Corneal opacities. May have cherry-red macular spots. Hearing loss. Large tongue. Upper airway obstruction. Short immobile neck. Laryngomalacia.

CHEST: Thoracic kyphosis. Pectus carinatum. Obstructive sleep apnea. Restrictive lung disease.

NEUROMUSCULAR

Type I: Progressive myoclonus worsened by smoking or related to the menstrual cycle. Seizures. Gait disturbances.

Type II: Mental retardation. Ataxia. Myoclonus.

ORTHOPEDIC: Scoliosis. Dysostosis of multiple bones.

GI:/GU: Hepatosplenomegaly. May have inguinal hernias.

ANESTHETIC CONSIDERATIONS

Patients with type I disease are likely taking anticonvulsant medications. Chronic use of anticonvulsant medication alters the metabolism of some anesthetic drugs. Anesthetic considerations for patients with type II disease have not been described but would presumably mirror those of the phenotypically related mucopolysaccharidoses. Because of the abnormal facies, a regular pediatric mask may not fit adequately, and it has been suggested that in these cases the mask be applied upside-down, with the narrower nasal bridge over the mouth. If there is redundant airway soft tissue, a nasal airway may be useful. Thickening of the soft tissues, an enlarged tongue, and a short, immobile neck may make laryngoscopy extremely difficult. Laryngoscopy may become more difficult with age. Regional anesthesia has been used successfully (2). Postoperative respiratory complications are common, and patients should be observed closely in the postanesthesia care unit for evidence of airway compromise.

Bibliography:

1. Rodriguez Criado G, Pshezhetsky AV, Rodriguez Becerra A, et al. Clinical variability of type II sialidosis by C808T mutation. *Am J Med Genet A* 2003;116:368–371.
2. Tran QHD, Kaufman I, Schricker T. Spinal anesthesia for a patient with type I sialidosis undergoing abdominal surgery. *Acta Anaesthesiol Scand* 2001;45:919–921.
3. Palmeri S, Villanova M, Malandrini A, et al. Type I sialidosis: a clinical, biochemical and neuroradiological study. *Eur Neurol* 2000;43: 88–94.

Sickle Cell Disease

MIM #: 603903

This archetypal molecular disease occurs when valine is substituted for glutamate at the sixth N-terminal position in the beta chain of hemoglobin, due to a substitution of thymine for adenine in the gene that encodes this protein. Sickle cell disease is inherited in an autosomal recessive fashion. It is most prevalent in people of African descent. The heterozygous state has been shown to confer some protection from malaria infection, which may account for the prevalence of this genetic defect in populations of African origin.

To maximize the oxygen-carrying capacity of the red blood cell and pack as much hemoglobin as possible into the red blood cell, hemoglobin must be extremely soluble. Desaturation of the sickle form of hemoglobin results in polymerization of hemoglobin, forming large aggregates called tactoids, which deform the red blood cells into the typical sickle shape. Homozygous (SS) cells begin to sickle at oxygen saturations below 85% (pO_2 of 40 to 50 mm Hg), and is complete at a saturation of 38%. The presence of fetal hemoglobin increases the minimum amount of hemoglobin needed for sickling, and is therefore protective, an effect seen until approximately 6 months of age. Sickling is exacerbated by cold, stasis, exertion, infection, dehydration, and hypoxemia. Heterozygous (AS) cells do not begin to sickle until oxygen saturation is below 40% (pO_2 of 25 to 30 mm Hg), well below saturations in venous blood, so sickling with sickle cell trait (the heterozygous state) is rarely if ever problematic without concomitant stasis.

At oxygen saturations less than 80% sickled hemoglobin has a decreased affinity for oxygen (a right-shifted oxygen–hemoglobin dissociation curve with a higher P_{50}). In addition, the Bohr effect is more pronounced in sickle hemoglobin, so that for a given drop in pH there is a greater decrease in oxygen affinity. Both of these effects facilitate unloading of oxygen to tissues, presumably allowing better organ function at low hematocrits. On the other hand, the higher P_{50} favors the formation of deoxyhemoglobin, which increases the polymerization of hemoglobin, particularly as the pH drops.

The pathophysiologic consequences of sickle cell disease are secondary to two main factors: small vessel obstruction in a wide variety of organs by sickle cells (vaso-occlusive events), and hemolytic anemia (the half-life of SS cells is approximately 12 days, compared with 120 days for normal red blood cells). Occlusive episodes can be extremely painful, and patients often have multiple hospital admissions for pain control.

The clinical severity of this disease can also be affected by the presence of other abnormalities in the hemoglobin gene. SC disease occurs when the patient has the gene for both sickle cell hemoglobin (valine at the sixth position) and hemoglobin C (lysine at the sixth position). These patients have a chronic mild hemolytic anemia and a peripheral blood smear similar to that seen in hemoglobin C disease (multiple target cells). Because the degree of hemolysis is less, the hematocrit is usually higher than in patients with SS disease. There is significant clinical variability, but potential complications of SC disease include all of those seen with SS disease. Elevated levels of fetal hemoglobin, hemoglobin F, also appear to be somewhat protective. Sickle beta-thalassemia occurs when an individual inherits both the genes for sickle cell disease and beta-thalassemia (see later). The severity of symptoms depends on the specific type of thalassemia.

HEENT/AIRWAY: Frontal bossing and prominent maxilla from increased marrow space. Eye changes are similar to those in diabetes, with neovascularization, microvascular retinopathy, vitreous hemorrhage, and retinal detachment. Eye changes are particularly common in SC disease. Functional asplenism is associated with hypertrophy of other lymphoid tissue, including the tonsils and adenoids. Obstructive sleep apnea.

CHEST: Pulmonary infarctions (acute chest syndrome). Bronchopulmonary anastomoses causing intrapulmonary right-to-left shunting. Inhaled nitric oxide has been used successfully in a limited series of patients with acute chest syndrome and resulted in decreased pulmonary hypertension and improved oxygenation (28). There is a suggestion that patients with sickle cell disease have an increased incidence of airway hyperreactivity (26).

CARDIOVASCULAR: Cardiomegaly that is usually secondary to the anemia, but may be due to congestive failure. Myocardial fibrosis from prior sickling. There can be pulmonary arterial hypertension secondary to pulmonary infarctions, increasing the risk of death.

NEUROMUSCULAR: May have findings ranging from transient ischemic attacks to true stroke. Young children are more prone to thrombotic strokes, whereas adults more commonly have hemorrhagic infarcts. A chronic transfusion program has been shown to lower central nervous system complications in children.

ORTHOPEDIC: Skeletal deformities from marrow hyperplasia and pain crises, particularly dactylitis (hand-foot syndrome), especially in children under 5 years of age. Multiple bone infarcts with arthropathies as sequelae. Thoracic kyphosis, lumbar lordosis. Aseptic necrosis, and leg ulcers. Aseptic necrosis of the hip is particularly common in SC disease. Growth failure, possibly related to zinc deficiency.

GI/GU: With time, there is complete infarction (autoinfarction) of the spleen with immune incompetence. However, before complete infarction, the spleen can suddenly enlarge and trap red blood cells and platelets—a splenic sequestration—with an acute drop in hematocrit that can be life threatening. Gallstones are common, and cholecystectomy is the most frequent surgical procedure in these patients. Liver function is spared, but intrahepatic sickling can cause painful hepatic enlargement. Transaminases are often slightly elevated.

Painful priapism may develop. Renal impairment begins in childhood and is common by adulthood. Renal involvement includes inability to concentrate urine (isosthenuria), polyuria, proteinuria, impaired potassium excretion, impaired acidification of urine, pyelonephritis, and glomerulonephritis. There can also be papillary necrosis and painless hematuria. Renal papillary necrosis is particularly common in SC disease.

OTHER: Hemolytic anemia. The peripheral blood smear always has sickle forms, and their presence is not diagnostic of a crisis. A variety of infections can be associated with an acute hemolytic crisis. Lack of splenic function renders patients particularly susceptible to infection with encapsulated organisms, such as pneumococci and *Hemophilus*. Patients should have received pneumococcal and *Hemophilus* vaccines, and older children may be receiving chronic antibiotic prophylaxis. Patients also are at increased risk for osteomyelitis and splenic abscess. Inflammation increases the expression of cell adhesion molecules on the endothelium, with increased adhesion of sickled cells and additional vascular occlusion.

Over 50% of pregnant women with SS disease have a crisis during the pregnancy, and many of those have a major complication. Preeclampsia with volume depletion and vasoconstriction favors sickling. Many signs of preeclampsia, such as abdominal pain, hypertension, renal dysfunction, and congestive heart failure, may be difficult to differentiate from complications of sickle cell disease. There is an increased incidence of preeclampsia (14% to 20% vs. 4%), placental abruption (4.5% vs. 0.3%), placenta previa (1.5% vs. 0.4%), and intrauterine growth retardation in pregnant patients with sickle cell disease. In general, however, pregnant patients with sickle cell disease have a good outcome. Pregnant patients with sickle cell trait should be similar to the general population, although a single intrapartum maternal death was reported, presumably due to aortocaval compression, with the sudden release of a large amount of hypoxemic, acidotic, sickled blood immediately after delivery (37).

Patients may be taking hydroxyurea, which has been shown to elevate fetal hemoglobin levels and decrease morbidity, at least in adults.

MISCELLANEOUS: The disease was first described by James Herrick in 1910. The second, following shortly, was from the University of Virginia. The ascertainment of an abnormal hemoglobin protein by Linus Pauling and colleagues in 1949 made this the first "molecular disease."

ANESTHETIC CONSIDERATIONS

Perioperative complications, such as painful crises and acute chest syndrome, are not uncommon. Routine preoperative investigations should include a hematocrit, plasma urea and creatinine, urine dipstick, and a chest radiograph (10). Factors known to enhance the likelihood of sickling must be avoided perioperatively: namely cold, stasis, exertion, infection, dehydration (as from a protracted preoperative fast), hypoxemia, and acidosis (2,9). Hypotension is more appropriately treated with fluids rather than with vasoconstrictors. Hypovolemia is poorly tolerated due to the renal concentrating defect. Avoidance of stasis should be the goal of positioning and padding. Also, efforts should be made to avoid compression of the inferior vena cava when the patient is prone. Pneumatic compression devices may help. The safety of tourniquets for orthopedic procedures is unclear. There does not seem to be any increased risk in patients with sickle cell trait, and the risk may be small in patients with sickle cell disease (11,27), although it has been suggested that a higher level of (protective) fetal hemoglobin in Hgb SS study patients accounted for the uneventful use of a tourniquet (9). Similarly, transient, uncomplicated clamping of major extremity vessels for femoropopliteal bypass has been reported (22), although that patient also had elevated levels of fetal hemoglobin. The incidence of postoperative complications is not necessarily diminished by regional (vs. general) anesthesia (32).

The development of an intraoperative crisis may be masked by general anesthesia. If muscle relaxants have not been used, there may be a change in the respiratory pattern or the development of seizures. Postoperative analgesics may mask the pain from painful crises. Postoperatively, acute chest syndrome may mimic aspiration pneumonitis, and back pain or neurologic problems may be attributed to regional anesthesia. Transfusion related acute lung injury (TRALI) can mimic acute chest syndrome, but resolves more rapidly (14). Acute chest syndrome occurs in up to 10% to 16% of patients after cholecystectomy or splenectomy, and typically involves the ipsilateral lower lobe (13). The treatment of acute chest syndrome includes increased fraction of inspired oxygen (FIO_2), continuous positive airway pressure (CPAP), mechanical ventilation if

necessary, bronchodilators, antibiotics, incentive spirometry, adequate hydration and sometimes nitric oxide.

During sickle crises, hemoglobin saturation measured by pulse oximetry tends to overestimate the true oxygen saturation. This is explained by the increase in carboxyhemoglobin found in hemolytic anemias.

The hemoglobin or hemoglobin S level required for elective or even urgent surgery was arbitrarily and dogmatically defined for many years (hemoglobin > 10 g/dL, hemoglobin S $< 30\%$), but currently there is no true consensus. Aggressive perioperative transfusion regimens have been associated with a high incidence of transfusion-related complications. Patients may have red blood cell antibodies from multiple transfusions, making cross-matching difficult. Excessive transfusion may actually increase the risk of sickling, because viscosity (and sludging) is increased, with still enough sickle hemoglobin around to sickle. Partial exchange transfusion can lower the concentration of sickle hemoglobin without increasing intravascular volume or inordinately increasing hematocrit. There are currently three principal approaches:

1. Fifteen mL/kg of packed red blood cells as a simple transfusion approximately 1 month before surgery. This increases hemoglobin from approximately 6 to 8 g/dL to approximately 10 to 12 g/dL, and decreases hemoglobin S from approximately 100% to approximately 65%. The shorter-lived SS cells die off, and the higher hematocrit inhibits new SS cell production. A second transfusion 2 weeks later maintains the hematocrit and decreases hemoglobin S to less than 40%. A final transfusion is given on the day before surgery, depending on the final laboratory results. Patients with the SC variant have higher baseline hematocrits and therefore may require a partial exchange transfusion rather than a simple transfusion.

2. Recommendations from the Perioperative Transfusion in Sickle Cell Disease Study Group (33) have by and large supplanted recommendation 1. These investigators examined a total of 604 surgeries performed on 551 sickle cell patients in a randomized, prospective, multicenter trial. Patients were randomly assigned either to the aggressive transfusion group, who were transfused preoperatively until they reached a hemoglobin S level of less than 30%, or to the conservative transfusion group, who were transfused preoperatively until their hemoglobin level was elevated to 10 g/dL, with no specific hemoglobin S level required. The frequency of serious complications was similar in both groups. However, there were twice as many transfusion-related complications in the aggressively transfused group than in the conservatively transfused group (14% vs. 7%). The results of this study indicate that there is no advantage to (and there is some risk in) aggressive preoperative transfusion. This study did not include a nontransfused control group.

3. Because the merits of preoperative transfusion have not been clearly demonstrated, and the real risks of

TABLE 5. *Potential misdiagnoses in sickle cell disease*

Pathology	Mistaken surgical diagnosis
Bone infarcts (often febrile)	Infective arthritis, osteomyelitis
Acute hemolysis	Surgical jaundice (biliary stones often present)
Sequestration with falling hemoglobin	Acute hemorrhage
Splenic infarct, pulmonary infarct, pneumonia	Acute abdomen

transfusion-related complications have been delineated, some practitioners advocate no routine preoperative transfusion. It seems likely that routine transfusions are unnecessary for short procedures with limited heat or fluid loss (3).

The use of cell savers is not recommended by manufacturers, but they have been used successfully without sequelae (36). Autologous transfusion has been used successfully with preoperative partial exchange transfusion.

Cardiopulmonary bypass is not problematic in patients with sickle cell trait, and there are routinely excellent results in patients with sickle cell disease. Good results have also been reported with SC disease. There are no consensus guidelines for intraoperative temperature, hematocrit, or hemoglobin S level (7, 8, 20, 23, 35). *In vitro* studies suggest that hypothermia may in fact be protective and prevent sickling.

Increased plasma tonicity can encourage sickling, so furosemide or mannitol, used in neurosurgical operations, might increase risks. Epidural anesthesia has been reported to resolve priapism in a single case report, and has also been shown to be useful for difficult-to-control abdominal pain.

Patients with sickle cell disease may be tolerant to the effects of narcotic medications because of long term use secondary to chronic pain. Larger doses of opioids may be necessary to control postoperative pain, and adjunctive pain control measures such as regional analgesia and nonopioid pain medications should be considered (1, 2). Achievement of adequate postoperative analgesia is critical for the success of incentive spirometry and early postoperative mobilization.

Medical complications of sickle cell disease may be misdiagnosed as surgical problems (see Table 5).

Bibliography:

1. Crawford MW, Galton S, Naser B. Postoperative morphine consumption in children with sickle-cell disease. *Paediatr Anaesth* 2006;16: 152–157.
2. Firth PG. Anaesthesia for peculiar cells—a century of sickle cell disease. *Br J Anaesth* 2005;95:287–299.
3. Fu T, Corrigan NJ, Quinn CT, et al. Minor elective surgical procedures using general anesthesia in children with sickle cell anemia without pre-operative blood transfusion. *Pediatr Blood Cancer* 2005;45:43–47.
4. Goodwin SR, Haberkern C, Crawford M, et al. Sickle cell and anesthesia: do not abandon well-established practices without evidence [Letter]. *Anesthesiology* 2005;103:205.
5. Park KW. Sickle cell disease and other hemoglobinopathies. *Int Anesthesiol Clin* 2004;42:77–93.
6. Tobin JR, Butterworth J. Sickle cell disease: dogma, science, and clinical care [Letter]. *Anesth Analg* 2004;98:283–284.
7. Hemming AE. Pro: Exchange transfusion is required for sickle cell trait patients undergoing cardiopulmonary bypass. *J Cardiothorac Vasc Anesth* 2004;18:663–665.
8. Messent M. Con: Exchange transfusion is not required for sickle cell trait patients undergoing cardiopulmonary bypass. *J Cardiothorac Vasc Anesth* 2004;18:666–667.
9. Sarjeant JM, Callum JL. The use of tourniquets in patients with sickle cell disease [Letter]. *Anesth Analg* 2004;99:630.
10. Firth PG, Head CA. Sickle cell disease and anesthesia. *Anesthesiology* 2004;101:766–785.
11. Al-Ghamdi AA. Bilateral total knee replacement with tourniquets in a homozygous sickle cell patient. *Anesth Analg* 2004;98:543–544.
12. Gladwin MT, Sachdev V, Jison ML, et al. Pulmonary hypertension as a risk factor for death in patients with sickle cell disease. *N Engl J Med* 2004;350:886–895.
13. Crawford MW, Speakman M, Carver ED, et al. Acute chest syndrome shows a predilection for basal lung regions on the side of upper abdominal surgery. *Can J Anaesth* 2004;51:707–711.
14. Firth PG, Tsuruta Y, Kamath Y, et al. Transfusion-related acute lung injury or acute chest syndrome of sickle cell disease?–A case report. *Can J Anaesth* 2003;50:895–899.
15. Marchant WA, Walker I. Anaesthetic management of the child with sickle cell disease. *Paediatr Anaesth* 2003;13:473–489.
16. Riddington C, Williamson L. Preoperative blood transfusions for sickle cell disease. *Cochrane Database Syst Rev* 2001;3:CD003149.
17. Frietsch T, Ewen I, Waschke KF. Anaesthetic care for sickle cell disease. *Eur J Anaesthesiol* 2001;18:137–150.
18. Labat F, Dubousset AM, Baujard C, et al. Epidural analgesia in a child with sickle cell disease complicated by acute abdominal pain and priapism. *Br J Anaesth* 2001;87:935–936.
19. Firth PG, Peterfreund RA. Management of multiple intracranial aneurysms: Neuroanesthetic considerations of sickle cell disease. *J Neurosurg Anesthesiol* 2000;12:366–371.
20. Djaiani GN, Cheng DC, Carroll JA, et al. Fast-track cardiac anesthesia in patients with sickle cell abnormalities. *Anesth Analg* 1999;89:598–603.
21. Vichinsky EP, Neumayr LD, Haberkern C, et al. The perioperative complication rate of orthopedic surgery in sickle cell disease: Report of the national sickle cell surgery study group. *Am J Hematol* 1999;62:129–138.
22. Vipond AJ, Caldicott LD. Major vascular surgery in a patient with sickle cell disease. *Anaesthesia* 1998;53:1204–1206.
23. Frimpong-Boateng K, Amoah AG, Barwasser HM, et al. Cardiopulmonary bypass in sickle cell anemia without exchange transfusion. *Eur J Cardiothorac Surg* 1998;14:527–529.
24. Burt N, Bailey M, Pinosky ML, et al. The perioperative management of patients with sickle cell disease: a survey of members of the Society for Pediatric Anesthesia. *Am J Anesthesiol* 1998;25:204–208.
25. Haberkern CM, Neumayr LD, Orringer EP, et al. Cholecystectomy in sickle cell anemia patients: perioperative outcome of 364 cases from the National Preoperative Transfusion Study. Preoperative Transfusion in Sickle Cell Disease Study Group. *Blood* 1997;89:1533–1542.
26. Leong MA, Dampier C, Varlotta L, et al. Airway hyperreactivity in children with sickle cell disease. *J Pediatr* 1997;131:278–283.
27. Adu-Gyamfi Y, Sankarankutty M, Marwa S. Use of a tourniquet in patients with sickle-cell disease. *Can J Anaesth* 1997;40:24–27.
28. Atz AM, Wessel DL. Inhaled nitric oxide in sickle cell disease with acute chest syndrome. *Anesthesiology* 1997;87:988–990.
29. Danzer BI, Birnbach DJ, Thys DM. Anesthesia for the parturient with sickle cell disease. *J Clin Anesth* 1996;8:598–602.
30. Oginni LM, Rufai MB. How safe is tourniquet use in sickle-cell disease? *Afr J Med Sci* 1996;25:3–6.
31. Hall JR, Clemency MV, Clarke G, et al. Effects of blood salvage and cell saver processing on sickle cell trait blood. *Anesthesiology* 1996;85:A405.
32. Koshy M, Weiner SJ, Miller ST, et al. Surgery and anesthesia in sickle cell disease. *Blood* 1995;86:3676–3684.
33. Vichinsky EP, Haberkern CM, Neumary L, et al. A comparison of conservative and aggressive transfusion regimens in the perioperative management of sickle cell disease. *N Engl J Med* 1995;333:206–213.
34. Gyamfi YA, Sankarankutty M, Marwa S. Use of a tourniquet in patients with sickle cell disease. *Can J Anaesth* 1993;40:24–27.

35. Balasundaram S, Duran CG, al-Halees Z, et al. Cardiopulmonary bypass in sickle cell anaemia: report of five cases. *J Cardiovasc Surg* 1991;32:271–274.
36. Cook A, Hanowell LH. Intraoperative autotransfusion for a patient with homozygous sickle cell disease. *Anesthesiology* 1990;73:177–179.
37. The Anaesthesia Advisory Committee to the Chief Coroner of Ontario. Intraoperative death during caesarian section in a patient with sickle-cell trait. *Can J Anaesth* 1987;34:67–70.

Siemerling-Creutzfeldt Disease

See Adrenoleukodystrophy

Simpson Dysmorphia Syndrome

See Simpson-Golabi-Behmel syndrome

Simpson-Golabi-Behmel Syndrome

SYNONYM: Simpson dysmorphia syndrome

MIM #: 312870

This X-linked recessive disorder was reported separately by Simpson et al. Golabi et al. and Behmel et al. The major clinical manifestations are hypertelorism, a broad, flat nose, and bony overgrowth abnormalities. Half of the affected patients have died of unknown causes by age 6 months. Female carriers sometimes have mild clinical manifestations. There is marked variability within and between families, and there is evidence of genetic heterogeneity. At least some cases have been ascribed to a defect in the *GPC3* gene, which encodes a proteoglycan, glypican 3, that plays a role in the control of growth of the embryonic mesodermal tissues.

HEENT/AIRWAY: Macrocephaly, coarse facies. Down-slanting palpebral fissures, hypertelorism, cataracts, retinal detachment, coloboma of optic disc. Cup-shaped ears, ear-lobe creases. Flat nasal bridge, short nose. Midline groove of lower lip, macrostomia. Macroglossia. Tethered tongue, perioral or palatal spotty pigmentation. High-arched palate, occasional cleft lip and palate. Large jaw. Short neck.

CHEST: Pectus excavatum, cervical ribs, 13 ribs. Congenital diaphragmatic hernia has been reported.

CARDIOVASCULAR: Conduction abnormalities, tachyarrhythmias. A variety of congenital cardiac defects (in approximately 30% of patients), including ventricular septal defect, pulmonic stenosis, transposition of the great arteries, and patent ductus arteriosus.

NEUROMUSCULAR: Intelligence is usually in the normal range. Clumsy.

ORTHOPEDIC: Tall stature. Broad, short hands and fingers, occasional postaxial polydactyly, syndactyly of second and third fingers and toes, nail hypoplasia, broad thumb and great toe. Fusion of C2-3 posteriorly. Six lumbar vertebrae, and sacral and coccygeal abnormalities. Occasional scoliosis.

GI/GU: Umbilical and inguinal hernias. Occasional pyloric stenosis, malrotation of the gut, choledochal cysts, splenomegaly. Occasional hypospadias, cryptorchidism, large kidneys, cystic kidneys.

OTHER: Neonatal hypoglycemia. Birth weight is high, as much as 5.8 kg. Supernumerary nipples, thickened or dark skin. Risk of embryonal tumors. Increased risk of neonatal and early infantile death.

MISCELLANEOUS: The first documented family described the look of its affected members as "bulldog"-like. Glypican 3 seems to form a complex with insulin-like growth factor 2 (IGF2). Interestingly, Beckwith-Wiedemann syndrome, another overgrowth syndrome, seems to be due to excessive IGF2.

ANESTHETIC CONSIDERATIONS
Difficult intubation has not been reported, but is a potential concern in these patients with macroglossia and cervical spine fusion which may limit neck mobility (2). Cardiac conduction abnormalities are common, and careful perioperative monitoring of cardiac rhythm is indicated. Patients with congenital heart disease require perioperative antibiotic prophylaxis as indicated.

Bibliography:
1. Mariani S, Iughetti L, Bertorelli R, et al. Genotype/phenotype correlations of males affected by Simpson-Golabi-Behmel syndrome with GPC3 gene mutations: patient report and review of the literature. *J Pediatr Endocrinol* 2003;16:225–232.
2. Tsuchiya K, Takahata O, Sengoku K, et al. Anesthetic management in a patient with Simpson-Golabi-Behmel syndrome [Japanese]. *Masui* 2001;50:1106–1108.
3. Lin AE, Neri G, Hughes-Benzie R, et al. Cardiac anomalies in the Simpson-Golabi-Behmel syndrome. *Am J Med Genet* 1999;83:378–381.
4. Verloes A, Massart B, Dehalleux I, et al. Clinical overlap of Beckwith-Wiedemann, Perlman and Simpson-Golabi-Behmel syndromes: a diagnostic pitfall. *Clin Genet* 1995;47:257–262.

Sjögren-Larsson Syndrome

MIM #: 270200

This autosomal recessive disorder is due to abnormal function of the enzyme fatty aldehyde dehydrogenase (FALDH). The disorder predominantly affects the skin and nervous system. There is clinical improvement with dietary fat restriction and supplementation with medium-chain triglycerides.

HEENT/AIRWAY: Pigmentary retinal degeneration, yellow-white dots on the retina. Photophobia.

NEUROMUSCULAR: Mental retardation, retardation of motor function, spastic quadriplegia, seizures.

ORTHOPEDIC: Short stature.

OTHER: Congenital ichthyosis, neonatal ecchymoses, hyperkeratosis with normal sweating. Normal hair and nails.

MISCELLANEOUS: This Sjögren is different from the Sjögren of Sjögren syndrome (keratoconjunctivitis sicca).

ANESTHETIC CONSIDERATIONS
Ichthyosis does not predominantly affect the dorsum of the hands and feet, leaving them available for vascular access. Patients with photophobia may be extremely sensitive to the bright lights in operating rooms. Chronic use of anticonvulsant medications may affect the metabolism of some anesthetic drugs.

Bibliography:
1. Willemsen MA, IJlst L, Steijlen PM, et al. Clinical, biochemical and molecular genetic characteristics of 19 patients with the Sjogren-Larsson syndrome. *Brain* 2001;124:1426–1437.
2. Willemsen MA, de Jong JG, van Domburg PH, et al. Sjogren-Larsson syndrome. *J Pediatr* 2000;136:261.

Sly Syndrome

SYNONYM: Mucopolysaccharidosis VII; Beta-glucuronidase deficiency

MIM #: 253220

This autosomal recessive mucopolysaccharidosis, due to a deficiency of the lysosomal enzyme beta-glucuronidase, may be clinically similar to Hurler syndrome, or may be milder (and without mental retardation). There is accumulation of heparan sulfate, keratan sulfate, chondroitin-4-sulfate, and chondroitin-6-sulfate. A neonatal form of Sly syndrome has been reported, with hydrops fetalis, dysostoses, and other findings of a lysosomal storage disease.

HEENT/AIRWAY: Coarse facies. Fine corneal opacities. Recurrent otitis media, conductive hearing loss.

CHEST: Pectus carinatum. Patients with a mucopolysaccharidosis are susceptible to pulmonary hemorrhage after bone marrow transplantation.

CARDIOVASCULAR: Mitral and aortic valve involvement with thickening and insufficiency. Aortic dissection. May have involvement of coronary arteries leading to coronary stenosis. Infiltration of the conduction system and complete heart block in a child with previously normal conduction was related to entry of a guidewire into the right ventricle (3).

NEUROMUSCULAR: Intelligence is usually normal, may have mild mental retardation.

ORTHOPEDIC: Odontoid hypoplasia and an unstable cervical spine have been reported in association with Sly syndrome (1). Short stature. Thoracolumbar gibbus deformity, progressive kyphoscoliosis. Multiple bone dysostoses, joint stiffness. Genu valgum.

GI/GU: Hepatosplenomegaly. Inguinal and umbilical hernias.

MISCELLANEOUS: The longest known survivor with Sly syndrome was 37 years old at the time of her death.

ANESTHETIC CONSIDERATIONS
The cervical spine should be evaluated preoperatively, or one should progress on the assumption of an unstable neck. Difficult laryngoscopy and tracheal intubation have not been reported with Sly syndrome, but have been reported in patients with other mucopolysaccharidoses. The laryngeal mask airway has been used successfully in other patients with mucopolysaccharidoses (1). Perioperative cardiac complications may occur as a result of valvular insufficiency, coronary artery stenosis and/or infiltration of the conducting system (3). Patients with cardiac valve involvement require perioperative antibiotic prophylaxis as indicated. Hemodynamic stability is crucial in patients with aortic dilatation or dissection.

Bibliography:
1. Dickerman RD, Colle KO, Bruno CA Jr, et al. Craniovertebral instability with spinal cord compression in a 17-month-old boy with the Sly syndrome (mucopolysaccharidosis type VII): a surgical dilemma. *Spine* 2004;29:e92–e94.
2. Schwartz I, Silva LR, Leistner S, et al. Mucopolysaccharidosis VII: clinical, biochemical and molecular investigation of a Brazilian family. *Clin Genet* 2003;64:172–175.
3. Toda Y, Tekeuchi M, Morita K, et al. Complete heart block during anesthetic management in a patient with mucopolysaccharidosis type VII. *Anesth Analg* 2001;95:1035–1037.
4. Walker RWM, Allen DL, Rothera MR. A fibreoptic intubation technique for children with mucopolysaccharidoses using the laryngeal mask airway. *Paediatr Anaesth* 1997;7:421–426.
5. Moores C, Rogers JG, McKenzie IM, et al. Anaesthesia for children with mucopolysaccharidoses. *Anaesth Intensive Care* 1996;24:459–463.
6. Walker RWM, Darowski M, Morris P. Anaesthesia and mucopolysaccharidoses: a review of airway problems in children. *Anaesthesia* 1994;49:1078–1084.
7. Diaz JH, Belani K. Perioperative management of children with mucopolysaccharidoses. *Anesth Analg* 1993;77:1261–1270.
8. Mahoney A, Soni N, Vellodi A. Anaesthesia and the mucopolysaccharidoses: a review of patients treated by bone marrow transplantation. *Paediatr Anaesth* 1992;2:317–324.
9. Sjögren P, Pedersen T, Steinmetz H. Mucopolysaccharidoses and anaesthetic risk. *Acta Anaesthesiol Scand* 1987;32:214–218.
10. King DH, Jones RM, Barrett MB. Anaesthetic considerations in the mucopolysaccharidoses. *Anaesthesia* 1984;39:126–131.
11. Kempthorne PM, Brown TCK. Anaesthesia and the mucopolysaccharidoses: a survey of techniques and problems. *Anaesth Intensive Care* 1983;11:203–207.
12. Baines D, Kenneally J. Anaesthetic management of the mucopolysaccharidoses: a fifteen-year experience in a children's hospital. *Anaesth Intensive Care* 1983;11:198–202.

Smith-Lemli-Opitz Syndrome

MIM #: 270400

The etiology of this autosomal recessive syndrome has been ascribed to abnormal function of 7-dehydrocholesterol reductase, an enzyme involved in the biosynthesis of cholesterol. This enzyme is the second-to-last sterol in the Kandutsch-Russell cholesterol biosynthetic pathway. Patients have elevated 7-dehydrocholesterol levels and low cholesterol levels. The main features of the syndrome are mental retardation, anteverted nostrils, ptosis, syndactyly of the second and third toes, and hypospadias and cryptorchidism in boys. Because of the block in cholesterol synthesis, dietary cholesterol might be an essential nutrient, but dietary cholesterol would not be expected to remedy the central nervous system manifestations because of the blood–brain barrier. Cholesterol is a component of some lipoproteins that have significant signaling functions. Some of the manifestations of this syndrome may be secondary to abnormal functioning of these proteins in the embryo. Some have suggested the existence of a type II disease, which includes the most severely affected patients, but it is likely that these patients merely represent the more severe end of a clinical spectrum.

HEENT/AIRWAY: Microcephaly, high, square forehead. Ptosis, epicanthal folds, strabismus, opsoclonus, demyelination of optic nerve, cataracts. Low-set ears. Short nose with anteverted nostrils. Small tongue, broad alveolar ridges, cleft palate. Micrognathia.

CHEST: Pulmonary hypoplasia, single-lobed lungs. Recurrent aspiration, pneumonia. Pneumonia is a leading cause of death.

CARDIOVASCULAR: Congenital heart disease, particularly tetralogy of Fallot and ventricular septal defect.

NEUROMUSCULAR: Moderate to severe mental retardation, variable muscle tone (hypotonic in infancy becoming hypertonic), seizures, demyelination of brain and peripheral nerves, hypoplasia and abnormal morphogenesis of various brain structures. Irritability with shrill screaming during infancy. Behavioral problems, including autism. May have holoprosencephaly.

ORTHOPEDIC: Prenatal growth retardation. Postaxial polydactyly, syndactyly of second and third toes, simian crease, flexed fingers, metatarsus adductus. Dislocated hips.

GI/GU: Feeding problems, vomiting, gastroesophageal reflux, pyloric stenosis, inguinal hernias, hepatic dysfunction, rectal atresia, Hirschsprung disease (see earlier). Hypospadias, cryptorchidism, ambiguity of external male genitalia with micropenis, bifid or hypoplastic scrotum,

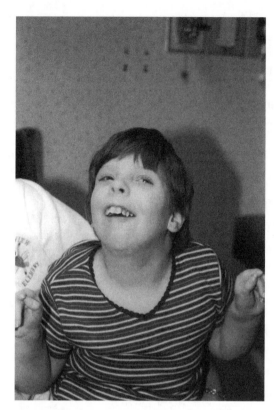

Smith-Lemli-Opitz syndrome. FIG. 1. This 9-year-old with Smith-Lemli-Opitz syndrome is 46 XY, but was born with micropenis and is being raised as a female.

male pseudohermaphroditism, renal hypoplasia, ureteropelvic junction obstruction, renal duplication, hydronephrosis, renal cysts.

OTHER: Failure to thrive. Photosensitivity. Usually have blond hair. May have adrenal insufficiency. Many are born in breech presentation. Stillbirths and early neonatal deaths may occur.

MISCELLANEOUS: Among white North Americans, the incidence of this syndrome places it only behind cystic fibrosis and phenylketonuria. It is probably the first multiple malformation syndrome for which a specific biochemical etiology was ascribed. David Smith was an American pediatrician and a pioneering dysmorphologist. His book, *Recognizable Patterns of Human Malformation,* is a classic reference known to all pediatricians and geneticists.

ANESTHETIC CONSIDERATIONS

Direct laryngoscopy and tracheal intubation may be difficult secondary to micrognathia and dysmorphic facial features. Fiberoptic intubation has been used as the initial technique for airway management in a number of anesthetics (5). The laryngeal mask airway (LMA) has also been used successfully to establish an airway (1, 3). Behavioral problems, particularly aggressive behavior, may complicate induction and postoperative care (5). Sedative medications

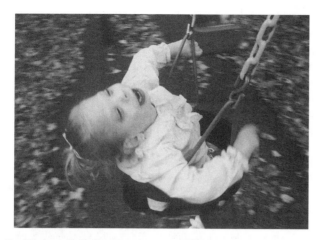

Smith-Lemli-Opitz syndrome. FIG. 2. A 6-year-old girl with Smith-Lemli-Opitz syndrome. She has many findings including a small mandible, crowded teeth, microcephaly, and bifid uvula. Her trachea had been intubated successfully, but it had been suggested to her parents that in the future a fiberoptic intubation be done with a smaller-than-normal endotracheal tube.

may be ineffectual (7). Consider preoperative evaluation of renal function in patients with a history of renal abnormalities which predispose to renal insufficiency. Vomiting and gastroesophageal reflux are common, and patients are at increased risk for perioperative aspiration. They may have chronic lung disease secondary to recurrent aspiration and pneumonia. Patients with congenital heart disease require perioperative antibiotic prophylaxis as indicated. Sensitivity to gender issues in intersex patients is important, although these patients may not have sufficient intellectual development to appreciate the issues.

Although there are two case reports of increased muscle rigidity after a volatile anesthetic (one with and one without succinylcholine) (9, 11), it is unlikely that this is a systematic response of patients with this syndrome or that this syndrome is associated with malignant hyperthermia (5, 8).

Bibliography:

1. Matveevskii A, Berman L, Sidi A, et al. Airway management of patient with Smith-Lemli-Opitz syndrome for gastric surgery: case report. *Paediatr Anaesth* 2006;16:322–324.
2. Goldenberg A, Wolf C, Chevy F, et al. Antenatal manifestations of Smith-Lemli-Opitz (RSH) syndrome: a retrospective survey of 30 cases. *Am J Med Genet A* 2004;124:423–426.
3. Sudou K, Shirotori T, Ichino T, et al. Anesthetic management of a patient with Smith-Lemli-Opitz syndrome complicated with thrombocytopenia [Japanese]. *Masui* 2003;52:1240–1242.
4. Jira PE, Waterham HR, Wanders RJ, et al. Smith-Lemli-Opitz syndrome and the DHCR7 gene. *Ann Hum Genet* 2003;67:269–280.
5. Quezado ZM, Veihmeyer J, Schwartz L, et al. Anesthesia and airway management of pediatric patients with Smith-Lemli-Opitz syndrome. *Anesthesiology* 2002;97:1015–1019.
6. Choi PT-L, Nowaczyk MJM. Anesthetic considerations in Smith-Lemli-Opitz syndrome. *Can J Anaesth* 2000;47:556–561.
7. Ryan AK, Bartlett K, Clayton P, et al. Smith-Lemli-Opitz syndrome: a variable clinical and biochemical phenotype. *J Med Genet* 1998;35:558–565.
8. Haji-Michael PG, Hatch DL. Smith-Lemli-Opitz syndrome and malignant hyperthermia [Letter]. *Anesth Analg* 1996;83:200.
9. Peterson WC, Crouch ER. Anesthesia-induced rigidity, unrelated to succinylcholine, associated with Smith-Lemli-Opitz syndrome and malignant hyperthermia. *Anesth Analg* 1995;80:606–608.
10. Opitz JM, Penchaszadeh VB, Holt MC, et al. Smith-Lemli-Opitz (RSH) syndrome bibliography: 1964–1993. *Am J Med Genet* 1994;50:339–343.
11. Mizushima A, Satoyoshi M. Unusual responses of muscle rigidity and hypothermia to halothane and succinylcholine: a case report of Smith-Lemli-Opitz (SLO) syndrome [Japanese]. *Masui* 1988;37:1118–1123.

Sneddon Syndrome

MIM #: 182410

This noninflammatory arteriopathy of medium-sized arteries is marked by livedo reticularis (a persistent purplish discoloration of the skin caused by blood vessel pathology) and cerebrovascular disease. It is likely inherited in an autosomal dominant fashion.

CARDIOVASCULAR: Multiple occlusion of medium-sized arteries. May be associated with rheumatic or other valvular disease. May have systemic arterial hypertension. May be predisposed to developing venous thrombosis.

NEUROMUSCULAR: Multiple strokes and transient ischemic attacks. Recovery from strokes is often complete. May have mental retardation. May have moyamoya-like pattern (see earlier). Arteriopathy involves meninges, superficial cortical vessels and the periventricular white matter. Headache and vertigo often precede other symptoms by a few years.

GI/GU: May have renal involvement.

OTHER: Livedo reticularis. Some patients have had lupus anticoagulant or antiphospholipid antibody.

MISCELLANEOUS: "Livedo reticularis" is used in the European literature to reflect this cutaneous vascular phenomenon when it disappears with skin warming; and "livedo racemosa" for the findings that persist after warming. American usage refers to "cutis marmorata" for the rash that disappears with warming, and "livedo reticularis" for the permanent change. Sneddon, despite being British, used the term livedo reticularis when describing the permanent skin changes associated with "his" syndrome.

ANESTHETIC CONSIDERATIONS

Note that patients may be on anticoagulant medications. Patients should be evaluated preoperatively for cardiac disease and systemic hypertension. Preoperative renal function should be evaluated. Patients (including children) should be managed perioperatively as if they have cerebrovascular disease, and the use of invasive monitoring may be justified. Chronic use of anticonvulsant medications may affect the metabolism of some anesthetic drugs. Measures should be taken perioperatively to prevent venous thrombosis. Patients with structural heart disease require perioperative antibiotic prophylaxis as indicated.

Bibliography:

1. Szmyrka-Kaczmarek M, Daikeler T, Benz D, et al. Familial inflammatory Sneddon syndrome-case report and review of the literature. *Clin Rheumatol* 2005;24:79–82.
2. Belena JM, Nunez M, Cabeza R, et al. Sneddon syndrome and anaesthesia. *Anaesthesia* 2004;59:622.
3. Hilton DA, Footitt D. Neuropathological findings in Sneddon syndrome. *Neurology* 2003;60:1181–1182.
4. Heesen M, Rossaint R. Anaesthesiological considerations in patients with Sneddon syndrome. *Paediatr Anaesth* 2000;10:678–680.

Sotos Syndrome

SYNONYM: Cerebral gigantism

MIM #: 117550

This disorder is marked by the prenatal onset of excessive growth. Most cases have been sporadic, but it has occurred in identical twins, and other familial cases have also been reported. It can be caused by a mutation in the *NSD1* gene, a coregulator of steroid receptors.

HEENT/AIRWAY: Excessive head growth in early infancy with macrocephaly, dolichocephaly, prominent forehead. Hypertelorism, strabismus, down-slanting palpebral fissures. High-arched palate, exostoses of the alveolar ridge, premature eruption of teeth. Prognathism.

CHEST: Recurrent pulmonary infections in infancy.

CARDIOVASCULAR: A variety of congenital cardiac defects has been reported.

NEUROMUSCULAR: The incidence of mild or borderline mental retardation is high, and children may be hyperactive or aggressive. Neonatal hypotonia. Mild hydrocephalus has been reported. May have seizures.

GU/GU: May have recurrent inguinal hernias.

ORTHOPEDIC: Bone age is advanced. Large hands and feet. Arm span greater than height. Congenital flexion contractures of the feet. Growth is rapid for the first few years of life, but final height may be normal. Kyphoscoliosis is reported, but uncommon.

OTHER: There may be glucose intolerance with increased somatomedin and growth hormone. Hyperthyroidism or hypothyroidism. Early menarche. May have reduced helper T-cells. These patients seem to be at increased risk for the development of a variety of benign and malignant tumors.

ANESTHETIC CONSIDERATIONS

There have been no reports of difficult intubations. A prominent occiput can make head positioning somewhat difficult.

Most children have needed an endotracheal tube sized appropriately for age, but one teenaged male has been reported who required a larger-than-normal tube. The smooth induction of anesthesia may be challenging if the patient exhibits significant behavioral problems. Behavioral expectations should be based on age and not size. Children with congenital cardiac defects require an appropriate anesthetic technique and perioperative antibiotic prophylaxis as indicated.

Bibliography:

1. Tatton-Brown K, Douglas J, Coleman K, et al. Genotype-phenotype associations in Sotos syndrome: an analysis of 266 individuals with NSD1 aberrations. *Am J Hum Genet* 2005;77:193–204.
2. Adhami EJ, Cancio-Babu CV. Anaesthesia in a child with Sotos syndrome. *Paediatr Anaesth* 2003;13:835–840.
3. Varvinski A, McGill FJ, Judd V, et al. Sotos' syndrome . . . a rare challenge? *Anaesthesia* 2001;56:809.
4. Mauceri L, Sorge G, Baieli S, et al. Aggressive behavior in patients with Sotos syndrome. *Pediatr Neurol* 2000;22:64–67.
5. Suresh D. Posterior spinal fusion in Sotos' syndrome. *Br J Anaesth* 1991;66:728–732.
6. Jones D, Doughty L, Brown K. Anaesthesia for a patient with Sotos syndrome [Letter]. *Anaesth Intensive Care* 1991;19:298–299.

Spherocytosis

See Hereditary spherocytosis

Spielmeyer-Vogt Disease

SYNONYM: Batten disease; Ceroid lipofuscinosis; Vogt-Spielmeyer disease

MIM #: 204200

This autosomal recessive disorder is one of several lipofuscinoses, which are lysosomal disorders with profound central nervous system degeneration secondary to lipofuscin accumulation in the brain. Others include Jansky-Bielschowsky disease (see earlier) and Santavuori-Haltia and Kuf disease (not described in text). Spielmeyer-Vogt disease is due to a mutation in the *CLN3* gene. Its product is a lysosomal enzyme, and its absence results in accelerated apoptosis of photoreceptors and neurons. Onset of symptoms is at about 4 to 10 years of age, and death is between 20 and 40 years of age.

HEENT/AIRWAY: Progressive visual loss with blindness by 6 to 14 years of age. Retinitis pigmentosa, macular degeneration, optic atrophy, abolished electroretinogram.

NEUROMUSCULAR: Psychomotor regression, mental retardation, dementia, extrapyramidal signs, cerebellar signs, seizures, dysarthria, cerebral atrophy. Behavioral changes. Lipofuscin accumulation in neuronal perikaryon.

OTHER: Vacuolated lymphocytes. Autonomic dysregulation, including abnormal thermal regulation.

ANESTHETIC CONSIDERATIONS

When meeting patients, recall that they are likely to be blind. Patients may be bedridden with muscle atrophy, so the use of succinylcholine may be associated with exaggerated hyperkalemia, although it has been used without incident in one patient (1). Autonomic dysregulation is common. Perioperative hypothermia can result from abnormal thermal regulation (3). Seizures can be difficult to control and can occur perioperatively. Chronic use of anticonvulsant medications may alter the metabolism of some anesthetic drugs.

Bibliography:

1. Gopalakrishnan S, Siddiqui S, Mayhew JF. Anesthesia in a child with Batten disease. *Paediatr Anaesth* 2004;14:890–891.
2. Haltia M. The neuronal ceroid-lipofuscinoses. *J Neuropathol Exp Neurol* 2003;62:1–13.
3. Yamada Y, Doi K, Sakura S, et al. Anesthetic management for a patient with Jansky-Bielschowsky disease. *Can J Anaesth* 2002;49:81–83.
4. Defalque RJ. Anesthesia for a patient with Kuf disease. *Anesthesiology* 1990;73:1041–1042.

Spinal Muscular Atrophy Types I and II

See Werdnig-Hoffmann disease

Spinal Muscular Atrophy Type III

See Kugelberg-Welander disease

Spinocerebellar Ataxia Type 3

See Joseph disease

Spondylocarpotarsal Synostosis Syndrome

MIM #: 272460

This relatively newly delineated, autosomal recessive syndrome involves primarily abnormalities of the hands, feet, and spine. It can be caused by a mutation in the gene encoding filamin B.

HEENT/AIRWAY: Broad, round face. Hypertelorism. May have retinal abnormalities, lens opacification. Sensorineural hearing loss, preauricular skin tags. Short nasal septum and broad nasal bridge. Cleft palate. Enamel hypoplasia.

CHEST: Restrictive lung disease from scoliosis.

ORTHOPEDIC: Short stature with predominantly short trunk. Odontoid hypoplasia. Failure of normal segmentation of thoracic vertebrae resulting in fused, or "block," vertebrae. If asymmetric, this causes progressive scoliosis or lordosis. The fused spine is difficult to identify in early childhood before it is adequately ossified. Synostosis of carpal and tarsal bones. Postaxial polydactyly. Decreased range of motion of elbows. Pes planus.

GI/GU: Inguinal hernias.

ANESTHETIC CONSIDERATIONS

Be sensitive to the fact that patients may have hearing loss. Patients with odontoid hypoplasia may have an unstable cervical spine. Patients with restrictive lung disease secondary to severe scoliosis are at increased risk for perioperative respiratory complications.

Bibliography:

1. Honeywell C, Langer L, Allanson J. Spondylocarpotarsal synostosis with epiphyseal dysplasia. *Am J Med Genet* 2002;109:318–322.
2. Seaver LH, Boyd E. Spondylocarpotarsal synostosis syndrome and cervical instability. *Am J Med Genet* 2000;91:340–344.

Spondyloepiphyseal Dysplasia Congenita

MIM #: 183900

This autosomal dominant dwarfing syndrome primarily involves the vertebral column and the epiphyses of long bones. Spondyloepiphyseal dysplasia congenita is due to a defect in the gene *COL2A1,* which encodes type II collagen. A variety of specific mutations have been described. Mutations in the *COL2A1* gene are also responsible for achondrogenesis, Kniest syndrome, and Stickler syndrome.

HEENT/AIRWAY: Normocephalic. Flat facies, malar hypoplasia. Myopia and retinal detachment. Sensorineural hearing loss has been reported. Occasional cleft lip. Cleft palate. Short neck with limited flexion.

CHEST: Restrictive lung disease from kyphoscoliosis. Pectus carinatum.

NEUROMUSCULAR: Hypotonia, weakness.

ORTHOPEDIC: Growth deficiency of prenatal onset. Odontoid hypoplasia with atlantoaxial or other cervical instability. Thoracic kyphoscoliosis and lumbar lordosis. Narrowed intervertebral disc spaces. Diminished mobility of elbows, knees, and hips. May have diaphyseal pseudoarthrosis-like lesions. Coxa vara, dislocated hips. Lack of ossification of os pubis, proximal femur, and proximal tibia. Clubfoot deformity.

GI/GU: Hypoplasia of abdominal muscles, abdominal and inguinal hernias.

OTHER: The small pelvis will require Caesarean section for delivery.

MISCELLANEOUS: While researching the lineage of an affected family he had identified at the Mayo Clinic, Stickler

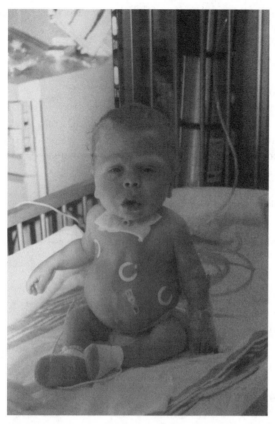

Spondyloepiphyseal dysplasia congenita. This young boy with spondyloepiphyseal dysplasia congenita was previously misdiagnosed as having hypochondrogenesis. He has required a tracheostomy for laryngotracheobronchomalacia.

discovered that the first affected family member had been seen by Charles Mayo himself nearly 100 years earlier.

ANESTHETIC CONSIDERATIONS

Direct laryngoscopy and tracheal intubation may be difficult secondary to a short neck and limited flexion (4). Patients may have cervical spine instability and there is a risk of cervical spine injury during laryngoscopy in these patients (2, 5, 6, 8). Preoperative flexion/extension radiographs and fiberoptic intubation should be considered (5). Because of their small stature, patients may require a smaller-than-expected endotracheal tube. Patients with restrictive lung disease are at increased risk of perioperative respiratory complications. Limitations in joint mobility may make intraoperative positioning difficult.

Epidural anesthesia (with decreased volume of local anesthetic) has been used successfully for cesarean section (3, 9).

Bibliography:

1. Miyoshi K, Nakamura K, Haga N, et al. Surgical treatment for atlantoaxial subluxation with myelopathy in spondyloepiphyseal dysplasia congenita. *Spine* 2004;29:e488–e491.
2. Tofield CE, Mackinnon CA. Cleft palate repair in spondyloepiphyseal dysplasia congenita: minimizing the risk of cervical cord compression. *Cleft Palate Craniofac J* 2003;40:629–631.
3. de Boer HD, Hemelaar A, van Dongen R, et al. Successful epidural anaesthesia for Caesarean section in a patient with spondyloepiphyseal dysplasia. *Br J Anaesth* 2001;86:133–134.
4. Watanabe N, Fukano N, Tamura M, et al. Anesthetic management for a patient with spondyloepiphyseal dysplasia congenital [Japanese]. *Masui* 2000;49:62–65.
5. Redl G. Massive pyramidal tract signs after endotracheal intubation: a case report of spondyloepiphyseal dysplasia congenita. *Anesthesiology* 1998;89:1262–1264.
6. Nakamura K, Miyoshi K, Haga N, et al. Risk factors of myelopathy at the atlantoaxial level in spondyloepiphyseal dysplasia congenita. *Arch Orthop Trauma Surg* 1998;117:468–470.
7. Mogera C, Muralidhar V. Spondyloepiphyseal dysplasia congenita syndrome: anesthetic implications. *Anesth Analg* 1996;83:433–434.
8. Reardon W, Hall CM, Shaw DG, et al. New autosomal dominant form of spondyloepiphyseal dysplasia presenting with atlanto-axial instability. *Am J Med Genet* 1994;52:432–437.
9. Rodney GE, Calander CC, Harmer M. Spondyloepiphyseal dysplasia congenita. *Anaesthesia* 1991;46:648–650.
10. Berkowitz ID, Raja SN, Bender KS, et al. Dwarfs: pathophysiology and anesthetic implications. *Anesthesiology* 1990;73:739–759.

Spondyloepiphyseal Dysplasia Tarda

MIM #: 184100, 313400

This form of short-trunk dwarfism is inherited in an autosomal dominant or X-linked fashion. The gene and gene product responsible for the autosomal dominant form are not known, but the disorder is not due to a defect in the type II collagen gene, which is responsible for spondyloepiphyseal dysplasia congenita. The X-linked form of spondyloepiphyseal dysplasia tarda has recently been mapped to Xp22. Patients with spondyloepiphyseal dysplasia tarda are radiographically and clinically normal at birth, with degenerative changes becoming apparent in the second decade of life.

HEENT/AIRWAY: Normocephalic, flattened facies. Short neck.

CHEST: Pectus carinatum.

ORTHOPEDIC: Short-trunk dwarfism. Odontoid hypoplasia occurs, but less frequently than in other dwarfism syndromes. Cervical subluxation. Cervical spine problems may worsen with age. Flattened, dysplastic vertebral bodies. Kyphoscoliosis, lumbar lordosis. Mild scoliosis. Extremities are shortened in proportion to the trunk. Degenerative changes in the femoral head. Eventually develop painful, stiff hips, shoulders, and cervical and lumbar spine. Arthritis often becomes disabling by late adulthood. Hip replacement often needed by 40 years of age.

GI/GU: Nephrotic syndrome has been reported in one family.

ANESTHETIC CONSIDERATIONS

Patients with odontoid hypoplasia may have an unstable cervical spine. Preoperative flexion/extension radiographs and fiberoptic intubation should be considered. Difficulty with intubation has not been reported, but is a concern given the cervical spine disease. Spine and joint disease may make prolonged positioning on the operating table uncomfortable.

Bibliography:

1. Savarirayan R, Thompson E, Gecz J. Spondyloepiphyseal dysplasia tarda (SEDL, MIM # 313400). *Eur J Hum Genet* 2003;11:639–642.
2. Whyte MP, Gottesman GS, Eddy MC, et al. X-linked recessive spondyloepiphyseal dysplasia tarda: clinical and radiographic evolution in a 6-generation kindred and review of the literature. *Medicine (Baltimore)* 1999;78:9–25.
3. Lama G, Marrone N, Majorana M, et al. Spondyloepiphyseal dysplasia tarda and nephrotic syndrome in three siblings. *Pediatr Nephrol* 1995;9: 19–23.
4. Berkowitz ID, Raja SN, Bender KS, et al. Dwarfs: pathophysiology and anesthetic implications. *Anesthesiology* 1990;73:739–759.

Spondylometaphyseal Dysplasia

SYNONYM: Kozlowski spondylometaphyseal dysplasia

MIM #: 184252

The main features of this autosomal dominant disorder are progressive short-trunk (short spine) dwarfism, irregular metaphyses, and pectus carinatum. At least seven subtypes of spondylometaphyseal dysplasia have been described, primarily based on radiographic differences. The Kozlowski type is the most common. All of the spondylometaphyseal dysplasias affect both the spine ("spondylo") and the metaphyses of the long bones.

HEENT/AIRWAY: Short neck. May have ophthalmologic abnormality.

CHEST: Pectus carinatum. Restrictive lung disease from kyphoscoliosis and diminished functional residual capacity from body habitus.

ORTHOPEDIC: Short stature, primarily due to a short trunk (short spine). Kyphoscoliosis. Odontoid hypoplasia with atlantoaxial instability. Irregular metaphyses, particularly in the long bones. Limited joint mobility by approximately 18 months of age. Contracted pelvis, coxa vara. Anterior narrowing of the thoracolumbar vertebrae on lateral radiographs.

ANESTHETIC CONSIDERATIONS
Patients may have atlantoaxial instability secondary to odontoid hypoplasia. Because of growth deficiency, patients may require a smaller-than-expected endotracheal tube, that also is not inserted as deeply as in normal adults. Patients must be carefully positioned secondary to limited joint mobility.

Bibliography:

1. Kozlowski K, Poon CC. Distinctive spondylometaphyseal dysplasia in two siblings. *Am J Med Genet A* 2003;116:304–309.
2. Nores JM, Dizien O, Remy JM, et al. Two cases of spondylometaphyseal dysplasia: literature review and discussion of the genetic inheritance of the disease. *J Rheumatol* 1993;20:170–172.

3. Berkowitz ID, Raja SN, Bender KS, et al. Dwarfs: pathophysiology and anesthetic implications. *Anesthesiology* 1990;73:739–759.
4. Benson KT, Dozier NJ, Coto H, et al. Anesthesia for cesarean section in patient with spondylometaphyseal dysplasia. *Anesthesiology* 1985;63:548–550.

Spondylothoracic Dysplasia

See Jarcho-Levin syndrome

Stargardt Disease

SYNONYM: Juvenile macular degeneration

MIM #: 248200

Stargardt disease is an autosomal recessive disorder associated with macular degeneration. The disease involves the accumulation of lipofuscin in the retinal epithelium. It is due to a mutation in the gene *ABCA4*, which encodes an ATP-binding cassette protein. This protein is a "flippase." It catalyzes a $180°$ rotation of a specific phospholipid and simultaneously moves it from the inner to the outer phospholipid bilayer. This protein is expressed in (at least) blue rod photoreceptors. This class of proteins is involved in the energy-dependent transfer of a wide variety of substrates across membranes.

HEENT/AIRWAY: Loss of central vision that is slowly progressive. Peripheral vision remains intact. Slow dark adaptation. There may be "pisciform" lesions seen throughout the fundus. The foveal reflex is absent or grayish, and there may eventually be depigmentation and chorioretinal atrophy of the macula. The degree of vision loss parallels the degree of macular involvement.

MISCELLANEOUS: This disease is also known as "fundus flavimaculatus," which historically has been used to refer to a disease with more pronounced peripheral involvement, whereas "Stargardt disease" has been used to refer to a disease with more pronounced macular involvement. They are currently thought to represent different parts of the spectrum of the same disease process.

ANESTHETIC CONSIDERATIONS
When meeting the patients preoperatively, recall that they may have significant vision loss.

Bibliography:

1. Oh KT, Weleber RG, Stone EM, et al. Electroretinographic findings in patients with Stargardt disease and fundus flavimaculatus. *Retina* 2004;24:920–928.
2. Rotenstreich Y, Fishman GA, Anderson RJ. Visual acuity loss and clinical observations in a large series of patients with Stargardt disease. *Ophthalmology* 2003;110:1151–1158.
3. Lois N, Holder GE, Bunce C, et al. Phenotypic subtypes of Stargardt macular dystrophy-fundus flavimaculatus. *Arch Ophthalmol* 2001;119:359–369.

Steinert Disease

See Myotonic dystrophy

Stickler Syndrome

MIM #: 108300

This autosomal dominant disorder exhibits extensive clinical variability. It was originally described as an arthroophthalmopathy. It is due to mutations in the gene *COL2A1,* which encodes type II collagen, a major component of cartilage, vitreous, and nucleus pulposus, all of which may be involved. These patients may also have associated Pierre Robin syndrome (see earlier). Mutations in the *COL2A1* gene are also responsible for achondrogenesis, Kniest syndrome, and spondyloepiphyseal dysplasia congenita (see earlier).

A second form of Stickler syndrome (type II) is due to a mutation in the gene *COL11A1.* A third form of Stickler syndrome (type III) is due to a mutation in the gene *COL11A2.* Type III Stickler syndrome does not include ocular abnormalities.

HEENT/AIRWAY: Flat facies. Epicanthal folds, myopia, dislocated lens, glaucoma, chorioretinal degeneration, retinal

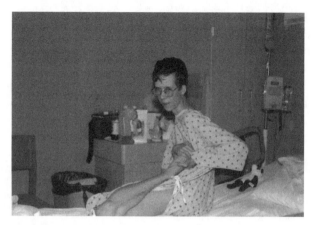

Stickler syndrome. FIG. 2. Additional demonstration of hyperextensible joints.

detachment, vision loss, cataracts. Sensorineural and conductive hearing loss. Anteverted nares, flat nasal bridge. Cleft palate, tooth anomalies. Stickler syndrome is a common cause of Pierre Robin syndrome (see earlier).

CHEST: Pectus excavatum.

CARDIOVASCULAR: Mitral valve prolapse.

NEUROMUSCULAR: Normal intelligence. Hypotonia.

ORTHOPEDIC: Marfanoid habitus. Hyperextensible joints, joint pains, arachnodactyly. Short stature, narrow long bones, abnormal leg epiphyses. Scoliosis, kyphosis, lumbar lordosis. Herniation of thoracic discs, flat vertebrae. Pes planus, genu valgus, hip subluxation, Legg-Calvé-Perthes disease (see earlier), clubfoot deformity. Arthritis in adulthood. May require total hip replacement in adulthood.

MISCELLANEOUS: This disorder has been suggested as a possible diagnosis for President Abraham Lincoln and his son Tad.

ANESTHETIC CONSIDERATIONS

Direct laryngoscopy and tracheal intubation may be very difficult in patients with a small mandible. Recall that patients may have vision loss. Some patients may have hearing loss. Patients must be carefully positioned intraoperatively secondary to joint laxity. Patients with mitral valve prolapse and insufficiency require perioperative antibiotic prophylaxis as indicated.

Bibliography:

1. Rose PS, Levy HP, Liberfarb RM, et al. Stickler syndrome: clinical characteristics and diagnostic criteria. *Am J Med Genet A* 2005;138:199–207.
2. Ahmad N, Richards AJ, Murfett HC, et al. Prevalence of mitral valve prolapse in Stickler syndrome. *Am J Med Genet A* 2003;116:234–237.
3. Stickler GB, Hughes W, Houchin P. Clinical features of hereditary progressive arthroophthalmopathy (Stickler syndrome): a survey. *Genet Med* 2001;3:192–196.

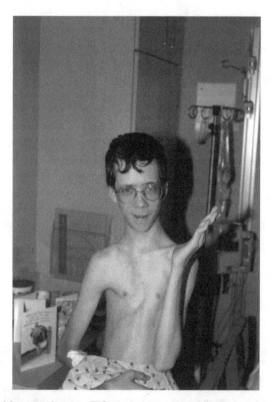

Stickler syndrome. FIG. 1. Hyperextensible joints in a 16-year-old boy with Stickler syndrome. He has had repair of pectus excavatum, and has a small mandible, a high-arched palate, mitral valve prolapse, and noncardiac chest pain.

4. Perkins JA, Sie KC, Milczuk H, et al. Airway management in children with craniofacial anomalies. *Cleft Palate Craniofac J* 1997;34:135–140.

Stiff-Baby Syndrome

SYNONYM: Hyperexplexia (hyperekplexia); Kok disease

MIM #: 149400

This autosomal dominant syndrome is due to a defect in the gene encoding the alpha₁ subunit of the glycine receptor. It is characterized by marked muscle rigidity immediately after birth, and an abnormal startle response. A mutation in the gene encoding the beta subunit of the glycine receptor has been implicated in the cause of an autosomal recessive form of stiff-baby syndrome.

NEUROMUSCULAR: There is flexion hypertonia while awake which resolves with sleep. There is an exaggerated startle response. This exaggerated startle response is sometimes accompanied by a generalized hypertonic response causing the patient to fall down. Muscle rigidity persists during infancy but gradually resolves during the first few years of life. Myoclonic jerks while asleep. The electromyogram shows continuous muscle activity even when resting quietly. Nerve conduction is normal. The hypertonic responses can be controlled with valproic acid or 5-hydroxytryptophan.

ORTHOPEDIC: Congenital hip dislocation.

GI/GU: Infants may have choking, vomiting, and dysphagia, which has been fatal. Inguinal and umbilical hernias.

MISCELLANEOUS: The symptoms are similar to those of the "stiff-man" syndrome of adults, which has multiple etiologies. This syndrome probably represents the hereditary form of the stiff-man syndrome.

It is possible, but unlikely, that the interestingly named "Jumping Frenchmen of Maine" syndrome is related. Interest in this latter syndrome inspired Gilles de la Tourette to investigate what later became his eponymous disease.

ANESTHETIC CONSIDERATIONS

One studied infant was relatively resistant to succinylcholine, and did not have an abnormal rise in serum potassium. Responses to pancuronium and neostigmine were normal (4). In another report, however, there was a marked train of four electromyographic fade (57%) following sevoflurane induction and resistance to succinylcholine neuromuscular blockade was not observed (3).

Bibliography:

1. Khasani S, Becker K, Meinck HM. Hyperekplexia and stiff-man syndrome: abnormal brainstem reflexes suggest a physiological relationship. *J Neurol Neurosurg Psychiatry* 2004;75:1265–1269.
2. Praveen V, Patole SK, Whitehall JS. Hyperekplexia in neonates. *Postgrad Med J* 2001;77:570–572.
3. Murphy C, Shorten G. Train of four fade in a child with stiff baby syndrome. *Paediatr Anaesth* 2000;10:567–569.
4. Cook WP, Kaplan RF. Neuromuscular blockade in a patient with stiff-baby syndrome. *Anesthesiology* 1986;65:525–528.

Sturge-Weber Syndrome

MIM #: 185300

The classic findings of this syndrome are capillary or cavernous hemangiomas (port-wine stain, nevus flammeus) in the cutaneous distribution of the trigeminal nerve, angiomas of the meninges of the ipsilateral hemisphere with a seizure disorder and mental retardation, and linear intracranial calcifications. Sturge-Weber syndrome does not appear to be genetic or familial. There are a large number of atypical cases. Patients may have Sturge-Weber syndrome along with manifestations of Klippel-Trenaunay-Weber syndrome (see earlier).

HEENT/AIRWAY: The hallmark finding is a facial port-wine stain, or angioma, in the distribution of the first or second division of the trigeminal nerve. Congenital glaucoma, retinal vessel varicosities, choroid hemangiomas, retinal detachment, optic atrophy. Angiomas can involve the mucous membranes of the lip, tongue, nose, palate, larynx, and trachea. There may be hypertrophy of the bones and soft tissues in the regions immediately adjacent to areas of facial angioma.

CHEST: Vascular abnormalities have been reported in the lung.

CARDIOVASCULAR: High-output heart failure is a rare consequence of shunting through intracranial angiomas. Vessels in the angiomas have an incidence of spontaneous bleeding and have abnormal autoregulation. Patients may be on antiplatelet drugs for recurrent thromboses.

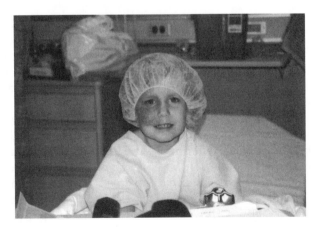

Sturge-Weber syndrome. FIG. 1. This 5-year-old is receiving laser treatment for the port wine stain. She has well-controlled seizures.

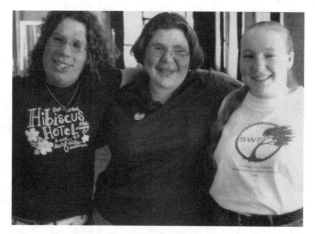

Sturge-Weber syndrome. FIG. 2. Three unrelated teenage girls with the Sturge-Weber syndrome. (Courtesy of The Sturge-Weber Foundation and Rick Guidotti of Positive Exposure.)

A variety of congenital heart defects have been reported in patients with Sturge-Weber syndrome, but it is unclear if this is a part of the syndrome or a chance association.

NEUROMUSCULAR: Vascular changes can be found in the meninges, brain, and pituitary. Leptomeningeal angiomas are ipsilateral to the facial port-wine stain. Many patients have seizures, which can be intractable and lead to mental retardation. Patients can also have hemiatrophy of the brain and hemiplegia. Progressive hemiparesis, focal seizures, and rarely cerebral hemorrhage. The classic radiologic findings are intracranial parallel "tram track" or "railroad track" calcifications, but rarely before 2 years of age. There may also be deep arteriovenous malformations.

GI/GU: Colonic ischemia and hematemesis from gastric bleeding have been reported.

OTHER: Angiomas can also be found on the trunk and extremities.

MISCELLANEOUS: Sturge first described the clinical features of the disease. Weber described the intracranial calcifications 50 years later. F. Parkes Weber was a British physician who had an interest in rare disorders and uncommon syndromes. Weber's father came from Germany to Britain (where he became physician to Queen Victoria), and Weber continued to pronounce his last name with the "W" pronounced as the Germanic "V." He had an encyclopedic knowledge of rare disorders. It is said that when, at a meeting of the Royal Society of Medicine, he first announced that he had not heard of a certain syndrome, such cheers and applause broke out from the audience that the meeting had to be abandoned. He wrote a total of 1,200 medical papers.

Sturge-Weber syndrome is one of the neuroectodermal disorders, or phakomatoses, along with neurofibromatosis, nevus sebaceus syndrome of Jadassohn, tuberous sclerosis, and von Hippel-Lindau syndrome. "Phakos" is Greek for a lentil or lens-shaped spot. It differs from the other phakomatoses by the absence of a cutaneous pigment abnormality, an absence of increased risk for the development of tumors, and lack of heritability.

ANESTHETIC CONSIDERATIONS
Angiomas of the mouth and upper airway may make mask ventilation difficult and may interfere with laryngoscopy and intubation. Rupture of an angioma can result in uncontrolled hemorrhage. Because these vessels have abnormal autoregulation, intraoperative blood pressure should be well controlled.

Scopolamine should be avoided in patients with glaucoma because of its mydriatic effect. Anticholinergic drugs used with anticholinesterases for reversal of neuromuscular blockade are acceptable. Succinylcholine also raises intraocular pressure transiently, but appears to be safe in patients with well controlled intraocular pressure. Succinylcholine is relatively contraindicated in patients with hemiplegia secondary to the risk of exaggerated hyperkalemia. Chronic use of anticonvulsant medications may affect the metabolism of some anesthetic drugs.

Bibliography:
1. Thomas-Sohl KA, Vaslow DF, Maria BL. Sturge-Weber syndrome: a review. *Pediatr Neurol* 2004;30:303–310.
2. Diaz JH. Perioperative management of children with congenital phakomatoses. *Paediatr Anaesth* 2000;10:121–128.
3. Ceyhan A, Cakan T, Basar H, et al. Anaesthesia for Sturge-Weber syndrome. *Eur J Anaesthesiol* 1999;16:339–341.
4. Sujansky E, Conradi S. Outcome of Sturge-Weber syndrome in 52 adults. *Am J Med Genet* 1995;57:35–45.
5. Batra RK, Gulaya V, Madan R, et al. Anaesthesia and the Sturge-Weber syndrome. *Can J Anaesth* 1994;41:133–136.
6. de Leon-Casasola OA, Lema MJ. Anesthesia for patients with Sturge-Weber disease and Klippel-Trenaunay syndrome. *J Clin Anesth* 1991;3:409–413.

Steroid 5α-Reductase 2 Deficiency

See 5α-reductase deficiency

Succinate-Coenzyme Q Reductase Deficiency

See Complex II deficiency

Sugarman Syndrome

Included in Oral-facial-digital syndrome, type I

Sulfite Oxidase Deficiency

Included in Molybdenum cofactor deficiency

Summitt Syndrome

Included in Carpenter syndrome

Swiss-Type Agammaglobulinemia

Included in Severe combined immunodeficiency syndrome

T

Tangier Disease

MIM #: 205400

This autosomal recessive disorder is characterized by a deficiency of high-density lipoproteins (HDL) and storage of cholesterol esters in multiple tissues. This disease is caused by a defect in apolipoprotein A-1. The structural gene for this protein is normal, and the defect is due to a mutation in the ATP-binding cassette-1 gene (*ABCA1* gene) which controls extrusion of the membrane lipid extracellularly. The lipid deposits are extralysosomal within foamy histiocytes. Familial HDL deficiency is due to abnormalities in the same gene, and so is allelic.

HEENT/AIRWAY: Facial diplegia. Ptosis, ocular muscle palsies, diplopia. Corneal infiltration, one fourth have corneal opacifications that do not impair vision. Ectropion and incomplete lid closure can cause eye injury from exposure. Two thirds have enlarged, orange tonsils secondary to cholesterol ester storage.

CARDIOVASCULAR: Can have lipid deposits on mitral and tricuspid valves, and in the pulmonary artery. There is a moderately increased incidence of premature coronary disease, which is further increased in the presence of other risk factors.

NEUROMUSCULAR: There can be one of three neuropathic syndromes: an asymmetric relapsing type that can involve cranial nerves; a symmetric, slowly progressive type primarily involving the lower extremities; and a syringomyelia-like type that is slowly progressive and presents with dissociated sensory and motor loss in the face and arms before extending to the lower extremities. The peripheral neuropathy is due to accumulation of storage material in Schwann cells. There can be muscle wasting. Loss of sensation to heat and pain can cause susceptibility to burns. Abnormalities in proprioception are uncommon.

ORTHOPEDIC: Hand muscle wasting.

GI/GU: Hepatomegaly (with normal function). Splenomegaly with hypersplenism. The rectal mucosa is routinely involved on biopsy. The ileum and colon, but not the jejunum, are also frequently involved, but only approximately 8% have intermittent diarrhea. Asymptomatic focal depositions in renal pelvis, ureter, and tunica albuginea of testes.

OTHER: Hemolytic anemia, thrombocytopenia, and platelet dysfunction have been reported. Circulating stomatocytes. Decreased circulating monocytes. Circulating chylomicronemia even in fasting patients. Deposition in histiocytes causes lymphoid tissue enlargement. Lymph nodes and thymus are also orange from cholesterol ester storage. Hypocholesterolemia and low levels of HDL. Hypertriglyceridemia. Focal depositions in skin.

MISCELLANEOUS: In this case, Tangier refers not to the city in Morocco but to Tangier Island in the Chesapeake Bay, where the first cases were described.

ANESTHETIC CONSIDERATIONS

The hematocrit and platelet count should be evaluated preoperatively in patients with hypersplenism. These patients are at risk for perioperative eye injury secondary to incomplete lid closure, and meticulous perioperative eye care is imperative. Patients can have decreased sensation to pain. Preexisting neuropathic abnormalities might interfere with the evaluation of complications of regional anesthesia. Succinylcholine may be contraindicated in patients with neuropathy and muscle atrophy secondary to the risk of exaggerated hyperkalemia.

Bibliography:
1. Mentis SW. Tangier disease. *Anesth Analg* 1996;83:427–429.
2. Francis GA, Knopp RH, Dram JF. Defective removal of cellular cholesterol and phospholipids by apolipoprotein A-I in Tangier disease. *J Clin Invest* 1995;96:78–87.

TAR Syndrome

See Thrombocytopenia-absent radii syndrome

Tarui Disease

Included in Glycogen storage disease type VII

Taybi Syndrome

See Otopalatodigital syndrome, type I

Tay-Sachs Disease

SYNONYM: GM$_2$ gangliosidosis, type I. (Includes Bernheimer-Seitelberger disease)

MIM #: 272800

Tay-Sachs disease is one of a group of disorders due to defective degradation and abnormal accumulation of GM_2 ganglioside. Defects can occur in the alpha subunit of hexosaminidase (Tay-Sachs disease, deficient hexosaminidase A isoenzyme), the beta subunit of hexosaminidase (Sandhoff disease, deficient hexosaminidase A and B, see earlier), or there can be a defect in the GM_2 activator protein (both isoenzymes are present, but hexosaminidase A is nonfunctional). Depending on the degree of severity of the enzyme deficiency caused by any one specific mutation, the disease can present as an infantile disease (classic Tay-Sachs disease), juvenile GM_2 gangliosidosis (**Bernheimer-Seitelberger disease**), or as adult-onset GM_2 gangliosidosis. However, there is significant clinical variability, and such classification schemes are arbitrary. The juvenile form may represent a compound heterozygote state: one Tay-Sachs gene and another different allelic mutation. In Tay-Sachs disease, accumulation of the GM_2 ganglioside occurs primarily in the lysosomes of neural tissue. The clinical manifestations are primarily neurologic. The disease is classically associated with visualization of a cherry-red spot on the retina. There is no hepatosplenomegaly, as is seen in Sandhoff disease. Death with the juvenile form is typically in the first 2 years of life.

Gangliosides have both a hydrophobic ceramide moiety and a hydrophilic oligosaccharide chain. They are components of the outer cell membrane, with the hydrophobic moiety anchoring it in the membrane and the hydrophilic chain extending into the extracellular space. Although their function is unknown, they have been implicated as binding sites for a variety of viruses, bacterial toxins, growth factors and interferons in the past.

HEENT/AIRWAY

Classic Tay-Sachs: Macrocephaly. The classic cherry-red spot in the area of the macula is normal macula surrounded by areas turned white by storage material. Progression to blindness. Discoordinated swallowing leads to difficulty handling oral secretions. Most require nasogastric or gastrostomy feeding.

Juvenile type: Cherry-red spot not as consistent a finding. Optic atrophy and retinitis pigmentosa. Loss of vision.

Adult type: Vision usually normal.

CHEST: Increased risk of recurrent aspiration. Poor cough. Recurrent infections.

NEUROMUSCULAR

Classic Tay-Sachs: Hypotonia, progressive weakness, psychomotor retardation, exaggerated startle response, eventual spasticity. Seizures. Both upper and lower motor neuron disease. Eventually an unresponsive, vegetative state.

Juvenile type: Similar, but later onset.

Adult type: Spinocerebellar, pyramidal tract, and lower motor neuron disease. Psychosis, particularly hebephrenic schizophrenia, episodic depression. Normal intelligence, which can be masked by severe dysarthria and other motor involvement. Early weakness or tremor. Anterior horn cell dropout and group atrophy.

GI/GU: There is no organomegaly.

MISCELLANEOUS: Warren Tay was a British ophthalmologist (and surgeon, pediatrician, and dermatologist, described as a "walking dictionary") who first described the bilateral cherry-red spots. Bernard "Barney" Sachs was an American neurologist who 6 years later independently described the clinical features of the disease, under the name "familial amaurotic idiocy."

ANESTHETIC CONSIDERATIONS

Difficult airways have not been reported in Tay-Sachs disease. Be aware that patients can have visual limitations. Patients are at increased risk for perioperative aspiration. Chronic use of anticonvulsant medications can affect the metabolism of some anesthetic drugs. Succinylcholine should be avoided in this disease with lower motor neuron involvement and muscle wasting because of the risk of exaggerated hyperkalemia.

Bibliography:
1. Fernandes Filho JA, Shapiro BE. Tay-Sachs disease. *Arch Neurol* 2004;61:1466–1468.
2. Mahoney A, Soni N, Vellodi A. Anaesthesia and the lipidoses: a review of patients treated by bone marrow transplantation. *Paediatr Anaesth* 1992;2:205–209.
3. Wark H, Gold P, Overton J. The airway of patients with a lipid storage disease. *Anaesth Intensive Care* 1984;12:343–344.

Telecanthus-Hypospadias Syndrome

See Hypertelorism-hypospadias syndrome

Tetrahydrobiopterin (BH4) Deficiency

Included in Phenylketonuria

Thalassemia

(Includes Cooley anemia, Hemoglobin H disease, Hemoglobin S-thalassemia)

MIM #: None

The thalassemias are a group of hereditary anemias caused by defective synthesis of either the alpha chain (alpha thalassemias) or beta chain (beta thalassemias) of hemoglobin. Heterozygotes have mild anemia. Homozygotes have severe anemia. The thalassemias represent the most common single gene disorders in the world.

Over 40 thalassemia variants have been described. Unbalanced synthesis of alpha and beta chains leads to unstable hemoglobin and early erythrocyte death, mostly in the marrow. Individuals can inherit the genes both for thalassemia and for a structurally abnormal hemoglobin, or for two different types of thalassemia, making for a diverse clinical presentation. Diseases in which there is no synthesis of the affected chain are noted by a superscript "zero," and those with diminished chain synthesis are noted by a superscript "+" There can be compensatory extramedullary hematopoiesis.

Beta Thalassemias: The heterozygous disease is known as thalassemia minor. The homozygous disease is known as thalassemia major, or **Cooley anemia.** In homozygous disease, unpaired alpha hemoglobin precipitates as inclusion bodies in early red cell precursor cells. These cause the intramedullary destruction of red cells and the ineffective erythropoiesis of this disorder. Excessive globin chains are apparently adequately lysed by proteolytic mechanisms. Severe anemia becomes apparent with the postnatal switch from fetal gamma chain production to beta chain production. Transfusions will decrease the excessive production of alpha hemoglobin, however it carries with it the risks of chronic iron overload.

Alpha Thalassemias: Alpha thalassemias are prevalent in Southeast Asia. There are normally four alpha chain genes, and alpha thalassemia results from the deletion of two or more genes. Absence of two genes is associated with an iron-unresponsive microcytic anemia. Absence of three genes results in **hemoglobin H disease,** a moderately severe anemia resembling thalassemia major (Cooley anemia). In hemoglobin H disease, there is a marked imbalance between alpha chain synthesis (which is reduced) and beta chain synthesis, resulting in the formation of hemoglobin H (four beta chains). In addition, approximately 10% of the total hemoglobin is hemoglobin Barts (four gamma chains). Hemoglobin H precipitates with red blood cell aging, and causes increased splenic uptake. Hemoglobin Barts and hemoglobin H have an increased affinity for oxygen (the oxygen dissociation curve is shifted to the left of normal) and therefore contribute less to oxygen transport. Hemoglobin H disease primarily results in hemolysis, with only mild impairment of erythropoiesis. Absence of all four alpha chain genes results in fetal hydrops; the dominant hemoglobin is hemoglobin Barts (four gamma chains). The altered oxygen dissociation properties of this hemoglobin makes oxygen unavailable to tissues, resulting in fetal demise.

A combination of the genes for sickle cell disease (see earlier) and thalassemia results in a disease more severe than either alone, known as **hemoglobin S-thalassemia.** In this disorder, there is moderately severe microcytic hemolytic anemia in addition to vaso-occlusive crises. On occasion, no hemoglobin A is present (hemoglobin S-beta-thalassemia).

HEENT/AIRWAY: Bone marrow hyperplasia secondary to extramedullary hematopoiesis results in characteristic changes, including frontal bossing, a prominent maxilla, and a relatively sunken nose. "Hair on end" appearance of the skull bones on radiographs.

CARDIOVASCULAR: There can be cardiac involvement from hemosiderosis secondary to chronic hemolysis or repeated transfusions. Cardiac failure, arrhythmias, or conduction disturbances can occur.

ORTHOPEDIC: Progressive bony changes from extramedullary hematopoiesis in thalassemia major. Osteoporosis with pathologic fractures. There is normal hematopoiesis in alpha thalassemias. Hypercoagulability.

GI/GU: Unconjugated hyperbilirubinemia in thalassemia major. Massive splenomegaly and hypersplenism in untransfused or undertransfused thalassemia major. Gallstones. Hemosiderosis from iron loading with chronic transfusions (controllable with chelation therapy). Hypogonadism.

OTHER

Thalassemia Minor: Mild hypochromic, microcytic anemia with hemoglobin levels 2 to 3 g/dL below normal for age. There are target cells, ovalocytes, and basophilic stippling. Hemoglobin A_2 levels are elevated.

Thalassemia Major: Profound anemia requiring chronic blood transfusions. Large numbers of circulating nucleated red blood cells.

Alpha Thalassemias: Hemoglobin synthesis (often hemoglobin H–four beta chains) proceeds at a normal pace in the marrow. There is, however, decreased red blood cell life span because of increased splenic uptake.

Increased risk of bacterial infections in all severe forms.

ANESTHETIC CONSIDERATIONS

The hematocrit must be evaluated preoperatively. Nucleated red blood cells can artifactually elevate the white blood cell count by automated methods. A thorough preoperative cardiac evaluation is indicated in patients who can have cardiac involvement from hemosiderosis (secondary to chronic hemolysis or repeated transfusions). The changes in facial bones from marrow hyperplasia have been reported to cause difficulties in visualizing the vocal cords. Elevated lactate dehydrogenase levels reflect the ineffective hematopoiesis. Splenomegaly may result in thrombocytopenia. Patients who have had a splenectomy can be at increased risk of infection with encapsulated organisms.

Infections and oxidant drugs can precipitate hemolysis in hemoglobin H disease. Anesthetic-related oxidant drugs include prilocaine, nitroprusside, sulfonamides, penicillin, vitamin K, and aspirin. Hemoglobin H precipitates with prolonged exposure to temperatures at or below 4°C, but there have been no reported problems with cold cardioplegia (5).

There is a single report of use of a cell saver in a patient with beta thalassemia. Although apparently successful, excessive hemolysis was noted and additional wash volume was required (3). Red blood cells do not show increased fragility during cardiopulmonary bypass.

Bibliography:
1. Rund D, Rachmilewitz E. β-thalassemia. *N Engl J Med* 2005;353: 1135–1146.
2. Venugopal K, Nair SG, Rao SG. Tetralogy of Fallot in a patient with β-thalassemia major. *J Cardiothorac Vasc Anesth* 2005;19:93–96.
3. Waters JH, Lukauskiene E, Anderson ME. Intraoperative blood salvage during cesarean delivery in a patient with β-thalassemia intermedia. *Anesth Analg* 2003;97:1808–1809.
4. Drew SJ, Sachs SA. Management of the thalassemia-induced skeletal facial deformity: case reports and review of the literature. *J Oral Maxillofac Surg* 1997;55:1331–1339.
5. Piomelli S. Recent advances in the management of thalassemia. *Curr Opin Hematol* 1995;2:159–163.
6. Rowbottom SJ, Sudhaman DA. Haemoglobin H disease and cardiac surgery. *Anaesthesia* 1988;43:1033–1034.

Thomsen Disease

See Myotonia congenita

Thoracic-Pelvic-Phalangeal Dystrophy

See Jeune syndrome

Thoracoabdominal Syndrome

See Pentalogy of Cantrell

Thrombocytopenia-Absent Radii Syndrome

SYNONYM: TAR syndrome

MIM #: 274000

This autosomal recessive disorder is distinct from the somewhat similar Fanconi anemia (see earlier). It may be allelic to pseudothalidomide syndrome (see earlier). Thrombocytopenia is worst in infancy, and can be precipitated by viral illness. Adults usually have no problems except menorrhagia. The responsible gene and gene product are not known.

HEENT/AIRWAY: Port-wine stain of forehead. Strabismus, ptosis. Small, upturned nose. Epistaxis. Can have micrognathia.

CARDIOVASCULAR: Congenital heart disease, most commonly tetralogy of Fallot, coarctation or atrial septal defect.

NEUROMUSCULAR: Can have sequelae of intracranial hemorrhage. Can have hypoplastic arm or shoulder musculature.

ORTHOPEDIC: All have bilateral absence of radii. Hypoplasia or unilateral or bilateral absence of ulnae. Despite radial abnormality, thumb always present. Abnormal humerus or shoulder. Dislocated hips, subluxation of knees, coxa valga, dislocated patella, femoral and tibial torsion, ankylosis of knee, small feet, abnormal toe placement, edema of the dorsum of the foot. Small stature. Arthritis of ankles and knees.

GI/GU: Pancreatic cysts, Meckel's diverticulum, hepatosplenomegaly. Renal anomalies including malrotation of the kidney.

OTHER: Thrombocytopenia at birth with diminished or absent megakaryocytes, eosinophilia, anemia, hypogammaglobulinemia. Dermatitis, excessive sweating. Cow's milk allergy is common and can precipitate thrombocytopenia, eosinophilia, or leukemoid reaction. Rare acute leukemia.

ANESTHETIC CONSIDERATIONS
The platelet count and hematocrit must be evaluated preoperatively. Patients may require perioperative platelet transfusions. Nasotracheal and nasogastric tubes are relatively contraindicated secondary to the risk of epistaxis. Limb anomalies may make vascular access more challenging, and might require careful positioning. Patients with congenital heart disease require perioperative antibiotic prophylaxis as indicated.

Bibliography:
1. Greenhalgh KL, Howell RT, Bottani A, et al. Thrombocytopenia-absent radius syndrome: a clinical genetic study. *J Med Genet* 2002;39:876–881.
2. Hall JG. Thrombocytopenia and absent radius (TAR) syndrome. *J Med Genet* 1987;24:79–83.

Thurston Syndrome

Included in Oral-facial-digital syndrome, type I

Tibial-Aplasia-Ectrodactyly Syndrome

MIM #: 119100

This is an autosomal dominant disorder with wide clinical variability. The responsible gene and gene product are unknown. The disorder has as its principal manifestations ectrodactyly ("lobster claw" deformity of the hand) and absence of the long bones of the arms and legs.

HEENT/AIRWAY: Cup-shaped ears.

CHEST: Bifid xiphoid.

ORTHOPEDIC: Ectrodactyly of the hand ("lobster claw" or "split" hand), also of the feet. Proximally placed thumbs, absent middle finger, syndactyly. Absence of fingers, tarsals, metatarsals, and toes. Extra preaxial digit. Absence of long bones of extremities, most commonly tibial aplasia or hypoplasia, also fibular or femoral aplasia or hypoplasia, and aplasia of radius, ulna, or humerus.

MISCELLANEOUS: A patient with this syndrome was described by Ambroise Paré, the great surgeon, in 1575.

ANESTHETIC CONSIDERATIONS

Limb abnormalities can complicate vascular access, particularly in infants.

Bibliography:
1. Hoyme HE, Jones KL, Nyhan WL, et al. Autosomal dominant ectrodactyly and absence of long bones of upper or lower limbs: further clinical delineation. *J Pediatr* 1987;111:538–543.

Toriello-Carey Syndrome

MIM #: 217980

The inheritance pattern for this dysmorphic syndrome remains uncertain. It is likely autosomal recessive, and the responsible gene and gene product are not currently known. It may represent a syndrome of midline structures. Death in early infancy can occur.

HEENT/AIRWAY: Telecanthus, short palpebral fissures. Abnormally shaped ears. Small nose with anteverted nostrils. Pierre Robin sequence, micrognathia, cleft palate. Laryngeal abnormalities. Redundant neck skin.

CARDIOVASCULAR: Congenital cardiac disease.

NEUROMUSCULAR: Agenesis of the corpus callosum. Hypotonia. Developmental delay.

ORTHOPEDIC: Short hands.

GI/GU: Anteriorly placed anus has been reported, as has a case with gastrointestinal dysmotility.

OTHER: Postnatal growth retardation.

ANESTHETIC CONSIDERATIONS

Laryngoscopy and intubation can be extremely difficult in these patients with (sometimes severe) micrognathia and laryngeal abnormalities. Patients with congenital cardiac disease will require appropriate antibiotic prophylaxis.

Bibliography:
1. Toriello HV, Carey JC, Addor MC, et al. Toriello-Carey syndrome: delineation and review. *Am J Med Genet A* 2003;123:84–90.
2. Auden SM. Additional techniques for managing the difficult airway. *Anesth Analg* 2000;90:878–880.

Tourette Syndrome

SYNONYM: Gilles de la Tourette syndrome

MIM #: 137580

This neurologic condition, occurring primarily in male patients, is characterized by motor and vocal tics with behavioral abnormalities. Onset is usually between 2 to 14 years of age, and about 10% of cases are familial. It is likely that the disease is mild in many people and does not come to medical attention. In 1885, de la Tourette noted that there were mildly affected family members of classically affected patients. The disorder can be due to mutations in the gene *SLITRK1*. It is thought that the underlying defect might be related to an abnormality of the dopaminergic system with disinhibition of the limbic system. This condition is most frequently treated with haloperidol and dopamine antagonists.

NEUROMUSCULAR: The disease begins with involuntary tic-like movements. These can include blinking, facial grimaces, shoulder shrugging, and head jerking. There can be complex sequences of coordinated motions, including bizarre gait, jumping, kicking, body gyrations, and seductive or obscene gestures. The tics wax and wane, and there is an irresistible urge before the tics, followed by relief after it. They may be temporarily suppressed. With progression there may be echolalia, grunting, coprolalia (verbalized obscenities), palilalia (repetition of a word or phrase more and more rapidly), and self-mutilation with aggressive or obsessive-compulsive behavior. Boys usually have more motor and vocal symptoms, whereas girls tend to have more obsessive-compulsive behavioral manifestations. A significant number of patients also have sleep disorders, and tics can occur during sleep. Sleep disorders include restlessness, insomnia, enuresis, sleep-walking, nightmares, and bruxism.

MISCELLANEOUS: Coprolalia, although the most noted symptom in the popular media, is relatively uncommon (approximately 8% of patients). It has been suggested that Samuel Johnson, the lexicographer, had Tourette syndrome. It has also been suggested that Mozart had Tourette syndrome, which would explain his predilection for cursing and his interest in nonsense words.

De la Tourette, a French neurologist, never saw the first patient he described (4). His interest in the area was raised by international interest in Beard's report of the Jumping Frenchmen of Maine. The first Tourette patient, the Marquise de Dampierre, was 26 years of age when she was reported by Itard in 1825 ("the case of the cursing marquise"). In 1885, de la Tourette selected her case as the paradigm of the syndrome. The syndrome was immediately named in honor of Tourette by his boss and mentor, the preeminent French neurologist of his day, Charcot, who was categorizing neurologic syndromes. De la Tourette differentiated this disorder from Sydenham and other choreas. Charcot preferred the euphonious eponym "Gilles de la Tourette syndrome," over using the last name only. Late in his career, de la Tourette was shot in the head in his consulting room by a distraught patient. Subsequently his behavior became increasingly erratic and he was confined to a mental hospital, where he died in 1904.

ANESTHETIC CONSIDERATIONS

The fear of losing control when confronted with a stressful situation (anesthesia and surgery) is of concern to many patients and their families. Time needs to be taken to discuss the anesthetic experience with patients, allow them to convey their specific concerns, and assure them that the anesthesia and operating teams are not uncomfortable with the patient's condition and are willing to tailor their approach to the patient's specific concerns. Midazolam has been reported to inhibit tics (1).

Bibliography:

1. Yoshikawa F, Takagi T, Fukayama H, et al. Intravenous sedation and general anesthesia for a patient with Gilles de la Tourette's syndrome undergoing dental treatment. *Acta Anaesthesiol Scand* 2002;46: 1279–1280.
2. Leckman JF. Tourette's syndrome. *Lancet* 2002;360:1577–1586.
3. Jankovic J. Tourette's syndrome. *N Engl J Med* 2001;345:1184–1192.
4. Kushner HI. Medical fictions: the case of the cursing Marquise and the (re)construction of Gilles de la Tourette's syndrome. *Bull Hist Med* 1995;69:225–254.
5. Morrison JE, Lockhart CH. Tourette syndrome: anesthetic complications. *Anesth Analg* 1986;65:200–202.
6. Critchley M. What's in a name? *Rev Neurol* 1986;142:865–866.

Townes-Brocks Syndrome

MIM #: 107480

This autosomal dominant dysmorphic syndrome is due to an abnormality of the *SALL1* gene, which encodes a transcription factor. There is significant clinical variability. Primary manifestations involve the external ear, the digits and the anus.

HEENT/AIRWAY: Microcephaly. External ear anomalies, occasional deafness.

CARDIOVASCULAR: Cardiac defects.

NEUROMUSCULAR: Occasional mental retardation.

ORTHOPEDIC: Hypoplastic, broad, bifid thumbs or triphalangeal thumbs. Preaxial polydactyly. Fusion of hand bones. Absent or hypoplastic third toe. Clinodactyly of fifth finger. Syndactyly of fingers and toes.

GI/GU: Stenotic, imperforate, or malplaced anus. Rectovaginal or rectoperineal fistula. Duodenal atresia. Renal hypoplasia, urethral valves, vesicoureteral reflux, hypospadias.

MISCELLANEOUS: In at least one species, and probably more, the homologous gene is regulated by the gene *sonic hedgehog.*

ANESTHETIC CONSIDERATIONS

Baseline renal function should be assessed. Hand abnormalities may complicate vascular access. Patients with cardiac defects require perioperative antibiotic prophylaxis as indicated.

Bibliography:

1. Powell CM, Michaelis RC. Townes-Brocks syndrome. *J Med Genet* 1999;36:89–93.
2. Newman WG, Brunet MD, Donnai D. Townes-Brocks syndrome presenting as end stage renal failure. *Clin Dysmorphol* 1997;6:57–60.

Transcobalamin II Deficiency

MIM #: 275350

Transcobalamin II is the major plasma transport protein for vitamin B_{12}. Its absence results in early and severe megaloblastic anemia. This autosomal recessive disease is due to a defect in the gene *TCN2* (*TC2*). There are several alleles. Transcobalamin II and intrinsic factor are required for the transport of B_{12} from the gut to the bloodstream. Serum cobalamin levels are normal, and B_{12} circulates attached instead to the R binder protein, whose function is not known. Patients are treated with supplemental cobalamin and sometimes also with folate.

NEUROMUSCULAR: Can be neurologically normal, or can have retarded intellectual development, ataxia, and pyramidal tract signs.

GI/GU: Diarrhea, vomiting, atrophy of intestinal mucosa, ulcerative stomatitis, intestinal disaccharidase deficiency.

OTHER: Neonatal failure to thrive. Hematologic disease consists of megaloblastic anemia, neutropenia, thrombocytopenia, and bleeding diathesis. Agammaglobulinemia and inadequate antibody response to antigens. Normal cellular immunity. Severe infections.

ANESTHETIC CONSIDERATIONS

The hematocrit must be evaluated preoperatively. Meticulous aseptic technique is indicated in patients with immune deficiency. Nitrous oxide should probably be avoided because it irreversibly inactivates the B_{12}-dependent enzyme methionine synthetase.

Bibliography:

1. Kaikov Y, Wadsworth LD, Hall CA, et al. Transcobalamin II deficiency: case report and review of the literature. *Eur J Pediatr* 1991;150:841–843.
2. Thomas PK, Hoffbrand AV, Smith IS. Neurological involvement in hereditary transcobalamin II deficiency. *J Neurol Neurosurg Psychiatry* 1982;45:74–77.

Trapezoidocephaly-Synostosis Syndrome

See Antley-Bixler syndrome

Treacher Collins Syndrome

SYNONYM: Mandibulofacial dysostosis; Franceschetti-Klein syndrome

MIM #: 154500

Treacher Collins syndrome is an autosomal dominant disorder, although most cases represent fresh mutations. There is significant clinical variability even within families. The involved gene has been sequenced and has been named both *TCOF1* and *treacle.* The gene may encode a nucleolar trafficking protein, and likely plays a critical role in early embryonic craniofacial development.

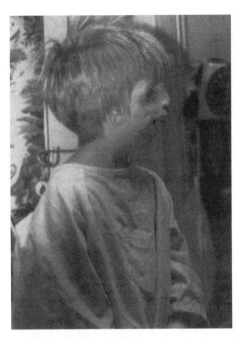

Treacher Collins syndrome. FIG. 2. Lateral view of the boy in figure 1, showing external ear deformity.

The major manifestations include malar hypoplasia, down-slanting palpebral fissures, colobomas of the lower eyelid, external ear abnormalities often involving hearing loss, and mandibular and pharyngeal hypoplasia. Patients commonly come to the operating room for plastic surgery.

HEENT/AIRWAY: Hypoplasia of the malar bones with or without cleft zygoma. Scalp hair spreading onto cheek. Down-sloping palpebral fissures, coloboma of the lower lid, partial to complete absence of the lower eyelashes, visual loss, microphthalmia. Low-set ears, often with atresia of the external canal and conductive deafness, preauricular blind fistulae. Absent parotid gland. Small mouth. High-arched palate, cleft lip or palate. Malocclusion of the teeth. Mandibular hypoplasia. Narrow airway due to pharyngeal hypoplasia, which can cause respiratory distress and necessitate a tracheostomy.

CHEST: Sleep apnea can develop.

CARDIOVASCULAR: Can have congenital cardiac defect.

NEUROMUSCULAR: Intelligence is usually normal.

GI/GU: Occasional cryptorchidism.

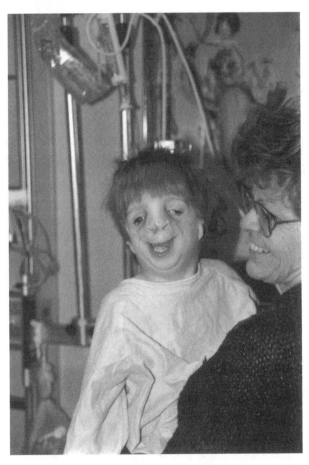

Treacher Collins syndrome. FIG. 1. This 3-year-old boy has had a cleft lip repaired but still has a cleft palate. He has bone conduction hearing and wears hearing aids on his mastoids. He has some speech. An experienced pediatric anesthesiologist had not been able to intubate his trachea previously. The current general anesthetic, for dental surgery, was done easily with a laryngeal mask airway.

MISCELLANEOUS: Edward Treacher Collins was one person, a British ophthalmologist. He used his mother's maiden name and his paternal family's name without a hyphen. Because Treacher Collins was one person, the syndrome is correctly Treacher Collins syndrome, not Treacher-Collins syndrome.

ANESTHETIC CONSIDERATIONS

Direct laryngoscopy and tracheal intubation may be extremely difficult or impossible secondary to severe mandibular hypoplasia, a small mouth, and a narrow airway. On occasion, laryngoscopy may obstruct an otherwise patent airway. Laryngoscopy may be more difficult with aging. The Bullard laryngoscope has been used successfully when other laryngoscopes failed (4). Laryngeal mask airways have been used successfully (1, 3, 5). Spontaneous ventilation may be improved by placing the patient prone so that the tongue does not fall posteriorly into the pharynx. Facial bone and pharyngeal growth during childhood may improve the airway.

Although patients may appear extremely dysmorphic, intelligence is usually normal. When talking with the patient, remember that he or she may have some hearing loss. Patients with congenital heart disease require perioperative antibiotic prophylaxis as indicated.

Bibliography:
1. Muraika L, Heyman JS, Shevchenko Y. Fiberoptic tracheal intubation through a laryngeal mask airway in a child with Treacher Collins syndrome. *Anesth Analg* 2003;97:1298–1299.
2. Perkins JA, Sie KC, Milczuk H, et al. Airway management in children with craniofacial anomalies. *Cleft Palate Craniofac J* 1997;34:135–140.
3. Inada T, Fujise K, Kazuya T, et al. Orotracheal intubation through the laryngeal mask airway in paediatric patients with Treacher-Collins syndrome. *Paediatr Anaesth* 1995;5:129–132.
4. Brown RE, Vollers JM, Rader GR, et al. Nasotracheal intubation in a child with Treacher Collins syndrome using the Bullard intubating laryngoscope. *J Clin Anesth* 1993;5:492–493.
5. Ebata T, Nishiki S, Masuda A. Anaesthesia for Treacher Collins syndrome using a laryngeal mask airway. *Can J Anaesth* 1991;38:1043–1045.
6. Rasch DK, Browder F, Barr M, et al. Anaesthesia for Treacher Collins and Pierre Robin syndromes: a report of three cases. *Can Anaesth Soc J* 1986;33:364–370.
7. Roa NL, Moss KS. Treacher-Collins syndrome with sleep apnea: anesthetic considerations. *Anesthesiology* 1984;60:71–73.
8. Maclennan FM, Robertson GS. Ketamine for induction and intubation in Treacher-Collins syndrome. *Anaesthesia* 1981;36:196–198.
9. Sklar GS, King BD. Endotracheal intubation and Treacher-Collins syndrome. *Anesthesiology* 1976;44:247–249.

Trichodentoosseous Syndrome

MIM #: 190320

This autosomal dominant disorder is marked by kinky hair, enamel hypoplasia and sclerotic bone. There appears to be abnormal synthesis of both keratin and enamel. The disorder is due to mutations in *DLX3*, the distal-less homeobox 3 gene. It has been suggested that there are two types of trichodentoosseous syndrome. Type II additionally includes microcephaly, obliterated mastoids and frontal sinuses, and thickened calvarium, with normal enamel and long bone density.

HEENT/AIRWAY: Dolichocephaly, partial craniosynostosis, thickened calvarium. Narrow external ear canals. Small, widely spaced teeth. Teeth have enlarged pulp chamber size [taurodontism (*tauro* = bull)], increased dental caries. Poor enamel. Teeth often become abscessed and are lost by the third decade. Square jaw.

ORTHOPEDIC: Increased bone density of skull, long bones, and spine. Brittle nails with peeling of nails.

OTHER: Hair is kinky at birth, but may straighten with age.

ANESTHETIC CONSIDERATIONS

Teeth are prone to premature loss. Dental abnormalities should be documented preoperatively, and extreme care should be exercised during laryngoscopy.

Bibliography:
1. Wright JT, Kula K, Hall K, et al. Analysis of the tricho-dento-osseous syndrome genotype and phenotype. *Am J Med Genet* 1997;72:197–204.
2. Kula K, Hall K, Hart T, et al. Craniofacial morphology of the tricho-dento-osseous syndrome. *Clin Genet* 1996;50:446–454.
3. Shapiro SD, Quattromani FL, Jorgenson RJ. Tricho-dento-osseous syndrome: heterogeneity or clinical variability. *Am J Med Genet* 1983;16:225–236.

Trichorhinophalangeal Syndrome, Type I

(Includes Trichorhinophalangeal syndrome, type III)

MIM #: 190350

Features of this autosomal dominant syndrome include characteristic facies with a bulbous nose and cone-shaped epiphyses. It is due to mutations in the gene *TRPS1*, which encodes a putative transcription factor. Langer-Giedion syndrome (see earlier), also known as trichorhinophalangeal syndrome, type II, is due to a deletion of at least two genes in the same area, including *TRPS1*. **Trichorhinophalangeal syndrome, type III**, also due to mutations in *TRPS1*, has as additional features brachydactyly and profound short stature.

HEENT/AIRWAY: Can have craniosynostosis. Protruding ears. Bulbous nose. Long, prominent philtrum. High-arched palate. Thin upper lip. Abnormal dentition with caries. Can have micrognathia. Horizontal groove on chin. Deep voice.

CHEST: Can have recurrent upper respiratory tract infections. Can have pectus carinatum.

NEUROMUSCULAR: Rare mental retardation, hypotonia in infancy.

ORTHOPEDIC: Mild growth deficiency. Cone-shaped epiphyses. Wide middle phalangeal joint with short metacarpals and metatarsals. Hypoplastic nails. Split distal radial epiphyses. Premature degenerative hip disease. Winged scapulae. Scoliosis. Lordosis. Type III disease has brachydactyly with short metacarpals and very short stature.

OTHER: Thin, sparse, relatively hypopigmented hair. Eyebrows thin laterally. Thin nails.

MISCELLANEOUS: *TRPS1* is overexpressed in breast cancer cells.

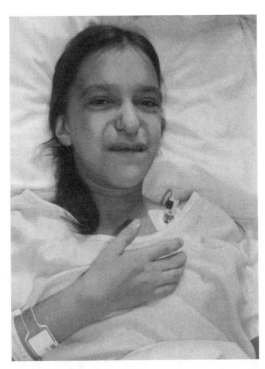

Trichorhinophalangeal syndrome, type I. This 14-year-old girl with trichorhinophalangeal syndrome, type I has poor dentition, thin hair, and a bulbous nose. Her chin groove is not well seen in this photo. She has multiple bone spurs.

ANESTHETIC CONSIDERATIONS

Can have recurrent upper respiratory tract infections, which may lead to cancellation of elective cases. Direct laryngoscopy and endotracheal intubation may be difficult secondary to micrognathia. Abnormal dentition may be more easily injured during laryngoscopy.

Bibliography:

1. Graybeal LS, Baum VC, Durieux ME. Anesthetic management of a patient with tricho-rhino-phalangeal syndrome [Letter]. *Eur J Anaesthesiol* 2005;22:400–402.
2. Buhler EM, Buhler UK, Beutler C, et al. A final word on the tricho-rhino-phalangeal syndromes. *Clin Genet* 1987;31:273–275.
3. Howell CJ, Wynne-Davies R. The tricho-rhino-phalangeal syndrome: a report of 14 cases in 7 kindreds. *J Bone Joint Surg Br* 1986;68:311–314.

Trichorhinophalangeal Syndrome, Type II

See Langer-Giedion syndrome

Triose Phosphate Isomerase Deficiency

MIM #: 190450

This disease, inherited in an autosomal dominant fashion, is due to a deficiency of triose phosphate isomerase. There are several alleles. Triose phosphate isomerase catalyzes the interconversion of dihydroxyacetone phosphate and glyceraldehyde-3-phosphate, a step in the glycolytic pathway. This enzyme is present in all tissues, and deficiency of the enzyme results in multisystem disease, unlike other enzyme defects of this pathway, which result in purely or primarily red blood cell hemolysis.

CARDIOVASCULAR: Sudden cardiac death, presumably secondary to arrhythmia.

NEUROMUSCULAR: Intelligence is usually normal. Weakness, hypotonia, absent limb reflexes, spasticity, myopathy, unintelligible speech. Lower motor neuron involvement, as well as pyramidal tract signs, tremor, dystonia, and dyskinesia from brainstem and basal ganglia involvement. Normal sensation.

ORTHOPEDIC: Fixed deformities of the hands and legs.

GI/GU: Splenomegaly. Cholelithiasis, cholecystitis.

OTHER: Moderately severe nonspherocytic hemolytic anemia. Neonatal hyperbilirubinemia. Increased susceptibility to infection. Hemolytic episodes precipitated by infections. Anemia in the chronic stage is generally mild. Sudden death without obvious cause.

ANESTHETIC CONSIDERATIONS

The hematocrit should be evaluated preoperatively. Metoclopramide can lead to extrapyramidal effects and probably should be avoided. Phenothiazines, butyrophenones, and other dopaminergic blockers may exacerbate movement disorders. Ondansetron should be safe as an antiemetic because it does not have antidopaminergic effects. Succinylcholine may be contraindicated in this disease with pronounced lower motor neuron involvement because of the risk of an exaggerated hyperkalemic response. Patients are at risk for sudden death, presumably secondary to arrhythmia.

Bibliography:

1. Schneider AS. Triosephosphate isomerase deficiency: historical perspectives and molecular aspects. *Best Pract Res Clin Haematol* 2000;13:119–140.
2. Hollan S, Fujii H, Hirono A, et al. Hereditary triosephosphate isomerase (TPI) deficiency: two severely affected brothers one with and one without neurological symptoms. *Hum Genet* 1993;92:486–490.

Trismus-Pseudocamptodactyly Syndrome

See Dutch-Kentucky syndrome

Trisomy 3p

MIM #: None

This disorder involves trisomy of a portion of the short arm of chromosome 3. It can be acquired as part of a balanced parental translocation or can arise *de novo*.

HEENT/AIRWAY: Brachycephaly, asymmetric skull with frontal bossing. Epicanthal folds. Low-set ears. Small nose, depressed nasal bridge. Short neck.

CARDIOVASCULAR: Can have congenital heart defects.

NEUROMUSCULAR: Developmental delay. Hypotonia. Febrile seizures.

GI/GU: Hypoplastic genitalia.

ANESTHETIC CONSIDERATIONS

Despite the facial features and short neck, a difficult airway was not a problem in the single case reported. That child did, however, require an endotracheal tube two sizes smaller than predicted for age because of a narrow glottis (1). Patients with congenital heart disease require perioperative antibiotic prophylaxis as indicated.

Bibliography:
1. Allen DL, Foster RN. Anaesthesia and trisomy 3p syndrome [Letter]. *Anaesth Intensive Care* 1996;24:615.
2. Reiss JA, Sheffield Li, Sutherland GR. Partial trisomy 3p syndrome. *Clin Genet* 1986;30:50–58.

Trisomy 4p

MIM #: None

This disorder involves trisomy of the short arm of chromosome 4. All affected people have severe mental retardation.

HEENT/AIRWAY: Microcephaly, small, flat forehead, prominent supraorbital ridges, eyebrows meet in midline (synophrys). Microphthalmia, uveal colobomas. Enlarged ears, thickened helix and antihelix. Flat nasal bridge. Cleft lip, macroglossia. Irregular teeth, small, poor dentition. Pointed mandible, short neck.

CHEST: Absent or additional ribs. Respiratory problems as a complication of feeding problems. Broad chest with aging. Widely spaced nipples.

CARDIOVASCULAR: May have cardiac defects.

NEUROMUSCULAR: Moderate to most likely severe mental retardation. Severe language delay. Behavioral problems. Hypertonic during infancy, then hypotonic. Seizures. Absence of corpus callosum.

ORTHOPEDIC: Prenatal-onset growth deficiency. Clinodactyly of fifth finger, camptodactyly, preaxial polydactyly, hypoplastic nails. Congenitally dislocated hips, clubfoot deformity, syndactyly of second and third toes. Kyphoscoliosis, vertebral anomalies, joint contractures. Stiff, unsteady gait.

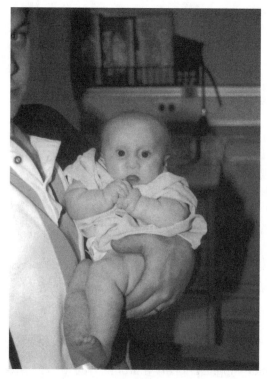

Trisomy 4p. A 6-month-old, 4.8 kg infant with trisomy 4p. The very puffy hands with redundant skin made venous access in the hands impossible.

GI/GU: Micropenis, cryptorchidism, hypospadias.

OTHER: Tend to be overweight. Puffy hands with redundant skin.

ANESTHETIC CONSIDERATIONS

Severe mental retardation or behavioral problems make the smooth induction of anesthesia a challenge. The large tongue and short neck might make direct laryngoscopy and tracheal intubation more difficult, particularly in infants. Puffy hands with redundant skin may make venous access difficult. Scoliosis and contractures may make optimal positioning more difficult. Chronic use of anticonvulsant medications may affect the metabolism of some anesthetic drugs. Patients with cardiac defects require perioperative antibiotic prophylaxis as indicated.

Bibliography:
1. Patel SV, Dagnew H, Parekh AJ, et al. Clinical manifestations of trisomy 4p syndrome. *Eur J Pediatr* 1995;154:425–431.
2. Kleczkowska A, Fryns JP, van den Berghe H. Trisomy of the short arm of chromosome 4: the changing phenotype with age. *Ann Genet* 1992;35:217–223.

Trisomy 8

MIM #: None

Patients with this syndrome are for the most part mosaic for trisomy 8/normal. There does not seem to be a correlation between the degree of impairment and the percentage of trisomic cells. The major manifestation is variable mental deficiency.

HEENT/AIRWAY: Strabismus, hypertelorism. Prominent, cupped ears with thickened helices, conductive hearing loss. Prominent nares. Everted lower lip, cleft lip, high-arched palate. Micrognathia. Short or webbed neck.

CHEST: Widely spaced nipples.

CARDIOVASCULAR: Can have cardiac defects.

NEUROMUSCULAR: Mild to severe mental retardation, clumsiness, seizures.

ORTHOPEDIC: Variable height, from short to tall. Camptodactyly of fingers and toes, deep creases on palms and soles, simian crease, abnormal nails. Dysplastic hips, absent patellas. Vertebral anomalies, scoliosis. Contractures of major joints.

GI/GU: Jejunal duplication, gastric leiomyosarcoma. Renal and ureteral anomalies, cryptorchidism.

OTHER: Anemia, factor VII deficiency. Mediastinal germ cell tumors.

MISCELLANEOUS: Acquired trisomy 8 is associated with myeloid malignancies and myelodysplastic syndrome.

ANESTHETIC CONSIDERATIONS

Micrognathia and a short neck may make laryngoscopy and tracheal intubation difficult. Consider evaluating the baseline hematocrit and clotting status. Major joint contractures may make intraoperative positioning more difficult. Chronic use of anticonvulsant medications may affect the metabolism of some anesthetic drugs. Patients with congenital heart disease require perioperative antibiotic prophylaxis as indicated.

Bibliography:
1. Kurtyka ZE, Krzykwa B, Piatkowska E, et al. Trisomy 8 mosaicism syndrome: two cases demonstrating variability in phenotype. *Clin Pediatr* 1988;27:557–564.

Trisomy 9

MIM #: None

Trisomy 9 can occur as a mosaic, or as a partial trisomy (trisomy 9p). The degree and severity of manifestations in mosaics are proportional to the number of cells with trisomy. Patients with the syndrome are typically neurologically devastated.

HEENT/AIRWAY

Mosaic: Sloping forehead, narrow bifrontal diameter. Narrow, up-slanting palpebral fissures, microphthalmia, absent optic tracts. Low-set, posteriorly rotated, misshapen ears. Short, prominent nasal bridge, slit-like nostrils. Prominent upper lip, cleft lip or palate. Micrognathia.

9p: Microcephaly, delayed closure of fontanelles and sutures. Hypertelorism, down-slanting palpebral fissures. Cup-shaped ears. Prominent nose. Down-turned corner of the mouth, cleft lip or palate. Micrognathia. Webbed neck.

CHEST

Narrow chest. Mosaic can have 13 ribs and thoracic vertebrae.

CARDIOVASCULAR

Can have congenital cardiac defects.

NEUROMUSCULAR

Severe mental retardation. Poor formation of gyri. Can have cysts of choroid plexus or arachnoid. Midline fusion defect of the cerebellum.

ORTHOPEDIC

Mosaic: Growth deficiency, primarily prenatal. Kyphoscoliosis, which can be congenital. Simian crease. Abnormal positioning or function of several joints. Hypoplastic sacrum and pelvis. Nonpitting edema of legs. Hypoplastic toes.

9p: Growth deficiency, primarily postnatal. Kyphoscoliosis, usually developing in adolescence. Short fingers and toes, small nails, clinodactyly of the fifth finger, simian crease. Congenital dislocation of the hip. Clubfoot deformity.

GI/GU: Bile duct proliferation, gastroesophageal reflux. Hypoplastic external genitalia. Cryptorchidism, hypospadias, micropenis. Renal anomalies. Delayed puberty.

OTHER: Severe failure to thrive.

ANESTHETIC CONSIDERATIONS

Micrognathia may make direct laryngoscopy and tracheal intubation difficult. Gastroesophageal reflux is common, and patients are at increased risk for perioperative aspiration. Intraoperative positioning may be complicated by abnormal joints and kyphoscoliosis. Patients with congenital heart disease require perioperative antibiotic prophylaxis as indicated.

Bibliography:
1. Cantu ES, Eicher DJ, Pai GS, et al. Mosaic vs. nonmosaic trisomy 9: report of a liveborn infant evaluated by fluorescence *in situ* hybridization and review of the literature. *Am J Med Genet* 1996;62:330–335.
2. Arnold GL, Kirby RS, Stern TP, et al. Trisomy 9: review and report of two new cases. *Am J Med Genet* 1995;56:252–257.

Trisomy 13

SYNONYM: Patau syndrome

MIM #: None

This syndrome is caused by trisomy of all or a large part of chromosome 13. Those affected have multiple craniofacial, cardiac, neurologic, and renal anomalies. Life expectancy is limited. Ninety-five percent die within the first 6 months. Five to 6% survive to age 1 or older and survival to over 5 years of age has been reported. Survival is somewhat better for girls and blacks. Clinical manifestations in patients who are mosaics or who are trisomic for only part of the chromosome are variable.

HEENT/AIRWAY: There is a characteristic occipital scalp defect. Microcephaly, wide sagittal suture and fontanelles. Capillary hemangioma of the forehead. Microphthalmia, anophthalmia, cyclopia, iris coloboma, hypertelorism, cataracts, retinal dysplasia, and optic nerve hypoplasia, limited vision. Low-set ears, abnormal helices, deafness (probably defects in organ of Corti). Broad, flat nose. Cleft lip, cleft palate, cleft tongue. Micrognathia. Loose skin over posterior neck.

CHEST: Pectus carinatum or short, barrel chest can develop in older children. Thin posterior ribs, may have missing ribs.

CARDIOVASCULAR: Over 80% have cardiac anomalies of a variety of types. The most common are ventricular septal defect, tetralogy of Fallot, and double-outlet right ventricle. Calcified pulmonary arterioles.

NEUROMUSCULAR: Apneic episodes in infancy are common. Holoprosencephaly with agenesis of the corpus callosum, absent olfactory nerves, cerebellar hypoplasia. Meningocele, meningomyelocele, other neural tube defects. Severe mental retardation, sometimes with seizures.

ORTHOPEDIC: Polydactyly, flexion deformities of the hands, retroflexible thumb, simian crease, camptodactyly, syndactyly. Can have radial aplasia. Prominent heel, rocker-bottom feet, clubfoot deformity. Thoracic kyphoscoliosis. Joint subluxation can develop in older children.

GI/GU: Inguinal and umbilical hernias common. Malrotation, omphalocele, large gallbladder, Meckel's diverticulum. Microscopic pancreatic dysplasia is a specific finding of trisomy 13. Most patients have renal anomalies, including unilateral renal agenesis, renal and urogenital duplication, hydronephrosis, and polycystic kidneys. Cryptorchidism, abnormal scrotum, hypospadias, bicornuate uterus, hypoplastic ovaries, abnormal insertion of fallopian tubes.

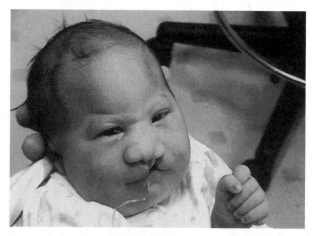

Trisomy 13. An infant with trisomy 13. The string from her mouth is attached to a retainer to aid in bottle feeding. She has required surgical repair of a cleft lip and palate and placement of a gastrostomy tube. She began to crawl at age 5 years. She is now 6 years old.

OTHER: Multiple capillary hemangiomas. High persistent levels of fetal hemoglobin.

MISCELLANEOUS: Probably first described by Bartholin in 1657; Patau recognized the syndrome to be due to a trisomy.

ANESTHETIC CONSIDERATIONS

The short neck, small mouth, and micrognathia may make direct laryngoscopy and tracheal intubation difficult. Patients are at risk for perioperative apnea, and must be monitored closely for respiratory adequacy. Radial anomalies may make placement of a radial arterial catheter more difficult. Flexion deformities and joint subluxation may make intraoperative positioning difficult. The lumbosacral area should be closely examined for cutaneous evidence of an underlying spinal dysraphism prior to caudal or epidural injections. Unexpected subarachnoid entry during attempted caudal anesthesia in a 4-year-old has been reported (1). Patients with renal insufficiency require careful titration of perioperative fluids and careful dosing of renally excreted medications. Patients with congenital heart disease require perioperative antibiotic prophylaxis as indicated.

Bibliography:
1. Cohen IT. Caudal block complication in a patient with trisomy 13. *Paediatr Anaesth* 2006;16:213–215.
2. Rasmussen SA, Wong L-YC, Yang Q, et al. Population-based analyses of mortality in trisomy 13 and trisomy 18. *Pediatrics* 2003;111:777–784.
3. Pollard RC, Beasley JM. Anaesthesia for patients with trisomy 13 (Patau's syndrome). *Paediatr Anaesth* 1996;6:151–153.
4. Martlew RA, Sharples A. Anaesthesia in a child with Patau's syndrome. *Anaesthesia* 1995;50:980–982.
5. Baty BJ, Jorde LB, Blackburn BL, et al. Natural history of trisomy 18 and trisomy 13: II. psychomotor development. *Am J Med Genet* 1994;49:189–194.
6. Baty BJ, Blackburn BL, Carey JC. Natural history of trisomy 18 and trisomy 13: I. growth, physical assessment, medical histories, survival, and recurrence risk. *Am J Med Genet* 1994;49:175–188.

Trisomy 18

SYNONYM: Edwards syndrome

MIM #: None

This syndrome is caused by trisomy of all or a large part of chromosome 18. Patients characteristically have severe mental retardation and a limited potential for survival, characteristic clenched hands noted at birth, and a short sternum. This is a relatively common genetic syndrome, with an incidence of 3 per 1,000 live births. The risk increases with older maternal age. For unknown reasons (higher intrauterine death rate for boys?), girls out-number boys by three to one. Most individuals with trisomy 18 die *in utero*. Of those born alive, most need resuscitation at birth and nonetheless die within the first week. Of those born alive, 13% have required surgery in the neonatal period. Ninety to 95% die within the first year of life. There are reports of survival into adolescence. Longer-term survivors usually have trisomy 18 mosaicism or have only partial trisomy.

HEENT/AIRWAY: Prominent occiput, narrow cranium. May have microcephaly, large fontanelles. Short palpebral fissures. May have epicanthal folds, ptosis, corneal opacity. Low-set, malformed ears. May have sensorineural hearing loss. Small mouth. High-arched palate. Can have cleft lip or palate. Micrognathia.

CHEST: Short sternum. Can have broad thorax with widely spaced nipples. Occasional diaphragmatic muscle hypoplasia with possible eventration. Can have absence or malformation of the right lung.

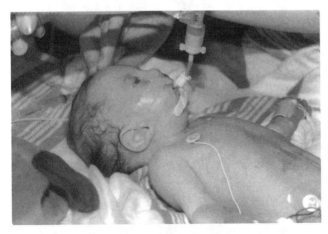

Trisomy 18. FIG. 1. This 4-month-old with trisomy 18 had surgery for volvulus at another hospital. Cardiac surgery for a ventricular septal defect was refused at that hospital due to the genetic defect. Micrognathia made tracheal intubation difficult and a fiberoptic intubation was done via a laryngeal mask airway. She weighs 2.6 kg and also has a rectovaginal fistula.

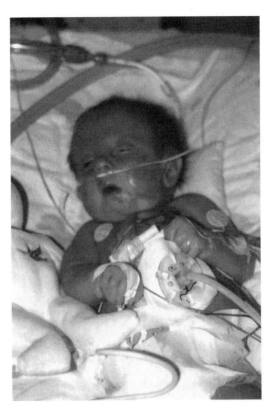

Trisomy 18. FIG. 2. This 1-month-old 2.3 kg infant is mosaic for trisomy 18. She has been operated on for malrotation of the gut.

CARDIOVASCULAR: The incidence of cardiac malformations is >95%. Multiple congenital cardiac lesions are possible, including ventricular septal defect, atrial septal defect, patent ductus arteriosus, bicuspid aortic valve, pulmonic valvular stenosis, and coarctation of the aorta. Can have aberrant subclavian artery. Conduction defects have also been reported.

NEUROMUSCULAR: Severe mental deficiency. Weak cry, hypotonia in the neonatal period. Recurrent apnea in the neonatal period. Hypertonia after the neonatal period. Can have holoprosencephaly.

ORTHOPEDIC: Characteristic clenched hands at birth, with index finger overlapping the third finger, and fifth finger sometimes overlapping the fourth. Short, hypoplastic, or absent thumb. Can have simian crease. Nail hypoplasia. Low-arch dermal ridge pattern on fingertips. Small, narrow pelvis, limited hip abduction. Can have clubfoot deformity, rocker-bottom feet, syndactyly of the second and third toes. Short stature.

GI/GU: Inguinal and umbilical hernias common. Cryptorchidism. Can have omphalocele, Meckel's diverticulum, malrotation, anal anomalies, ectopic pancreatic or splenic tissue. Can have renal anomalies, including ectopic kidney, horseshoe kidney, polycystic kidney, hydronephrosis, duplication of the collecting system.

OTHER: Failure to thrive. Redundant skin. Cutis marmorata. Decreased muscle mass, subcutaneous tissue, and fat.

ANESTHETIC CONSIDERATIONS

Neonates are at high risk for perioperative apnea. Direct laryngoscopy and tracheal intubation may be difficult in these patients who have small mouths and micrognathia. Placement of a subclavian intravenous catheter may be contraindicated because an aberrant subclavian artery may be present. Decreased subcutaneous tissue may make intraoperative temperature regulation more difficult. Patients with renal insufficiency require careful titration of perioperative fluids and careful dosing of renally excreted drugs. Patients with congenital heart disease require perioperative antibiotic prophylaxis as indicated.

Bibliography:

1. Courrèges P, Nieuviarts R, Lecoutre D. Anaesthetic management for Edward's [sic] syndrome. *Paediatr Anaesth* 2003;13:267–269.
2. Rasmussen SA, Wong L-YC, Yang Q, et al. Population-based analyses of mortality in trisomy 13 and trisomy 18. *Pediatrics* 2003;111:777–784.
3. Baty BJ, Jorde LB, Blackburn BL, et al. Natural history of trisomy 18 and trisomy 13: II. psychomotor development. *Am J Med Genet* 1994;49:189–194.
4. Baty BJ, Blackburn BL, Carey JC. Natural history of trisomy 18 and trisomy 13: I. growth, physical assessment, medical histories, survival, and recurrence risk. *Am J Med Genet* 1994;49:175–188.
5. Bailey C, Chung R. Use of the laryngeal mask airway in a patient with Edward's syndrome [Letter]. *Anaesthesia* 1992;47:713.

Trisomy 21

See Down syndrome

Tuberous Sclerosis

MIM #: 191100

This autosomal dominant disorder is characterized by the classic triad of mental retardation, seizures, and adenoma sebaceum (fibroangiomas). Tuberous sclerosis is one of the most common autosomal dominant diseases. New mutations are relatively common. There is wide variability in the clinical manifestations. There is progression of the clinical disease with aging. Four separate genes (*TSC1* and *2*, which encode hamartin and tuberin, and the uncommon *TSC 3* and *4)* at different locations have been associated with tuberous sclerosis. *TSC 1* and *2*, at least, are tumor suppressor genes. The *TSC2* gene is located adjacent to the polycystic kidney disease-1 gene, which might account for the renal cysts which can develop in some tuberous sclerosis patients.

HEENT/AIRWAY: Adenoma sebaceum (more correctly, fibroangiomas), typically on the malar areas of the face.

Multiple retinal astrocytomas, choroid hamartomas, hypopigmented lesions of the iris. Pitting of tooth enamel. Oral tumors, fibromas, or papillomas.

CHEST: Pulmonary involvement is rare and tends to occur in women in the third or fourth decade. The features are similar to pulmonary lymphangiomyomatosis with cystic changes. Can have diffusion defects and airway obstruction. Pulmonary or pleural hamartomas can develop. Patients can have dyspnea, spontaneous pneumothorax, hemoptysis, and respiratory failure.

CARDIOVASCULAR: Cardiac rhabdomyomas are almost pathognomonic. They may be single or multiple and in any chamber, may result in obstruction to blood flow, arrhythmias, or heart block, and can rarely embolize. These tumors are very common during fetal life and most involute or become relatively smaller with postnatal growth. Wolff-Parkinson-White syndrome (see later) has also been reported. Abdominal aortic aneurysms have been reported in infants and children. Can have aneurysms or narrowing of other major arteries.

NEUROMUSCULAR: Mental retardation is common. Seizures occur in most patients. Infantile spasms, a particular type of seizure ("salaam seizures"), are particularly common. Autism and other behavioral problems are common. Mental

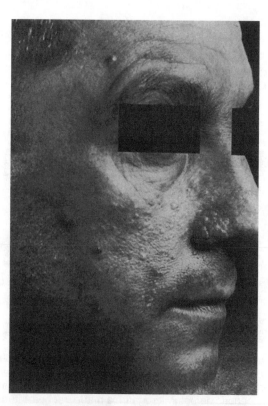

Tuberous sclerosis. FIG. 1. Typical adenoma sebaceum on the face. (Courtesy of Dr. Kenneth E. Greer, Department of Dermatology, University of Virginia Health System.)

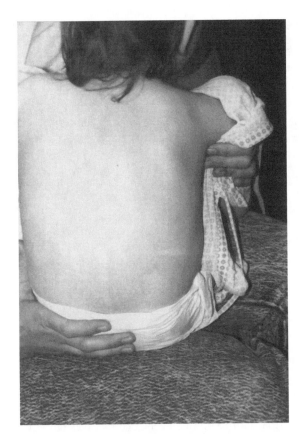

Tuberous sclerosis. FIG. 2. Typical lens-shaped, hypopigmented, mountain ash leaf spots in a young boy with a history of seizures, cardiac rhabdomyoma with supraventricular tachycardia, hypertension, and renal angiolipoma.

retardation, seizures, and behavioral problems are particularly associated with mutations in *TSC2*. Brain lesions include giant cell astrocytomas and subependymal periventricular nodules, which can calcify or cause hydrocephalus. Tubers (hence "tuberous sclerosis") are focal areas of loss of normal brain architecture, often surrounded by gliosis, and are apparent on MRI scanning. Sacrococcygeal chordomas.

ORTHOPEDIC: Periungual fibromas around the fingertips are particular to this disease. Separation of periosteum from underlying bone can cause palpable cysts in the phalanges and long bones.

GI/GU: Tumors can involve the gastrointestinal tract at many levels, including the mouth, esophagus, stomach, intestines, pancreas, or liver. Adrenal angiolipomas can develop. Renal angiomyolipomas, often multiple and bilateral. The combination of renal angiomyolipomas and cysts is characteristic of the disease, and is usually asymptomatic, although renal failure or hematuria may occur. Renal carcinomas can develop. Spontaneous hemorrhage into angiolipomas or rupture can lead to retroperitoneal bleeding, which can worsen with intraoperative manipulation. Growth

of renal tumors appears to be accelerated during pregnancy, increasing the risk of rupture or hemorrhage.

OTHER: The cutaneous manifestations also include shagreen patches (roughened skin likened to shark skin), typically over the lower trunk, and hypopigmented, elliptical or lenticular-shaped ("mountain ash leaf") macules that are particularly well seen under ultraviolet light (Wood's lamp). Can have café au lait spots. A wide variety of endocrinopathies have been described, including the otherwise uncommon papillary adenoma of the thyroid.

MISCELLANEOUS: The "tuberous" in tuberous sclerosis likens the cerebral tumors to tubers, such as the potato. "Adenoma sebaceum" is not actually an adenoma, and the sebaceous glands are involved only secondarily. Tuberous sclerosis is one of the phakomatoses, or neurocutaneous diseases. Other phakomatoses include neurofibromatosis, nevus sebaceus syndrome of Jadassohn, Sturge-Weber syndrome and von Hippel-Lindau syndrome. "Phakos" is Greek for a lentil or lens-shaped spot.

ANESTHETIC CONSIDERATIONS

Oropharyngeal or laryngeal tumors may hinder tracheal intubation. Patients deserve a baseline cardiac assessment to evaluate the potential complications of cardiac rhabdomyomas. Obstructive cardiomyopathy from rhabdomyomas can occur. Chronic use of anticonvulsant medications may alter the metabolism of some anesthetic drugs.

Bibliography:
1. Shenkman Z, Rockoff MA, Eldredge EA, et al. Anaesthetic management of children with tuberous sclerosis. *Paediatr Anaesth* 2002;12:700–704.
2. Diaz JH. Perioperative management of children with congenital phakomatoses. *Paediatr Anaesth* 2000;10:121–128.
3. Tsukui A, Noguchi R, Honda T, et al. Aortic aneurysm in a four-year-old child with tuberous sclerosis. *Paediatr Anaesth* 1995;5:67–70.
4. Lee JJ, Imrie M, Taylor V. Anaesthesia and tuberous sclerosis. *Br J Anaesth* 1994;73:421–425.
5. Schweiger JW, Schwartz RE, Stayer SA. Anaesthetic management of the patient with tuberous sclerosis complex. *Paediatr Anaesth* 1994;4:339–342.

Turcot Syndrome

MIM #: 276300

This autosomal recessive disorder is characterized by malignant tumors of the central nervous system and adenomatous polyposis of the colon. Turcot syndrome can be due to a defect in one of three genes: the adenomatous polyposis coli (*APC*) gene (associated with medulloblastoma formation), or the mismatch repair genes *MLH1* or *PMS2*. It has been suggested that Turcot syndrome is just one manifestation of Gardner syndrome (see earlier). Presentation has been reported in a previously healthy 67-year-old.

NEUROMUSCULAR: Gliomas, astrocytomas, glioblastoma multiforme.

GI/GU: Adenomatous colonic polyps, colon adenocarcinoma. Gastric carcinoma. Focal nodular hyperplasia of the liver.

OTHER: Café au lait spots. Multiple lipomas. Multiple basal cell carcinomas. Leukemia. Papillary carcinoma of the thyroid. Radiosensitivity.

MISCELLANEOUS: Turcot, a French Canadian, pronounced his name with a silent final "t."

ANESTHETIC CONSIDERATIONS

There are no specific anesthetic considerations in the absence of critically placed central nervous system tumors. Marginally indicated radiologic studies should be avoided in these radiosensitive patients.

Bibliography:

1. Hamilton SR, Liu B, Parsons RE, et al. The molecular basis of Turcot's syndrome. *N Engl J Med* 1995;332:839–847.
2. Mastronardi L, Ferrante L, Lunardi P, et al. Association between neuroepithelial tumor and multiple intestinal polyposis (Turcot's syndrome): report of a case and critical analysis of the literature. *Neurosurgery* 1991;28:449–452.

Turner Syndrome

SYNONYM: XO syndrome

MIM #: None

This well known syndrome in girls is due to a single X chromosome (45, XO). However, more than half of the patients with Turner syndrome are mosaics (45, XO/46, XX). Mosaics usually have fewer or milder clinical manifestations. Short stature, webbed neck, and gonadal dysgenesis are the most universal features. Treatment with growth hormone has been used recently and can apparently increase final adult height by approximately 4 inches. The paternal X chromosome is the one most likely to be missing.

HEENT/AIRWAY: Low posterior hairline. Strabismus, amblyopia, ptosis, inner canthal folds, cataracts. Red-green color blindness with the same frequency as normal males. Protruding external ear, recurrent otitis media, progressive sensorineural hearing loss. High-arched palate. Palatal dysfunction can be worsened by adenoidectomy. Micrognathia. Short, webbed neck (a residuum of fetal lymphedema).

CHEST: Broad, "shield-like" chest. Mild pectus excavatum.

CARDIOVASCULAR: Coarctation of the aorta and bicuspid aortic valve. Aortic dissection in adults even without coarctation, although almost always associated with coarctation, bicuspid aortic valve or systemic arterial hypertension. Even though coarctation and bicuspid aortic valve are most commonly associated with the syndrome, the relative risk (vs. the

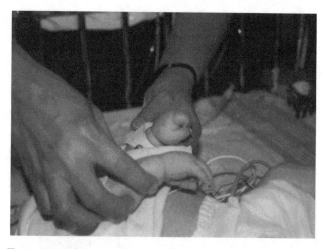

Turner syndrome. FIG. 1. Puffy hands in a 6-week-old infant with Turner syndrome (2.9 kg product of a full-term pregnancy) admitted to the hospital for a sepsis work-up. It can be easily appreciated that the puffiness might make venous access challenging.

general population) of partial anomalous pulmonary venous return is actually higher, although the absolute incidence is lower than that of the other two lesions. Hypertension.

NEUROMUSCULAR: Intelligence normal or slightly diminished. Motor delays.

ORTHOPEDIC: Short stature [mean adult height of 55 inches (140 cm)]. Increased carrying angle of the elbows (cubitus valgus), short fourth metacarpal or metatarsal, narrow or deeply set nails. Dislocated hips, tibial exostoses, prominent medial tibial and femoral condyles causing knee pain. Scoliosis, kyphosis. Puffy hands and feet (a residuum of fetal lymphedema). This can become more prominent with growth hormone or estrogen therapy. Dislocation of the patella. Madelung deformity of the radial head, seen in Leri-Weill dyschondrosteosis (see earlier), is uncommonly found.

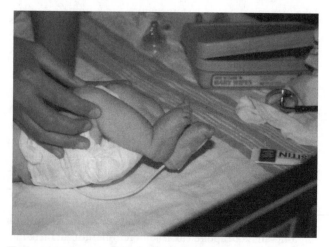

Turner syndrome. FIG. 2. Puffy feet in same infant.

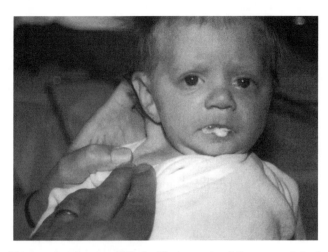

Turner syndrome. FIG. 3. Photograph of the same infant showing the webbed neck.

GI/GU: Increased incidence of Crohn's disease and ulcerative colitis. Gonadal dysgenesis or agenesis with streak ovaries, absent thelarche and menarche. Most will require hormone therapy to initiate puberty. Can have dyspareunia from a small vagina or an atrophic vaginal lining. Fertility is rare and occurs mostly in women who are mosaics, but there is an increased incidence of spontaneous fetal loss and aneuploidy in fetuses carried to term. Older patients will be on long-term estrogen and progestin replacement therapy. Renal anomalies, including horseshoe kidney, but renal function is usually normal. A small number can develop obstructive uropathy from a duplicated collecting system.

OTHER: Small for gestational age. Tend to be overweight. Patients may be receiving chronic growth hormone treatment. Insulin resistance with type 2 diabetes. Hypothyroidism (Hashimoto thyroiditis, associated with antithyroid antibodies). Increased incidence of keloid formation and pigmented nevi. Mosaics are at increased risk for development of gonadoblastoma. A recent study suggested that patients with Turner syndrome have an increased risk for development of neuroblastoma and related tumors. Hypercholesterolism.

MISCELLANEOUS: Although patients with Turner syndrome are said to have widely spaced nipples, careful measurement showed that they have only the appearance of widely spaced nipples.

Henry Turner was an endocrinologist who was the Professor of Medicine at the University of Oklahoma. The syndrome was actually described in the literature by Ullrich several years before Turner. In fact, Morgagni appears to have described a case in the 17th century.

ANESTHETIC CONSIDERATIONS
Patients should be spoken to in a manner appropriate for their chronologic age, not their height age. The short, webbed neck may make direct laryngoscopy and tracheal intubation more difficult. Patients have been reported with short tracheal lengths, making appropriate location of the tip of a normal length endotracheal tube difficult. Hypothyroidism, when present, could result in delayed gastric emptying, alterations in drug metabolism and impaired temperature regulation. Puffy hands and feet can make venous access challenging. Adult patients can be hypertensive, and are at risk for aortic dissection. Patients with congenital heart disease require antibiotic prophylaxis as indicated.

Bibliography:
1. Mashour GA, Sunder N, Acquadro MA. Anesthetic management of Turner syndrome: a systematic approach. *J Clin Anesth* 2005;17:128–130.
2. Sybert VP, McCauley E. Turner's syndrome. *N Engl J Med* 2004;351:1227–1238.
3. Saenger P. Turner's syndrome. *N Engl J Med* 1996;335:1749–1754.
4. Divekar VM, Kothari MD, Kamdar BM. Anaesthesia in Turner's syndrome. *Can Anaesth Soc J* 1983;30:417–418.

Tyrosinemia I

MIM #: 276700

Tyrosinemia I is an autosomal recessive disorder due to a deficiency of fumarylacetoacetate hydrolase. In the past it has been called "tyrosinosis," "hereditary tyrosinemia," and "congenital tyrosinosis." It is also known as hepatorenal tyrosinemia. This enzyme is involved in a final stage of tyrosine catabolism, where it catalyzes the conversion of fumarylacetoacetic acid to fumaric acid and acetoacetic acid. Acute and chronic forms have been described even within the same family, and are thought to be due to the amount of residual enzyme activity. A variety of specific mutations in the gene have been described.

Diminished enzyme activity leads to the accumulation of metabolites of another, unaffected degradation pathway. Succinylacetate is structurally similar to maleic acid, an inhibitor of renal tubular function, and may be responsible for the renal tubular dysfunction. Succinylacetone is structurally related to delta-aminolevulinic acid, which inhibits porphobilinogen synthetase (delta-aminolevulinic acid dehydratase), leading to elevated levels of delta-aminolevulinic acid and symptoms of porphyria (see earlier). Succinylacetone also inhibits renal tubular transport of glucose and amino acids. Other compounds that are produced in excess are capable of inhibiting methionine synthetase.

In addition to liver transplantation, treatment has included NTBC, an inhibitor of 4-hydroxyphenylpyruvate dioxygenase, which prevents the formation of maleylacetoacetate and fumarylacetoacetate. Early treatment has apparently removed the risk of hepatocellular carcinoma and neurologic decompensation.

HEENT/AIRWAY: Epistaxis. Severe bruxism. Macroglossia has been reported.

CHEST: Mechanical ventilation may be required for weakness during an acute exacerbation.

CARDIOVASCULAR: Can have hypertrophic cardiomyopathy, systemic arterial hypertension.

NEUROMUSCULAR: Polyneuropathy. There are episodes of vomiting, and peripheral neuropathy with severe pain, extensor hypertonia, muscle weakness and self-mutilation. Hypertonia can be misidentified as seizures or opisthotonus. Episodes can include autonomic findings and paralysis. Episodes often follow an infection. There usually is normal neurologic function between episodes. Can exhibit developmental delay, but development is usually normal, and level of consciousness is normal during neurologic crisis.

ORTHOPEDIC: Hypophosphatemic rickets.

GI/GU: Episodes of abdominal pain, vomiting, diarrhea, and paralytic ileus. Hepatic failure. Hepatomegaly, chronic liver disease (chronic active hepatitis with fatty infiltration), cirrhosis, ascites. Hepatocellular carcinoma can develop in young childhood. Can have acute episodes of hepatic failure associated with infection or other catabolic stress. Painful abdominal crises similar to those seen with porphyria. In some hepatocytes in many patients mutations revert to the normal sequence, and these cells form nodules with normal enzyme activity. These can be difficult to differentiate non-invasively from nodules of hepatocellular carcinoma. Hyperplastic pancreatic islets. Melena. Renal tubular acidosis. Hypophosphatemic rickets. Fanconi syndrome (see earlier), renal swelling, hematuria. Can develop renal failure.

OTHER: Failure to thrive. An odor similar to boiled cabbage. Intermittent fever. Normocytic anemia, possible thrombocytosis, prolonged prothrombin time. Coagulopathy, which is in excess of other liver function abnormalities, can be symptomatic and is not correctable by vitamin K. Hypocholesterolemia. There can be hypoglycemia unresponsive to glucagon. Hypoproteinemia. Can have edema and ecchymoses of skin.

MISCELLANEOUS: NTBC was originally developed as an herbicide.

ANESTHETIC CONSIDERATIONS
Abdominal pain may be misdiagnosed as a surgical abdomen. May require mechanical ventilation during a neurologic crisis. Can have bleeding dyscrasia. Clotting parameters should be evaluated prior to regional anesthesia. Coagulopathy will not be vitamin K responsive. There are no reports of the anesthetic management of a patient with tyrosinemia I. However, given the biochemical similarity with porphyria, it would seem prudent to use the same precautions (see Porphyria, earlier). During acute episodes, adequate calories to prevent or minimize catabolism should be supplied. Pain associated with neurologic crises may require narcotic analgesics. Renal output may not closely reflect intravascular volume status. See Fanconi syndrome (earlier) for renal metabolic consequences. Serum glucose levels should be monitored perioperatively, and patients should receive glucose supplementation as needed. Patients may have hypertrophic cardiomyopathy or hypertension. Nitrous oxide can also inhibit methionine synthetase, and probably should be avoided in this disorder.

FIGURE: See **Appendix B**

Bibliography:
1. Russo PA, Mitchell GA, Tanguay RM. Tyrosinemia: a review. *Pediatr Dev Pathol* 2001;4:212–221.
2. Grompe M. The pathophysiology and treatment of hereditary tyrosinemia type 1. *Semin Liver Dis* 2001;21:563–571.

Tyrosinemia II

SYNONYM: Richner-Hanhart syndrome

MIM #: 276600

This oculocutaneous syndrome is due to an autosomal recessive deficiency of hepatic tyrosine aminotransferase, the rate-limiting first enzyme in tyrosine catabolism. Some families have been reported with skin lesions, but no eye lesions, and vice versa. In general, eye lesions predate the skin lesions. Ocular and cutaneous lesions respond to a protein-restricted or phenylalanine-restricted diet.

HEENT/AIRWAY: Lacrimation, photophobia, redness, mild herpetiform corneal lesions, dendritic ulcers, and rarely corneal and conjunctival plaques. Neovascularization. Corneal scarring, nystagmus, glaucoma. Hyperkeratosis of the tongue.

NEUROMUSCULAR: Mental retardation, self-mutilation or fine motor abnormalities.

OTHER: Hyperkeratotic lesions of the palms and soles, which can be painful. Tyrosinemia. Growth retardation. Untreated maternal disease may be deleterious to the fetus, which can have abnormal neurologic development.

MISCELLANEOUS: The association of this clinical syndrome with tyrosinemia was suggested 35 years after its description by Richner and later by Hanhart. A similar disease occurs in minks.

ANESTHETIC CONSIDERATIONS
Consideration should be given to patients with photophobia in brightly lit operating rooms. Dietary limitations (protein or phenylalanine restrictions) should be maintained perioperatively. An orogastric tube or throat packs should be placed for surgery with the potential for oral or intestinal bleeding

because blood aspirated into the gastrointestinal tract after oral or nasal surgery might present an excessive protein load.

FIGURE: See **Appendix B**

Bibliography:
1. Rabinowitz LG, Williams LR, Anderson CE, et al. Painful keratoderma and photophobia: hallmarks of tyrosinemia type II. *J Pediatr* 1995;126:266–269.

Tyrosinemia III

SYNONYM: 4-hydroxyphenylpyruvic acid dioxygenase (oxidase) deficiency

MIM #: 276710

This autosomal recessive disorder of tyrosine metabolism is due to deficient activity of 4-hydroxyphenylpyruvic acid dioxygenase, which is also known as 4-hydroxyphenylpyruvate acid oxidase. The responsible gene has been sequenced and named the *HPD* gene. Three disorders have been linked to abnormalities in this gene: tyrosinemia III, hawkinsinuria, and transient tyrosinemia of the newborn. Hawkinsinuria results from a heterozygous mutation. Transient tyrosinemia is caused by an immature enzyme in concert with high dietary phenylalanine and tyrosine and relative ascorbate deficiency. The clinical findings are limited to the nervous system.

HEENT/AIRWAY: There are no eye findings.

NEUROMUSCULAR: Acute intermittent ataxia, lethargy. Psychomotor development may be abnormal, mild mental retardation. Can have seizures.

GI/GU: Hepatic function is normal.

ANESTHETIC CONSIDERATIONS
Any dietary restrictions should be continued perioperatively. Chronic use of anticonvulsant medications may affect the metabolism of some anesthetic drugs.

FIGURE: See **Appendix B**

Bibliography:
1. Ellaway CJ, Holme E, Standing S, et al. Outcome of tyrosinaemia type III. *J Inherit Metab Dis* 2001;24:824–832.

Tyrosinosis

MIM #: 276800

There is some confusion over the terms "tyrosinosis" and "tyrosinemia." It has been suggested that "tyrosinosis" be reserved for a rare condition that involves an autosomal recessive defect in liver tyrosine transaminase. It is likely that patients carrying the diagnosis of tyrosinosis will in fact have tyrosinemia (see Tyrosinemia I, II, or III, earlier).

U

Ubiquinone-Cytochrome *c* Oxidoreductase Deficiency

See Complex III deficiency

Uhl Anomaly

SYNONYM: Arrhythmogenic right ventricular dysplasia

MIM #: 107970

This peculiar autosomal dominant defect consists of the absence of muscle in the right ventricle with few, if any myocardial cells, forming a thin "parchment paper-like" right ventricle. The disorder is due to abnormalities in the gene *TGFB3*, which encodes a transforming growth factor. The term arrhythmogenic right ventricular dysplasia encompasses a larger number of lesions than Uhl anomaly, which represents a single type. Brugada syndrome, for example, would be another type.

CARDIOVASCULAR: The right ventricular anterior wall is preferentially affected, with replacement of normal muscle with fat and fibrous tissue. There can be recurrent, sustained ventricular tachycardia, with a left bundle branch configuration. Associated cardiac defects are uncommon, although there can be associated tricuspid insufficiency. Right-to-left shunting through a patent foramen ovale can result in cyanosis. There is often impressive cardiomegaly on the chest radiograph. The electrocardiogram shows large P waves and a small QRS, particularly over the right precordial leads.

GI/GU: There can be hepatomegaly secondary to congestion, and severe involvement with ascites has been reported.

MISCELLANEOUS: Appropriate attachment of the tricuspid valve annulus differentiates this entity from Ebstein anomaly (see earlier) on echocardiography.

ANESTHETIC CONSIDERATIONS
Efforts should be made to minimize pulmonary vascular resistance. Patients should receive perioperative antibiotic prophylaxis as indicated. With significant congestion, hepatic function can be abnormal, which could affect coagulation and drug metabolism. Surgical options include a so-called one and one-half ventricle repair (utilizing a Glenn anastomosis) with or without volume reduction of the right ventricle.

Several postoperative deaths after noncardiac surgery in previously undiagnosed adolescents have been reported, and were not thought related to anesthetic technique as they occurred hours postoperatively. Although it has been suggested that halothane be avoided, there are no data suggesting inherent safety of any particular anesthetic drug.

Bibliography:
1. Houfani B, Meyer P, Merckx J, et al. Postoperative sudden death in two adolescents with myelomeningocele and unrecognized arrhythmogenic right ventricular dysplasia. *Anesthesiology* 2001;95:257–259.
2. Fontaine G, Gallais Y, Fornes P, et al. Arrhythmogenic right ventricular dysplasia/cardiomyopathy. *Anesthesiology* 2001;95:250–254.
3. Uhl HS. Uhl's anomaly revisited. *Circulation* 1996;93:1483–1484.

Urbach-Wiethe Disease

See Lipoid proteinosis

Uridine Diphosphate Galactose Epimerase Deficiency

MIM #: 230350

This autosomal recessive disorder is due to deficient activity of uridine diphosphate (UDP) galactose epimerase, which catalyzes the conversion of UDP-galactose to UDP-glucose, in the interconversion pathway of galactose to glucose, and in the synthesis of galactose when only glucose is available. This enzyme deficiency is occasionally included in the term "galactosemia."

There are two forms of this disorder. One form is benign and affects only red and white blood cell enzyme activity. Patients are asymptomatic. The other, more rare form, has findings that are similar to those of galactose-1-phosphate uridyltransferase deficiency, the defect in classic galactosemia. The enzyme deficiency here is more generalized. However, recent work suggests that these disorders represent a spectrum rather than two distinct entities. The treatment of this defect differs somewhat from that of the other two disorders causing galactosemia. Galactose cannot be synthesized from glucose with deficiency of UDP galactose epimerase, so some dietary galactose is required. Galactose is required for the synthesis of complex carbohydrates and galactolipids.

HEENT/AIRWAY: Sensory deafness. May be at risk for cataracts.

NEUROMUSCULAR: Delayed intellectual and motor development. Hypotonia.

GI/GU: Jaundice, vomiting, hepatosplenomegaly.

OTHER: Failure to thrive. Generalized aminoaciduria. May have elevated blood galactose.

MISCELLANEOUS: Abnormal urine levels of galactose are not identified by current urine test strips because they use glucose oxidase, which is specific for glucose. Older tablet techniques identified all reducing sugars, including galactose.

ANESTHETIC CONSIDERATIONS
There are no specific anesthetic concerns with this disorder. Perioperative temperature maintenance may be difficult in these small, thin children. May be on a galactose-limited diet.

Bibliography:
1. Openo KK, Schulz JM, Vargas CA, et al. Epimerase-deficiency galactosemia is not a binary condition. *Am J Hum Genet* 2006;68:89–102.

Urticaria–Deafness–Amyloidosis Syndrome

SYNONYM: Muckle-Wells syndrome

MIM #: 191900

This autosomal dominant disorder has as its primary manifestations progressive cochlear deafness, urticaria, and renal amyloidosis. The disorder seems to be due to mutations in the gene *NALP3* (*CIAS1*). This gene is predominantly expressed in peripheral leukocytes. It is considered an autoinflammatory disease–one in which the inflammatory episode is unprovoked. Treatment with an interleukin-1 receptor antagonist has met with preliminary success.

HEENT/AIRWAY: Conjunctivitis. Absent organ of Corti, cochlear nerve atrophy.

ORTHOPEDIC: Arthralgias.

GI/GU: Amyloid infiltration of the kidney. Nephrotic syndrome.

OTHER: Urticaria. Periodic fever. Can have candidiasis of the mouth and perineum. Elevated erythrocyte sedimentation rate. Increased sensitivity to cold.

ANESTHETIC CONSIDERATIONS
When meeting with the patient before surgery, recall that he or she may have hearing loss. Baseline renal function should be assessed preoperatively. There are no guidelines regarding the safety of histamine-releasing drugs in this disease that involves urticaria, and there is no information regarding the effects of intraoperative hypothermia, as the urticarial lesions can be induced by cold air but not by ice cubes or cold water.

Bibliography:
1. Haas N, Kuster W, Zuberbier T, et al. Muckle-Wells syndrome: clinical and histological skin findings compatible with cold air urticaria in a large kindred. *Br J Dermatol* 2004;151:99–104.

V

VACTERL Association

See VATER association

Valproate

See Fetal valproate syndrome

van der Woude Syndrome

SYNONYM: Lip pit-cleft lip syndrome

MIM #: 119300

This autosomal dominant disorder, due to a mutation in the gene encoding interferon regulatory factor 6, is an association of cleft lip or palate with pits of the lower lip, which represent accessory salivary glands. There is some clinical heterogeneity, and some family members may have cleft lip, whereas others do not. The accessory salivary glands can produce an annoying watery discharge, and so may be surgically removed. This disorder is allelic with popliteal pterygium syndrome (see earlier).

HEENT/AIRWAY: Cleft lip, cleft palate, cleft uvula. Lower lip pits (accessory salivary glands). Hypotonic lower lip can produce lip asymmetry and protruding lower lip. Hypodontia with missing incisors, canines, or bicuspids. Syngnathia, an adhesion of the maxilla and the mandible, has been reported, as have other oral synechiae.

MISCELLANEOUS: Single-nucleotide polymorphisms in interferon regulatory factor 6 are thought to be a major

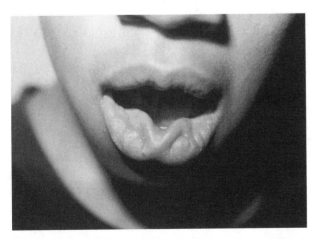

van der Woude syndrome. Typical lower lip in a boy with van der Woude syndrome. (Courtesy of Dr. K. Lin and the Craniofacial Anomalies Clinic, University of Virginia Health System.)

contributor to the development of cleft lip with or without cleft palate.

ANESTHETIC CONSIDERATIONS
Dental abnormalities should be documented preoperatively to avoid mistakenly assuming that teeth have been dislodged intraoperatively. Oral synechiae and syngnathism have resulted in markedly limited mouth opening which required nasal intubation and caused postoperative obstructive apnea in a neonate (1).

Bibliography:
1. Denion E, Capon N, Martinot V, et al. Neonatal permanent jaw constriction because of oral synechiae and Pierre Robin sequence in a child with van der Woude syndrome. *Cleft Palate Craniofac J* 2002;39:115–119.
2. Kulkarni ML, Sureshkumar C, Venkataramana V, et al. Van der Woude syndrome. *Ann Dent* 1995;54:34–35.

Varadi-Papp Syndrome

Included in Oral-facial-digital syndrome, type I

VATER Association

(Includes VACTERL association)

MIM #: 192350

VATER stands for **V**ertebral anomalies, **A**nal atresia, **T**racheoesophageal fistula, **E**sophageal atresia, and **R**adial and renal dysplasia, any combination of which can be present in a particular patient. The association of these diverse anomalies is sporadic and the etiology of the association is unknown, although there is an increased incidence in children of diabetic mothers. VATER association can also occur as part of a larger pattern of malformations, such as in trisomy 18. The VATER association has also been referred to as the **VACTERL** association (**V**ertebral anomalies, **A**nal atresia, **C**ardiac malformations, **T**racheoesophageal fistula, **E**sophageal atresia, **R**enal anomalies, **L**imb anomalies).

A separate entity, VATER with hydrocephalus from aqueductal stenosis, has been described as having both autosomal and X-linked inheritance.

HEENT/AIRWAY: Corneal anesthesia with secondary corneal injury has been reported. Laryngeal stenosis, tracheal atresia. Can have choanal atresia.

CHEST: Tracheoesophageal fistula. Respiratory distress from an ectopic bronchus has been reported. Esophageal atresia.

CARDIOVASCULAR: A variety of congenital cardiac defects can occur.

Orthopedic: Vertebral anomalies such as hemivertebrae, dysplastic vertebrae, vertebral fusion. Radial dysplasia. Can have dysplastic thumb. Preaxial polydactyly, syndactyly.

Gi/Gu: Esophageal atresia with tracheoesophageal fistula, duodenal atresia, imperforate anus with or without fistula. Renal anomalies. Defects of external genitalia.

Other: Single umbilical artery.

ANESTHETIC CONSIDERATIONS

Infants with tracheoesophageal fistula should have a cardiac examination to exclude congenital heart disease as part of the association. The anesthetic management of tracheo-esophageal fistula is complicated, particularly with respect to positioning the endotracheal tube to ventilate both lungs adequately without distending the stomach through the fistula. Many techniques exist to accomplish this (2–4).

Baseline renal status should be assessed preoperatively. Limb anomalies may limit options for vascular access. Radial anomalies may make placement of a radial arterial catheter more difficult. Patients with congenital heart disease require perioperative antibiotic prophylaxis as indicated. Successful epidural anesthesia has been reported in a parturient with known but unspecified vertebral anomalies.

Bibliography:
1. Chhibber AK, Hengerer AS, Fickling KB. Unsuspected subglottic stenosis in a two-year-old. *Paediatr Anaesth* 1997;7:65–67.
2. Reeves ST, Burt N, Smith CD. Is it time to reevaluate the airway management of tracheoesophageal fistula? *Anesth Analg* 1995;81:866–869.
3. Block EC, Filston H. A thin fiberoptic bronchoscope as an aid to occlusion of the fistula in infants with tracheoesophageal fistula. *Anesth Analg* 1988;67:791–793.
4. Borland LM, Reilly JS, Smith SD. Anesthetic management of tracheal esophageal fistula with distal tracheal stenosis. *Anesthesiology* 1987;67:132–133.
5. Lubinsky M. VATER and other associations: historical perspectives and modern interpretations. *Am J Med Genet* 1986;2:S9–S16.
6. Bleicher MA, Melmed AP, Bogaerts XV, et al. VATER association and unrecognized bronchopulmonary foregut malformation complicating anesthesia. *Mt Sinai J Med* 1983;50:435–438.

Velocardiofacial Syndrome

Synonym: Shprintzen syndrome

MIM #: 192430

This autosomal dominant syndrome is due to the same defect as the DiGeorge syndrome (see earlier), namely, a microdeletion of chromosome 22 (22q11), and the two syndromes have significant clinical overlap. Velocardiofacial syndrome has been ascribed to the *TBX1* gene, which resides in the center of the DiGeorge deletion region. T-box genes encode transcription factors involved in the regulation of developmental processes. This has also been called the CATCH-22 syndrome (see earlier). The syndrome consists of cleft palate, typical facies, cardiac anomalies, and learning disabilities.

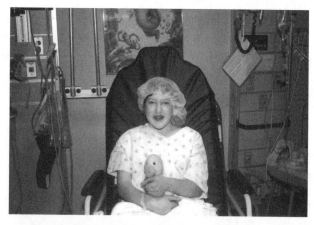

Velocardiofacial syndrome. This 14-year-old girl with velocardiofacial syndrome has had a laryngeal web and cleft, and a vascular ring. She has an asymmetric face and residual subglottic stenosis.

HEENT/AIRWAY: Microcephaly. Myopathic facies. Narrow palpebral fissures, small optic discs, tortuous retinal vessels, cataracts. Minor external ear anomalies. Prominent nose with bulbous tip and deficient alae nasi. Small, open mouth, pharyngeal hypotonia, cleft palate, velopharyngeal insufficiency with nasal speech. Decreased pharyngeal lymphoid tissue. Micrognathia, retrognathia.

CARDIOVASCULAR: Congenital heart disease, in particular conotruncal defects such as tetralogy of Fallot. Medial displacement of internal carotid arteries.

NEUROMUSCULAR: Learning disabilities, mental retardation. Blunt or inappropriate affect, psychiatric illness.

ORTHOPEDIC: Short stature. Thin hands and feet, hyperextensible hands and fingers.

Gi/Gu: Umbilical and inguinal hernias.

OTHER: Neonatal hypocalcemia, thymic aplasia with T-cell immunodeficiency, hypothyroidism.

ANESTHETIC CONSIDERATIONS

Micrognathia or retrognathia can make laryngoscopy and tracheal intubation very difficult. The serum calcium level should be evaluated in neonates preoperatively. Blood for transfusion should be irradiated because patients often have T-cell defects, leaving them at risk for graft-versus-host disease. Hypothyroidism, when present, could result in delayed gastric emptying, alterations in drug metabolism, and impaired temperature regulation. Patients with congenital heart disease need perioperative antibiotic prophylaxis as indicated. This region of chromosome 22 also includes the gene encoding catechol-*O*-methyltransferase (*COMT*), responsible for degrading catecholamines. A patient has been reported with unexpected tachycardia from epinephrine containing local analgesic given during dental surgery, possibly from being hemizygous for *COMT*.

Bibliography:

1. Passariello M, Perkins R. Unexpected postoperative tachycardia in a patient with 22q11 deletion syndrome after multiple dental extractions [Letter]. *Paediatr Anaesth* 2005;15:1145–1151.
2. Vogels A, Fryns JP. The velocardiofacial syndrome: a review. *Genet Couns* 2002;13:105–113.
3. Perez E, Sullivan KE. Chromosome 22q11.2 deletion syndrome (DiGeorge and velocardiofacial syndromes). *Curr Opin Pediatr* 2002;14: 678–683.
4. Goldberg R, Motzkin B, Marion R, et al. Velo-cardio-facial syndrome: a review of 120 patients. *Am J Med Genet* 1993;45:313–319.

Very-Long-Chain Acyl-CoA Dehydrogenase Deficiency

MIM #: 201475

This inborn error of metabolism is an autosomal recessive disease caused by a defect in the gene for very-long-chain acyl-CoA dehydrogenase, one of several acyl-CoA dehydrogenases, which are mitochondrial enzymes required for the beta-oxidation of fatty acids. The major clinical manifestations are hypertrophic cardiomyopathy, pericardial effusion, steatosis, and hypoglycemia. Treatment by supplying most of the dietary fat as medium-chain triglycerides has improved survival (4). Children may also be on carbohydrate-rich diets low in long-chain fatty acids and consuming frequent meals.

Fatty acids are oxidized in mitochondria. After mobilization from adipose tissue, they are taken up by the liver and other tissues, and converted to acyl-CoA esters in the cytoplasm. They enter mitochondria as carnitine esters, and become reesterified as acyl-CoA esters. Beta-oxidation results in the liberation of electrons. As beta-oxidation proceeds, the acyl chain is gradually shortened, and this first step in the oxidation process is catalyzed by acyl-CoA dehydrogenases with differing, but overlapping, chain-length specificities. These are very-long-chain, long-chain, medium-chain, and short-chain acyl-CoA dehydrogenases.

The phenotype is somewhat variable, with three general subtypes. An early, severe form with cardiomyopathy and early death presenting in infancy, a less severe form presenting in childhood and an adult-onset myopathic form which lacks cardiomyopathy. Episodes of acute decompensation can be initiated by fasting, viral illnesses, exercise, cold or emotional distress, including the prospect of surgery (1).

CARDIOVASCULAR: Essentially all patients except those with adult-onset disease have cardiomyopathy, including hypertrophic cardiomyopathy. Pericardial effusion. Cardiomyopathy is a common cause of death, and can regress with appropriate treatment.

NEUROMUSCULAR: Exercise-induced rhabdomyolysis and myoglobinuria, preventable by dietary carbohydrates before exercise. Elevated serum creatine kinase during acute decompensations. Muscle pains and stiffness in older patients.

GI/GU: Hepatocellular disease, steatosis. Elevated liver enzymes during acute decompensation.

OTHER: Hypoketotic hypoglycemia. Lactic acidosis. Marked lipid accumulation in many tissues. Decreased plasma carnitine.

ANESTHETIC CONSIDERATIONS

Perioperative fasting must be avoided, and patients should receive perioperative glucose supplementation. Perioperative fasting was believed to be the cause of death in a child with previously unrecognized disease (2). During periods of stress and metabolic decompensation, patients may need a very large amount of intravenous glucose (up to 10 to 15 mg/kg/minute). The degree and type of myocardial involvement should be delineated before surgery.

Propofol vehicle contains predominantly long-chain fatty acids, mainly C18, and propofol may inhibit mitochondrial entry of long-chain fatty acids and inhibit the respiratory chain. Interestingly, the propofol infusion syndrome in children sedated with propofol in the intensive care unit has many similarities with this syndrome. Propofol is probably contraindicated. Ringer's lactate should be avoided in cases of metabolic decompensation with lactic acidosis.

Bibliography:

1. Steiner LA, Studer W, Baumgartner ER, et al. Perioperative management of a child with very-long-chain acyl-coenzyme A dehydrogenase deficiency. *Paediatr Anaesth* 2002;12:187–191.
2. Roe CR, Wiltse HE, Sweetman L, et al. Death caused by perioperative fasting and sedation in a child with unrecognized very long chain acyl-coenzyme A dehydrogenase deficiency. *J Pediatr* 2000:136:397–399.
3. Straussberg R, Harel L, Varsano I, et al. Recurrent myoglobinuria as a presenting manifestation of very long chain acyl coenzyme A dehydrogenase deficiency. *Pediatrics* 1997;99:894–896.
4. Brown-Harrison MC, Nada MA, Sprecher H, et al. Very long chain acyl-CoA dehydrogenase deficiency: successful treatment of acute cardiomyopathy. *Biochem Mol Med* 1996;58:59–65.

Vitamin D-Resistant Rickets

SYNONYM: X-linked hypophosphatemic rickets

MIM #: 307800

Vitamin D-resistant rickets is the most common form of hereditary rickets. The primary defect is an inability to reabsorb filtered phosphate by the proximal renal tubule brush border membrane. This results in phosphate wasting and severe hypophosphatemia. There is also impaired regulation of 1α-hydroxylase activity, causing lower than appropriate levels of 1,25-dihydroxy vitamin D_3. In most patients the defect is due to mutations in the phosphate-regulating endopeptidase gene (*PHEX*). There are several other entities which also produce hypophosphatemic rickets.

An autosomal dominant form is due to abnormalities in the fibroblast growth factor gene *FGF23,* and oncogenic osteomalacia, associated with small, primitive tumors, in which elevated levels of fibroblast growth factor or other phosphaturic substances are considered paraneoplastic. Removal of the tumor is curative.

Treatment is with oral phosphorus supplementation and 1,25-dihydroxy vitamin D_3 (calcitriol). Complications of this therapy can include hypercalcemia, hypercalciuria, nephrocalcinosis, and secondary or tertiary hyperparathyroidism.

HEENT/AIRWAY: Craniosynostosis with frontal bossing. Craniotabes in infants (a ping-pong ball-like effect elicited by pressure on the parietal bones). Sensorineural deafness. Abnormal dentin formation and tooth pulp abscesses.

CHEST: Rachitic rosary (prominent rib costochondral junctions).

CARDIOVASCULAR: Hypertension and left ventricular hypertrophy have been reported in treated adults. Cardiac calcifications have been reported in cases of tertiary hyperparathyroidism and hypercalcemia.

NEUROMUSCULAR: Spinal stenosis from ossification of the ligamentum flavum and thickening of the laminae with cord compression has been reported in both untreated and treated patients.

ORTHOPEDIC: Rickets in children, osteomalacia in adults. Short stature, bowed legs, waddling gait. Extraskeletal ossification, particularly of tendons and ligaments. Painful degenerative joint disease similar to ankylosing spondylitis in adulthood. Metaphyseal widening, particularly of the lower extremities.

OTHER: Hypophosphatemia from renal phosphate wasting. Calcium levels are normal or low-normal, unlike other types of rickets. 1,25-dihydroxy vitamin D_3 levels are low despite hypophosphatemia.

ANESTHETIC CONSIDERATIONS
Serum calcium and phosphorus levels must be evaluated in patients on phosphate and vitamin D therapy. Older patients who may have osteomalacia must be carefully positioned perioperatively. Neuraxial anesthesia may be technically difficult when there is calcification of the ligamentum flavum.

Bibliography:

1. Carpenter TO. New perspectives on the biology and treatment of X-linked hypophosphatemic rickets. *Pediatr Clin North Am* 1997;44:443–466.
2. Scriver CR, Tenenhouse HS, Glorieux FH. X-linked hypophosphatemia: an appreciation of a classic paper and a survey of progress since 1958. *Medicine (Baltimore)* 1991;70:218–228.

Vogt-Spielmeyer Disease

See Spielmeyer-Vogt disease

von Gierke Disease

SYNONYM: Glycogen storage disease type I; Glucose-6-phosphatase deficiency

MIM #: 232200, 232220

Type I glycogen storage disease is the most commonly recognized of the glycogenoses. This autosomal recessive disease is due to a lack of hepatic and renal glucose-6-phosphatase (type IA). Glucose-6-phosphatase catalyzes the interconversion of glucose-6-phosphate and glucose in the Embden-Meyerhof pathway. This enzyme is crucial for allowing the production of glucose from glycogen stores (glycogenolysis) or from gluconeogenesis. The glucose-6-phosphate that is formed in the absence of the glucose-6-phosphatase enzyme is instead eventually converted to lactate. Decreased phosphatase causes decreased hepatic adenosine triphosphate, which in turn affects purine synthesis and causes hyperuricemia. Lactate itself also competitively inhibits renal tubular secretion of urate. Hypophosphatemia can occur secondary to excessive cellular accumulation of phosphorus as glucose-6-phosphate.

Type IB disease, also autosomal recessive, is due to deficiency of the carrier protein that transports glucose-6-phosphate across the microsomal membrane to the enzyme in hepatocytes and leukocytes. The enzyme itself is intact. Clinical findings are the same as for type IA, with additional findings as indicated.

Patients with von Gierke disease are treated with frequent high-carbohydrate feedings during the day and nasogastric or gastrostomy carbohydrate feedings overnight to maintain adequate serum glucose levels. Hypoglycemia is often very well tolerated, suggesting that these patients can use alternative substrates to supply brain glucose.

HEENT/AIRWAY: Lipemia retinalis. Gouty tophi. Nosebleeds. Oral lesions in type IB, including hyperplastic gingiva.

CARDIOVASCULAR: Hypertension in adults. Pulmonary hypertension has been reported.

NEUROMUSCULAR: Poorly controlled disease with recurrent hypoglycemia can result in neurologic injury.

ORTHOPEDIC: Osteopenia.

GI/GU: Hepatomegaly. Benign hepatic adenomatous nodules can cause massive bleeding, and uncommonly undergo malignant degeneration. Hepatic adenomas have developed in adults who have been treated appropriately for many years. Crohn's disease, chronic inflammatory bowel disease, and perianal abscesses in type IB. Rarely, pancreatitis as a complication of hyperlipidemia. Renal enlargement, renal calcification, uric acid stones, and nephropathy. Adult patients can have proteinuria, hematuria, or decreased creatinine clearance with progressive renal insufficiency. Delayed puberty. Polycystic ovaries.

OTHER: Life-threatening hypoglycemia, associated with metabolic acidosis, occurs even after brief periods of fasting. Hypoglycemia is more likely to occur with an unstable diet or with intercurrent illness. Hypophosphatemia, hyperuricemia. Hyperuricemic gout. Hypertriglyceridemia and hypercholesterolemia. Platelet dysfunction with a bleeding diathesis mirrors the clinical state. Platelet dysfunction is not due to an absence of glucose-6-phosphatase in the platelets, and improves as biochemical derangements are corrected. Xanthomas. Poorly controlled patients have growth failure. Intermittent severe neutropenia and recurrent infections in type IB. Symptoms can be exacerbated during pregnancy.

MISCELLANEOUS: Edgar von Gierke was a prominent German pathologist. Patients with von Gierke disease are resistant to the inebriating effects of ethanol, due to its accelerated metabolism. This was the first metabolic defect for which an enzymatic defect was identified.

ANESTHETIC CONSIDERATIONS

A preoperative fast without supplemental glucose must be avoided. Serum glucose should be monitored perioperatively and perioperative intravenous fluids should contain glucose. Intravenous fluids containing lactate should be avoided in patients with chronic lactic acidosis. Infants can be obese as the result of frequent demand and nocturnal feedings, which might increase the aspiration risk and make vascular access challenging. Renal function should be established preoperatively, particularly in adult or poorly controlled patients. Poorly controlled patients can have symptomatic platelet dysfunction. Platelet function has been reported to improve with both intensive glucose therapy for 24 to 48 hours and desmopressin (DDAVP). Propofol may increase urinary uric acid excretion (1), and this may be a consideration during longer cases using propofol anesthesia or sedation.

FIGURES: See **Appendix E**

Bibliography:

1. Miyazawa N, Takeda J, Izawa H. Does propofol change uric acid metabolism? *Anesth Analg* 1998;86:S486.
2. Shenkman Z, Golub Y, Meretyk S, et al. Anaesthetic management of a patient with glycogen storage disease type lb. *Can J Anaesth* 1996;43:467–470.
3. Talente GM, Coleman RA, Alter C, et al. Glycogen storage disease in adults. *Ann Intern Med* 1994;120:218–226.
4. Chen YT, Coleman RA, Scheinman JI, et al. Renal disease in type I glycogen storage disease. *N Engl J Med* 1988;318:7–11.
5. Bevan JC. Anaesthesia in Von Gierke's disease: current approach to management. *Anaesthesia* 1980;35:699–702.

von Hippel-Lindau Syndrome

MIM #: 193300

This autosomal dominant disease is characterized by multiple hemangioblastomas of the retina, central nervous system, and viscera. The hemangioblastomas lack a tight junction and so are prone to leak plasma. The von Hippel-Lindau gene, *VHL*, functions as a recessive tumor suppressor gene, and it is thought that inactivation of both alleles of *VHL* is critical for the development of tumors. One copy of the gene is inherited as a genetic mutation from a parent, and loss of activity of the second gene copy probably occurs as an acquired mutation or chromosomal rearrangement. The protein product of *VHL* posttranslationally modifies hypoxia-inducing factor (HIF) in an oxygen-dependent manner. Thus, with the loss of this gene product there is excessive production of HIF and gene products targeted by HIF, such as a variety of growth factors and erythropoietin. Approximately half the people carrying the defective gene have only one symptomatic lesion and are unlikely to be diagnosed as having the syndrome.

Two types have been described. Families with type I disease do not have pheochromocytoma, while families with type II disease are at risk for developing pheochromocytoma. Type II mutations are missense mutations.

HEENT/AIRWAY: Retinal vascular hamartomas are distinctive for this disease and are typically its earliest manifestation in type I patients. Capillary hemangiomas, exudative retinopathy, retinal detachment. Tumors of the endolymphatic sac of the ear leading to hearing loss, tinnitus, vertigo and seventh nerve dysfunction.

CHEST: Pulmonary cysts, oat cell carcinoma.

CARDIOVASCULAR: Cerebellar tumors can produce episodic hypertension similar to that seen with pheochromocytoma.

NEUROMUSCULAR: Cerebellar, medullary, and spinal cord hemangioblastomas. Spinal cord involvement has been reported in up to 100% of patients. Cord lesions are typically single, cervicothoracic, and asymptomatic, but can be lumbosacral or involve the cauda equina. Half of these patients have meningeal varicosities. Hemangioblastomas have also been found in nerve roots and in vertebrae. Intramedullary tumors are associated with syringomyelia in most. Spinal cord hemangiomas can bleed if patients develop hypertension. Cerebellar tumors typically present with signs of increased intracranial pressure, and only uncommonly with subarachnoid hemorrhage.

GI/GU: Hepatic adenomas, hepatocellular carcinoma. Pancreatic cysts, islet cell tumors. Renal cysts, ovarian cysts. Hypernephromas and renal cell carcinomas are common. Can have adenomas of the adrenals and bilateral cystadenomas of the epididymis.

OTHER: Erythrocytosis. Although the hemangioblastomas are benign, they can cause damage based on their location. Pheochromocytomas develop in 7% to 19% overall and can be the presenting finding in type II patients. Symptoms can develop, or become exacerbated, with pregnancy.

MISCELLANEOUS: von Hippel described the retinal lesions. Lindau recognized the association of retinal angiomas (von Hippel disease) and similar tumors of the cerebellum and elsewhere in the central nervous system. Actually, Treacher Collins was the first to recognize the angiomatous nature of the retinal lesions, several years before von Hippel reported his patients. The term "Lindau's disease" was coined by Harvey Cushing.

von Hippel-Lindau syndrome is one of the neuroectodermal disorders, or phakomatoses, along with neurofibromatosis, nevus sebaceous syndrome of Jadassohn, Sturge-Weber syndrome and tuberous sclerosis. "Phakos" is Greek for a lentil or lens-shaped spot.

ANESTHETIC CONSIDERATIONS

Spinal cord involvement is usually in the cervicothoracic region, well above the level at which a lumbar catheter would be placed. In fact, epidural anesthesia has been used successfully for cesarean section (4, 8) and neurosurgery (to limit the cerebrovasodilatory effects of general anesthetics) (5). However, the incidence of spinal cord involvement would indicate caution in the use of epidural or spinal anesthesia. Preoperative magnetic resonance imaging can delineate the location and extent of spinal hemangiomas. Patients with cerebellar involvement can have increased intracranial pressure, in which case precautions must be taken to avoid further increases in pressure. Cerebellar tumors can produce episodic hypertension similar to that seen with pheochromocytoma. Since pheochromocytomas are not uncommon and can be undiagnosed, unexpected and otherwise unexplained intraoperative hypertension should at least raise the suspicion of pheochromocytoma.

Bibliography:

1. Boker A, Ong BY. Anesthesia for Cesarean section and posterior fossa craniotomy in a patient with von Hippel-Lindau disease. *Can J Anaesth* 2001;48:387–390.
2. Diaz JH. Perioperative management of children with congenital phakomatoses. *Paediatr Anaesth* 2000;10:121–128.
3. Couch V, Lindor NM, Karnes PS, et al. von Hippel-Lindau disease. *Mayo Clin Proc* 2000;7:265–272.
4. Wang A, Sinatra RS. Epidural anesthesia for cesarean section in a patient with von Hippel-Lindau disease and multiple sclerosis. *Anesth Analg* 1999;88:1083–1084.
5. Mugawar M, Rajender Y, Purohit AK, et al. Anesthetic management of von Hippel-Lindau syndrome for excision of cerebellar hemangioblastoma and pheochromocytoma surgery. *Anesth Analg* 1998;86:673–674.
6. Joffe D, Robins R, Benjamin A. Cesarean section and phaeochromocytoma resection in a patient with von Hippel Lindau disease. *Can J Anaesth* 1993;40:870–874.
7. Maher ER, Yates JR, Harries R, et al. Clinical features and natural history of von Hippel-Lindau disease. *Q J Med* 1990;77:1151–1163.
8. Matthews AJ, Halshaw J. Epidural anaesthesia in von Hippel-Lindau disease: management of childbirth and anaesthesia for cesarean section. *Anaesthesia* 1986;41:853–855.

von Recklinghausen Disease

See Neurofibromatosis

von Voss-Cherstvoy Syndrome

See DK-phocomelia syndrome

von Willebrand Disease

MIM #: 193400

von Willebrand disease is the most common inherited bleeding disorder in humans. The most common symptom is mucocutaneous bleeding. von Willebrand factor (vWF) serves as the first link between platelets and injured blood vessels by binding to platelet receptors GpIb and GpIIb-IIIa and to ligands within the exposed vessel wall. It is also the carrier in plasma for factor VIII, localizing it to the initial platelet plug. Type 1 disease, the most common variant, has low amounts of normal vWF. In type 2 disease there is abnormal structure and/or function of vWF. This can be due to diminished synthesis or secretion, or increased peripheral proteolysis. Type 2N is associated with mutations in the factor VIII binding domain of vWF, resulting in a mild hemophilia A–like disorder. Type 2A results in selective loss of the largest vWF multimers. Type 2B results from mutations in the platelet binding domain, resulting in excessive platelet binding and circulating thrombocytopenia. Type 3, the least common and the most severe, is associated with very low or undetectable levels of vWF.

Type 1 is autosomal dominant. Type 2 is autosomal dominant, although rare cases of recessive disease have been reported. Type 3 has been inconsistently reported as autosomal recessive. There is significant clinical variability within type 1, even within families, and laboratory and clinical findings can be discrepant even within an individual. Patients with mild or moderate type 1 disease may experience amelioration of symptoms in the second or third decade of life.

Type 1 disease can often be treated successfully with desmopressin (DDAVP), which induces vWF and factor VIII secretion from endothelial cells and which increases plasma vWF levels by a factor of 2 to 3. Types 2 and 3 do not respond to DDAVP and require treatment with plasma or factor VIII concentrate containing large amounts of vWF.

HEENT/AIRWAY: Epistaxis, gingival bleeding.

ORTHOPEDIC: Hemarthroses rare and usually only with major joint trauma, more common in type 3 disease. Muscle hematomas in type 3 disease.

GI/GU: Can have gastrointestinal bleeding. Menorrhagia.

OTHER: Easy bruising. Prolonged bleeding time. Thrombocytopenia in type 2B, during times of increased vWF synthesis, such as pregnancy, as a neonate, or postoperatively, but thrombocytopenia is rarely low enough to result in excessive bleeding.

MISCELLANEOUS: The first described patient, a young girl, died from hemorrhage in adolescence when she began menstruating.

ANESTHETIC CONSIDERATIONS

Excessive bleeding with trauma and dental extractions. Can have delayed bleeding after tonsillectomy. Treatment is with DDAVP in type 1 patients, DDAVP and vWF-containing concentrates such as Humate-P and Alphanate in types 2A and 2B, and vWF-containing concentrates in types 2N and 3. DDAVP can potentially worsen type 2B disease as the high molecular weight vWF released from storage has high affinity for GpIb binding sites and can worsen thrombocytopenia. Type 2N patients generally do not respond to DDAVP. Approximately 80% of type 1 patients will respond to DDAVP, and response to one dose predicts responses to future doses. DDAVP is administered 1 hour preoperatively and then every 12 hours for 2 to 4 doses, after which the clinical response is lost. DDAVP therapy is associated with a risk of dilutional hyponatremia, particularly at the extremes of age. It may be relatively contraindicated in patients with coronary artery disease due to a possible increased risk of coronary artery thrombosis.

It is suggested that in patients requiring treatment with concentrates, goals for activity are approximately 50% to 80% in major trauma, surgery or central nervous system hemorrhage, >50% for childbirth, >30% to 50% for dental extractions or minor surgery and 20% to 80% for mucous membrane bleeding or menorrhagia. Antifibrinolytics are also commonly used. Autologous red cells, plasma, and platelets can be collected prior to elective surgery with expected significant blood loss. Multidisciplinary planning with hematologists and surgeons should precede elective surgery.

vWF levels generally rise during pregnancy. However, because of this, type 2B may worsen during pregnancy (1). Because of the general improvement during gestation, neuraxial analgesia has been reported in a very few parturients, but because of the variability in clinical type and degree of symptoms in all, it should be undertaken after discussions with the patient's hematologist to weigh the risks and advantages. The risk of neonatal disease is not an indication for cesarean section.

Bibliography:
1. Hepner D, Tsen L. Severe thrombocytopenia, type 2B von Willebrand disease and pregnancy. *Anesthesiology* 2004;101:1465–1467.
2. Lee JW. Von Willebrand disease, hemophilia A and B and other factor deficiencies. *Int Anesthesiol Clin* 2004;42:59–76.
3. Bolan C, Rick ME, Polly DW Jr. Transfusion medicine management for reconstructive spinal repair in a patient with von Willebrand's disease and a history of heavy surgical bleeding. *Spine* 2001;26:E552–E556.

W

Waardenburg Syndrome

(Includes Klein-Waardenburg syndrome and Shah-Waardenburg syndrome)

MIM #: 193500

This autosomal dominant disorder is a well known clinical syndrome that classically consists of congenital deafness and a white forelock as a sign of partial albinism. It is one of several auditory-pigmentary syndromes. Four types have been described: type 1, due to mutations in the *PAX3* gene, has lateral displacement of the inner canthi of the eyes. *PAX* genes encode transcription factors. Numerous distinct mutations in this gene have been described. The gene product is thought to be involved in early neuronal development. Type 2 is heterogeneous and does not have this lateral displacement. Some cases of type 2 are due to mutations in the gene *MITF*, which encodes a transcription factor important for melanocyte differentiation. Type 3, known as **Klein-Waardenburg syndrome**, is uncommon and has the manifestations of type I plus dysplasia of the upper limbs and muscles. This type probably represents either an allelic mutation of the *PAX3* gene or involvement of a contiguous gene. Type 4 is due to mutations in one of several genes and is associated with Hirschsprung disease. Type 4 is sometimes referred to as **Shah-Waardenburg syndrome**. There is some clinical heterogeneity, and some patients are not deaf.

HEENT/AIRWAY: White forelock, which can be present at birth and then become pigmented, or which can persist. Lateral displacement of the inner canthi, short palpebral fissures, medial flaring of bushy eyebrows, synophrys, hypopigmented fundus, hypochromic pale blue iris, heterochromic irises. Congenital cochlear deafness, unilateral or usually bilateral, with aplasia of the posterior semicircular canal. Hypoplastic alae nasi. Smooth philtrum. Cleft lip and palate have been reported. Broad prognathic mandible.

CHEST: Supernumerary ribs.

NEUROMUSCULAR: Spina bifida.

ORTHOPEDIC: Scoliosis. Supernumerary vertebrae.

GI/GU: Hirschsprung disease (see earlier) in type 4. Esophageal or anal atresia. Absent vagina and adnexae.

OTHER: Premature graying, hypopigmented skin lesions.

MISCELLANEOUS: Described independently by Petrus Waardenburg and David Klein. Waardenburg was a Dutch ophthalmologist who made contributions in the field of genetic ophthalmology. He was the first to suggest that Down syndrome was due to a chromosomal abnormality (1932). His last medical paper was published when he was 84 years old.

The association of pigmentary abnormalities and deafness is known in many animal species, and its occurrence in cats was commented upon by Darwin. Neural tube defects are also found in the "splotch" mouse, which carries a mutation in the homologous gene.

ANESTHETIC CONSIDERATIONS
When meeting patients before surgery, recall that they may have significant hearing loss.

Bibliography:
1. Dourmishev AL, Dourmishev LA, Schwartz RA, et al. Waardenburg syndrome. *Int J Dermatol* 1999;38:665–663.
2. Read AP, Newton VE. Waardenburg syndrome. *J Med Genet* 1997;34: 656–665.
3. Liu XZ, Newton VE, Read AP. Waardenburg syndrome type II: phenotypic findings and diagnostic criteria. *Am J Med Genet* 1995;55:95–100.

WAGR Syndrome

See Aniridia-Wilms tumor association

Walker-Warburg Syndrome

SYNONYM: Warburg syndrome; HARD(E) syndrome

MIM #: 236670

This autosomal recessive disorder is a muscular dystrophy with brain and eye manifestations. It has multiple names, including the acronym HARD for **H**ydrocephalus, **A**gyria, **R**etinal **D**ysplasia, or HARDE (the **E** for "encephalocele"). All patients have lissencephaly, retinal malformations, mental retardation, and a muscular dystrophy. It is often fatal within the first few months of life. It is similar to muscle-eye-brain disease (see earlier). Walker-Warburg syndrome is due to defects the gene encoding protein O-mannosyltransferase (*POMT 1*). This enzyme is involved with the glycosylation of alpha-dystroglycan, one of the proteins in the complex which links dystrophin to the cell membrane. Limb-girdle muscular dystrophy type 2A is an allelic disorder. Another phenotypically similar disorder is Fukuyama muscular dystrophy (not included in this text). Fukuyama muscular dystrophy is due to abnormalities in the gene *FCMD*, which encodes fukutin. Abnormal glycosylation of alpha-dystroglycan is a feature of these syndromes also.

HEENT/AIRWAY: Almost all have malformations of the anterior chamber, including cataracts, corneal clouding and/or glaucoma. All have retinal defects, including microphthalmia, hyperplastic vitreous causing a retrolental mass, coloboma or retinal detachment. Microtia, absent external auditory canals. Cleft lip or palate. Can have micrognathia.

NEUROMUSCULAR: All have a muscular dystrophy. Brain malformations, including lissencephaly, with prominent agyria and scattered areas of microgyria, thickened cortex, absent or hypoplastic corpus callosum or septum pellucidum. Cerebellar malformations, Dandy-Walker malformation, occipital encephalocele, hydrocephalus. Profound mental retardation in those who survive the first year. Seizures develop with aging.

ORTHOPEDIC: Congenital contractures.

GI/GU: Imperforate anus. Genital anomalies. Renal dysplasia.

OTHER: Intrauterine growth retardation.

ANESTHETIC CONSIDERATIONS
Micrognathia can make laryngoscopy difficult. Patients can have elevated intracranial or intraocular pressure, in which case precautions should be taken to avoid further elevations in pressure. Renal function should be evaluated preoperatively. Contractures can make intraoperative positioning difficult. Succinylcholine is contraindicated in patients with a myopathy because of the risk of an exaggerated hyperkalemic response. Seizures, poor airway control, and swallowing difficulties make close observation for postoperative respiratory complications important.

Bibliography:
1. Sahajananda H, Meneges J. Anaesthesia for a child with Walker-Warburg syndrome. *Paediatr Anaesth* 2003;13:624–628.
2. Dobyns WB, Pagon RA, Armstrong D, et al. Diagnostic criteria for Walker-Warburg syndrome. *Am J Med Genet* 1989;32:195–210.

Warburg Syndrome

See Walker-Warburg syndrome

Warfarin

See Fetal warfarin syndrome

Watson Syndrome

MIM #: 193520

This autosomal dominant syndrome was originally described by Watson as involving pulmonic stenosis, dull intelligence, and café au lait spots. The clinical syndrome has been expanded since Watson's original description. The disorder is due to a mutation in the neurofibromatosis gene (*NF1*). Clinically, the syndrome overlaps with neurofibromatosis (see earlier), although there are significant differences.

HEENT/AIRWAY: Relative macrocephaly. Lisch nodules of the iris are uncommon.

CARDIOVASCULAR: Valvar pulmonary stenosis, which may be severe. Ectasia of the coronary arteries.

NEUROMUSCULAR: Low normal intelligence. Watson syndrome is not thought of as having the neurologic manifestations of neurofibromatosis, although one family with central nervous system involvement on magnetic resonance imaging scan has been reported.

ORTHOPEDIC: Short stature. Limited knee and ankle movement.

GI/GU: Retroperitoneal or visceral neurofibromas.

OTHER: Café au lait spots, small numbers of neurofibromas, axillary freckling.

ANESTHETIC CONSIDERATIONS
Patients must be carefully positioned secondary to limited lower extremity movement. Isolated pulmonic stenosis is usually well tolerated. Patients with pulmonic stenosis require perioperative antibiotic prophylaxis as indicated.

Bibliography:
1. Leao M, da Silva ML. Evidence of central nervous system involvement in Watson syndrome. *Pediatr Neurol* 1995;12:252–254.
2. Conway JB, Posner M. Anaesthesia for cesarean section in a patient with Watson's syndrome. *Can J Anaesth* 1994;41:1113–1116.

Weaver Syndrome

SYNONYM: Weaver-Smith syndrome

MIM #: 277590

The hallmarks of this autosomal dominant syndrome are accelerated growth, abnormal facies, and camptodactyly. At least some cases are due to mutations in the gene *NSD1*, which encodes a coregulator of the androgen receptor. This gene is also mutated in most patients with Sotos syndrome (see earlier). Like Sotos syndrome, Weaver syndrome is one of overgrowth.

HEENT/AIRWAY: Macrocephaly, flat occiput. Hypertelorism, epicanthal folds, strabismus, down-slanting palpebral fissures. Large ears. Depressed nasal bridge, long philtrum. Underdeveloped teeth. Large, thick tongue. Relative micrognathia (retrognathia). Prominent chin. Short, broad neck with excessive fat. Low-pitched, hoarse voice with dysarthric speech.

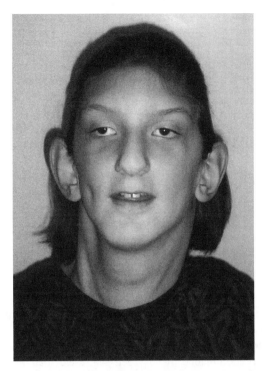

Weaver syndrome. This girl has the typical facies of Weaver syndrome with prominent ears.

NEUROMUSCULAR: Developmental delay, usually mild. Tantrums and behavioral problems. Hypertonia, seizures. Abnormal cerebral vessels.

GI/GU: Can have inguinal and umbilical hernias. Can have cryptorchidism.

ORTHOPEDIC: Accelerated growth and maturation, beginning prenatally. Advanced bone age. Weight is increased more than height. Camptodactyly, broad thumbs, prominent finger pads, hyperextensible fingers, deeply set nails. Limited extension of elbows and knees. Foot deformities. Kyphosis. Scoliosis. Unstable upper cervical spine has been reported.

GI/GU: Inguinal or umbilical hernias. Cryptorchidism.

OTHER: Loose skin, thin hair. Neoplasia has been reported in some.

ANESTHETIC CONSIDERATIONS
The bull neck and small mandible (relative to the large head) make visualization of the larynx very difficult. Based on 2 cases, it has been suggested that the difficulty in laryngoscopy might improve with age (1). Behavioral problems can make smooth induction of anesthesia a challenge. Excessive fat on the limbs can make intravenous access difficult. Chronic use of anticonvulsant medications may affect the metabolism of some anesthetic drugs. An unstable cervical spine is not generally considered to be a part of this syndrome, but has been reported.

Bibliography:
1. Crawford MW, Rohan D. The upper airway in Weaver syndrome. *Paediatr Anaesth* 2005;15:893–896.
2. Celebioglu B, Yener F. Anaesthesia for open-heart surgery in a patient with Weaver's syndrome [Letter]. *Eur J Anaesthesiol* 2002;19:897–898.
3. Opitz JM, Weaver DW, Reynolds JF Jr. The syndromes of Sotos and Weaver. *Am J Med Genet* 1998;79:294–304.
4. Cole TR, Dennis NR, Hughes HE. Weaver syndrome. *J Med Genet* 1992;29:332–337.
5. Turner DR, Downing JW. Anaesthetic problems associated with Weaver's syndrome. *Br J Anaesth* 1985;57:1260–1263.

Weaver-Smith Syndrome

See Weaver syndrome

Weber-Christian Disease

MIM #: None

This chronic disease involves relapsing fever and panniculitis. The etiology of this disease is unknown, and there can be a variety of systemic manifestations. There is a female predominance. It has been suggested that this is an autoimmune disease, and a number of patients have gone on to acquire other autoimmune disorders. Steroid and other immunosuppressive treatments have been used with variable success.

HEENT/AIRWAY: Orbital involvement with panniculitis of the retrobulbar fat with proptosis.

CHEST: Pleural panniculitis.

CARDIOVASCULAR: Myocardial involvement with heart failure. There can be vascular fragility.

NEUROMUSCULAR: Myalgias.

ORTHOPEDIC: Arthritis and arthralgias.

GI/GU: Ileal and colonic perforations have been reported secondary to focal disease. Acalculous cholecystitis. Pancreatic or adrenal involvement. Splenic vein occlusion with the development of varices from intraabdominal disease has been reported. Ureteral obstruction from retroperitoneal fibrosis. Membranous glomerulonephritis associated with circulating immune complexes.

OTHER: Erythematous lesions of the arms and legs from involvement of subcutaneous fat are usually the earliest manifestation, followed by subcutaneous atrophy. Mammary calcifications on mammography. Fever and edema are common. Anemia, leukopenia, and hypocomplementemia. Circulating immune complexes.

MISCELLANEOUS: See Sturge-Weber syndrome for a discussion of Weber. Henry Christian, a native of Virginia, was the first physician-in-chief at the Peter Bent Brigham Hospital in Boston.

ANESTHETIC CONSIDERATIONS

The manifestations of this disease are protean, and perioperative care must be tailored (as always) to the individual. The hematocrit should be evaluated preoperatively. Trauma to fat by heat, cold, or pressure should be avoided. Myocardial depressant agents should be used with care if there is evidence of myocardial involvement. Patients taking immunosuppressive drugs can have electrolyte abnormalities. Patients who have been taking steroids require perioperative stress doses. A history of relapsing fever can complicate the interpretation of postoperative fever.

Bibliography:
1. Lemley DE, Ferrans VJ, Fox LM, et al. Cardiac manifestations of Weber-Christian disease: report and review of the literature. *J Rheumatol* 1991;18:756–760.
2. Panush RS, Yonker RA, Dlesk A, et al. Weber-Christian disease: analysis of 15 cases and review of the literature. *Medicine (Baltimore)* 1985;64:181–191.

Weill-Marchesani Syndrome

MIM #: 277600, 608328

This disorder can be autosomal recessive or autosomal dominant. The recessive form is due to abnormalities in the gene *ADAMTS10*. The dominant form is due to mutations in the gene *FBN1*, which encodes fibrillin. Abnormalities in this gene are also responsible for Marfan syndrome. The hallmark features are ectopia lentis, short stature, and brachydactyly.

HEENT/AIRWAY: Brachycephaly. Lens dislocation, small round lens, myopia, glaucoma, cataract, blindness. Depressed nasal bridge. Mild maxillary hypoplasia with narrow palate. Malformed, malaligned teeth.

CARDIOVASCULAR: Can have subvalvar aortic stenosis or other cardiac defects.

NEUROMUSCULAR: Usually normal intelligence, may have mild mental retardation.

ORTHOPEDIC: Proportionate short stature. Brachydactyly, broad phalanges. Carpal tunnel syndrome. Stiff joints (particularly hands). Scoliosis. Thick skin.

ANESTHETIC CONSIDERATIONS

When meeting the patient before surgery, recall that he or she may have vision loss, and intelligence will be appropriate for chronological age, not height age. Glaucoma can be induced by provoking mydriasis. Endotracheal intubation can be difficult due to limited mouth opening. A laryngeal mask airway (LMA) has been used successfully. Endotracheal tube depth should be appropriate for patient height. Patients with cardiac disease require perioperative antibiotic prophylaxis as indicated.

Bibliography:
1. Dal D, Şahin A, Aypas U. Anesthetic management of a patient with Weill-Marchesani syndrome. *Acta Anaesthesiol Scand* 2003;47:369–370.
2. Karabiyik L. Airway management of a patient with Weill-Marchesani syndrome. *J Clin Anesth* 2003;15:214–216.

Werdnig-Hoffmann disease

SYNONYM: Spinal muscular atrophy type I. (Includes Spinal muscular atrophy type II)

MIM #: 253300, 253550

This autosomal recessive disease of anterior horn cells and cranial nerve nuclei involves a defect in the telomeric gene *SMN1* (survival of motor neuron 1). This same gene is affected in spinal muscular atrophy types I, II, and III, and these disorders are allelic. The gene product is involved with RNA processing. Several clinical phenotypes have been described, and the clinical manifestations can vary within a given family. Disease severity can be modified by changes in expression of the centromeric copy of the gene, termed *SMN2*. Approximately half of SMA I patients and 20% of

SMA II patients have abnormalities in the gene *NAIP*, the gene encoding neuronal apoptosis inhibitory protein, which may play a role in disease modification.

Spinal muscular atrophy type I (acute Werdnig-Hoffmann disease, acute infantile spinal muscle atrophy) presents in the first 6 months of life. One third present *in utero* with decreased fetal movement. Survival beyond 2 years of age is uncommon.

Spinal muscular atrophy type II (chronic Werdnig-Hoffmann disease, intermediate spinal muscle atrophy) presents at approximately 6 months of age when, after previously normal development, motor milestones become delayed. The trunk and proximal limb muscles are predominantly involved. There can be periods of stability in the progression of the disease, and some patients can have a stable course after an initial period of progressive weakness. Survival until adulthood is possible. The muscle biopsy tends to show fewer atrophic muscle fibers than in type I, but there is significant overlap, and the muscle biopsy does not correlate with prognosis.

Spinal muscular atrophy type III (juvenile spinal muscle atrophy) is known as Kugelberg-Welander disease (see earlier).

HEENT/AIRWAY

Type I: Difficulty with swallowing and handling secretions. Atrophy and visible fasciculations of the tongue. Extraocular and facial muscles are spared.

Type II: Difficulties with chewing and swallowing are rare. Tongue fasciculations and atrophy in approximately one half of patients.

CHEST

Type I: Respiratory distress. Shallow respirations, paradoxical respiratory pattern with diaphragmatic breathing. Death is often from pulmonary infection with respiratory failure. Infants who present with decreased movement *in utero* have decreased lung volumes.

Type II: Respiratory embarrassment from severe scoliosis. Recurrent infections.

NEUROMUSCULAR

Type I: Hypotonia, profound weakness, absent deep tendon reflexes. Normal intelligence and development (except for motor skills). No sensory loss.

Type II: Fine tremor of the hands. Deep tendon reflexes diminished or absent. Normal intelligence. No sensory loss.

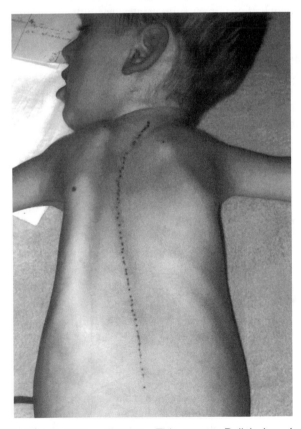

Werdnig-Hoffman disease. This young Polish boy has Werdnig-Hoffman disease. The muscle wasting is evident and he is developing scoliosis.

ORTHOPEDIC

Type II: Kyphoscoliosis. Late contractures. Can have pseudohypertrophy of the calves.

GI/GU

Type I: Feeding problems.

OTHER

Type II: Pregnancy can be associated with worsening of symptoms and premature labor. Restrictive lung disease can also be exacerbated by the enlarging uterus.

MISCELLANEOUS: The disorder was described independently by Werdnig and Hoffmann.

ANESTHETIC CONSIDERATIONS

Remember that these children have normal intelligence, and interactions with them should be age appropriate. Patients with bulbar disease may be at increased risk for perioperative aspiration. Intraoperative positioning may be difficult secondary to severe kyphoscoliosis. Patients may need protracted postoperative ventilation or chest physiotherapy. Succinylcholine is contraindicated because of the risk of exaggerated hyperkalemia. Nondepolarizing muscle relaxants should be titrated and given only as needed.

Bibliography:
1. Bush A, Fraser J, Jardine E, et al. Respiratory management of the infant with type 1 spinal muscular atyrophy. *Arch Dis Child* 2005;90:709–711.
2. Habib AS, Helsley SE, Millar S, et al. Anesthesia for cesarean section in a patient with spinal muscular atrophy. *J Clin Anesth* 2004;16:217–219.
3. Samaha FJ, Buncher CR, Russman BS, et al. Pulmonary function in spinal muscular atrophy. *J Child Neurol* 1994;9:326–329.
4. Thomas NH, Dubowitz V. The natural history of type I (severe) spinal muscular atrophy. *Neuromuscul Disord* 1994;4:497–502.

Werner Syndrome

MIM #: 277700

This autosomal recessive disorder is one of apparent premature aging. The disorder is due to abnormalities in the gene *RECQL2*, which encodes a helicase. Helicases regulate DNA synthesis, and its gene product catalyzes DNA unwinding. Some patients with "atypical Werner" syndrome have their disorder due to abnormalities in the gene *LMNA*, which encodes a nuclear lamin. Lamins are proteins which determine the size and shape of the nucleus. Cells from Werner patients are capable of only about one-third of the doublings when cultured *in vitro* compared to normal cells. Children are normal until a failure of the pubertal growth spurt, and other signs and symptoms then follow. The mean age at death is 47 years, with cancer the most common cause.

HEENT/AIRWAY: Prematurely aged face. Cataracts. Beaked nose. Premature loss of teeth. Vocal cord atrophy with high-pitched, hoarse voice.

CARDIOVASCULAR: Premature atherosclerosis with calcification, hypertension.

NEUROMUSCULAR: Muscle hypoplasia. Organic brain syndrome with calcification of the media (Monckeberg arteriosclerosis).

ORTHOPEDIC: Short stature [mean height in Caucasian populations of 5 ft. 1 in. (157 cm) in males and 4 ft. 9 in. (146 cm) in females]. Normal as children, but do not have an adolescent growth spurt. Thin, spindly extremities, small hands and feet. Atrophy of distal extremities. Osteoporosis.

GI/GU: Hypogonadism. Adrenal atrophy.

OTHER: Loss of subcutaneous fat. Patches of stiffened scleroderma-like skin on face and lower legs, ulcerations of skin, thin dermis. Hyperkeratotic palms and soles. Sparse hair. Premature graying and balding. Type II diabetes. Metastatic calcifications. Hypercholesterolemia and hypertriglyceridemia. Increased incidence of a wide variety of malignancies. Mild hyperthyroidism. Increased sensitivity to DNA-damaging drugs, such as chemotherapeutic drugs.

MISCELLANEOUS: Werner reported this disorder as his doctoral thesis in 1904. He was a German general practitioner.

ANESTHETIC CONSIDERATIONS

Teeth should be inventoried preoperatively because of premature loss. Loss of subcutaneous fat may make intraoperative temperature maintenance difficult. There is a risk of perioperative cardiac ischemia. It is not clear whether drug metabolism mirrors that of elderly patients, although this would be a reasonable assumption. Insulin resistance is treatable with drugs which sensitize insulin action. Cataract surgery has been complicated by wound dehiscence.

Bibliography:
1. Nehlin JO, Skovgaard GL, Bohr VA. The Werner syndrome. A model for the study of human aging. *Ann NY Acad Sci* 2000;908:167–179.
2. Duvic M, Lemak NA. Werner's syndrome. *Dermatol Clin* 1995;13:163–168.

Whelan Syndrome

Included in Oral-facial-digital syndrome, type I

Whistling Face Syndrome

SYNONYM: Freeman-Sheldon syndrome; Craniocarpotarsal dysplasia

MIM #: 193700

This usually autosomal dominant disorder is thought to be due to a slowly progressive myopathy. It is considered to be a distal arthrogryposis, of which nine types have been delineated. Increased muscle tone leads to many of the features of this syndrome, including masklike "whistling" facies, ulnar deviation of the hands, and clubfoot deformity. Autosomal dominant inheritance is possible, but autosomal recessive inheritance has also been described.

HEENT/AIRWAY: Full forehead and prominent supraorbital ridges. Can have microcephaly. Increased tone and fibrosis of the facial muscles causes an immobile, masklike facial expression. Strabismus. Can have epicanthal folds, ptosis, telecanthus, blepharophimosis. Hearing loss. Broad nasal bridge. Small nose. Hypoplastic alae nasi with notching. Long philtrum. Fibrotic bands around the mouth result in microstomia, pursed lips and the "whistling face" appearance. High-arched palate. Small tongue and limited palatal movement, which results in nasal speech. Small mandible. Mound of subcutaneous tissue demarcated by "H"-shaped dimple on the chin. Muscle contractures cause cephalad positioning of the larynx. Pharyngeal muscle myopathy can lead to chronic airway obstruction, and children requiring tracheostomy have been rarely reported. Can have short neck.

CHEST: Intercostal myopathy and abnormal development of the bony thorax (pectus excavatum). Dysphagia and recurrent vomiting can lead to aspiration pneumonia. Kyphosis, often presenting later in life, can cause restrictive lung disease. Sleep disordered breathing.

CARDIOVASCULAR: Cor pulmonale can develop secondary to chronic airway obstruction.

NEUROMUSCULAR: Intelligence is usually normal, but mental retardation in approximately one-third. Generalized myopathy. Increased muscle tone. Can have spina bifida occulta. Can have seizures.

ORTHOPEDIC: Kyphoscoliosis develops with time at congenitally malformed vertebrae. Multiple joint contractures can develop. Camptodactyly. Ulnar deviation of the hands. Flexion contractures of the fingers. Adduction of the thumbs. Clubfoot deformity and toe contractures. Can have hip dislocation.

GI/GU: Can have dysphagia and recurrent vomiting. Inguinal hernias. Cryptorchidism.

MISCELLANEOUS: Ernest Freeman was a British orthopedic surgeon. Joseph Sheldon was a British physician who later became the president of the International Association of Gerontologists. The patient in the original case report by Freeman and Sheldon in 1938 had postoperative pneumonia and empyema.

ANESTHETIC CONSIDERATIONS

The fixed microstomia is not relieved by muscle relaxants. The combination of microstomia, micrognathia, neck shortening, and cephalad positioning of the larynx may make direct laryngoscopy and visualization of the vocal cords extremely difficult or impossible. A laryngeal mask airway (LMA) has been used successfully as a primary airway (6) and to guide fiberoptic intubation (8). The small mouth may not accept an LMA (5), but the LMA can be folded to fit in the small mouth (3).

Chronic airway obstruction can be present in patients with pharyngeal muscle myopathy. Chronic lung disease may have developed in patients with a history of recurrent aspiration pneumonia. Acute aspiration is a risk in those patients with dysphagia and vomiting. There is an increased incidence of postoperative respiratory complications, in part due to intercostal muscle myopathy and abnormal development of the bony thorax.

Deformities of the hands and feet can make peripheral vascular access more difficult. Patients require careful positioning because of kyphoscoliosis and extremity contractures. Spina bifida occulta can occur and should be considered prior to utilizing a caudal or epidural block. Although there are no data, succinylcholine should be used with caution in this myopathy because of the risk of exaggerated hyperkalemia. However, we are aware of its use without hyperkalemic complications in a relatively large number of patients (Berry FA, University of Virginia, personal communication).

Whistling face syndrome has been associated with muscle rigidity after the administration of anesthetic agents (particularly halothane), but has not been associated with malignant hyperthermia (10–13).

Bibliography:

1. Stevenson DA, Carey JC, Palumbos J, et al. Clinical characteristics and natural history of Freeman-Sheldon syndrome. *Pediatrics* 2006;117:754–762.
2. Kim JS, Park SY, Min SK, et al. Awake nasotracheal intubation using fiberoptic bronchoscope in a pediatric patient with Freeman-Sheldon syndrome. *Paediatr Anaesth* 2005;15:790–792.
3. Chen A, Lai H-Y, Lee Y, et al. Anesthesia for Freeman-Sheldon syndrome using a folded laryngeal mask airway [Letter]. *Anesth Analg* 2005;101:606–615.
4. Agritmis A, Unlusoy O, Karaca S. Anesthetic management of a patient with Freeman-Sheldon syndrome. *Paediatr Anaesth* 2004;14:874–877.
5. Okawa M, Kinouchi K, Kitamura S, et al. Anesthetic management of an infant with Freeman-Sheldon syndrome [Japanese]. *Masui* 2002;51:659–662.
6. Cruickshanks GF, Brown S, Chitayat D. Anesthesia for Freeman-Sheldon syndrome using a laryngeal mask airway. *Can J Anaesth* 1999;46:783–787.
7. Vas L, Naregal P. Anaesthetic management of a patient with Freeman-Sheldon syndrome. *Paediatr Anaesth* 1998;8:175–177.
8. Munro HM, Butler PJ, Washington EJ. Freeman-Sheldon (whistling face) syndrome: anaesthetic and airway management. *Paediatr Anaesth* 1997;7:345–348.
9. Ohyama K, Susami T, Kato Y, et al. Freeman-Sheldon syndrome: case management from age 6 to 16 years. *Cleft Palate Craniofac J* 1997;34:151–153.
10. Mayhew JF. Anesthesia for the patient with Freeman-Sheldon syndrome [Letter]. *Anesthesiology* 1993;78:408.
11. Jones R, Dolcourt JL. Muscle rigidity following halothane anesthesia in two patients with Freeman-Sheldon syndrome. *Anesthesiology* 1992;77:599–600.
12. Duggar RG, DeMars PD, Bolton VE. Whistling face syndrome: general anesthesia and early postoperative caudal anesthesia. *Anesthesiology* 1989;1989:545–547.
13. Laishley RS, Roy WL. Freeman-Sheldon syndrome: report of three cases and anaesthetic implications. *Can J Anaesth* 1986;33:388–393.

14. Tateishi M, Imaizumi H, Namiki A, et al. Anesthetic management of a patient with Freeman-Sheldon ("whistling face" syndrome) [Japanese]. *Masui* 1986;35:1114–1118.

2. Hughes PJ, Davies PT, Roche SW, et al. Wildervanck or cervico-oculo-acoustic syndrome and MRI findings. *J Neurol Neurosurg Psychiatr* 1991;54:503–504.

Wiedemann-Rautenstrauch Syndrome

See Neonatal progeroid syndrome

Wildervanck Syndrome

SYNONYM: Cervicooculoacoustic syndrome

MIM #: 314600

This sporadic syndrome consists primarily of Klippel-Feil sequence (fused cervical vertebrae), abducens palsy with a retracted globe (Duane syndrome) and congenital deafness. The etiology of this syndrome is unknown. Because most patients have been female, the possibility of X-linked dominant inheritance with lethality in boys has been raised, although it is more likely that inheritance is multifactorial. Patients can have severe torticollis, which exacerbates the craniofacial abnormalities.

HEENT/AIRWAY: Asymmetric facies with a low hairline. Abducens palsy with retraction of the eye and narrowing of the palpebral fissure of the affected eye on adduction. Pseudopapilledema. Epibulbar dermoids. Deafness due to bony abnormalities of the inner ear. Preauricular pits and skin tags. Can have cleft palate. Very short neck, Klippel-Feil sequence (fused cervical vertebrae). Torticollis.

CHEST: Sprengel deformity (winged scapulae). Can have cervical ribs.

CARDIOVASCULAR: Can have cardiac defects.

NEUROMUSCULAR: Intelligence is usually normal. Can have occipital meningocele or other craniospinal abnormalities and brainstem abnormalities including low cranial nerve abnormalities.

ORTHOPEDIC: Can have growth deficiency.

GI/GU: Rare cholelithiasis or absent kidney.

ANESTHETIC CONSIDERATIONS
Consider having an interpreter present perioperatively to ease communication with those patients who are deaf. Diminished neck mobility secondary to the Klippel-Feil sequence or torticollis can make laryngoscopy and intubation extremely difficult.

Bibliography:
1. Gupte G, Mahajan P, Shreenivas VK, et al. Wildervanck syndrome (cervico-oculo-acoustic syndrome). *J Postgrad Med* 1992;38:180–182.

Williams-Beuren Syndrome

See Williams syndrome

Williams Syndrome

SYNONYM: Williams-Beuren syndrome

MIM #: 194050

This autosomal dominant disorder classically involves "elfin" facies, supravalvar aortic stenosis, and neonatal hypercalcemia. It is a continuous gene disorder, and the phenotype is due, at least in part, to a deletion of the elastin gene. However, as a continuous gene disorder, involvement of several other nearby genes in developing the clinical phenotype would account for the clinical heterogeneity.

HEENT/AIRWAY: "Elfin" facies. Puffy eyes. Lacy, stellate iris pattern. Hyperacusis. Depressed nasal bridge, anteverted nares. Enamel hypoplasia. Small teeth. Harsh or brassy voice. A patient with bilateral vocal cord paralysis has been described.

CARDIOVASCULAR: Aortic stenosis, typically supravalvar but also valvar and rarely subvalvar. Can have bicuspid aortic valve, mitral valve prolapse, mitral insufficiency, left coronary artery stenosis, myocardial ischemia. Distorted aortic valve leaflets can obstruct either main coronary artery ostium. In the case of supravalvar aortic stenosis, the coronary arteries arise from the proximal, hypertensive aorta, and can develop dysplastic, thickened walls with luminal narrowing. Multiple areas of peripheral pulmonary artery stenosis. Abdominal aortic coarctation and narrowing of celiac, mesenteric, and renal arteries have been reported. Recent carotid ultrasound data showing increased wall thickness also suggest a diffuse arteriopathy. Hypertension. There is an overall 3% incidence of sudden death with a 30-year follow-up. Cardiovascular disease is more common and more severe in males.

NEUROMUSCULAR: Mild mental retardation. Specifically, there appears to be poor visuomotor integration. Attention deficit disorder. Language development is normal, and some components of language, such as social uses of language, can be relatively advanced, so mental retardation is easily overlooked. Patients often have musical ability. Infantile hypotonia. Hypertonicity later. Cerebral artery stenoses with ischemic events.

ORTHOPEDIC: Short stature. The pubertal growth spurt occurs earlier in both girls and boys. Hypoplastic nails. Hallux valgus. Progressive joint limitation.

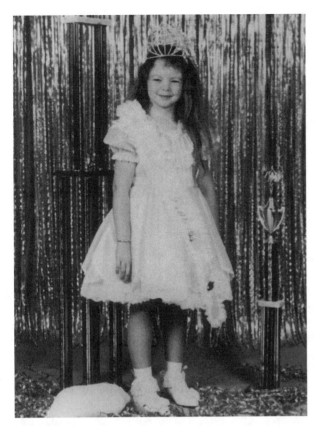

Williams syndrome. A young girl with Williams syndrome posing with her beauty pageant trophies. Her friendly personality is evident. (Courtesy of Dr. Sharon Hostler, University of Virginia Health System.)

GI/GU: Chronic constipation, diverticulosis, inguinal hernias. Nephrocalcinosis, urinary anomalies or stenoses with recurrent urinary tract infections. A variety of renal structural anomalies. Renal artery stenosis.

OTHER: Neonatal hypercalcemia, although hypercalcemia can persist until adulthood. Early menarche. Can have hypothyroidism.

MISCELLANEOUS: Socially gregarious, friendly children, described as having a "cocktail party" personality, are said to be musically talented, and can have perfect pitch.

Born in New Zealand, Williams also spent time working in London. Presumably on his way to accept a job at the Mayo Clinic in the United States, Williams disappeared and was not heard from again. An unclaimed suitcase of his was discovered in a luggage office in London.

ANESTHETIC CONSIDERATIONS

Sudden death has been reported, outside of the hospital as well as during cardiac catheterization and during anesthesia (2, 3). The risk of sudden death is thought to be related to the severity of the vascular stenoses or ischemic coronary disease, even in young children. Patients with biventricular outflow obstruction or evidence of ischemic disease are thought to be at particular risk. Impairment in cardiac supply-demand can be related to ventricular hypertrophy (demand) or hypotension, tachycardia or coronary artery disease (main coronary artery orifice obstruction from thickened aorta; adhesion of aortic valve leaflet obstructing orifice; coronary vessel abnormalities from chronic hypertension or primary arteriopathy) (supply). Baseline electrocardiogram and echocardiogram should be obtained. Ketamine is not optimal for patients with coronary artery involvement (2). The approach should generally mirror that taken for an adult with real or suspected coronary artery disease. Patients with congenital heart disease require perioperative antibiotic prophylaxis as indicated. Patients, particularly neonates, should be evaluated preoperatively for hypercalcemia.

Bibliography:

1. Medley J, Russo P, Tobias JD. Perioperative care of the patient with Williams syndrome. *Paediatr Anaesth* 2005;15:243–247.
2. Horowitz PE, Akhtar S, Wulff JA, et al. Coronary artery disease and anesthesia-related death in children with Williams syndrome. *J Cardiothorac Vasc Anesth* 2002;16:739–741.
3. Bird LM, Gillman GF, Lacro RV, et al. Sudden death in Williams syndrome: report of ten cases. *J Pediatr* 1996;129:926–931.
4. Kececioglu D, Kotthoff S, Vogt J. Williams-Beuren syndrome: a 30-year follow-up of natural and postoperative course. *Eur Heart J* 1993;14:1458–1464.
5. Patel J, Harrison MJ. Williams syndrome: masseter spasm during anesthesia. *Anaesthesia* 1991;46:115–116.

Wilson Disease

SYNONYM: Hepatolenticular degeneration

MIM #: 277900

This autosomal recessive disorder of copper metabolism results in the intracellular accumulation of copper initially in the eye and the liver, and eventually in many other tissues throughout the body, when copper overloaded hepatic cells die and release copper into the circulation. Children tend to present with hepatic disease, clinically similar to chronic active hepatitis. Older patients present with predominantly neurologic disease.

The responsible gene *ATP7B* encodes a cation-transporting ATPase. The gene product is thought to be similar to that causing Menkes kinky hair syndrome in that both have the characteristics of a copper-transporting adenosine triphosphatase. The Wilson disease gene product is involved with the export of copper out of cells, whereas the Menkes kinky hair syndrome gene product is involved with the transport of copper into cells.

Patients may be treated with a chelating agent. Treatment with penicillamine is associated with inhibition of pyridoxine-dependent enzymes requiring pyridoxine supplementation, zinc deficiency requiring zinc supplementation, fever, urticaria, systemic lupus erythematous, hemolytic anemia, Goodpasture syndrome, and a syndrome resembling myasthenia gravis. Another chelating drug that has been used is trientine (triethylenetetramine dihydrochloride). Zinc supplementation has also been used therapeutically. The disease is fatal if untreated. Liver transplantation is curative.

HEENT/AIRWAY: Kayser-Fleischer rings are pathognomonic—may require slit-lamp examination to identify. These are copper deposits in the Descemet membrane of the cornea. Kayser-Fleischer rings mirror neurologic involvement. Patients with hepatic disease only do not have them. "Sunflower" cataracts from copper deposition in the lens.

CARDIOVASCULAR: Cardiomyopathy.

NEUROMUSCULAR: Copper accumulation in the brain, particularly the basal ganglia. Neurologic problems prominent in adolescents and adults. Degeneration of the basal ganglia, extrapyramidal signs. Dysarthria, dystonia, choreoathetosis, tremors, ataxia, peripheral neuropathy, seizures, Parkinsonism. Intellectual impairment and pseudobulbar palsy occur late. Can have behavioral and psychiatric problems.

ORTHOPEDIC: Osteoarthropathy, chondrocalcinosis. Fingernails can exhibit "azure lunulae" (discoloration from copper).

GI/GU: Hepatic failure, which can be the presenting finding. Onset is gradual, but there can be acute episodes of hepatorenal failure with hemolysis (often fatal). Cirrhosis. Rarely hepatocellular carcinoma. Portal hypertension. Patients can have difficulty swallowing late in the disease. Calcified, pigmented gallstones. Pancreatic disease. Can have hypercalciuria, nephrocalcinosis with renal stones, renal tubular acidosis, Fanconi syndrome (see earlier).

OTHER: Acute hemolytic episodes. Anemia, neutropenia, thrombocytopenia. Hypoparathyroidism.

MISCELLANEOUS: Samuel Wilson was a neurologist at the National Hospital, Queen Square, London. Seen by some as arrogant and insensitive, he once instructed a patient to "see to it that I get your brain when you die." Wilson's paper describing the disease introduced the term "extrapyramidal."

ANESTHETIC CONSIDERATIONS

This disease can affect numerous organ systems, and anesthesia care needs to be tailored (as always) to the individual patient. A preoperative baseline hematocrit and platelet count should be obtained, particularly in patients taking penicillamine. Hypoalbuminemia from liver failure can alter the binding of some anesthetic drugs. Hepatic biopsy specimens must be specially handled to avoid copper contamination. Anticonvulsant medications need to be continued (or a parenteral form substituted), and can affect the metabolism of some anesthetic drugs. Metoclopramide can cause extrapyramidal effects and probably should be avoided. Phenothiazines, butyrophenones, and other dopaminergic blockers can exacerbate movement disorders. Ondansetron should be safe as an antiemetic because it does not have antidopaminergic effects.

Bibliography:
1. El-Youssef M. Wilson disease. *Mayo Clin Proc* 2003;78:1126–1136.
2. Gitlin JD. Wilson disease. *Gastroenterology* 2003;125:1868–1877.
3. Walshe JM. Treatment of Wilson's disease: the historical background. *Q J Med* 1996;89:553–555.

Wiskott-Aldrich Syndrome

MIM #: 301000

The primary manifestations of this X-linked recessive immune deficiency disease are eczema, thrombocytopenia with small platelets, B-cell lymphomas and recurrent infection. The gene product of the responsible gene, called WASP for Wiskott-Aldrich syndrome protein, is involved in the organization of the actin cytoskeleton. T-cells from these patients have deficient surface microvillus projections. WASP is only found in blood cells. A variety of mutations in the gene have been described. The gene product may interfere with Cdc42 signaling. Cdc42 is a cell division cycle protein that is a member of the rho family of guanosine triphosphate-binding proteins. In addition, deficits in the cell membrane glycoprotein sialophorin have been described. Wiskott-Aldrich syndrome has been reported in girls, due to nonrandom inactivation of X chromosomes. Bone marrow or umbilical cord blood transplantation is curative.

HEENT/AIRWAY: Recurrent oral infections can result in early tooth loss. Recurrent otitis media, sinusitis. Epistaxis.

CHEST: Recurrent pulmonary infections.

CARDIOVASCULAR: An autoimmune vasculitis can affect the coronary arteries.

NEUROMUSCULAR: Intracranial hemorrhage. An autoimmune vasculitis can affect the cerebral arteries.

GI/GU: Bloody diarrhea. Patients may require a splenectomy to control thrombocytopenia. Renal insufficiency.

OTHER: Eczema. Thrombocytopenia, small platelet size (which normalizes after splenectomy), bleeding diathesis. Increased incidence of autoimmune disorders. There are many varieties of autoimmune disease, including Coombs positive hemolytic anemia, a juvenile rheumatoid arthritis-like disease, vasculitis which may affect coronary and cerebral vessels, and a superimposed idiopathic thrombocytopenic purpura-like thrombocytopenia that may become apparent only after splenectomy. Increased incidence of malignancies, particularly lymphoreticular. The most common malignancies are non-Hodgkin lymphoma and brain cancer. There is often a widespread peripheral lymphadenopathy.

These nodes remain tumor free (unless widespread disseminated cancer develops).

Immune deficiency. The immune defects are selective, rather than global. There is variable immunoglobulin deficiency. The most common pattern is normal IgG, elevated IgA, and decreased IgM. Increased metabolism of immunoglobulins and albumin. Antibody responses are normal to some antigens, and absent to others. There is absent antibody formation to all of the polysaccharide antigens, with low or absent isohemagglutinins and an inability to make antibody to capsular polysaccharides of *Hemophilus* or pneumococci. Selective T-cell abnormalities are present, and there is cutaneous anergy. Abnormal function of monocytes. Neutrophils have abnormal chemotactic, but normal bacteriocidal function. Patients are at particular risk from overwhelming chickenpox. Other infectious agents include *Streptococcus pneumoniae, Hemophilus influenzae, Candida albicans*, cytomegalovirus, herpes simplex, and *Pneumocystis carinii*. Disseminated vaccinia was a cause of death after receiving smallpox vaccination.

MISCELLANEOUS: Wiskott, a German, described the disease 17 years before Aldrich, an American. Wiskott called it Werlhof's disease, the eponymous designation of thrombocytopenic purpura.

ANESTHETIC CONSIDERATIONS
Meticulous aseptic technique is imperative. The platelet count should be evaluated preoperatively, and platelet transfusion may be indicated. Neuraxial analgesia may be contraindicated with low platelet count. The hematocrit should be evaluated preoperatively. All transfused blood products must be irradiated to prevent graft-versus-host disease. Baseline renal function should be evaluated preoperatively. Patients who are taking steroids should receive perioperative stress doses of steroids.

Bibliography:
1. Snapper SB, Rosen FS. A family of WASPs. *N Engl J Med* 2003;384:350–351.
2. Parolini O, Ressmann G, Haas OA, et al. X-linked Wiskott-Aldrich syndrome in a girl. *N Engl J Med* 1998;38:291–295.
3. Kirchhausen T, Rosen FS. Disease mechanism: unraveling Wiskott-Aldrich syndrome. *Curr Biol* 1996;6:676–678.

Wolf-Hirschhorn Syndrome

See 4p- syndrome

Wolff-Parkinson-White Syndrome

MIM #: 194200

Wolff-Parkinson-White syndrome (WPW) is an electrophysiologic syndrome due to the presence of Kent fibers, which are conduction fibers that run along the lateral margins of the atrioventricular valves, bypassing the atrioventricular node to enter the ventricular myocardium directly. Bypass of the atrioventricular node leads to a short PR interval (the normal atrioventricular node delay is bypassed) and the initial slow upstroke of the QRS, secondary to initial cell-to-cell transmission of the electrical impulse, until the normally conducted impulse finally gets through the atrioventricular node and depolarizes the ventricles rapidly through the His-Purkinje system. The presence of Kent fibers creates a potential reentry circuit increasing the risk for the development of paroxysmal supraventricular tachycardia. It is thought that these bypass tracts represent persistence of a normal fetal structure. WPW is most common in the neonatal period, and many cases spontaneously regress by approximately 6 months of age, when chronic treatment often can be stopped. Familial cases have been described, and a gene which encodes the gamma-2 regulatory subunit of AMP-activated protein kinase has been identified as the responsible gene. Ablation of the bypass tract in the catheterization laboratory is curative.

There are two types of WPW, diagnosed electrocardiographically. Type A represents a left-sided bypass tract, and type B a right-sided bypass tract.

CARDIOVASCULAR: Wolff-Parkinson-White syndrome can be associated with a variety of congenital cardiac defects, such as Ebstein anomaly of the tricuspid valve.

Type A: The electrocardiogram shows a short PR interval (<120 msec) and a delta wave at the onset of the QRS. There is a delta wave and a prominent R wave in lead V1.

Type B: Negative delta wave and a prominent S wave in lead V1.

MISCELLANEOUS: One of us had the opportunity to speak with the patient who was case number two in the original case report of Wolff-Parkinson-White syndrome. He had been at that time a swimmer on the Yale swim team and confided that he had been unsure if he could trust young Dr. White (Paul Dudley White), a Harvard doctor.

Interestingly, Kent actually described Mahaim fibers (similar specialized conducting fibers, but nodoventricular) and Mahaim described Kent fibers. John Parkinson of Wolff-Parkinson-White syndrome is distinct from James Parkinson of Parkinson's disease.

ANESTHETIC CONSIDERATIONS
Episodes of reentrant tachycardia can be induced by sympathetic stimulation, so good preoperative sedation would seem reasonable. Perioperative increases in vagal tone, such as from drugs or gagging, may inhibit normal antegrade conduction through the atrioventricular node, and unmask conduction down the bypass tract, with preexcitation (short PR interval and delta wave) becoming suddenly visible (11). Similarly, 1.0 mg of neostigmine (without an anticholinergic)

has converted hemodynamically stable atrial fibrillation with a narrow QRS complex into hemodynamically unstable atrial fibrillation with a more rapid ventricular response and a wide QRS, presumably on the basis of increased vagal tone, enhancing accessory pathway conduction (1). Atropine produces normal atrioventricular conduction and can cause the delta wave to disappear. Atrial fibrillation can develop during the increase in sympathetic tone during emergence from general anesthesia. Episodes of tachycardia have also occurred for the first time in a patient with concealed Wolff-Parkinson-White syndrome during spinal anesthesia (8) and have been induced by passing a central venous guidewire.

Isoflurane has been used without apparent problems during electrophysiologic mapping or radiofrequency catheter ablation (5, 6), and it appears that sevoflurane can also be used for these procedures (3). Propofol and fentanyl have been used uneventfully for general anesthesia (2, 6). Patients with associated structural heart disease need perioperative antibiotic prophylaxis as indicated.

Drugs and maneuvers that can be used intraoperatively to convert paroxysmal supraventricular tachycardia are the same as for paroxysmal supraventricular tachycardia not associated with WPW, namely adenosine, verapamil, beta blockade, amiodarone or overdrive pacing [transesophageal pacing has been used successfully (9)]. Drugs used to terminate tachycardia (adenosine or beta blockers) can exacerbate reactive airway disease (4). Beta$_2$ agonists such as albuterol should not induce arrhythmias (7).

Verapamil and digoxin (without quinidine) are contraindicated for the treatment of atrial flutter or fibrillation in patients with WPW because they can accelerate the rate of conduction through the bypass tract and induce ventricular fibrillation. Procainamide may be useful for atrial fibrillation in this setting. Concurrent verapamil and propranolol (and possibly other combinations of calcium channel blockers and beta blockers) can cause significant bradycardia. Chronic therapy with amiodarone can cause hypothyroidism or pulmonary fibrosis.

Bibliography:

1. Kadoya T, Seto A, Aoyama K, et al. Development of rapid atrial fibrillation with a wide QRS complex after neostigmine in a patient with intermittent Wolff-Parkinson-White syndrome. *Br J Anaesth* 1999;83:815–818.
2. Yamaguchi S, Nagao M, Mishio M, et al. Anesthetic management using propofol and fentanyl of a patient with concealed Wolff-Parkinson-White syndrome [Japanese]. *Masui* 1998;47:730–733.
3. Sharpe MD, Cuillerier DJ, Lee JK, et al. Sevoflurane has no electrophysiological effects during reciprocating tachycardia in Wolff-Parkinson-White (WPW) patients. *Anesth Analg* 1998;86:5101.
4. Abraham EL, Jahr JS, Gitlin MC. Anesthetic management of a child with Wolff-Parkinson-White syndrome and bronchial asthma. *Am J Anesth* 1997;24:151–153.
5. Chang RK, Stevenson WG, Wetzel GT, et al. Effects of isoflurane on electrophysiological measurements in children with the Wolff-Parkinson-White syndrome. *Pacing Clin Electrophysiol* 1996;19:1082–1088.
6. Lavoie J, Walsh EP, Burrows FA, et al. Effects of propofol or isoflurane anesthesia on cardiac conduction in children undergoing radiofrequency catheter ablation for tachydysrhythmias. *Anesthesiology* 1995;82:884–887.
7. Bonnin AJ, Richmond GW, Musto PK. Repeated inhalation of nebulized albuterol did not induce arrhythmias in a patient with Wolff-Parkinson-White syndrome and asthma. *Chest* 1993;103:1892–1894.
8. Nishikawa K, Mizoguchi M, Yukioka H, et al. Concealed Wolff-Parkinson-White syndrome detected during spinal anaesthesia. *Anaesthesia* 1993;48:1061–1064.
9. Stevenson GW, Schuster J, Kross J, et al. Transoesophageal pacing for perioperative control of neonatal paroxysmal supraventricular tachycardia. *Can J Anaesth* 1990;37:672–674.
10. Richmond MN, Conroy PT. Anesthetic management of a neonate born prematurely with Wolff Parkinson White syndrome. *Anesth Analg* 1988;67:477–478.
11. Lubarsky D, Kaufman B, Turndorf H. Anesthesia unmasking benign Wolff-Parkinson-White syndrome. *Anesth Analg* 1988;68:172–174.
12. Vidaillet HJ, Pressley JC, Henke E, et al. Familial occurrence of accessory atrioventricular pathways (preexcitation syndrome). *N Engl J Med* 1987;317:65–69.
13. Sadowski AR, Moyers JR. Anesthetic management of the Wolff-Parkinson-White syndrome. *Anesthesiology* 1979;51:553–556.

Wolfram Syndrome

See DIDMOAD syndrome

Wolman Disease

(Includes Cholesterol ester storage disease)

MIM #: 278000

This autosomal recessive disorder is due to deficient activity of lysosomal acid lipase (cholesterol ester hydrolase), which is encoded by the gene *LIPA*. The major function of this enzyme is the hydrolysis of cholesterol esters in various lipoproteins. Wolman disease results in widespread deposition of cholesterol esters and triglycerides in lysosomes, with secondary fibrosis. Wolman disease has profound manifestations in infancy, and is usually fatal in the first year of life.

Different alleles result in both Wolman disease and the milder disease, **cholesterol ester storage disease** (cholesteryl ester storage disease). Cholesterol ester storage disease is associated with hepatomegaly and may not present until adulthood. It is sometimes associated with cirrhosis, portal hypertension, intestinal involvement, and hypercholesterolemia and hypertriglyceridemia, which can respond to treatment with statin drugs.

CARDIOVASCULAR: Pulmonary hypertension has been reported. Lipid deposition in vessels without gross atherosclerosis, perhaps due to early deaths.

NEUROMUSCULAR: Normal at birth, with deterioration within a few weeks.

GI/GU: Diarrhea, vomiting, steatorrhea, abdominal distension. Hepatic deposition of cholesterol esters and triglycerides, abnormal liver function tests, portal fibrosis. Hepatosplenomegaly, which can be massive. Esophageal varices. Involvement of small bowel mucosa, particularly the proximal small bowel. Adrenal gland deposition with enlargement and finely stippled calcification.

OTHER: Malabsorption, malnutrition. Failure to thrive. Anemia. Persistent low-grade fever. Foam cells in bone marrow, vacuolated lymphocytes.

MISCELLANEOUS: The first reported case was, in retrospect, that of Alexander, who reported what he called a case of Niemann-Pick disease with adrenal calcification.

ANESTHETIC CONSIDERATIONS
The hematocrit should be evaluated preoperatively. Hepatic insufficiency can affect the binding of some anesthetic drugs. The presence of esophageal varices is a relative contraindication to placement of a nasogastric tube.

Bibliography:
1. Wolman M. Wolman disease and its treatment. *Clin Pediatr* 1995;34: 207–212.
2. D'Agostino D, Bay L, Gallo G, et al. Cholesterol ester storage disease: clinical, biochemical, and pathological studies of four new cases. *J Pediatr Gastroenterol Nutr* 1988;7:446–450.

X

Xanthine Dehydrogenase Deficiency

Included in Molybdenum cofactor deficiency

Xanthinuria

SYNONYM: Hereditary xanthinuria

MIM #: 278300, 603592

This autosomal recessive disorder is due to deficient activity of xanthine dehydrogenase (xanthine oxidoreductase). This enzyme catalyzes the conversion of xanthine and hypoxanthine to uric acid, the last step in purine catabolism. A significant number of patients are asymptomatic, and are discovered fortuitously by low serum uric acid. Combined deficiency of xanthine oxidase and sulfite oxidase, due to a molybdenum cofactor deficiency (see earlier), is not uncommon. There are two biochemically distinct forms of xanthinuria. In xanthinuria type I, only xanthine dehydrogenase activity is deficient. In xanthinuria type II, there is deficiency of both xanthine dehydrogenase and aldehyde oxidase, purportedly due to an abnormality in molybdenum cofactor sulfurase. The only clinical difference is that type I patients can metabolize allopurinol, while type II patients cannot.

NEUROMUSCULAR: Myopathy with crystalline deposits of xanthine and hypoxanthine causing muscle pain and cramps

has been reported. These may have been caused by exercise, which increases nucleotide turnover.

GI/GU: Hyperxanthinuria. Xanthine renal stones (brown, radiolucent), hydronephrosis, renal colic, recurrent urinary tract infections, renal failure. Stones can occur during infancy. Infants can have intermittent hematuria and occasional orange-brown staining of diapers.

OTHER: Decreased serum uric acid.

MISCELLANEOUS: Hypoxanthine and xanthine accumulate during ischemia, and oxidants are produced upon reperfusion. Tissue injury from reperfusion injury can be ameliorated by inactivation of xanthine dehydrogenase (the enzyme also functions as an oxidase).

ANESTHETIC CONSIDERATIONS
Renal failure (if present) affects perioperative fluid management and the metabolism of some anesthetic drugs. Perioperative fluid administration must be adequate to maintain a diuresis and prevent further concentration of xanthine in the urine. Xanthine is somewhat more soluble at an alkaline pH. Methylxanthines such as theophylline and caffeine are not metabolized by xanthine oxidase, and are not contraindicated. Fluids and medications should be titrated carefully in patients with renal failure.

Bibliography:
1. Badertscher E, Robson WL, Leung AK, et al. Xanthine calculi presenting at 1 month of age. *Eur J Pediatr* 1993;152:252–254.
2. Fildes RD. Hereditary xanthinuria with severe urolithiasis occurring in infancy as renal tubular acidosis and hypercalciuria. *J Pediatr* 1989;115:277–280.

X-Associated Tremor/Ataxia Syndrome

Included in Fragile X syndrome

Xeroderma Pigmentosum

MIM #: 194400, 278700, 278720, 278730, 278740, 278750, 278760, 278780, 278810

This disorder, of which there are many subtypes, is an autosomal recessive defect in the repair of ultraviolet-induced damage to DNA. The defect can be identified prenatally in cultured fibroblasts obtained by amniocentesis. de Sanctis-Cacchione syndrome (see earlier) is a subtype of xeroderma pigmentosum. Most of the clinical findings are related to excessive sensitivity to sunlight, including eye changes, atrophic and pigmentary skin changes, and actinic skin tumors. The severity of eye and skin lesions is related to the degree of sun exposure. Some subtypes involve neurologic abnormalities. Death is often secondary to cancer.

Patients with xeroderma pigmentosum have been classified into ten complementation groups (A through I, plus a variant). It may be that groups D and H are the same. These divisions are based on the ability of cells from one group to correct the defect when hybridized with cells from the other groups. Clinical findings vary somewhat among the groups. Groups A, C, and D are the most common. Neurologic problems are usually found in groups A and D patients, and they have the lowest level of DNA repair. Group C patients have the highest level of DNA repair, and have a longer life expectancy. Readers are directed to other sources, such as *Mendelian Inheritance in Man*, for a discussion of the various genes, gene products, and biochemical pathophysiologies involved in the various types.

HEENT/AIRWAY: Can have microcephaly. Photophobia, conjunctival injection, corneal clouding or vascularization from exposure. Conjunctival, corneal and lid tumors. Ectropion. Occasional sensorineural hearing deficit. Atrophic skin around the mouth sometimes limits mouth opening. Squamous cell carcinoma of tip of tongue, gingiva, or palate.

NEUROMUSCULAR: Progressive central nervous system deterioration with cerebral atrophy, choreoathetosis, ataxia, spasticity. Brain tumors may develop.

OTHER: Skin abnormalities typically begin during early childhood. Excessive sensitivity to sunlight with severe sunburn, freckling, atrophy with irregular pigmentation, telangiectasis, angiomas, keratoses, basal cell and squamous cell carcinomas in sun-exposed areas. Skin cancers are of several types, but basal cell and squamous cell carcinomas are most frequent. Less common are keratoacanthoma, adenocarcinoma, melanoma, neuroma, sarcoma, or angiosarcoma. The median age for the development of the first skin cancer is 8 years. Nonskin cancers such as brain or lung cancer or leukemia can develop. Can have frequent infections.

MISCELLANEOUS: Xeroderma pigmentosum was first described by Moritz Kaposi (born Moritz Kohn). DNA repair mechanisms are abnormal in four other inherited diseases: ataxia-telangiectasia, Fanconi anemia, Bloom syndrome, and Cockayne syndrome.

ANESTHETIC CONSIDERATIONS
Perioperative radiographic studies are indicated only when absolutely necessary because these patients are sensitive to irradiation. Consideration should be given to patients with photophobia in brightly lit operating rooms. Limited mouth opening has not been reported to hinder laryngoscopy and tracheal intubation.

Bibliography:
1. Brunner T, Jöhr M. Anesthetic management of a child with xeroderma pigmentosum. *Paediatr Anaesth* 2004;14:697–698.
2. Rapin I, Lindenbaum Y, Dickson DW, et al. Cockayne syndrome and xeroderma pigmentosum. *Neurology* 2000;55:1442–1449.
3. Lambert WC, Kuo HR, Lambert MW. Xeroderma pigmentosum. *Dermatol Clin* 1995;13:169–209.
4. Kraemer KH, Lee MM, Scotto J. Xeroderma pigmentosa: cutaneous, ocular, and neurologic abnormalities in 830 published cases. *Arch Dermatol* 1987;123:241–250.
5. Meyer RJ. Awake blind nasal intubation in a patient with xeroderma pigmentosum. *Anaesth Intensive Care* 1982;10:64–66.

X-Linked Alpha-Thalassemia/Mental Retardation Syndrome

See ATR-X syndrome

X-Linked Hydrocephalus Syndrome

See MASA syndrome

X-Linked Hypophosphatemic Rickets

See Vitamin D-resistant rickets

XO Syndrome

See Turner syndrome

XXXXX Syndrome

See Penta X syndrome

XXY Syndrome

See Klinefelter syndrome

XXXY Syndrome

Included in Klinefelter syndrome

XXXXY

Included in Klinefelter syndrome

XXYY Syndrome

Included in Klinefelter syndrome

XYY Syndrome

MIM #: None

This disorder is due to an extra Y chromosome. These boys are 47, XYY. Most people with XYY are asymptomatic and are not diagnosed.

HEENT/AIRWAY: Prominent glabella (the part of the forehead just above the nose). Long ears. Shallow palate, large teeth.

CHEST: Mild pectus excavatum.

CARDIOVASCULAR: First-degree atrioventricular block.

NEUROMUSCULAR: Intelligence within the normal range, but usually less than siblings. Speech delay and learning disabilities. Behavioral problems with easy distractibility, hyperactivity, and temper tantrums. Aggressiveness is usually controllable by patients as they age, and behavioral problems are usually not significant for these boys as they get older. Relatively weak, with poor fine motor control and sometimes fine tremor. Psychiatric problems (schizophrenia) have been reported.

ORTHOPEDIC: Relatively long and thin body habitus with long fingers. Size is usually normal until a growth spurt at approximately 5 to 6 years of age. Radioulnar synostosis.

GI/GU: Cryptorchidism, small penis, hypospadias. Several case reports suggest an association with renal agenesis or dysplasia and the Potter syndrome (see earlier) with XYY syndrome.

OTHER: Severe acne during adolescence.

ANESTHETIC CONSIDERATIONS
Preoperative management may be challenging in patients with behavioral problems, particularly if they are hyperactive or aggressive. Baseline renal function should be evaluated as indicated.

Bibliography:
1. Robinson A, Bender BG, Linden MG. Summary of clinical findings in children and young adults with sex chromosome anomalies. *Birth Defects* 1990;26:225–228.

Y

Yunis-Varon Syndrome

MIM #: 216340

Yunis-Varon syndrome is an autosomal recessive disorder primarily involving growth failure and orthopedic abnormalities. Survival is poor beyond the neonatal period. The specific gene and gene product are not known. A case has been reported in which a muscle biopsy showed characteristics of a lysosomal storage disease.

HEENT/AIRWAY: Microcephaly. Thin scalp hair, eyebrows, and eyelashes. Wide sutures and fontanelles. Short, up-slanting palpebral fissures, cataracts. Low-set ears. Anteverted nares, short philtrum, thin lips. Micrognathia. Loose neck skin. Premature loss of deciduous teeth.

CHEST: Hypoplastic or aplastic clavicles. Absent nipples.

CARDIOVASCULAR: Tetralogy of Fallot was described in one patient.

NEUROMUSCULAR: Severe developmental delay. Agenesis of the corpus callosum, abnormal cerebellar vermis.

ORTHOPEDIC: Hypoplasia or agenesis of thumbs and great toes, short, tapered fingers with nail hypoplasia, hypoplasia or agenesis of middle and distal phalanges of fingers and toes, syndactyly, simian crease. Abnormal scapulae, absent sternal ossification. Dislocated hips. Growth retardation.

GI/GU: A patient has been reported with atrophy of the left lobe of the liver with a hepatic vascular anomaly. Abnormal external genitalia.

OTHER: Prenatal growth deficiency with postnatal failure to thrive.

ANESTHETIC CONSIDERATIONS
Experiences with anesthesia have not been reported with this syndrome. Micrognathia may complicate direct laryngoscopy and tracheal intubation. A single child with upper airway obstruction with obstructive sleep apnea has been reported. Abnormalities of the clavicles make placement of a subclavian venous catheter more difficult.

Bibliography:
1. Dworzak F, Mora M, Borroni C, et al. Generalized lysosomal storage in Yunis Varon syndrome. *Neuromuscul Disord* 1995;5:423–428.
2. Hennekam RCM, Vermeulen-Meiners C. Further delineation of the Yunis-Varon syndrome. *J Med Genet* 1989;26:55–58.

Z

Zellweger Syndrome

SYNONYM: Cerebrohepatorenal syndrome

MIM #: 214100

This autosomal recessive disorder is associated with generalized peroxisomal dysfunction and an absence of peroxisomes. It has been suggested that the same gene [peroxin-1 (*PEX1*)], the functioning of which is required for transportation of proteins into peroxisomes, is involved in infantile Refsum disease, neonatal adrenoleukodystrophy, and Zellweger syndrome. These three disorders represent a continuum, with Zellweger syndrome being the most severe, neonatal adrenoleukodystrophy intermediate, and infantile

Refsum disease being the least severe. In addition, the Zellweger phenotype can be caused by defects in a variety of other genes encoding peroxisomal proteins, including *PEX2, PEX3, PEX5, PEX6, PEX12* and others. Life expectancy is approximately 6 months.

HEENT/AIRWAY: High forehead. Large fontanelles with open metopic suture. Long, flat face, shallow, flat supraorbital ridges. Epicanthal folds, puffy lids, corneal opacities, cataracts, glaucoma, Brushfield spots of the iris, gliosis of the optic nerve, retinitis pigmentosa. Abnormal external ears. High-arched palate, cleft palate. Micrognathia. Extra neck skinfolds.

CHEST: Respiratory insufficiency secondary to hypotonia, apnea.

CARDIOVASCULAR: Patent ductus arteriosus, septal defects, aortic abnormalities.

NEUROMUSCULAR: Hypotonia. Retarded psychomotor development. Poor suck. Microgyria, failure of myelination and white matter development. Seizures. The electroretinogram, brainstem auditory evoked response, and somatosensory evoked response are grossly abnormal or not elicitable at all.

ORTHOPEDIC: Simian crease, camptodactyly. Contractures, particularly of knees and fingers. Cubitus valgus, metatarsus adductus, talipes equinovarus. Punctate epiphyseal calcifications of a variety of flat bones.

GI/GU: Hepatomegaly, jaundice, cirrhosis, albuminuria. Cryptorchidism. Renal cortical cysts. Impaired adrenal cortical function or adrenal atrophy.

OTHER: Marked failure to thrive.

MISCELLANEOUS: Zellweger syndrome is a good example of a disease that was originally thought to be a dysmorphic "multiple congenital anomaly" but was later found to have a clear physiologic and genetic basis. Rhizomelic chondrodysplasia punctata, which also results in punctate calcifications, is also a peroxisomal disorder.

Hans Zellweger, originally Swiss, spent 1937 to 1939 with Albert Schweitzer in Lambarene, Gabon.

ANESTHETIC CONSIDERATIONS
Contractures may make intraoperative positioning more difficult. There may be altered binding of some anesthetic drugs in patients with hepatic disease. Renal function can be impaired. Adrenal response to stress may be inadequate, and patients may require perioperative stress doses of steroids. Patients with congenital heart disease require perioperative antibiotic prophylaxis as appropriate.

Bibliography:
1. Moser HW. Peroxisomal disorders. *Semin Pediatr Neurol* 1996;3: 298–304.
2. FitzPatrick DR. Zellweger syndrome and associated phenotypes. *J Med Genet* 1996;33:863–868.
3. Palosaari PM, Kilponen JM, Hiltunen JK. Peroxisomal diseases. *Ann Med* 1992;24:163–166.

Appendix A

Steroid Biosynthesis

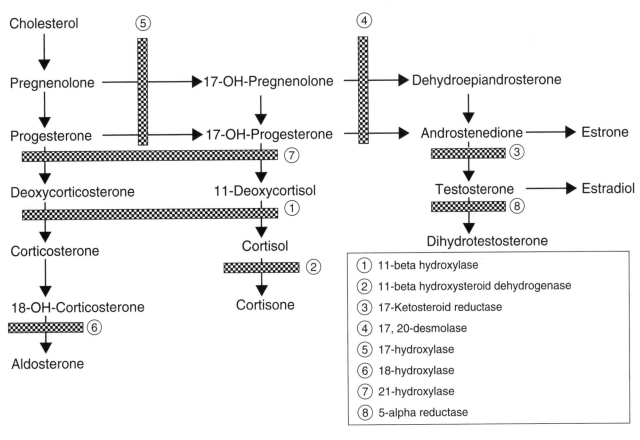

1. 11-beta hydroxylase
2. 11-beta hydroxysteroid dehydrogenase
3. 17-Ketosteroid reductase
4. 17, 20-desmolase
5. 17-hydroxylase
6. 18-hydroxylase
7. 21-hydroxylase
8. 5-alpha reductase

Appendix B

Tyrosine Metabolism

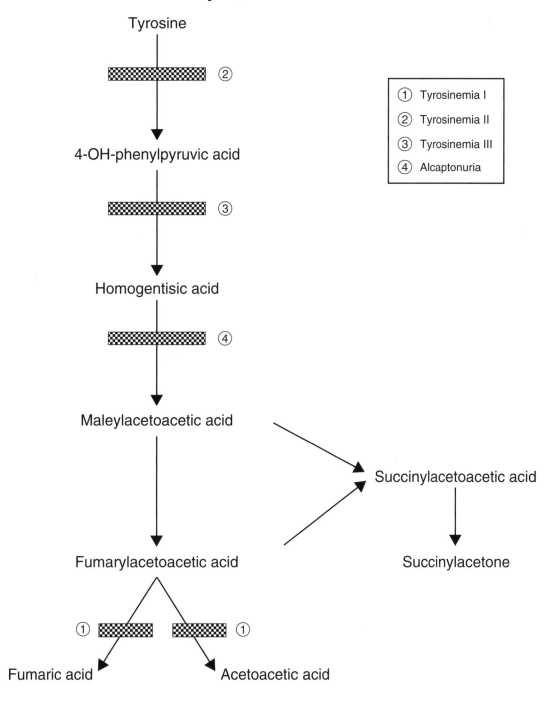

Tyrosine

②

4-OH-phenylpyruvic acid

③

Homogentisic acid

④

Maleylacetoacetic acid → Succinylacetoacetic acid

Fumarylacetoacetic acid

Succinylacetone

① ①

Fumaric acid   Acetoacetic acid

① Tyrosinemia I
② Tyrosinemia II
③ Tyrosinemia III
④ Alcaptonuria

Appendix C

Simplified Urea Cycle

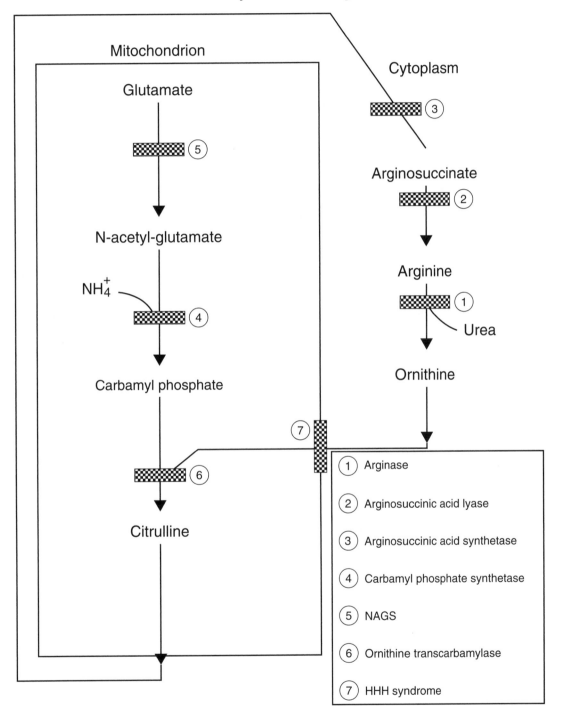

Appendix D

Metabolism of Branched-Chain Amino Acids

Valine → 2-Oxo-isovalericacid → Isobutyryl-CoA → Methacrylyl-CoA → 3-OH-isobutyryl-CoA → 3-OH-isobutyric acid → Methylmalonyl semialdehyde

Isoleucine → 2-Oxo-3-methylvalerate → 2-Methylbutyryl-CoA → Tiglyl-CoA → 2-Methyl-3-OH-butyryl-CoA → 2-Methylacetoacetyl-CoA ①

Leucine → 2-Oxoisocaproic acid ④ → Isovaleryl-CoA ③ → 3-Methylcrotonyl-CoA → 3-Methylglutaconyl-CoA → 3-OH-3-methylglutaryl-CoA ② → Acetoacetate

Propionyl-CoA ⑤ → Methylmalony-CoA ⑤ → Succinyl-CoA

Acetyl-CoA ⑥ → Malonyl-CoA → Acetyl-CoA

① Beta-ketothiolase
② Hydroxymethylglutaric aciduria
③ Isovaleric acidemia
④ Maple syrup urine disease
⑤ Methylmalonic acidemia
⑥ Propionic acidemia

411